Oxford Textbook of

Psoriatic Arthritis

Titles in the Oxford Textbooks in Rheumatology series

Oxford Textbook of
Psoriatic Arthritis

Edited by

OLIVER FITZGERALD

DAFNA GLADMAN

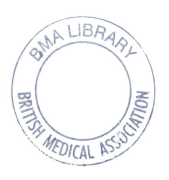

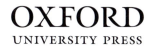

OXFORD

UNIVERSITY PRESS

OXFORD
UNIVERSITY PRESS

Great Clarendon Street, Oxford, OX2 6DP,
United Kingdom

Oxford University Press is a department of the University of Oxford.
It furthers the University's objective of excellence in research, scholarship,
and education by publishing worldwide. Oxford is a registered trade mark of
Oxford University Press in the UK and in certain other countries

Published in the United States of America by Oxford University Press
198 Madison Avenue, New York, NY 10016, United States of America

British Library Cataloguing in Publication Data
Data available

Library of Congress Control Number: 2017962136

ISBN 978-0-19-873758-2

Printed in Great Britain by
Bell & Bain Ltd., Glasgow

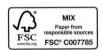

This book is dedicated to the memory of Dr Ignazio Olivieri (died July 2017) who contributed the excellent chapter on 'Dactylitis' to this textbook. Dr Olivieri published several seminal papers on the subject of Psoriatic Arthritis during his long career. He will be much missed by his many friends and colleagues.

Contents

List of contributors

Frank Behrens, CIRI, Rheumatology & Fraunhofer TMP, Goethe-University, Frankfurt, Germany

Tristan Boyd, St Joseph's Hospital, London, Ontario, Canada

Juan D. Cañete, Arthritis Unit, Rheumatology Department, Hospital Clínic and IDIBAPS, Barcelona, Spain

Francesco Caso, Rheumatology Unit, Department of Clinical Medicine and Surgery, University Federico II, Naples, Italy

Alberto Cauli, Department of Rheumatology, University of Cagliari, Sardinia, Italy

Vinod Chandran, Centre for Prognosis Studies in Rheumatic Diseases, Krembil Research Institute, University Health Network, Toronto, Ontario, Canada

Laura Coates, Nuffield Department of Orthopaedics, Rheumatology, and Musculoskeletal Sciences, University of Oxford, Oxford, UK

Luisa Costa, Rheumatology Unit, Department of Clinical Medicine and Surgery, University Federico II, Naples, Italy

Salvatore D'Angelo, Rheumatology Department of Lucania, San Carlo Hospital of Potenza and Madonna delle Grazie Hospital of Matera, Potenza, Italy

Kurt de Vlam, Department of Rheumatology, Louvain University Hospital, Leuven, Belgium

Maarten de Wit, Department of Medical Humanities, VU University, Amsterdam, The Netherlands

Nicola Matteo Dario Di Minno, Department of Clinical and Experimental Medicine, University Federico II, Naples, Italy

Lihi Eder, Women's College Hospital, University of Toronto, Toronto, Ontario, Canada

James T. Elder, University of Michigan, Department of Dermatology, Ann Arbor, Michigan, USA

Iris Eshed, Department of Diagnostic Imaging, Sheba Medical Center, Sackler School of Medicine, Tel-Aviv University, Tel Aviv, Israel

Laura Acosta Felquer, Rheumatology Section, Medical Services, Hospital Italiano de Buenos Aires, Buenos Aires, Argentina

Camille Figueiredo, Division of Rheumatology, Universidade des Sao Paulo, Sao Paulo, Brazil

Oliver FitzGerald, St Vincent's University Hospital and Conway Institute for Biomolecular Research, University College Dublin, Ireland

George E. Fragoulis, Institute of Infection, Immunity and Inflammation, University of Glasgow, Glasgow, UK

Joel M. Gelfand, Department of Dermatology, University of Pennsylvania Perelman School of Medicine, Philadelphia, USA

Dafna Gladman, Toronto Western Hospital, Krembil Research Institute, University of Toronto, Toronto, Canada

Laure Gossec, Department of Rheumatology, Pitié Salpêtrière Hospital, Paris, France

Alice Gottlieb, Department of Dermatology, New York Medical College, Metropolitan Hospital, New York, NY, USA

Tania Gudu, Department of Rheumatology, Pitié Salpêtrière Hospital, Paris, France

Caely A. Hambro, Department of Dermatology, University of Michigan Medical School, Ann Arbor, Michigan

Muhammad Haroon, Department of Medicine, Waterford Regional Hospital, Waterford, Ireland

Philip Helliwell, Rheumatology and Rehabilitation Research Unit, University of Leeds, Leeds, UK

Elaine Husni, Department of Rheumatic and Immunologic Diseases, Cleveland Clinic, Cleveland, Ohio, USA

Deep Joshipura, Department of Dermatology, Tufts Medical Center, Boston, MA, USA

Gurjit Kaeley, Division of Rheumatology, University of Florida College of Medicine, Jacksonville, Florida, USA

Arthur Kavanaugh, Division of Rheumatology Allergy and Immunology, UCSD, San Diego, California, USA

Brian Kirby, Department of Dermatology, St Vincent's University Hospital, Elm Park, Dublin, Ireland

Bruce Kirkham, Rheumatology Department, Guy's and St Thomas' NHS Foundation Trust, London, UK

Michaela Koehm, CIRI, Rheumatology & Fraunhofer TMP, Goethe-University, Frankfurt, Germany

Rik Lories, Division of Rheumatology, University Hospitals Leuven, Belgium

Ennio Lubrano, Academic Rheumatology Unit, Department of Health Sciences, University of Molise, Italy

Dennis McGonagle, The Leeds Institute of Rheumatic and Musculoskeletal Medicine, Leeds, UK

Neil McHugh, Royal National Hospital for Rheumatic Diseases, Royal United Hospitals Bath NHS Foundation Trust, UK

Iain McInnes, Institute of Infection, Immunity and Inflammation, University of Glasgow, Glasgow, UK

Philip Mease, Swedish Medical Center, Seattle, Washington, USA

Madonna Michael, Department of Rheumatic and Immunologic Diseases, Cleveland Clinic, Cleveland, Ohio, USA

Darren D. O'Reilly, Research Scientist, Faculty of Medicine, Memorial University of Newfoundland, Newfoundland and Labrador, Canada

Katerina Oikonomopoulou, Centre for Prognosis Studies in Rheumatic Diseases, Krembil Research Institute, University Health Network, Toronto, Ontario, Canada

Ignazio Olivieri[†], Rheumatology Department of Lucania, San Carlo Hospital of Potenza and Madonna delle Grazie Hospital of Matera, Potenza, Italy

Angela Padula, Rheumatology Department of Lucania, San Carlo Hospital of Potenza and Madonna delle Grazie Hospital of Matera, Potenza, Italy

Carlo Palazzi, Rheumatology Department of Lucania, San Carlo Hospital of Potenza and Madonna delle Grazie Hospital of Matera, Potenza, Italy

Michael J. Pamham, Fraunhofer Institute for Molecular Biology and Applied Ecology IME, Frankfurt, Germany

Rosario Peluso, Department of Clinical and Experimental Medicine, University Federico II, Naples, Italy

Proton Rahman, St Clare's Mercy Hospital, Memorial University of Newfoundland, St John's, Newfoundland, Canada

Julio Ramírez, Arthritis Unit, Rheumatology Department, Hospital Clínic, Barcelona, Spain

Christopher Ritchlin, Center for Musculoskeletal Medicine, University of Rochester Medical Center, New York, USA

Cheryl F. Rosen, Division of Dermatology, Toronto Western Hospital, University of Toronto, Toronto, Canada

Ami Saraiya, Department of Dermatology, Tufts Medical Center, Boston, MA, USA

Enrico Scarano, Radiology Department, San Carlo Hospital of Potenza, Potenza, Italy

Raffaele Scarpa, Department of Clinical and Experimental Medicine, University Federico II, Naples, Italy

Georg Schett, Rheumatology and Immunology, University of Erlangen-Nuremberg, Erlangen, Germany

Enrique R. Soriano, Rheumatology Section, Medical Services, Hospital Italiano de Buenos Aires, Buenos Aires, Argentina

Philip E. Stuart, Department of Dermatology, University of Michigan Medical School, Ann Arbor, Michigan

Junko Takeshita, Department of Dermatology, University of Pennsylvania Perelman School of Medicine, Philadelphia, USA

William Taylor, Rehabilitation Teaching and Research Unit, Department of Medicine, Wellington School of Medicine, University of Otago, New Zealand

William Tillett, Royal National Hospital for Rheumatic Diseases, Royal United Hospitals Bath NHS Foundation Trust, UK

Lam C. Tsoi, Department of Dermatology, University of Michigan Medical School, Ann Arbor, Michigan

Filip Van den Bosch, Department of Rheumatology, Ghent University Hospital, Ghent, Belgium

Robert Winchester, Division of Rheumatology, Department of Medicine, Columbia University College of Physicians and Surgeons, New York, USA

Abbreviations

AU	acute anterior uveitis
anti-CCP	anticyclic citrullinated peptide antibodies
anti-MCVs	anti-mutated citrullinated vimentin
aOR	adjusted odds ratio
AS	ankylosing spondylitis
ASAS	Assessment of SpondyloArthritris International Society
AUC	area under the receiver operating curve
BASRI	Bath Ankylosing Spondylitis Radiology Index
BB-UVB	broadband UVB
BMI	body mass index
BMPs	bone morphogenetic protein
BSA	body surface area
CAD	coronary artery disease
CCP	cyclic citrullinated peptide
CD	Crohn's disease
CHD	coronary heart disease
CI	confidence interval
C-IMT	carotid intimal medial thickness
CIR	controlled ileal release
CKD	chronic kidney disease
CPDAI	Composite Psoriatic Disease Activity Index
cPLA2	phospholipase A2
CREB	cAMP responsive element binding protein
CsA	cyclosporin
CT	computed tomography
CVD	cardiovascular disease
Cyclic AMP	cAMP
DAS28	Disease Activity Score in 28 joints
DC	dendritic cell
DC-STAMP	dendritic cell-specific transmembrane protein
DIP	distal interphalangeal
DLQI	Dermatology Quality of Life Index
DMARD	disease-modifying antirheumatic drug
DMF	dimethylfumarate
DSMIV	Diagnostic and Statistical Manual of Mental Disorders
DZ	dizygotic
ESR	erythrocyte sedimentation rate
ESRD	end-stage renal disease
ESSG	European Spondylarthropathy Study Group
EULAR	European League Against Rheumatism
FDA	US Food and Drug Administration
FLS	fibroblast-like synoviocytes
FM	fibromyalgia
GFR	glomerular filtration rate
GI	gastrointestinal
GPP	generalized pustular psoriasis
GRAPPA	Group for Research and Assessment of Psoriasis and Psoriatic Arthritis
GUESS	Glasgow Ultrasound Enthesitis Scoring System
GWAS	genome wide association studies
HDL	high-density lipoprotein
HIF	hypoxia-inducible factor
HIV	human immunodeficiency virus
HLA	human leucocyte antigen
HR	hazard ratio
HRQOL	health-related quality of life
IBD	inflammatory bowel disease
IBP	inflammatory back pain
ICAM1	intercellular adhesion molecule 1
IFN	interferon
IHD	ischaemic heart disease
ILC	innate lymphoid cells
IMID	immune-mediated inflammatory disease
INSPIRE	International Spondyloarthritis Inter-rater Reliability Exercise
IR	insulin resistance
IRR	incidence rate ratios
KIR	killer immunoglobulinlike receptor
LD	linkage disequilibrium
LEF	leflunomide
LEI	Leeds Enthesitis Index
LOS	longitudinal observational studies
MACE	major adverse cardiovascular events
MAF	minor allele frequency
MAIT	mucosa-associated invariant T cells
MASEI	MAdrid Sonographic Entheseal Index
MASES	Maastricht Ankylosing Spondylitis Enthesis Score
MCAM	melanoma cell adhesion molecule
MCP-1	monocyte chemoattractant protein-1
MCSF	monocyte-colony stimulating factor
mDCs	myeloid dendritic cells
MetS	metabolic syndrome
MHC	major histocompatibility complex
MI	myocardial infarction

MIP1α	macrophage inflammatory protein 1α	PsA	psoriatic arthritis
MMP	metalloproteinases	PsC	cutaneous-only psoriasis
mNY	modified New York	PsO	psoriasis
MR1	MHC class I-related protein	PsV	psoriasis vulgaris
MRM	multiple reaction monitoring	RA	rheumatoid arthritis
m-SASSS	modified Stoke Ankylosing Spondylitis Spine Score	RASSS	Radiographic Ankylosing Spondylitis Spinal Score
MTX	methotrexate	RF	rheumatoid factor
MZ	monozygotic	ROC	receiver operating characteristic
NAFLD	non-alcoholic fatty liver disease	RR	relative risk or risk ratio
NASH	non-alcoholic hepatic steatosis	SEC	synovial–entheseal complex
NB-UVB	narrowband	SF	synovial fluid
NCAMs	neural cell adhesion molecules	sIgA	serum secretory immunoglobulin A
NFκ-B	nuclear factor kappa-light-chain-enhancer of activated B cells	SIJ	sacroiliac joint
		SIR	standardized incidence ratio
NK	natural killer	SLE	systemic lupus erythematosus
NKG2A	natural killer group 2 member A	SM	synovial membrane
NRS	numeric rating scale	S-MAPA	simple measure for assessing psoriasis activity
NSAIDs	nonsteroidal anti-inflammatory drugs	SMD	standardized mean difference
OCPs	osteoclast precursors	SNPs	single nucleotide polymorphisms
OPG	osteoprotegerin	SpA	spondyloarthritis
OR	odds ratio	SPARCC	Spondyloarthritis Research Consortium of Canada
PASDAS	Psoriatic Arthritis Disease Activity Score	SSZ	sulfasalazine
PASI	Psoriasis Area Severity Index	TCR	T-cell receptors
PASRI	Psoriatic Arthritis Spondylitis Radiology Index	TGFβ	transforming growth factor beta
PBC	peripheral blood cells	TNF-α	tumor necrosis factor
PBMC	peripheral blood mononuclear cells	UC	ulcerative colitis
pDCs	plasmacytoid dendritic cells	uSpA	undifferentiated SpA
PDE	phosphodiesterases	UTE	ultra-short echo time
PDGF	platelet-derived growth factor	UVA	ultraviolet A
PDUS	power Doppler ultrasound	UVB	ultraviolet B
PIP	proximal interphalangeal	VAS	visual analogue scales
PMN	polymorphonuclear leukocyte	VEGF	vascular endothelial growth factor
POPP	psoriatic onychopachydermoperiostitis		

Introduction

CHAPTER 1

Introduction

Dafna Gladman and Oliver FitzGerald

When we were approached to edit a textbook on psoriatic arthritis we questioned whether it was really necessary. The Group for Research and Assessment of Psoriasis and Psoriatic Arthritis (GRAPPA) had just embarked on a GRAPPA book on psoriasis and psoriatic arthritis, and we were not convinced that another book was required. However, because of recent advances in the recognition of psoriatic arthritis, its outcome, its pathogenesis, and the development of several novel therapeutic approaches, we agreed that such an in depth textbook would be very timely indeed.

This book thus provides the most up-to-date information on advances in the field of psoriatic arthritis. These advances include the development of classification criteria, and with that the recognition that psoriatic arthritis is more common than was previously thought. Psoriatic arthritis is recognized as a complex disease which manifests in several domains, including peripheral joints, axial disease, dactylitis, and enthesitis, in addition to skin and nail lesions. The pathogenesis of psoriatic arthritis is still evolving, but further evidence for genetic contribution as well as immunologic aberrations of both the innate and adaptive immunity has emerged. This has led to novel therapeutic interventions. Moreover, new mechanisms of bone destruction and bone formation which occur in psoriatic arthritis have been identified, and these too may lead to novel therapeutic interventions. At the same time new methods of assessment of the disease and outcome measures to be used in clinical trials and clinical practice were developed. These new measures have now been incorporated into clinical trials. New imaging techniques have been developed and are at various stages of validation in psoriatic arthritis. It is now clear that psoriatic disease is associated with a number of comorbidities and their relationship to the disease process has been investigated. In addition to the conventional disease-modifying anti-rheumatic medications which have been used, albeit not very successfully, in psoriatic arthritis, we now have novel therapies in the form of anti-cytokines and small molecules which have been proven effective for most domains of the disease.

This book was structured to address these advances. We begin with chapters on epidemiology of skin and joint disease, followed by an overview of pathogenesis. Then there are individual chapters dedicated to specific pathogenetic factors including genetics, immunology including cytokines, and mechanism of bone destruction.

We then follow with the description of the domains of psoriatic arthritis beginning with a chapter on psoriasis and nail disease, followed by chapters on peripheral arthritis, axial disease, enthesitis, dactylitis, and extra-articular extra-cutaneous features occurring in patients with psoriatic arthritis. We also have a chapter dedicated to the comorbidities of psoriatic arthritis.

A section on imaging follows with chapters detailing plain radiography, ultrasound, MRI, and microCT.

Next we have chapters on clinical course and outcome as well as biomarkers for a number of disease outcomes including damage.

The development of outcome measures is described in chapters on domains and instruments, patient reported outcomes, and composite measures.

Treatment chapters include treatment of psoriasis, followed by an approach to the management of psoriatic arthritis, with detailed chapters on synthetic disease-modifying anti-rheumatic drugs, anti-tumour necrosis factor (TNF) agents, non-TNF biologic agents, and small molecules. These are followed by a chapter on treatment algorithms as well as the treat-to-target approach.

We conclude the book with a chapter on future directions.

We hope you enjoy reading this book and that it is useful as a reference book for managing your patients with psoriatic arthritis.

Epidemiology

CHAPTER 2

Epidemiology of psoriasis

Junko Takeshita and Joel M. Gelfand

Prevalence

Prevalence represents the number of people or percentage of a population that is affected by a condition at a given time. Psoriasis is a chronic, multisystem, inflammatory disease of the skin and sometimes joints that is estimated to affect approximately 125 million people worldwide [1] with a global prevalence ranging from 0.91 to 8.5% in the adult population [2]. Most studies of psoriasis have been performed among Western adult populations with prevalence estimates ranging from 2 to 4% [3, 4]. Psoriasis is suggested to be more prevalent among Caucasians but has not been well-studied in non-Caucasian populations. A single United States population-based study of psoriasis among African Americans found the prevalence of psoriasis to be 1.3% in African Americans compared with 2.5% in Caucasians [5].

Psoriasis affects men and women equally and may present at any age but is uncommon under the age of 9 with prevalence estimates of up to 0.55% [2]. The prevalence of psoriasis tends to increase with age with two major peaks around ages 20–40 [2] and 50–70 [6, 7], after which the prevalence declines [2]. The specific prevalence of psoriasis in the paediatric and elderly populations has not been as extensively studied. Existing studies from Europe and Asia suggest paediatric (less than 18 years old) psoriasis prevalence to range from 0 to 2.1% [2]. A single study of the prevalence of psoriasis among the US Medicare population, including the disabled and those aged 65 and older, estimated the administrative claims-based psoriasis prevalence to range from 0.51 to 1.23% [8]. Additional studies are needed to confirm these findings.

The majority of patients with plaque psoriasis—the most common type of psoriasis—have mild disease that is defined by the National Psoriasis Foundation as having less than 3% of their body surface area (BSA) affected. Moderate (3–10% BSA) and severe (greater than 10% BSA) plaque psoriasis, affects nearly 25% of patients [1]. Though it is an indication for treatment with phototherapy or systemic medication, up to nearly 40% of patients with moderate to severe disease remain untreated [9, 10].

Incidence

Incidence is defined by the number of people in a population that newly develop a condition during a given time period. The incidence of psoriasis has not been widely studied with only seven studies having examined psoriasis incidence in the general population (one in the paediatric population, three in the adult population, and three across all ages). Incidence rates of psoriasis vary depending on the populations studied. Population-based estimates of age- and sex- adjusted incidence rates of psoriasis in the US range from 60.4 [11] to 78.9 [12] per 100,000 person-years. European estimates derived from primary care databases report psoriasis incidence rates of 120 to 140 per 100,000 person-years [13, 14]. In a single study of psoriasis incidence among children in the United States from 1970 to 1999, the incidence was estimated to be 40.8 per 100,000 person-years with incidence rates successively increasing during the observed time period [15]. Among adults, estimates of psoriasis incidence were similar in two US studies—78.9 [12] and 82 [16] per 100,000 person-years—but higher in an Italian study at 230 per 100,000 person-years [17]. Psoriasis incidence among adults was observed to increase over a 30-year period (1970 to 2000), similar to what was observed among children [12].

All studies of psoriasis incidence reported similar trends of increasing psoriasis incidence with age up to 39 years with a second peak of increasing incidence around 50–69 years of age [2].

Principal causes

Psoriasis is a complex disorder caused by a combination of genetic, immunologic, and environmental factors, each of which plays a variable role in the development of the disease. The genetics and immunology of psoriasis are discussed in Chapters 5 and 7, respectively.

Environmental and behavioural risk factors

Of the several potential non-genetic risk factors for psoriasis, obesity [16, 18, 19] and smoking [19–21] have been identified as having stronger associations with psoriasis. In the case of obesity, large population-based prospective studies of incident psoriasis among US women found that 30% of new psoriasis cases were attributable to obesity. Importantly, each one unit increase in body mass index was associated with a 5% increased risk of psoriasis [16, 18]. With regard to smoking, men and women with new onset psoriasis were more likely to have a positive smoking history (previous or current smoker) [21], and smoking has a particularly strong association with the development of pustular psoriasis [19].

Other potential risk factors for psoriasis include alcohol use [22, 23], infections (particularly streptococcal pharyngitis as a risk factor for guttate psoriasis) [24, 25], and psychological stress [19, 26]. However, these and other emerging potential risk factors, such as periodontal disease [27] and obstructive sleep apnoea [28], require further study for confirmation.

Natural history and prognosis

Psoriasis is generally a chronic disease with waxing and waning course with variable periods of quiescence. Estimates of spontaneous disease clearance rates differ depending on the study and defined length of remission. In one study of 5,600 patients with psoriasis, approximately 39% reported spontaneous clearance at any time for durations ranging from 1 to 54 years [29]. Furthermore, before the introduction of biologic therapy, it was estimated that at least 50% of psoriasis patients with moderate to severe disease persisted with the same level of disease severity after 10 years regardless of treatment [29]. The main exception to this is guttate psoriasis which, particularly when present in children or adolescents, often runs a self-limited course with only occasional recurrences.

Comorbid diseases in psoriasis

In the last decade, major advances in psoriasis research have contributed to the recognition of psoriasis as a disorder with important health implications that extend beyond the skin. Excluding psoriatic arthritis, the epidemiology of which is discussed in Chapter 3, the first observation of comorbid disease in psoriasis patients was made in 1897 by Strauss [30] who reported an association between psoriasis and diabetes. In 1961, Reed et al. [31] described a high prevalence of heart disease including coronary thrombosis and myocardial infarction (MI) in postmortem examinations of psoriasis patients with psoriatic arthritis. Subsequently, in 1978, McDonald et al. [32] observed an increased prevalence of venous and arterial vascular disease in hospitalized psoriasis patients. Now many years later, a quickly evolving body of literature using modern epidemiological techniques has demonstrated that

psoriasis, particularly more severe disease, is associated with an increased risk of mortality, resulting in an average of 5 years of life lost, primarily due to comorbid disease, namely cardiovascular disease [33, 34].

Cardiometabolic disease

Cardiometabolic disorders have long been recognized to be associated with psoriasis, though only in more recent years have large epidemiologic studies emerged that support greater prevalence of cardiovascular risk factors (including obesity, hypertension, diabetes, dyslipidaemia, and metabolic syndrome) among patients with psoriasis compared with patients without the skin disease. Findings from these studies have been summarized in multiple systematic reviews and meta-analyses (Table 2.1). More severe psoriasis (identified either indirectly via receipt of phototherapy or systemic therapies used to treat more severe disease or directly via measures of BSA involvement by psoriasis) is generally associated with a greater likelihood of cardiometabolic diseases than mild psoriasis. For example, in a population-based study in the UK, greater BSA involvement in by psoriasis was associated with a significantly greater likelihood of metabolic syndrome in a dose-dependent relationship: adjusted odds ratio (aOR) for mild (≤2% BSA) 1.22, 95% confidence interval (CI) 1.11–1.35; moderate (3–10% BSA) 1.56, 95% CI 1.38–1.76); and severe (>10% BSA) psoriasis 1.98, 95% CI 1.62–2.43 [35]. Similarly, in the same UK population, increasing

Table 2.1 Summary of systematic reviews and meta-analyses assessing the association between psoriasis and cardiovascular disease risk factors

Study	Study design	Study dates	Total number of patients		Number of studies included	CV risk factor	Composite measure of association (95% CI)
			Psoriasis	No psoriasis			
Armstrong et al.[90]	Systematic review and meta-analysis	1 January 1980–1 January 2012	201,831	2,119,329	Total: 16 Severity Assessment: 5 Incidence: 1	Obesity	Overall: OR 1.66 (1.46–1.89) Mild: OR 1.46 (1.17–1.82) Severe: OR 2.23 (1.63–3.05) Incidence: HR 1.18 (1.14–1.23)
Armstrong et al.[91]	Systematic review and meta-analysis	1 January 1980–1 January 2012	309,469	2,384,229	Total: 24 Severity Assessment: 5 Incidence: 2	Hypertension	Overall: OR 1.58 (1.42–1.76) Mild: OR 1.30 (1.15–1.47) Severe: OR 1.49 (1.20–1.86) Incidence: HR 1.09 (1.05–1.14) RR 1.17 (1.06–1.30)
Armstrong et al.[37]	Systematic review and meta-analysis	1 January 1980–1 January 2012	404,494	4,640,847	Total: 27 Severity Assessment: 5 Incidence: 5	Diabetes	Overall: OR 1.59 (1.38–1.83) Mild: OR 1.53 (1.16–2.04) Severe: OR 1.97 (1.48–2.62) Incidence: RR 1.27 (1.16–1.40)
Ma et al.[92]	Systematic review	1 January 1980–1 January 2012	265,685	2,167,198	Total: 25 Severity Assessment: 5 Incidence: 1	Dyslipidemia	Overall OR: 1.04–5.55 Mild OR: 1.10–3.38 Severe OR: 1.26–5.55
Armstrong et al.[93]	Systematic review and meta–analysis	1 January 1980–1 January 2012	41,853	1,357,324	Total: 12 Severity Assessment: 3	Metabolic Syndrome	Overall OR: 2.26 (1.70–3.01) Mild OR: 1.22 (1.11–1.35)[a] Moderate OR: 1.56 (1.38–1.76)[a] Severe OR: 1.98 (1.62–2.43)[a]

OR, odds ratio

[a]Reported from single study by Langan et al.[35]

psoriasis severity was also significantly associated with a greater likelihood of poor blood pressure control among patients with diagnosed hypertension [36].

The directionality of association between psoriasis and cardiovascular risk factors has not yet been well established except in the cases of obesity and diabetes. As summarized earlier in this chapter (see Environmental and behavioral risk factors), data suggest that, not only are psoriasis patients more likely to be obese, but obesity seems to also be a risk factor for psoriasis [16, 18]. Regarding diabetes, multiple longitudinal studies suggest psoriasis to be a risk factor for diabetes, independent of traditional risk factors, with a pooled relative risk (RR) of 1.27 (95% CI 1.16–1.40) according to a meta-analysis of five studies [37]. Furthermore, in a population-based study in the UK, patients with severe psoriasis and incident diabetes were more likely to be treated with systemic diabetic therapy compared with patients with incident diabetes who did not have psoriasis (RR 1.55 [95% CI 1.15–2.10]) [38]. Psoriasis patients with diabetes have also been suggested to be more likely to develop microvascular (hazard ratio [HR] 1.14 [95% CI 1.06–1.23]) and macrovascular (HR 1.13 [95% CI 1.05–1.22]) complications in a single study using US administrative claims data [39].

In addition to being associated with cardiovascular risk factors, observational studies also suggest psoriasis to be associated with an increased risk of major adverse cardiovascular events (MACE) including myocardial infarction [40], stroke [41], and cardiovascular mortality [42]. Importantly, this relationship is independent of the increased prevalence of traditional cardiovascular risk factors noted among patients with psoriasis. Since the publication of the initial studies that found positive associations between psoriasis and cardiovascular outcomes, numerous subsequent epidemiologic studies have found similar results with few exceptions [43–46]. To date, eight meta-analyses assessing the association between psoriasis and various cardiovascular outcomes confirm psoriasis to be an independent risk factor for MACE (Table 2.2) [47–54]. More practically interpretable measures of the increased RR of MACE associated with psoriasis were evaluated and reported in two studies [55, 56]. In a cohort study of patients with severe psoriasis in the UK, the attributable risk of severe psoriasis on MACE over a 10-year period was found to be 6.2% [56]. Additionally, in a Dutch population-based study, the increased risk of a composite cardiovascular outcome (myocardial infarction, stroke, and cardiovascular mortality) among patients with severe psoriasis was found to be nearly identical to that conferred by diabetes alone [55].

In sum, psoriasis, especially more severe disease, is associated with significant cardiometabolic disease burden and is suggested to be an independent risk factor for MACE. Future studies aimed at identifying any causal relationships between psoriasis and cardiometabolic diseases are needed to guide the education of and medical care for patients with psoriasis.

Malignancy

Due to the chronic inflammatory nature of psoriasis, it has been hypothesized that patients with psoriasis may be at increased risk of developing cancer. Malignancy is a major cause of death after cardiovascular disease and infection among patients with psoriasis who are receiving therapies for moderate to severe disease [34]. A meta-analysis of 11 observational studies evaluating the risk of malignancy among patients with psoriasis suggests that the overall risk of cancer, excluding non-melanoma skin cancers, is increased in patients with psoriasis with an overall standardized incidence ratio (SIR) for cancer of 1.16 (95% CI 1.07–1.25) [57]. While Pouplard et al.'s [57] meta-analysis also assessed the risks of specific malignancies among psoriasis patients and suggested increased risks of upper aerodigestive tract, respiratory tract, liver, pancreas and urinary tract cancers, and lymphoma, the level of heterogeneity among the included studies was high, making interpretation challenging. Furthermore, lack of adjustment for important confounding factors such as smoking and drinking and/or accounting for psoriasis treatment effects on the risk of subsequent malignancy call into question the validity of attributing the increased risk of cancer to psoriasis, alone. In the case of lymphoma, however, three studies [58–60] performed analyses of lymphoma risk in psoriasis patients with and without exposure to systemic treatment and found a persistently increased risk of lymphoma (between 1.3 and 2-fold increased risk) among psoriasis patients without a history of immunosuppressive therapy, though absolute risk remained low. Furthermore, in Brauchli et al.'s [58] study, the association between psoriasis and lymphoma risk persisted after accounting for potential confounding factors such as smoking and drinking habits. Of the specific lymphoma types, Gelfand et al. [60] found the association between psoriasis and cutaneous T cell lymphoma to be the strongest (HR 5.84 [95% CI 3.61–9.44]). Additional studies clarifying the risk of malignancy attributable to psoriasis versus its immunosuppressive therapies are necessary.

Gastrointestinal disease

Nonalcoholic fatty liver disease

Non-alcoholic fatty liver disease (NAFLD) refers to a spectrum of liver disorders from mild hepatic steatosis to non-alcoholic steatohepatitis (NASH) which can lead to cirrhosis and, in severe cases, hepatocarcinoma. Considering the relationship between psoriasis and metabolic syndrome, the latter of which is an established risk factor for NAFLD, associations between psoriasis and NAFLD have also been suggested and reported in the literature. A meta-analysis of seven observational studies assessing the association between psoriasis and NAFLD found an overall OR of 2.15 (95% CI 1.57–2.94) for NAFLD among psoriasis patients [61]; though, the majority of included studies did not adjust for potential confounding factors such as metabolic syndrome. In a single population-based cross-sectional study of elderly (>55 years old) Rotterdam residents, psoriasis was found to be independently associated with NAFLD after adjusting for traditional risk factors such as metabolic syndrome (aOR 1.7 [95% CI 1.1–2.6]) [62], suggesting that the observed association is at least partially attributable to psoriasis. The directionality of association between psoriasis and NAFLD remains to be elucidated.

Inflammatory bowel disease

Inflammatory bowel disease (IBD) encompasses both ulcerative colitis (UC) and Crohn's disease (CD). Common genetic and inflammatory pathways have been implicated in psoriasis and IBD [63, 64] but the epidemiology of the relationship between psoriasis and IBD has not been well defined. Several cross-sectional studies have observed increased prevalences of IBD among patients with psoriasis and vice versa [65–68], though existing studies report varying degrees of association between the two diseases, and a Taiwanese study suggests an absence of association [69]. Cohen et al. [66] observed psoriasis to be more strongly associated with

Table 2.2 Summary of systematic reviews and meta-analyses assessing the association between psoriasis and major adverse cardiovascular events

Study	Study design	Study dates	Number of studies included	Total number of patients		Outcome	Composite measure of association (95% CI)	
				Psoriasis	No psoriasis			
Armstrong et al.[47]	Systematic review and meta-analysis	1 January 1980– 1 January 2012	9	Mild: 201,239 Severe: 17,415	9,914,799	Major adverse CV events (MACE): MI, stroke, CV mortality	Mild	Severe
							MI	
							RR 1.29 (1.02–1.63)	RR 1.70 (1.32–2.18)
							Stroke	
							RR 1.12 (1.08–1.16)	RR 1.56 (1.32–1.84)
							CV mortality	
							RR 1.03 (0.86–1.25)	RR 1.39 (1.11–1.74)
Gaeta et al.[48]	Meta-analysis	NR	13	1,862,297	43,407,300	CV risk: MI, vascular disease, mortality	Overall CV risk	
							RR 1.24 (1.18–1.31)	
							MI	
							RR 1.24 (1.11–1.39)	
							Vascular disease	
							RR 1.27 (1.12–1.43)	
							Mortality	
							RR 1.41 (0.97–2.04)	
Gu et al.[49]	Meta-analysis	1966–October 2012	15	Total (psoriasis + no psoriasis): 6,230,774		MI Stroke CVD CV mortality	MI	
							RR 1.32 (1.13–1.55)	
							Stroke	
							RR 1.26 (1.12–1.41)	
							CVD	
							RR 1.47 (1.30–1.60)	
							CV mortality	
							RR 1.33 (1.00–1.77)	
Horreau et al.[50]	Systematic review and meta-analysis	1980–December 2011	33	324,650	5,309,087	MI CAD Stroke	MI	
							RR Cohort: 1.25 (1.03–1.52) Cross-sectional: 1.57 (1.08–2.27)	
							CAD	
							RR Cohort: 1.20 (1.13–1.27) Case-control: 1.84 (1.09–3.09) Cross-sectional: 1.19 (1.14–1.24)	
							Stroke	
							Cohort: 1.02 (0.92–1.14) Cross-sectional: 1.14 (1.08–1.19)	

Table 2.2 Continued

Study	Study design	Study dates	Number of studies included	Total number of patients — Psoriasis	Total number of patients — No psoriasis	Outcome	Composite measure of association (95% CI)		
Miller et al.[51] 2013[a]	Systematic review and meta-analysis	Prior to October 25, 2012	75	503,686	29,686,694	CVD IHD Cerebrovascular disease CV mortality	CVD OR 1.4 (1.2–1.7) IHD OR 1.5 (1.2–1.9) Cerebrovascular disease 1.1 (0.9–1.3) CV mortality 0.9 (0.4–2.2)		
Pietrzak et al.[94]	Meta-analysis	1960–2011	14	367,358	9,199,656	CV events (MI, IHD, cerebral ischemic stroke, sudden cardiac death)	OR 1.28 (1.18–1.38)		
Samarasekera et al.[53]	Systematic review and meta-analysis	1974–2012	14	All: 488,315 Mild: 327,418 Severe: 12,854	10,024,815	MI Stroke CV mortality	**All** MI HR/IRR 1.40 (1.03–1.89) Stroke HR/IRR 1.13 (1.01–1.26) CV mortality NR	**Mild** MI HR/IRR 1.34 (1.07–1.68) Stroke HR/IRR 1.15 (0.98–1.35) SMR 1.03 (0.86–1.25)	**Severe** MI HR/IRR 3.04 (0.65–14.35) Stroke HR/IRR 1.59 (1.34–1.89) SMR 1.37 (1.17–1.60) HR 1.57 (1.26–1.96)
Xu et al.[54]	Meta-analysis	Database inception–March 2012	7	326,598	5,230,048	Composite of MI & stroke	Composite RR 1.20 (1.10–1.31) MI RR 1.22 (1.05–1.42) Stroke RR 1.21 (1.04–1.40)		

RR, relative risk or risk ratio; HR, hazard ratio; IRR, incidence rate ratio; OR, odds ratio; SMR, standardized mortality ratio

CAD, coronary artery disease; CHD, coronary heart disease; CVD, cardiovascular disease; IHD, ischaemic heart disease; MI, myocardial infarction

[a]Systematic review and meta-analysis of the association between psoriasis and cardiovascular disease and cardiovascular risk factors. Total numbers of studies and patients included are as reported in the full systematic review and meta-analysis, a subset of which is specifically relevant to psoriasis and cardiovascular disease.

CD than UC (OR 2.49 and 1.64, respectively). Similarly, in a longitudinal cohort study of US women, an increased risk of CD among patients with psoriasis was observed (RR 3.86 [95% CI 2.23–6.67]) while the risk of UC was attenuated and not statistically significant (RR 1.17 [95% CI 0.41–3.36]) [70]. Lastly, in a Danish nationwide cohort study of incident psoriasis and IBD, increased risks of CD and UC were observed among patients with psoriasis and vice versa [71]. Additional studies are necessary to better understand the nature and strength of association between psoriasis and IBD.

Psychiatric disorders

Psoriasis has a major impact on patients' physical and emotional health-related quality of life comparable to other major illnesses [72] that may predispose patients to the development of psychiatric disorders such as depression, anxiety, and suicidality.

Psychiatric disorders, particularly depression, are suggested to be more prevalent in patients with psoriasis than in the general population with the prevalence of depression among psoriasis patients estimated to be up to 62% depending on the study and definition of depression used [73]. In a meta-analysis of 98 studies, most of which were cross-sectional, examining the association between psoriasis and depression, patients with psoriasis had more depressive symptoms (pooled standardized mean difference [SMD] 1.16; 95% CI 0.67–1.66) and were more than at least one and a half times more likely to experience depression (pooled OR 1.57; 95% CI 1.40–1.76) than patients without psoriasis [73]. Most studies included in the meta-analysis defined depression based on validated questionnaires assessing depressive symptoms, whereas larger studies using secondary databases utilized diagnostic codes for depression and/or antidepressant use; very few studies defined depression based on the 4th edition of the *Diagnostic and Statistical Manual of Mental Disorders* (DSM-IV). Importantly, in studies of 217 patients with psoriasis, Gupta et al. [74, 75] found that 10% of patients reported a desire to be dead, 5.5% of patients reported active suicidal ideation, and hospitalized psoriasis patients had an approximately 2- to 3-fold higher prevalence of suicidal ideation than outpatients and general medical patients.

The risk of depression in psoriasis has been specifically evaluated in two cohort studies: one population-based study in the UK [76] and another among US women [77]. In the UK study, Kurd et al. [76] found patients with psoriasis to have increased risks of depression (HR 1.39; 95% CI 1.37–1.41), anxiety (HR 1.31; 95% CI 1.29–1.34), and suicidality (HR 1.44; 95% CI 1.32–1.57), and the findings were robust to several sensitivity analyses including adjustment for comorbid conditions. Furthermore, the risk of depression was greatest among patients receiving therapies for severe psoriasis (HR 1.72; 95% CI 1.57–1.88). Similarly, Dommasch et al. [77] found psoriasis in women to be associated with a nearly 30% increased risk of depression (RR 1.29; 95% CI 1.10–1.52), independent of age, body mass index (BMI), lifestyle factors, and comorbid conditions. These findings highlight the importance of being aware of psychiatric disorders among patients with psoriasis.

Chronic kidney disease

The concept of 'psoriatic nephropathy' is relatively new and was first introduced in the literature based on case reports of glomerulonephritis in patients with psoriasis [78]. To further elucidate any relationship between psoriasis and renal disease, a population-based cohort study in the UK was performed and was the first to report an increased risk of moderate to advanced chronic kidney disease (CKD) among patients with psoriasis (HR 1.05; 95% 1.02–1.07), independent of traditional risk factors for CKD [79]. Patients receiving therapies for severe psoriasis were found to be particularly at risk with a nearly two-fold greater risk of CKD compared with patients without psoriasis (HR 1.93; 95% CI 1.79–2.08). Furthermore, in a nested analysis of psoriasis patients with documented BSA involvement to define psoriasis severity, more severe skin disease was confirmed to be significantly associated with increasing prevalence of CKD (HR for mild 0.89; 95% CI 0.72–1.10; moderate 1.36; 95% CI 1.06–1.74; and severe psoriasis 1.58; 95% CI 1.07–2.34) [79], suggesting that the findings were not entirely attributable to psoriasis therapies. Confirming Wan et al.'s [79] novel observations, a subsequent Taiwanese population-based study also found increased risks of CKD and end-stage renal disease (ESRD) among patients with severe psoriasis as defined by receipt of phototherapy or systemic therapies (HR for CKD 1.90; 95% CI 1.33–2.70; and HR for ESRD 2.97; 95% CI 1.72–5.11) [80]. Future studies confirming and characterizing the associations between psoriasis and kidney disease will be important in furthering our understanding of this newly identified relationship.

Other emerging comorbidities

Additional emerging comorbid conditions that have been suggested to be associated with psoriasis include chronic obstructive pulmonary disease [81–83], peptic ulcer disease [82, 84], serious infection [85, 86], sexual dysfunction [87], and obstructive sleep apnoea [28, 88, 89] among others. Further characterization of known comorbidities and identification of new comorbid disease associations with psoriasis are anticipated as research efforts continue to focus on the epidemiology of psoriasis and its comorbid diseases.

References

1. National Psoriasis Foundation. http://www.psoriasis.org/research/science-of-psoriasis/statistics. Accessed September 1, 2014.
2. Parisi R, Symmons DP, Griffiths CE, et al. Global epidemiology of psoriasis: a systematic review of incidence and prevalence. J Invest Dermatol 2013;133(2):377–85.
3. Kurd SK, Gelfand JM. The prevalence of previously diagnosed and undiagnosed psoriasis in US adults: results from NHANES 2003-2004. J Am Acad Dermatol 2009;60(2):218–24.
4. Rachakonda TD, Schupp CW, Armstrong AW. Psoriasis prevalence among adults in the United States. J Am Acad Dermatol 2014;70(3):512–6.
5. Gelfand JM, Stern RS, Nijsten T, et al. The prevalence of psoriasis in African Americans: results from a population-based study. J Am Acad Dermatol 2005;52(1):23–6.
6. Smith AE, Kassab JY, Rowland Payne CM, Beer WE. Bimodality in age of onset of psoriasis, in both patients and their relatives. Dermatology 1993;186(3):181–6.
7. Henseler T, Christophers E. Psoriasis of early and late onset: characterization of two types of psoriasis vulgaris. J Am Acad Dermatol 1985;13(3):450–6.
8. Takeshita J, Gelfand JM, Li P, et al. Psoriasis in the U.S. Medicare population: prevalence, treatment, and factors associated with biologic use. J Invest Dermatol 2015; 135(12):2955–63.
9. Armstrong AW, Robertson AD, Wu J, Schupp C, Lebwohl MG. Undertreatment, treatment trends, and treatment dissatisfaction among patients with psoriasis and psoriatic arthritis in the United

States: findings from the National Psoriasis Foundation surveys, 2003-2011. JAMA Dermatol 2013;149(10):1180–5.

10. Horn EJ, Fox KM, Patel V, Chiou CF, Dann F, Lebwohl M. Are patients with psoriasis undertreated? Results of National Psoriasis Foundation survey. J Am Acad Dermatol 2007;57(6):957–62.

11. Bell LM, Sedlack R, Beard CM, Perry HO, Michet CJ, Kurland LT. Incidence of psoriasis in Rochester, Minn, 1980-1983. Arch Dermatol 1991;127(8):1184–7.

12. Icen M, Crowson CS, McEvoy MT, Dann FJ, Gabriel SE, Maradit Kremers H. Trends in incidence of adult-onset psoriasis over three decades: a population-based study. J Am Acad Dermatol 2009;60(3):394–401.

13. Donker GA, Foets M, Spreeuwenberg P, van der Werf GT. [Management of psoriasis in family practice is now in closer agreement with the guidelines of the Netherlands Society of Family Physicians]. Ned Tijdschr Geneeskd 1998;142(24):1379–83.

14. Huerta C, Rivero E, Rodriguez LA. Incidence and risk factors for psoriasis in the general population. Arch Dermatol 2007;143(12):1559–65.

15. Tollefson MM, Crowson CS, McEvoy MT, Maradit Kremers H. Incidence of psoriasis in children: a population-based study. J Am Acad Dermatol 2010;62(6):979–87.

16. Setty AR, Curhan G, Choi HK. Obesity, waist circumference, weight change, and the risk of psoriasis in women: Nurses' Health Study II. Arch Intern Med 2007;167(15):1670–5.

17. Vena GA, Altomare G, Ayala F, et al. Incidence of psoriasis and association with comorbidities in Italy: a 5-year observational study from a national primary care database. Eur J Dermatol 2010;20(5):593–8.

18. Kumar S, Han J, Li T, Qureshi AA. Obesity, waist circumference, weight change and the risk of psoriasis in US women. J Eur Acad Dermatol Venereol 2013;27(10):1293–8.

19. Naldi L, Chatenoud L, Linder D, et al. Cigarette smoking, body mass index, and stressful life events as risk factors for psoriasis: results from an Italian case-control study. J Invest Dermatol 2005;125(1):61–7.

20. Setty AR, Curhan G, Choi HK. Smoking and the risk of psoriasis in women: Nurses' Health Study II. Am J Med 2007;120(11):953–9.

21. Li W, Han J, Choi HK, Qureshi AA. Smoking and risk of incident psoriasis among women and men in the United States: a combined analysis. Am J Epidemiol 2012;175(5):402–13.

22. Naldi L, Peli L, Parazzini F. Association of early-stage psoriasis with smoking and male alcohol consumption: evidence from an Italian case-control study. Arch Dermatol 1999;135(12):1479–84.

23. Qureshi AA, Dominguez PL, Choi HK, Han J, Curhan G. Alcohol intake and risk of incident psoriasis in US women: a prospective study. Arch Dermatol 2010;146(12):1364–9.

24. Naldi L, Peli L, Parazzini F, Carrel CF, Psoriasis Study Group of the Italian Group for Epidemiological Research in D. Family history of psoriasis, stressful life events, and recent infectious disease are risk factors for a first episode of acute guttate psoriasis: results of a case-control study. J Am Acad Dermatol 2001;44(3):433–8.

25. Gudjonsson JE, Thorarinsson AM, Sigurgeirsson B, Kristinsson KG, Valdimarsson H. Streptococcal throat infections and exacerbation of chronic plaque psoriasis: a prospective study. Br J Dermatol 2003;149(3):530–4.

26. Dominguez PL, Han J, Li T, Ascherio A, Qureshi AA. Depression and the risk of psoriasis in US women. J Eur Acad Dermatol Venereol 2013;27(9):1163–7.

27. Nakib S, Han J, Li T, Joshipura K, Qureshi AA. Periodontal disease and risk of psoriasis among nurses in the United States. Acta Odontol Scand 2013;71(6):1423–9.

28. Cohen JM, Jackson CL, Li TY, Wu S, Qureshi AA. Sleep disordered breathing and the risk of psoriasis among US women. Arch Dermatol Res 2015;307(5):433–8.

29. Farber EM, Nall ML. The natural history of psoriasis in 5,600 patients. Dermatologica 1974;148(1):1–18.

30. Strauss H. Zur Lehre von der neurogenen und der thyreogenen Glykosurie. Dtsch Med Wochenschr. 1897;20:309–12.

31. Reed WB, Becker SW, Rohde R, Heiskell CL. Psoriasis and arthritis. Clinicopathologic study. Arch Dermatol 1961;83:541–8.

32. McDonald CJ, Calabresi P. Psoriasis and occlusive vascular disease. Br J Dermatol 1978;99(5):469–75.

33. Gelfand JM, Troxel AB, Lewis JD, et al. The risk of mortality in patients with psoriasis: results from a population-based study. Arch Dermatol 2007;143(12):1493–9.

34. Abuabara K, Azfar RS, Shin DB, Neimann AL, Troxel AB, Gelfand JM. Cause-specific mortality in patients with severe psoriasis: a population-based cohort study in the U.K. Br J Dermatol 2010;163(3):586–92.

35. Langan SM, Seminara NM, Shin DB, et al. Prevalence of metabolic syndrome in patients with psoriasis: a population-based study in the United Kingdom. J Invest Dermatol 2012;132(3 Pt 1):556–62.

36. Takeshita J, Wang S, Shin DB, et al. Effect of psoriasis severity on hypertension control: a population-based study in the United Kingdom. JAMA Dermatol 2015;151(2):161–9.

37. Armstrong AW, Harskamp CT, Armstrong EJ. Psoriasis and the risk of diabetes mellitus: a systematic review and meta-analysis. JAMA Dermatol 2013;149(1):84–91.

38. Azfar RS, Seminara NM, Shin DB, Troxel AB, Margolis DJ, Gelfand JM. Increased risk of diabetes mellitus and likelihood of receiving diabetes mellitus treatment in patients with psoriasis. Arch Dermatol 2012;148(9):995–1000.

39. Armstrong AW, Guerin A, Sundaram M, et al. Psoriasis and risk of diabetes-associated microvascular and macrovascular complications. J Am Acad Dermatol 2015;72(6):968–77.

40. Gelfand JM, Neimann AL, Shin DB, Wang X, Margolis DJ, Troxel AB. Risk of myocardial infarction in patients with psoriasis. JAMA 2006;296(14):1735–41.

41. Gelfand JM, Dommasch ED, Shin DB, et al. The risk of stroke in patients with psoriasis. J Invest Dermatol 2009;129(10):2411–8.

42. Mehta NN, Azfar RS, Shin DB, Neimann AL, Troxel AB, Gelfand JM. Patients with severe psoriasis are at increased risk of cardiovascular mortality: cohort study using the General Practice Research Database. Eur Heart J 2010;31(8):1000–6.

43. Brauchli YB, Jick SS, Miret M, Meier CR. Psoriasis and risk of incident myocardial infarction, stroke or transient ischaemic attack: an inception cohort study with a nested case-control analysis. Br J Dermatol 2009;160(5):1048–56.

44. Dowlatshahi EA, Kavousi M, Nijsten T, et al. Psoriasis is not associated with atherosclerosis and incident cardiovascular events: the Rotterdam Study. J Invest Dermatol 2013;133(10):2347–54.

45. Parisi R, Rutter MK, Lunt M, et al. Psoriasis and the risk of major cardiovascular events: cohort study using the Clinical Practice Research Datalink. J Invest Dermatol 2015;35(9):2189–97.

46. Wakkee M, Herings RM, Nijsten T. Psoriasis may not be an independent risk factor for acute ischemic heart disease hospitalizations: results of a large population-based Dutch cohort. J Invest Dermatol 2010;130(4):962–7.

47. Armstrong EJ, Harskamp CT, Armstrong AW. Psoriasis and major adverse cardiovascular events: a systematic review and meta-analysis of observational studies. J Am Heart Assoc 2013;2(2):e000062.

48. Gaeta M, Castelvecchio S, Ricci C, Pigatto P, Pellissero G, Cappato R. Role of psoriasis as independent predictor of cardiovascular disease: A meta-regression analysis. Int J Cardiol 2013;168(3):2282–8.

49. Gu WJ, Weng CL, Zhao YT, Liu QH, Yin RX. Psoriasis and risk of cardiovascular disease: a meta-analysis of cohort studies. Int J Cardiol 2013;168(5):4992–6.

50. Horreau C, Pouplard C, Brenaut E, et al. Cardiovascular morbidity and mortality in psoriasis and psoriatic arthritis: a systematic literature review. J Eur Acad Dermatol Venereol 2013;27 Suppl 3:12–29.

51. Miller IM, Ellervik C, Yazdanyar S, Jemec GB. Meta-analysis of psoriasis, cardiovascular disease, and associated risk factors. J Am Acad Dermatol 2013;69(6):1014–24.

52. Pietrzak A, Bartosinska J, Chodorowska G, Szepietowski JC, Paluszkiewicz P, Schwartz RA. Cardiovascular aspects of psoriasis: an updated review. Int J Dermatol 2013;52(2):153–62.

53. Samarasekera EJ, Neilson JM, Warren RB, Parnham J, Smith CH. Incidence of cardiovascular disease in individuals with psoriasis: a systematic review and meta-analysis. J Invest Dermatol 2013;133(10):2340–46.

54. Xu T, Zhang YH. Association of psoriasis with stroke and myocardial infarction: Meta-analysis of cohort studies. Br J Dermatol 2012;167(6):1345–50.

55. Ahlehoff O, Gislason GH, Charlot M, et al. Psoriasis is associated with clinically significant cardiovascular risk: a Danish nationwide cohort study. J Intern Med 2011;270(2):147–57.

56. Mehta NN, Yu Y, Pinnelas R, et al. Attributable risk estimate of severe psoriasis on major cardiovascular events. Am J Med 2011;124(8):775 e771–6.

57. Pouplard C, Brenaut E, Horreau C, et al. Risk of cancer in psoriasis: a systematic review and meta-analysis of epidemiological studies. J Eur Acad Dermatol Venereol 2013;27 Suppl 3:36–46.

58. Brauchli YB, Jick SS, Miret M, Meier CR. Psoriasis and risk of incident cancer: an inception cohort study with a nested case-control analysis. J Invest Dermatol 2009;129(11):2604–12.

59. Margolis D, Bilker W, Hennessy S, Vittorio C, Santanna J, Strom BL. The risk of malignancy associated with psoriasis. Arch Dermatol 2001;137(6):778–83.

60. Gelfand JM, Shin DB, Neimann AL, Wang X, Margolis DJ, Troxel AB. The risk of lymphoma in patients with psoriasis. J Invest Dermatol 2006;126(10):2194–201.

61. Candia R, Ruiz A, Torres-Robles R, Chavez-Tapia N, Mendez-Sanchez N, Arrese M. Risk of non-alcoholic fatty liver disease in patients with psoriasis: a systematic review and meta-analysis. J Eur Acad Dermatol Venereol 2015;29(4):656–62.

62. van der Voort EA, Koehler EM, Dowlatshahi EA, et al. Psoriasis is independently associated with nonalcoholic fatty liver disease in patients 55 years old or older: Results from a population-based study. J Am Acad Dermatol 2014;70(3):517–24.

63. Najarian DJ, Gottlieb AB. Connections between psoriasis and Crohn's disease. J Am Acad Dermatol 2003;48(6):805–21; quiz 822–04.

64. Skroza N, Proietti I, Pampena R, et al. Correlations between psoriasis and inflammatory bowel diseases. Biomed Res Int 2013;2013:983902.

65. Yates VM, Watkinson G, Kelman A. Further evidence for an association between psoriasis, Crohn's disease and ulcerative colitis. Br J Dermatol. 1982;106(3):323–30.

66. Cohen AD, Dreiher J, Birkenfeld S. Psoriasis associated with ulcerative colitis and Crohn's disease. J Eur Acad Dermatol Venereol 2009;23(5):561–5.

67. Bernstein CN, Wajda A, Blanchard JF. The clustering of other chronic inflammatory diseases in inflammatory bowel disease: a population-based study. Gastroenterology. 2005;129(3):827–36.

68. Lee FI, Bellary SV, Francis C. Increased occurrence of psoriasis in patients with Crohn's disease and their relatives. Am J Gastroenterol 1990;85(8):962–3.

69. Tsai TF, Wang TS, Hung ST, et al. Epidemiology and comorbidities of psoriasis patients in a national database in Taiwan. J Dermatol Sci 2011;63(1):40–6.

70. Li WQ, Han JL, Chan AT, Qureshi AA. Psoriasis, psoriatic arthritis and increased risk of incident Crohn's disease in US women. Ann Rheum Dis 2013;72(7):1200–5.

71. Egeberg A, Mallbris L, Warren RB, et al. Association between psoriasis and inflammatory bowel disease—a Danish nationwide cohort study. Br J Dermatol 2016;175(3):487–92.

72. Rapp SR, Feldman SR, Exum ML, Fleischer AB, Jr., Reboussin DM. Psoriasis causes as much disability as other major medical diseases. J Am Acad Dermatol 1999;41(3 Pt 1):401–7.

73. Dowlatshahi EA, Wakkee M, Arends LR, Nijsten T. The prevalence and odds of depressive symptoms and clinical depression in psoriasis patients: a systematic review and meta-analysis. J Invest Dermatol 2014;134(6):1542–51.

74. Gupta MA, Schork NJ, Gupta AK, Kirkby S, Ellis CN. Suicidal ideation in psoriasis. Int J Dermatol 1993;32(3):188–90.

75. Gupta MA, Gupta AK. Depression and suicidal ideation in dermatology patients with acne, alopecia areata, atopic dermatitis and psoriasis. Br J Dermatol 1998;139(5):846–50.

76. Kurd SK, Troxel AB, Crits-Christoph P, Gelfand JM. The risk of depression, anxiety, and suicidality in patients with psoriasis: a population-based cohort study. Arch Dermatol 2010;146(8):891–5.

77. Dommasch ED, Li T, Okereke OI, Li Y, Qureshi AA, Cho E. Risk of depression in women with psoriasis: a cohort study. Br J Dermatol 2015;173(4):975-80.

78. Singh NP, Prakash A, Kubba S, et al. Psoriatic nephropathy–does an entity exist? Ren Fail 2005;27(1):123–7.

79. Wan J, Wang S, Haynes K, Denburg MR, Shin DB, Gelfand JM. Risk of moderate to advanced kidney disease in patients with psoriasis: population based cohort study. BMJ 2013;347:f5961.

80. Chi CC, Wang J, Chen YF, Wang SH, Chen FL, Tung TH. Risk of incident chronic kidney disease and end-stage renal disease in patients with psoriasis: A nationwide population-based cohort study. J Dermatol Sci 2015;78(3):232–8.

81. Dreiher J, Weitzman D, Shapiro J, Davidovici B, Cohen AD. Psoriasis and chronic obstructive pulmonary disease: a case-control study. Br J Dermatol 2008;159(4):956–60.

82. Yeung H, Takeshita J, Mehta NN, et al. Psoriasis severity and the prevalence of major medical comorbidity: a population-based study. JAMA Dermatol 2013;149(10):1173–9.

83. Chiang YY, Lin HW. Association between psoriasis and chronic obstructive pulmonary disease: a population-based study in Taiwan. J Eur Acad Dermatol Venereol 2012;26(1):59–65.

84. Yang YW, Keller JJ, Lin HC. Medical comorbidity associated with psoriasis in adults: a population-based study. Br J Dermatol 2011;165(5):1037–43.

85. Wakkee M, de Vries E, van den Haak P, Nijsten T. Increased risk of infectious disease requiring hospitalization among patients with psoriasis: a population-based cohort. J Am Acad Dermatol 2011;65(6):1135–44.

86. Kao LT, Lee CZ, Liu SP, Tsai MC, Lin HC. Psoriasis and the risk of pneumonia: a population-based study. PLoS ONE 2014;9(12):e116077.

87. Molina-Leyva A, Jimenez-Moleon JJ, Naranjo-Sintes R, Ruiz-Carrascosa JC. Sexual dysfunction in psoriasis: a systematic review. J Eur Acad Dermatol Venereol 2015;29(4):649–55.

88. Papadavid E, Vlami K, Dalamaga M, et al. Sleep apnea as a comorbidity in obese psoriasis patients: a cross-sectional study. Do psoriasis characteristics and metabolic parameters play a role? J Eur Acad Dermatol Venereol 2013;27(7):820–26.

89. Yang YW, Kang JH, Lin HC. Increased risk of psoriasis following obstructive sleep apnea: a longitudinal population-based study. Sleep Med 2012;13(3):285–9.

90. Armstrong AW, Harskamp CT, Armstrong EJ. The association between psoriasis and obesity: a systematic review and meta-analysis of observational studies. Nutr Diabetes 2012;2:e54.

91. Armstrong AW, Harskamp CT, Armstrong EJ. The association between psoriasis and hypertension: a systematic review and meta-analysis of observational studies. J Hypertens 15 2012.

92. Ma C, Harskamp CT, Armstrong EJ, Armstrong AW. The association between psoriasis and dyslipidaemia: a systematic review. Br J Dermatol 2013;168(3):486–95.

93. Armstrong AW, Harskamp CT, Armstrong EJ. Psoriasis and metabolic syndrome: A systematic review and meta-analysis of observational studies. J Am Acad Dermatol 2013;68(4):654–62.

94. Pietrzak A, Bartosinska J, Chodorowska G, Szepietowski JC, Paluszkiewicz P, Schwartz RA. Cardiovascular aspects of psoriasis: An updated review. Int J Dermatol 2013;52(2):153–62.

CHAPTER 3

Epidemiology of psoriatic arthritis

Elaine Husni and Madonna Michael

Introduction

Epidemiological studies of the incidence and prevalence of psoriatic arthritis (PsA) are quite challenging to interpret as our understanding of the disease is still evolving. As knowledge of case definitions of psoriatic diseases matures, the epidemiology of this disease may be more uniformly documented. There is evidence that psoriatic disease is influenced by both genetics and environmental factors, adding to its complexity. However, in general, our understanding of many rheumatic diseases, including PsA, has been greatly advanced by data obtained from epidemiologic studies. In this chapter, we will review the main epidemiologic studies to date regarding PsA.

PsA is a unique chronic, inflammatory joint disease, associated with cutaneous psoriasis. The diverse and unique characteristics of PsA distinguish this disease from other types of inflammatory arthritis. Apart from joint involvement, PsA also commonly affects surrounding musculoskeletal structures such as tendons and ligaments leading to dactylitis or enthesitis. In addition, PsA can affect the nails, causing nail pitting and onycholysis. There are also multiple comorbidities seen in PsA including cardiovascular disease, uveitis, osteoporosis, and subclinical bowel inflammation. Due to this heterogeneity in the disease itself and other methodological issues, the ability to accurately define the epidemiology of PsA has been an ongoing challenge to investigators.

Classification of PsA was previously achieved by the Moll and Wright criteria, which were developed in 1973, but more recently an updated classification scheme, known as the CASPAR criteria, was developed in 2006 [1, 2]. Prompt diagnosis and treatment may alleviate joint pain and inflammation, ultimately preventing disease progression. Accurately diagnosing PsA, especially in the early stages of the disease, continues to remain challenging due to the disease heterogeneity, and overlapping clinical picture resembling other inflammatory joint diseases. Patients presenting with cutaneous psoriasis and arthritis raise clinical suspicion and these presentations may aid in establishing a diagnosis. However, in 10% to 15% of PsA patients, joint symptoms appear prior to skin manifestations of psoriasis (referred to as 'psoriatic arthritis sine psoriasis'), and often times there may be a delay in diagnosis. An extensive review of past medical history, thorough physical examination, laboratory tests and advanced imaging may aid in evaluating and accurately diagnosing patients with PsA earlier.

Treatments with anti–tumour necrosis factor (TNF) inhibitors and IL-17 inhibitors have been a remarkable breakthrough in the management of this disease. In addition to the large improvement in the peripheral synovial disease and cutaneous psoriasis, there is significant benefit in alleviating axial disease, dactylitis, and enthesitis symptoms in comparison to traditional nonbiologic disease-modifying therapies.

Epidemiology

PsA prevalence is reported in up to 1% of the worldwide general population, and more specifically in 0.3% to 1% of the US population, with a range of 7% to 42% in patients with known psoriasis [3–6] (Table 3.1). For the last several decades, studies conducted from around the world reported wide ranges of PsA incidence and prevalence in different countries, ranging from 0.1 to 23.0/100,000, and 0.001 to 0.42%, respectively, making interpretation difficult (Table 3.1). Some of the wide range and variation in PsA epidemiology may be due to ethnic and geographical distribution along with age and gender as real contributing factors while lack of precise case definition and sample size account for methodological variability within the studies [7–10].

The literature continues to demonstrate some debate in stratifying true incidence rates of PsA. A 30-year prospective study in Olmsted County, Minnesota, USA, conducted by Wilson et al., identifies 147 patients fulfilling the CASPAR criteria and demonstrates an increase in incidence of PsA over time. Results displayed age- and sex-adjusted incidence of PsA/100,000 increased from 3.6 (95% confidence interval [CI] 2.0–5.2) in the decade of the 1970s to 9.8 (95% CI 27.7–11.9) in the 1990s [11]. A 30-year cross-sectional, multi-centre study in Europe, conducted by Christophers et al., identified 1,560 patients with plaque psoriasis, of which 126 patients had PsA. Results of a survival analysis reflects stable PsA incidence (less than 1%) and an increase in prevalence of 20.5% through the 30-year period reviewed [12].

A 6-year, prospective, health management organization-based study from Buenos Aires, Argentina, conducted by Soriano et al., including adults (>18 years) meeting the CASPAR criteria, reports estimates of PsA incidence of 6.26 (95% CI 4.2–8.3) cases/100,000 person-years, and prevalence of 74 (95% CI 5–94) cases/100,000 members. Soriano et al. conclude that the calculated PsA incidence and prevalence rates in the study are similar to other studies from the United States and Europe [13]. A 14-year cross-sectional study from England by Ogdie et al., involving 4.8 million adults (18–90 years old), where primary care derived data was collected through THIN (The Health Improvement Network) database, using diagnostic

Table 3.1 PsA epidemiology according to countries

Country	Incidence (1/100,000)	Prevalence (%)	Study
USA	7.2	0.16–0.25	[11]
Central Norway	41.3	0.67	[16]
Japan	—	0.001	[29]
England	—	0.19	[14]
Argentina	6.3	0.07	[13]
Southern Sweden	8.0	0.25	[21, 30]
Greece	3.02	0.17	[19, 31]
Finland	23.0	—	[32]
Iceland	—	0.14	[22]

codes to identify PsA patients, displayed a PsA prevalence rate of 0.19% (95% CI 0.185–0. 193) overall, and 8.6% (95% CI 7.7–9.5) in patients with psoriasis [14].

A prospective Canadian study with over 400 patients with psoriasis (PsO) followed for onset of PsA demonstrated an incidence rate of 2.7 (95% CI 2.1–3.6) cases/100 psoriasis patients [15].

A 9-year population-based study known as the HUNT 3 (Nord-Trøndelag Health) from Central Norway, conducted by Hoff et al., collected information on 1,238 patients with known or at high risk of PsA using patient questionnaires and a brief medical examination. PsA diagnosis was then identified by reviewing medical records from 2000–2008 and applying CASPAR criteria. This study demonstrated a PsA incidence of 41.3 (95% CI 35.8–47.6) cases/ 100,000 person-years, and prevalence of 6.7 (95% CI 5.9–7.4) cases/ 1,000 members [16].

Several studies attempt to correlate the variation of PsA epidemiology, with geographical distribution. Two systematic reviews of multiple studies on psoriatic disease from Europe, the Americas (USA, Argentina, Mexico), Asia, and Australia, suggest lower prevalence and incidence in Asia and specifically Japan in comparison to the Americas and Europe [7, 8]. A more recent study conducted in Japan suggested, however, that PsA prevalence in psoriasis patients is similar to that of Western countries and more than that previously reported in Asia [17]. It was difficult to interpret and summarize these systematic reviews, given the wide range of PsA incidence and prevalence. Some differences could be attributed to using a population-based vs cohort-based study which may underestimate or overestimate its true incidence or prevalence [7, 8].

A recent study by Haroon et al., comprised of 100 patients with known skin psoriasis followed in a dermatology clinic, had patients complete PsA screening questionnaires and an extensive musculoskeletal evaluation by rheumatologists who were blinded to the questionnaires results. This study concluded that 29% of patients with skin psoriasis were diagnosed with PsA for the first time [18].

PsA may occur at any age, commonly presenting in both males and females between the ages of 40 to 50 years [8, 19, 20]. Unlike other types of inflammatory arthritis with a larger female predominance, PsA seems to affect men equally or even at a slightly greater rate [8]; however, there are some smaller geographically focused studies that have reported a female predominance [21, 22]. There are only a few studies regarding ethnicity. An interesting cross-sectional study of 146 patients with PsA with varying ethnic backgrounds demonstrated that PsA was seen more commonly in Caucasians (58.3%) than in South Asians (18.5%; P < 0.001) or African/Afro-Caribbean (7.3%; P < 0.002) individuals [23].

Screening

PsA can be underdiagnosed and under treated and significant effort has been directed towards earlier detection of PsA. Since approximately 30% of psoriasis patients develop PsA, it seems prudent to screen for PsA in psoriasis on a more consistent basis. Many studies have focused on multidisciplinary collaborations between dermatologists and rheumatologists, in which psoriasis patients were either managed simultaneously or with some variation of comanagement. Through this type of dual management approach, researchers identified a high percentage of psoriasis patients who were unaware of their underlying diagnosis of PsA. This collaborative effort reflects the ability to achieve an earlier diagnosis of PsA, through early screening and better evaluation of patients with psoriasis [18, 24].

Several screening methods have been developed to aid in early identification of patients with PsA, especially in general practitioners and dermatology outpatient clinics. The most commonly used screening tools are the Psoriasis Arthritis Screening and Evaluation Questionnaire (PASE), the Psoriasis Epidemiology Screening Tool (PEST), and the Toronto Psoriatic Arthritis Screen (ToPAS), with reported sensitivity of 93%, 92%, and 87%, and specificity of 75%, 78%, and 93%, respectively. Of note, these patient questionnaires were used in various medicine disciplines with some used in internal medicine populations while other screening tools were used in dermatology populations, thus making it difficult to compare them directly [18, 25–27]. A more recent study suggested that adding axial involvement to the ToPAS questionnaire increases the sensitivity of the test as a screening tool as axial disease is more likely to be part of the PsA spectrum [28].

Conclusion

Despite recent efforts to improve upon the reporting of PsA epidemiology, the true incidence and prevalence of PsA may continue to be underestimated. Caregivers should maintain a high level of suspicion in patients with pre-existing psoriasis. Early screening and management of PsA may likely increase the recognition and diagnosis of this disease and be able to better define the true incidence and prevalence with greater precision. Furthermore, a multidisciplinary approach between primary care physicians (PCPs), dermatologists, and rheumatologists should be encouraged in the diagnosis and management of PsA as this heterogeneous disease is best cooperatively managed.

References

1. Zlatkovic-Svenda M, Kerimovic-Morina D, Stojanovic RM. Psoriatic arthritis classification criteria: Moll and Wright, ESSG and CASPAR—a comparative study. Acta Reum Port 2013;38(3):172–8.
2. Coates LC, Conaghan PG, Emery P, et al. Sensitivity and specificity of the classification of psoriatic arthritis criteria in early psoriatic arthritis. Arthritis Rheum 2012;64(10):3150–5.
3. Gladman DD, Antoni C, Mease P, Clegg DO, Nash P. Psoriatic arthritis: epidemiology, clinical features, course, and outcome. Ann Rheum Dis 2005;64 Suppl 2:ii14–7.

4. Mease PJ, Armstrong AW. Managing patients with psoriatic disease: the diagnosis and pharmacologic treatment of psoriatic arthritis in patients with psoriasis. Drugs 2014;74(4):423–41.

5. Gottlieb A, Korman NJ, Gordon KB, et al. Guidelines of care for the management of psoriasis and psoriatic arthritis: section 2. Psoriatic arthritis: overview and guidelines of care for treatment with an emphasis on the biologics. J Am Acad Dermatol 2008;58(5):851–64.

6. Gelfand JM, Gladman DD, Mease PJ, et al. Epidemiology of psoriatic arthritis in the population of the United States. J Am Acad Dermatol 2005;53(4):573.

7. Chandran V, Raychaudhuri SP. Geoepidemiology and environmental factors of psoriasis and psoriatic arthritis. J Autoimmun 2010;34(3):J314–21.

8. Liu J-T, Yeh H-M, Liu S-Y, Chen K-T. Psoriatic arthritis: epidemiology, diagnosis, and treatment. World J Orthop 2014;5(4):537.

9. Parisi R, Symmons DPM, Griffiths CEM, Ashcroft DM. Global epidemiology of psoriasis: a systematic review of incidence and prevalence. J Invest Dermatol 2012;133(2):377–85.

10. Löfvendahl S, Theander E, Svensson Å, Carlsson KS, Englund M, Petersson IF. Validity of diagnostic codes and prevalence of physician-diagnosed psoriasis and psoriatic arthritis in southern Sweden–a population-based register study. PLoS One 2014;9(5):e98024.

11. Wilson FC, Icen M, Crowson CS, McEvoy MT, Gabriel SE, Kremers HM. Time trends in epidemiology and characteristics of psoriatic arthritis over three decades: a population-based study. J Rheumatol 2009;36(2):361–7.

12. Christophers E, Barker JNWN, Griffiths CEM, et al. The risk of psoriatic arthritis remains constant following initial diagnosis of psoriasis among patients seen in European dermatology clinics. J Eur Acad Dermatol Venereol 2010;24(5):548–54.

13. Soriano ER, Rosa J, Velozo E, et al. Incidence and prevalence of psoriatic arthritis in Buenos Aires, Argentina: a 6-year health management organization-based study. Rheumatology (Oxford) 2011;50(4):729–34.

14. Ogdie A, Langan S, Love T, et al. Prevalence and treatment patterns of psoriatic arthritis in the UK. Rheumatology (Oxford) 2013;52(3):568–75.

15. Eder L, Haddad A, Rosen CF, et al. The incidence and risk factors for psoriatic arthritis in patients with psoriasis—a prospective cohort study. Arthritis Rheumatol (Hoboken, NJ) Arthritis Rheumatol. 2016;68(4):915–23.

16. Hoff M, Gulati AM, Romundstad PR, Kavanaugh A, Haugeberg G. Prevalence and incidence rates of psoriatic arthritis in central Norway: data from the Nord-Trøndelag health study (HUNT). Ann Rheum Dis 2015;74(1):60–4.

17. Ohara Y, Kishimoto M, Takizawa N, et al. Prevalence and clinical characteristics of psoriatic arthritis in Japan. J Rheumatol 2015;42(8):1439–42.

18. Haroon M, Kirby B, FitzGerald O. High prevalence of psoriatic arthritis in patients with severe psoriasis with suboptimal performance of screening questionnaires. Ann Rheum Dis 2013;72(5):736–40.

19. Alamanos Y, Voulgari P V, Drosos AA. Incidence and prevalence of psoriatic arthritis: a systematic review. J Rheumatol 2008;35(7):1354–8.

20. Eder L, Thavaneswaran A, Chandran V, Gladman DD. Gender difference in disease expression, radiographic damage and disability among patients with psoriatic arthritis. Ann Rheum Dis 2013;72(4):578–82.

21. Haglund E, Bremander AB, Petersson IF, et al. Prevalence of spondyloarthritis and its subtypes in southern Sweden. Ann Rheum Dis 2011;70(6):943–8.

22. Love TJ, Gudbjornsson B, Gudjonsson JE, Valdimarsson H. Psoriatic arthritis in Reykjavik, Iceland: prevalence, demographics, and disease course. J Rheumatol 2007;34(10):2082–8.

23. Ciurtin C, Roussou E. Cross-sectional study assessing family members of psoriatic arthritis patients affected by the same disease: differences between Caucasian, South Asian and Afro-Caribbean populations living in the same geographic region. Int J Rheum Dis 2013;16(4):418–24.

24. Mease PJ, Gladman DD, Papp KA, et al. Prevalence of rheumatologist-diagnosed psoriatic arthritis in patients with psoriasis in European/North American dermatology clinics. J Am Acad Dermatol 2013;69(5):729–35.

25. Khraishi M, Mong J, Mugford G, Landells I. The electronic Psoriasis and Arthritis Screening Questionnaire (ePASQ): a sensitive and specific tool to diagnose psoriatic arthritis patients. J Cutan Med Surg 2011;15(3):143–9.

26. Ibrahim GH, Buch MH, Lawson C, Waxman R, Helliwell PS. Evaluation of an existing screening tool for psoriatic arthritis in people with psoriasis and the development of a new instrument: the Psoriasis Epidemiology Screening Tool (PEST) questionnaire. Clin Exp Rheumatol 2009;27(3):469–74.

27. Gladman DD, Schentag CT, Tom BDM, et al. Development and initial validation of a screening questionnaire for psoriatic arthritis: the Toronto Psoriatic Arthritis Screen (ToPAS). Ann Rheum Dis 2009;68(4):497–501.

28. Tom BDM, Chandran V, Farewell VT, Rosen CF, Gladman DD. Validation of the Toronto Psoriatic Arthritis Screen Version 2 (ToPAS 2). J Rheumatol 2015;42(5):841–6.

29. Hukuda S, Minami M, Saito T, et al. Spondyloarthropathies in Japan: nationwide questionnaire survey performed by the Japan Ankylosing Spondylitis Society. J Rheumatol 2001;28(3):554–9.

30. Söderlin MK, Börjesson O, Kautiainen H, Skogh T, Leirisalo-Repo M. Annual incidence of inflammatory joint diseases in a population based study in southern Sweden. Ann Rheum Dis 2002;61(10):911–5.

31. Trontzas P, Andrianakos A, Miyakis S, et al. Seronegative spondyloarthropathies in Greece: a population-based study of prevalence, clinical pattern, and management. The ESORDIG study. Clin Rheumatol 2005;24(6):583–9.

32. Savolainen E, Kaipiainen-Seppänen O, Kröger L, Luosujärvi R. Total incidence and distribution of inflammatory joint diseases in a defined population: results from the Kuopio 2000 arthritis survey. J Rheumatol 2003;30(11):2460–8.

Pathogenesis

CHAPTER 4

Overview of psoriatic arthritis pathogenesis

Kurt de Vlam

Introduction

Psoriatic arthritis (PsA) is a chronic inflammatory arthritis occurring in patients with psoriasis presenting with different subtypes. Some subtypes, such as the oligoarticular and axial subtypes can be classified as spondyloarthritis (SpA). An enthesitis-based model has been proposed to unify skin and joint manifestation in some of the subtypes, and to differentiate PsA from other rheumatic diseases such as rheumatoid arthritis (RA) and osteoarthritis but it is unclear if this model can explain all different manifestations [1]. The aetiology and pathogenesis is still subject of intensive research since it is poorly understood. Moreover until recently the concept of PsA was heavily debated. However, the occurrence of arthritis amongst the patients with psoriasis is more common than one would expect by random co-occurrence of an inflammatory arthritis and psoriasis in the same individual, supporting the concept of PsA as a separate entity. The existence of patients with psoriasis, arthritis, and rheumatoid factor, and/or anti-cyclic citrullinated peptide (CCP) antibodies is a real challenge for the concept and the understanding of the aetiopathogenesis of PsA.

The development of PsA results from the interplay of genes, the immune response, and different environmental factors. The fact that more than 80% of patients with PsA have precedent or simultaneous psoriasis suggests that the skin disease is almost a 'conditio sine qua non' for the development of PsA. Data from an animal model suggest that epidermal alterations are sufficient to initiate both skin lesions (psoriasis) and arthritis. The induction of an epidermal deletion of JunB and its functional companion c-Jun in adult mice results in the development of psoriasis and specific arthritic involvement within two weeks [2]. Insight into the pathogenesis of psoriasis may lead to better understanding of the development of PsA.

In PsA different phases can be distinguished during the disease process. Clinically, there is a preclinical stage, an early (inflammatory) stage, and a chronic/established stage with or without damage. Different stages are also recognized in disease pathogenesis: initiation, amplification, and effector stages. In each of these stages different cell types and molecules play an important role (Figure 4.1).

Is psoriatic arthritis an autoimmune disease or autoinflammatory disease?

Autoimmune diseases are mainly mediated by the adaptive/acquired immune system and refer to diseases where high titres of organ-specific and non-organ-specific autoantibodies may predate disease by years. MHC class II associations and extra-articular manifestations are common. Immunopathology primarily relates to aberrant B and T cells and dendritic cell responses in primary and secondary lymphoid organs resulting in breaking of tolerance. RA, primary biliary cirrhosis, Hashimoto's thyroiditis, and systemic lupus erythematosus are classic examples. These diseases can be induced in animal models by injection of specific autoantigens.

Autoinflammatory diseases are principally mediated by the innate immune system without ostensible adaptive immune responses contributing to immunopathology. Tissue damage is due to excessive activation of innate immune cells, including macrophages and neutrophils and non-immune cells. Local factors at the predisposed site lead to innate immune cell activation evolving in self-directed inflammation. Hereditary periodic fevers are a typical example.

Finally, a group of diseases shows characteristics of both and have a strong adaptive and innate immune overlaps. This group of disorders provides evidence for tissue-specific factors that contribute to disease; their immunopathology is related to subsequent adaptive immune responses and best exemplified by the MHC class-1-associated diseases. There is a striking clinical overlap with the autoinflammatory diseases [3].

PsA has previously been viewed as an archetypical autoimmune disorder and by extension psoriasis and psoriatic nail disease also. But in PsA, tissue-specific autoantibodies have not yet been identified (Figure 4.2). Psoriasis and PsA are associated with MHC Class 1 alleles. PsA cannot be induced by injection by autoantigens in animal models but rather by overexpression or deletion of specific growth factors, cytokines or proteins in specific signalling pathways. Therefore it cannot be viewed as an autoimmune disease and is best classified as an autoinflammatory condition.

Aetiology of psoriatic arthritis

The actual disease model proposes a tissue-specific dysregulation (skin and/or joint) that culminates in a secondary inflammatory response. It is believed that there is a genetic basis for the inflammatory process.

A 40-fold increase of recurrence rate in first-degree relatives of patients with PsA suggests a strong and complex genetic susceptibility component along with an important environmental contribution [4]. Additional evidence of the genetic basis for PsA arises from association studies demonstrating class-I human leukocyte antigens

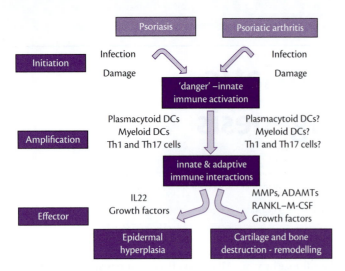

Figure 4.1 Parallels between psoriasis and psoriatic arthritis. In both diseases, initiation, amplification, and effector phases can be distinguished. Innate immune mechanisms appear essential in the initiation of the cascades, but in the further development of the chronic inflammatory reaction, adaptive immune mechanisms also contribute. In the effector phase, tissue specificity of the reaction may be a critical factor in determining the outcome of disease. ADAMTS, a disintegrin-like metalloproteinase with thrombospondin motifs; DC, dendritic cell; IL, interleukin; M-CSF, monocyte colony-stimulating factor; MMP, matrix metalloproteinase; RANKL, receptor activator of nuclear factor-κB ligand; Th, T-helper cell.

(HLA), non-HLA major histocompatibility complex (MHC) genes and validated genetic associations outside the MHC region [5]. Genome wide association studies (GWAS) revealed common genes in psoriasis and PsA but also genes exclusively linked to PsA [6, 7].

Genes may contribute at different levels of the disease process: initiation and magnitude of the inflammatory process, clinical presentation, outcome with or without damage, and co-morbidities. Among environmental triggers infections, trauma, stress, and, recently, the microbiome have been studied.

Immunogenetics

Genes involved in different aspects and stages of the inflammatory and immune response have been identified in psoriasis and PsA.

Genes involved in antigen presentation may alter signalling pathways. In GWAS different genes have been identified either crucial for antigen presentation such as HLA-B and HLA-C or in function and generation of CD8+ cells. The earliest association studies showed a consistent and dominant effect of genes located on chromosome 6p21.3 within the MHC region. Different HLA genes are associated with PsA: HLA–Cw0602 but to a lower extent than in psoriasis, HLA-B*13, HLA-B*27, HLA-B*38/39, HLA-B*57 and HLA-DRB1*04. A more in depth association study shows different haplotypes, such as HLA-C*12/B*38, HLA-B*27, and HLA-C*06/B*57, to be robustly associated with PsA. However, it remains difficult to determine whether the primary association is with arthritis or psoriasis [8, 9].

Recently specific HLA association related to the clinical phenotype in PsA and psoriasis have been identified [10]. HLA-C*0602 is notably lower in PsA than in psoriasis. HLA-B*2705 and HLA-B*3902 are susceptibility alleles for arthritis but not for psoriasis while HLA-B*0801 in PsA is protective for the development of

psoriasis. HLA-B*2705 is associated with symmetrical sacroiliitis while asymmetric sacroiliitis is associated with the HLA-B*08:01-C07:01 haplotype.

Enthesitis and dactylitis are associated with the HLA-B*2705-C01:02 haplotype [11]. The underlying mechanisms for these associations are not clear yet.

Also genes outside the MHC region are associated with PsA and psoriasis. A RunX3 variant is found in PsA and psoriasis. Interestingly, RunX3 is also associated with ankylosing spondylitis, but is different from the allelic variant in PsA. RunX3 is involved in CD8+ differentiation pointing to PsA as a T-cell-mediated disease and underlining the role of the adaptive immune system in PsA and psoriasis [12]. PTPN22 is solely associated with the susceptibility to PsA but not to psoriasis. This shows evidence for a specific PsA risk locus [6]. PTPN22 is a potent inhibitor of T cell activation but may have a differential effect between the different T cell populations. The functional role of this association has yet to be elucidated.

Genes related to innate immunity dealing with interferon (IFN), tumour necrosis factor (TNF)-α, and nuclear factor kappa-light-chain-enhancer of activated B cells (NFκ-B) signalling are associated in both PsA and psoriasis. Genetic variation in the IFN signalling may lead to accumulation of pro-inflammatory cytokines contributing to the psoriatic disease. Up to eight genes coding for proteins essential for TNF signalling have been identified but only one reached genome-wide significance for PsA: Tyk2 [7]. Although TNF-α is identified as a key pro-inflammatory cytokine in psoriasis and PsA, GWAS initially failed to detect any association with psoriatic arthritis. A meta-analysis showed a significant association between TNF-α-238A/G and TNF-α-857 T/C polymorphism and susceptibility [13]. Most genes found to be associated with psoriasis interfere with NFκ-B signalling and four of them also reached significance for PsA: TNIP1, REL, FBXL19 and TYK2.

Finally genes involved in the adaptive immune response are also associated with psoriasis and PsA [5]. The emerging role of IL-17 and-IL-17 promoting cytokines in the pathogenesis of psoriatic disease directed the interest to the Th17 signalling pathway and the genes involved. Several associated genes have been identified in the interleukin-23 (IL-23) pathway for psoriasis and PsA. In PsA candidate gene approaches revealed variation in IL-23A, IL-23R and STAT3. GWAS only showed significance for IL-12β. The finding of a Tyk2 association is of interest since Tyk2 binds to the IL-12Rβ and is critical for IL-23 signalling and Th17 differentiation. TRAF3IP2 which is significantly associated with PsA and codes for Act-1 involved in Il17 signalling.

Genes involved in IL-1β signalling were initially reported but not confirmed. Up until now, no genes have been found to be associated with either the TGB-β and IL-6 signalling pathways.

Environmental factors

The initiating factors of the psoriatic disease are still an enigma. Several factors are hypothesized to induce the inflammatory process on a susceptible genetic background. Trauma, infection, and microbiome interactions are now considered as possible candidates.

Trauma

Mechanical stress per se or microtrauma with subsequent inflammation may initiate arthritis in psoriasis patients with the susceptible genetic background. More than 40 years ago, Moll and Wright

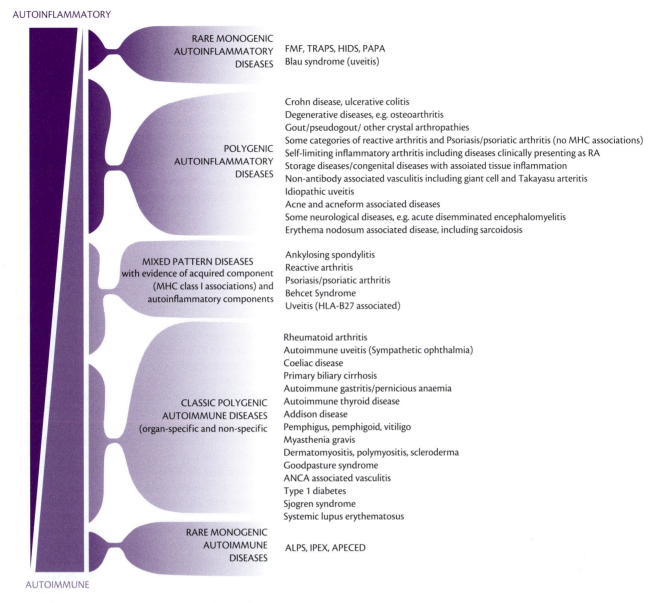

AUTOINFLAMMATORY

RARE MONOGENIC AUTOINFLAMMATORY DISEASES
FMF, TRAPS, HIDS, PAPA
Blau syndrome (uveitis)

POLYGENIC AUTOINFLAMMATORY DISEASES
Crohn disease, ulcerative colitis
Degenerative diseases, e.g. osteoarthritis
Gout/pseudogout/ other crystal arthropathies
Some categories of reactive arthritis and Psoriasis/psoriatic arthritis (no MHC associations)
Self-limiting inflammatory arthritis including diseases clinically presenting as RA
Storage diseases/congenital diseases with assoiated tissue inflammation
Non-antibody associated vasculitis including giant cell and Takayasu arteritis
Idiopathic uveitis
Acne and acneform associated diseases
Some neurological diseases, e.g. acute disemminated encephalomyelitis
Erythema nodosum associated disease, including sarcoidosis

MIXED PATTERN DISEASES with evidence of acquired component (MHC class I associations) and autoinflammatory components
Ankylosing spondylitis
Reactive arthritis
Psoriasis/psoriatic arthritis
Behcet Syndrome
Uveitis (HLA-B27 associated)

CLASSIC POLYGENIC AUTOIMMUNE DISEASES (organ-specific and non-specific
Rheumatoid arthritis
Autoimmune uveitis (Sympathetic ophthalmia)
Coeliac disease
Primary biliary cirrhosis
Autoimmune gastritis/pernicious anaemia
Autoimmune thyroid disease
Addison disease
Pemphigus, pemphigoid, vitiligo
Myasthenia gravis
Dermatomyositis, polymyositis, scleroderma
Goodpasture syndrome
ANCA associated vasculitis
Type 1 diabetes
Sjogren syndrome
Systemic lupus erythematosus

RARE MONOGENIC AUTOIMMUNE DISEASES
ALPS, IPEX, APECED

AUTOIMMUNE

Figure 4.2 The immunological disease continuum, with examples.

The monogenic 'autoinflammatory' diseases may be exclusively determined by local tissue-specific factors. For rare monogenic 'autoimmune' conditions, the disease localization appears to be determined predominantly by the adaptive immune response. The clinical heterogeneity within immunological diseases, both among patients and between populations, may reflect the variable expression of autoinflammatory and autoimmune factors in disease causation. For example, in humans, there is considerable genetic and molecular evidence for uveitis falling into all of the disease categories, with the exception of the rare monogenic autoimmune diseases. There is also considerable overlap between polygenic autoinflammatory diseases and MHC class 1-associated diseases, but to simplify classification, these are split up into different categories. This figure does not include all immunologically recognized diseases because there are so many.
Reproduced from McGonagle D, McDermott MF. A proposed classification of the immunological diseases. PLoS Med. 2006 Aug;3(8):e297 under the Creative Commons license CC by 2.0 UK.

described different cases of trauma preceding arthritis onset with subsequent development of arthritis mutilans [14]. This event was termed the deep Koebner phenomenon in reference to the Koebner phenomenon observed in some patients with skin psoriasis. The Koebner phenomenon is the formation of psoriatic lesions in uninvolved skin of psoriatic patients after cutaneous trauma and is described as early as in 1876 by Heinrich Koebner. It is not exclusively linked to psoriasis but is also described in other cutaneous diseases such as vitiligo and lichen planus. The pathogenesis is unknown but cytokines, stress proteins, adhesion molecules, and autoantigens

may be involved. As the Koebner phenomenon is well recognized in psoriasis it has become more and more clear that a similar phenomenon, the deep Koebner phenomenon, may also exist in PsA. Asymptomatic entheseal or bone abnormalities, documented by ultrasound or MRI, have been frequently described in patients with psoriasis. A recent study found that 40% of subclinical entheseal involvement evolves to overt disease over a period of 3 years [15]. Psoriasis patients without PsA show clear signs of enthesophyte formation at mechanically exposed sites on the joint while this phenomenon is absent in healthy controls [16].

Furthermore, the development of PsA following a fracture or occupations such as heavy lifting is also described [17–20]. Recent data showed that the thumbnail of the dominant hand is most involved, pointing towards local factor involved, such as injury. The evidence for links between trauma and the development of arthritis in humans is circumstantial. For many decades, the links between joint and skin were viewed in relation with the synovial inflammation, but a plausible explanation was lacking. Only recently it was demonstrated that the early phase in PsA and other SpA-related disease are associated with subclinical enthesitis and osteitis in the same joint [21, 22]. Further suggestions are derived from MRI studies in degenerative diseases. Mechanical problems and degenerative arthritis show the same patterns of involvement on MRI as in PsA [23]. After extreme exercises, elite soldiers show bone oedema patterns on MRI comparable to that seen in PsA [24]. These MRI observations suggest that entheses and adjacent bone are involved. Entheses and the adjacent bone are subject to high mechanical loading with subsequent microtrauma and microinflammation even in apparently normal entheses; Ultrasound has confirmed the microdamage at the enthesis fibrocartilage in both healthy subjects and SpA patients [25]. The unifocal development of PsA in identical twins following a site-specific trauma supports evidence for biomechanical triggering in genetically susceptible individuals [26]. However, microtrauma does not explain all patterns of joint involvement in PsA.

Formal proof is difficult to obtain in humans but, based on the knowledge of the synovial entheseal organ, the mechanical stress paradigm has been tested in animal models. Mechanical stress is involved in the development of enthesitis in the TNFΔARE model. In this model dysregulated production of TNFα induces enthesitis, sacroiliitis, and Crohn's-like ileitis. The disease starts with inflammation of the Achilles tendon and spreads subsequently to the adjacent tissues. Furthermore, the enthesis fibroblasts are the key players in the initiation of the enthesitis [27]. Hind limb unloading can efficiently prevent enthesitis development at the Achilles tendon [28]. Mechanical stress exerted on fibroblasts induces a variety of intracellular signalling responses such as the activation of the MAPK and p38 kinases, which can induce IL-23 overexpression at the entheseal site. At least in mice, this IL-23 overexpression is dependent on the presence of a novel population of innate lymphoid-like cells at the enthesis [29]. Blockade of the MAPkinase ErK delays the enthesitis onset in the TNFΔARE mice [28].

Infection

Infection is another possible inciting factor. The association of guttate psoriasis and streptococcal infection of the upper respiratory airways strengthens this suggestion. Elevated levels of antibodies to streptococcal exotoxin anti-deoxyribonuclease-B in PsA were found while absent in patients with psoriasis without arthritis [30]. The presence of streptococci-specific ribosomal RNA was described in the peripheral blood of patients with PsA and also in some synovial fluids but not in the blood of patients with RA [31]. Also an association of infections requiring antibiotic therapy was reported in patients with psoriasis who subsequently developed PsA [19]. The presence of bacteria-related antigens could not be found in a large number of joints examined from patients with PsA. A more recent study could not confirm a disease-specific role of synovial T lymphocytes when compared between RA, PsA, and osteoarthritis. In all three diseases, T cell clones proliferated in a similar way in response to group A streptococci [32]. It remains unclear if streptococci and, by extension, bacteria in general play a specific role in the pathogenesis of PsA leading to a form of reactive arthritis or if it is just an ubiquitous trigger of PsA.

An increased incidence of serological markers for hepatitis C has been reported in patients with PsA compared to patients with RA but is not confirmed [33, 34]. Finally the advent of HIV and the *de novo* appearance of psoriasis and PsA in a population with previously low incidence and prevalence such as the sub-Saharan population renewed interest in the dysregulation of innate immunity due to infection [35, 36].

But a clear-cut contribution of an infectious pathogen, either bacterial or viral, to the pathogenesis and development of PsA remains elusive.

Environment–host interaction: the role of the microbiome

The skin and the gut are the largest physical barriers of defence in the human body towards the outside world. They are both complex and dynamic ecosystems harbouring an extensive number of microorganisms. Disruption of these physical barriers is hypothesized to contribute to the development of psoriasis and PsA.

There is evidence of inflammation in the gut and the skin in patients with psoriasis and PsA.

Functional and genetic studies implicate the role of certain genes in the barrier function of the skin and in innate and adaptive immune system. There is also an increasing role for the IL-23/IL-17 axis in the pathogenesis of psoriasis and PsA. This points towards a central role of the Th17 subset of T cells. Local microbiota seem to be important in driving the Th17 cell repertoire and are important for maintaining the balance between regulatory T cells and Th17 cells in the gut. Animal models support the role for microbiota interactions with Th17 cells and indicate that resident commensals are necessary for optimal skin immune fitness [37]. The study of the skin microbiome symbiotic relationship with host and microbe is ongoing in psoriasis. The microbiome can be studied using cultivation-dependent or cultivation-independent methods.

For psoriasis the microbial biota has not been defined using cultivation-dependent methods, but the cultivation-independent approach shows overrepresentation of some phyla such as Firmicutes (46.2%) compared to normal skin of patients and healthy persons while others such as Actinobacteria showed underrepresentation. Finally, some are underrepresented in affected psoriatic skin and at intermediate level in non-affected skin of these patients but still much lower than on the skin of healthy persons. Thus psoriasis is associated with substantial alteration in the composition and representation of the cutaneous bacterial biota [38, 39, 40].

As PsA develops in patients with psoriasis, the study of the microbiome of the skin and the gut in those patients with psoriasis with or without arthritis may be of interest. Patients with PsA and psoriasis had a lower relative abundance of multiple intestinal bacteria compared to normal healthy persons but significant differences between PsA and psoriasis patients were noticed. In PsA, *Akkermansia* and *Ruminococcus* were decreased compared to psoriasis patients and in psoriasis there was a relative underrepresentation of *Bacteroides* and *Coprobacillus*. None of the bacterial taxa were overrepresented in PsA. Interestingly the reduction of *Ruminococcus* and *Akkermansia* are also reported in the intestinal microbiome in IBD [41].

The alteration of the microbial community in the gut was associated with a differential local immune response, measured by the concentration of luminal serum secretory immunoglobulin A (sIgA): sIgA was increased in PsA and conversely faecal RANK-ligand was decreased; furthermore the reduced production of medium-chain fatty acids by the intestinal microbial population reflects the altered microbial population [41].

It is still unclear if the observed state of dysbiosis is causative or rather a consequence of chronic inflammation. Many factors, including medications and diet may influence results.

Inflammatory process in psoriatic disease: the histopathology of psoriatic arthritis

An important distinction must be made in the natural history of both psoriasis and PsA by identifying two phases: an initiation phase where inflammation starts and a maintenance phase that perpetuates the inflammatory process. This distinction is actually clearer in psoriasis than in PsA. This conceptual distinction can help identify cellular and molecular events that initiate and trigger the disease and those which induce a self-perpetuating inflammatory process.

Immunopathology in PsA can be studied by analysing the immunopathologic differences between inflammation in the psoriatic skin and synovitis. Organ-specific reactions between skin and synovial tissue can partly explain these differences. An alternative approach compares the key differences between PsA and RA, a different inflammatory arthritis. Further, comparison of involved and uninvolved joints in the same patients could reveal clues to subclinical involvement. Finally, comparing joints before and after treatment can reveal patterns of treatment success or failure [42].

The inflammatory process in PsA is not limited to the synovial membrane, as in RA, but can also affects the entheses, juxtaarticular bone, tendon sheaths, and fat pads. It is suggested that, at least in some patients, the primary lesions are found in the entheses.

Synovitis

Synovitis is characterized by inflammation in the synovial tissue compartment and by the production of synovial fluid. The key features of synovitis in PsA are increased vascularity, tissue proliferation, and infiltration by inflammatory cells.

Angiogenesis is a prominent early event in psoriasis and PsA. It is a fundamental and necessary step in synovial inflammation. Dysregulated angiogenesis facilitates synovial membrane vessel infiltration, persistent leucocyte infiltration, and lining layer hyperplasia capable of destroying adjacent cartilage and bone. Macroscopically PsA synovitis is characterized by tortuous hypervascularity, hyperaemic villi and to some extent thin fibrinoid deposits. In contrast, arthroscopic evaluation in RA shows a straight vessel pattern but has a higher degree of vascularity. The elongated and tortuous vessels in PsA are a specific feature and suggest dysregulated angiogenesis. Factors associated with angiogenesis such as vascular endothelial growth factor (VEGF), transforming growth factor beta (TGFβ), and angiopoietins are present in the synovial fluid, synovial tissue, and skin of PsA patients [43, 44]. The levels of VEGF are similar in the synovial fluid of PsA compared to RA, but there is less VEGF, mRNA, and Ang2 mRNA in the perivascular regions of PsA synovium [45, 46, 47]. VEGF, Ang, platelet-derived growth factor (PDGF) and neural cell adhesion molecules (NCAMs) all regulate vessel stability but also induce fibroblast invasion.

Hypoxia seems to be the key driving force for angiogenesis and activation of inflammatory cells and vascular remodelling. In PsA low levels of synovial tissue pO2 are associated with increased vascularity and blood vessel instability in the inflamed joint and alter the responsiveness to TNF inhibitors. Hypoxia-inducible factor (HIF)-1α is expressed in synovial tissue in chronic arthritis. *In vitro* hypoxia induces the expression of HIF1-α, key angiogenic factors, chemokines, and metalloproteinases (MMP) in synovial cell cultures. Recent studies showed that the effects of hypoxia and subsequent increase of reactive oxygen species are mediated by the NOX-2 protein in inflammatory arthritis [48].

Hypertrophy of cellular layers is recognized in both psoriasis and PsA. Hypertrophy of the synovial layer is omnipresent in PsA but to a lesser extent than in RA [49]. p53 is a marker associated with synovial hypertrophy and is also over-expressed in PsA in the lining, sublining, and the endothelial layer although at a significantly lower level than in RA. In contrast to RA, the expression of p53 in PsA is not associated with joint damage [50].

In PsA, a marked *infiltration* of mononuclear cells (T and B lymphocytes as well as macrophages and plasma cells) and polymorphonuclear cells is found in the synovial tissue. (Figure 4.3) The cellular infiltrate is predominantly in the perivascular regions and may migrate to the lining layers of the joint. Follicular aggregates of lymphocytes, both of T cells and B cells, resembling lymphoid follicles are a marked feature of RA but have also been described in PsA. More extensive analysis of synovial tissue in PsA showed frequent ectopic lymphoid neogenesis with typical highly organized structure responding upon effective treatment [51].

Synovial fluid

The cellular compartment of the synovial fluid in PsA contains an increased number of clonally expanded CD8+ T-cells while clonally expanded CD4+ T-cells are fewer in number [52, 53]. VLA-1 integrin expressing T-cells isolated from synovial fluids, in particular, display an oligoclonal repertoire [54].

High levels of TNF-α, TNF-α receptors, IL-1, IL-6, IL-8, IL-13, and other pro-inflammatory cytokines are found in the synovial fluid, but not as much as those in RA synovium [55, 56].

Also IL-22 levels are significantly elevated in synovial fluids. IL-22 induces proliferation of fibroblast-like synoviocytes (FLS) and has a synergistic effect on the proliferation of FLS from PsA patients in the presence of TNF-α [57]. IL-22 also enhances the expression of MMP-1 and MMP-3 [58]. A specific anti IL-22R antibody can successfully inhibit the IL-22-induced FLS proliferation. IL -22 is a downstream effector of IL-23 suggesting an important role for the IL-17/IL-23 pathway in the local synovial pathology in PsA.

CCL22 production was significantly increased in the synovial fluids of PsA patients [59, 60]. CXC chemokines attract neutrophil granulocytes and T-cells. CXCL9, CXCL10, and CCL2 may contribute to the presence of neutrophils in the inflamed tissue in PsA.

The roles of MMP-2 and MMP-9 in angiogenesis have been investigated. Synovial fluid MMP-9 levels were significantly increased in early PsA patients compared to early RA patients. In PsA patients, MMP-2 was detected in the latent form only, while MMP-9 was present in both latent and active forms. Both gelatinases and tissue inhibitors of metalloproteinases, such as TIMP-1 and TIMP-2, were more concentrated in synovial fluid than in serum [61, 62].

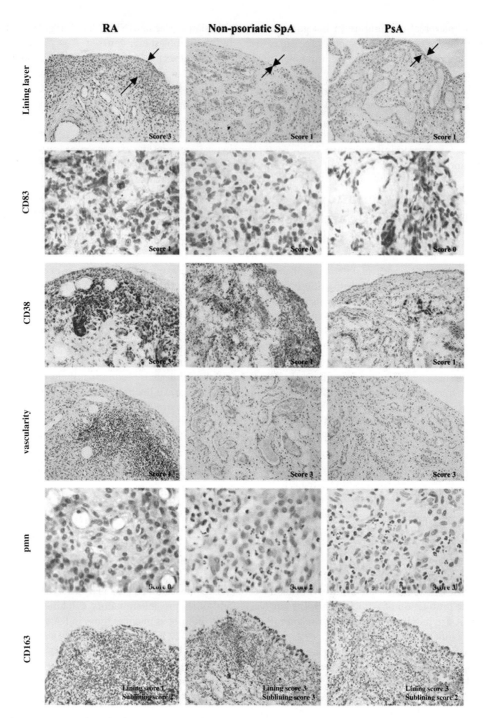

Figure 4.3 Synovial histology in patients with RA (RA), psoriatic arthritis (PsA) and non-psoriatic spondyloarthropathy (ankylosing spondylitis [AS] + undifferentiated spondyloarthropathy [USpA]).
Synovial biopsies from RA, PsA, and spondyloarthropathy (SpA; AS/USpA) patients were scored on a semiquantitative scale (0–3) by two independent observers. Representative sections of RA and PsA and non-psoriatic SpA synovium are shown, and the corresponding semiquantitative score for each picture is indicated.
The evaluated parameters included synovial lining layer thickness, CD83+ dendritic cells, CD38+ plasma cells, degree of vascularity, number of neutrophils (polymorphonuclear neutrophils [pmn]) and CD163+ macrophages

Reprinted from Kruithof E et al. Synovial histopathology of psoriatic arthritis, both oligo- and polyarticular, resembles spondyloarthropathy more than it does rheumatoid arthritis (2005) Arthritis Research and Therapy 7:R569 under Creative Commons license CC by 2.0 http://www.arthritis-research.com/content/7/3/R569.

Enthesitis

The enthesis is the anatomic site of ligamentous or capsular attachment to the bone and is of great importance in the understanding of the pathophysiology of PsA and SpA. Recently, the concept has broadened to the synovio-entheseal complex and entheseal organ [63]. This concept may explain some of the particular features of PsA differentiating PsA from RA. The pathological features of enthesitis are hardly studied in PsA. The few available materials originate mostly from patients with SpA, including some specimens from PsA patients.

Synovio-entheseal complex

Enthesitis is an important feature in PsA. Recent studies have suggested that inflammation in PsA may arise at the enthesis based on imaging and anatomical data and might be present in the subclinical phase of the disease [64]. In the earliest clinical phase, perientheseal oedema has been demonstrated on MRI. Inflammation at the enthesis might be accompanied by an exuberant repair response that results in new bone formation or even ankylosis. Biopsy samples from the Achilles tendon or anterior cruciate entheses have shown disruption of the normal entheseal architecture within the fibrous part with disorganization of the normal fibrillar architecture, increased vascularity, and cellular infiltration [65]. While this is an important hypothesis, it does not explain all features of PsA.

Histological analysis shows that the entheseal architecture is abnormal in the SpA group, with increased vascularity in the fibrous part of the enthesis and cellular infiltration compared with normal subjects. On immunohistochemical analysis, the predominant immune cells at the enthesis were CD68+ macrophages, mainly found at the sites of increased vascularity and cellularity. Neither the fibrous part of the enthesis nor the fibrocartilaginous parts were infiltrated by lymphocytes (either CD3 or CD8) but T lymphocytes could be detected in the bone marrow near the enthesis (predominantly CD8) [65, 66] (Figure 4.4).

Osteitis and juxta-articular bone involvement

In PsA, there are different manifestations of dynamic bone involvement including large eccentric erosions, tuft resorption,

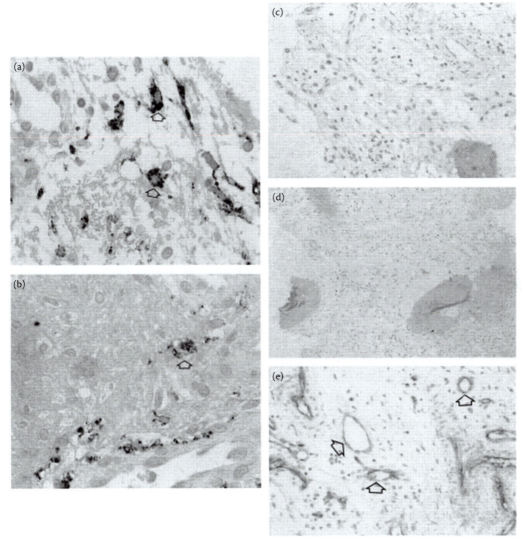

Figure 4.4 Immunohistochemistry using the ABC method showing the presence of macrophages in fibrous tissue at the enthesis (open arrows) (a) and in the entheseal fibrocartilage (b) with prominent CD68 positive staining. There is no CD3 (c) or CD8 (d) positive lymphocytic infiltration at these sites. The increased vascularity within the enthesis is demonstrated by CD34 positivity (open arrows) (e).
Reproduced from McGonagle D, Marzo-Ortega H, O'Connor P, et al. Histological assessment of the early enthesitis lesion in spondyloarthropathy Annals of the Rheumatic Diseases 2002;61:534-537 with permission from BMJ Publishing Group Ltd.

periostitis, ankylosis, and acro-osteolysis. Two striking features of peripheral involvement in PsA are subchondral peri-entheseal oedema and diffuse bone oedema, which are not present in RA [67, 68].

In RA, oedema is considered to be a pre-erosive lesion. It is not clear if bone oedema in PsA reflects the same process or might be related to osteoproliferation as seen in the spontaneous arthritis model in caged DBA1 mice. This model shows some striking characteristics of PsA such as ankylosing enthesitis, dactylitis, and onychoperiostitis. The morphological changes in this model are driven by bone morphogenetic proteins [69].

The subchondral bone adjacent to the joint or enthesis is almost unexplored in PsA. The few available materials originate mostly from patients with SpA, including some specimens from PsA patients.

The sub-entheseal bone is disorganized with increased vascularity. Hyperosteoclastic erosive lesions are found. The bone marrow shows oedema and inflammatory cellular infiltrate including T cells (CD4+ and CD8+), CD68+ macrophages, and proliferating fibroblasts. There is an increased expression of TNFα and TGFβ mRNA. In less destructive areas, cellular hyperplasia and fibrillation of the chondroid matrix occurs in the cartilaginous zone. Fibrous tissue proliferation is observed in some cases [65, 66].

Bone remodelling in PsA: specific tissue responses in PsA

PsA is characterized by bone destruction (erosions) but also by new bone formation (candle wax spurs, enthesophytes, and ankylosis). Both processes can occur simultaneously in the same patient, even in the same digit. The bone formation can be seen at sites different to the erosions, suggesting an uncoupling between the osteoblast–osteoclast homeostasis, seen in physiological bone turn-over and bone formation. Bone anabolic changes, including bone formation, progress despite effective suppression of inflammation and the formation of erosions by methotrexate or TNF blockade [70]. The uncoupling between inflammation and repair was previously described in ankylosing spondylitis [71]. The bone formed is mainly endochondral bone but the presence of appositional bone also suggests membranous bone formation. Several pathways are involved in these types of bone formation: the Wingless, transforming growth factor (TGF-beta), bone morphogenetic proteins, and prostaglandins.

Spur formation in PsA occurs at a typical localization of the entheseal region while in hand osteoarthritis, another bone-forming condition, bone spurs typically emerge at the cartilage–bone interphase and the joint margins [72].

Levels of serum osteocalcin and bone alkaline phosphatase are not increased in patients with PsA compared to healthy controls and psoriasis if corrected for gender and disease activity [73]. However, PsA patients had higher levels of bone alkaline phosphatase but not of osteocalcin compared to RA patients [74]. The levels of osteoprotegerin, a decoy receptor for RANKL are equal or higher than the controls [75, 76, 77]. Bone morphogenetic proteins, including BMP2,4,6 are not increased [78].

Cellular and molecular compartments involved in psoriatic arthritis

Cellular compartment

Lymphocytes

T lymphocytes

T lymphocytes are the most frequent cellular population in both psoriasis and PsA. In both cases, there is a prominent lymphocytic infiltrate, localized to the dermal papillae in skin and to the sub-lining layer stroma in the joint [49]. However, the role of T lymphocytes is somewhat controversial. While T lymphocytes are present in the synovial tissue in PsA among other cell types, some groups reported a lower prevalence than in RA. Oligo-clonal T-cell expansions have been demonstrated in the synovium, suggesting that an antigen-driven T-cell response could be promoting ongoing inflammation [79, 80]. It remains to be elucidated which antigen may be driving these T cells. CD4+ cells are the most frequent population in skin and synovial tissue but in synovial fluid and enthesis the CD8+ population is more predominant. Possibly CD8+cells are the driving force in PsA. This is supported by the known association of PsA with MHC class 1 molecules and the increased frequency of PsA in HIV patients upon CD4 depletion. Recent findings about a new subset of T lymphocytes originating from CD4+ cells are shedding a new light on their role in PsA.

From clinical trials, it is clear that T-cell-targeted therapies may be beneficial but far less effective than recent cytokine-targeted approaches. This does not mean that T cells may not be important. A specific subset could still promote the inflammatory process and T regulatory cells may play a role in controlling the inflammatory process. Recent findings about the role of Th17 cells may support this hypothesis.

B lymphocytes

Interestingly, the skin of patients with PsA compared to the skin of those with psoriasis alone showed differences in the presence of B-lymphocytes and there were significantly more DR+ cells in the PsA epidermis compared with psoriasis alone [81]. With B cells also abundant in synovial tissue, the exact role of B cells in PsA and psoriasis remains to be elucidated since auto-antibodies are not found in PsA.

Th17 lymphocytes

A new subset of T cells, Th17, has been characterized recently. Th17 may shed new light on the role and importance of T cells in the inflammatory process in PsA. Th17 are a new type of effector T lymphocytes producing IL-17, TNF-α, IL-21, and IL-22 upon stimulation with IL-23. The latter is abundantly present in the psoriatic skin lesions. Th17 cells develop from naïve CD4 cells upon stimulation by IL-23 in the presence of IL-6 and TGF-β [82]. Activated Th17 cells migrate to inflamed tissue. They over-express CCL2 and its receptor CCR 6 attracting neutrophils to the site of inflammation [83].

Increased frequencies of IL-17+ and IL-22+ CD4+ T cells are seen in peripheral blood of patients with PsA and psoriasis. A higher proportion of the CD4+ cells making IL-17 or IL-22 expressed IL-23R. Frequencies of IL-17+, CCR6+, and CCR4+ T cells are elevated in patients with psoriasis and PsA, IL-23R+T cell numbers are also elevated in synovial fluid compared to peripheral blood [84].

Comparing PsA with RA showed that in the synovial fluid of PsA patients both the IL-17+CD8+ and IL-17+CD4+ compartments are enriched compared to the peripheral blood whereas in the synovial fluid of RA patients only an increase in IL-17+CD4+ T cells was observed compared to the peripheral blood. In PsA, these T cell subsets also correlated with disease activity and erosion status after 2 years of treatment [83].

Dendritic cells

In psoriatic skin, the dendritic cell (DC] population overall is increased in the epidermis and dermis. Different types of DC are present in the dermis: myeloid DCs, plasmacytoid DCs, and slan DCs (6-sulfo LacNAc dendritic cells, a less common type of DC].

Microbial infection, autoantigens, such as LL37, and mechanical stress are known inducers of DCs and innate immune mechanisms.

LL37 may be the missing link between the innate immune reaction and the adaptive immune reaction in psoriasis [85]. The aggregation of LL37 with autogenous DNA activates Toll-like receptor-9 on plasmacytoid DCs resulting in production of TNF α, IL-23, IL-6, and IFN-gamma by myeloid DCs. Together with cytokines produced by macrophages, this promotes Th17 polarization and naïve CD4 cells [86].

DCs in synovial tissue in PsA are poorly studied. They are equally present in the synovial fluid of RA and PsA patients but almost absent in the synovial fluid of osteoarthritis patients [87]. DCs are more prevalent in the synovial tissue of RA patients than PsA [45]. In PsA, mostly plasmacytoid DCs are present but they seem to be in an immature state [88].

Macrophages

There is some controversy about the role and presence of macrophages. Initially immunohistologic analysis showed fewer macrophages invading the stroma and migrating to the lining layer in PsA synovial membrane than in RA synovial membrane [49]. More recent analysis, however, showed that macrophages are abundantly present in the synovial tissue in PsA compared to RA. Both CD68+ and CD163+ macrophages are present. Recent data especially show a clear increase in the CD163+ subset in PsA compared to RA [45, 49].

Macrophages are the source of pro-inflammatory cytokines such as TNF-α and synergize the effect of myeloid DCs promoting the polarization of Th17 cells. The activated monocyte/macrophage system may be responsible for the increased levels of S100A8/A9 in PsA, thereby reflecting disease activity [89].

Osteoclasts/pre osteoclasts

Altered bone remodelling is a key feature of PsA but can present with varying degrees in the individual patient. The altered bone remodelling is a combination of bone formation and bone resorption, represented by the presence of bone erosions. Those erosions result from bone resorption by osteoclasts [90].

Blood samples from PsA patients, particularly those with bone erosions visible on plain radiographs, exhibit a marked increase in osteoclast precursors (OCPs) compared with those from healthy controls. Moreover, PsA peripheral blood monocytes readily formed osteoclasts *in vitro* without exogenous receptor activator of NF-κB ligand (RANKL) or monocyte-colony stimulating factor. Blocking osteoprotegerin (OPG) and TNF-α with their specific antibodies inhibits osteoclast (OC) formation. OC formation in PsA patients is supported by data showing the production of osteoclastogenic cytokines, such as RANKL, TNF-α, and IL-7 by lymphocytes and fibroblasts [91].

Immunohistochemical analysis of subchondral bone and synovium revealed RANK-positive perivascular mononuclear cells and osteoclasts in PsA specimens. RANKL expression was dramatically up-regulated in the synovial lining layer, while OPG immunostaining was restricted to the endothelium. These results suggest a model for understanding the pathogenesis of aggressive bone erosions in PsA.

OCPs arise from CD14+ mononuclear cell lineage upon stimulation with RANK and fibroblasts from synovial fluid and express the CD16+ marker. The expression of CD16+ is associated with a higher bone erosion score [92]. Monocytes need to express DC-stamp in order to differentiate into OCPs. The bone marrow of patients with PsA harbours a subset of DC-STAMP+CD45intermediate monocytes which was absent in the blood. In general, more OCPs are found in the BM than in the peripheral blood supporting the BM as the major source of circulating OCPs [93].

In vivo, OCP frequency, correlates with joint scores and disability scores and declined substantially in PsA patients following treatment with anti-TNF agents [94].

Molecular compartment

The pro-inflammatory cytokines such as TNF-α, IL-1, IL-15, and IL-10, are increased in psoriatic skin and in the synovial tissue and fluid of PsA patients. Analysis of cytokine and nuclear factor κB expression in the synovial membrane of PsA patients and in lesional and perilesional areas of psoriasis skin reveals that these pro-inflammatory cytokines are produced by macrophages and suggests that the same cytokines trigger the inflammation in the skin and the joint.

Recently, other cytokines such as IL-17 and IL-23, important in the innate immunity cascade, have also been demonstrated in skin and synovial membrane in psoriasis and PsA [95].

Tumour necrosis factor-α

The evidence for the role of TNF-α in psoriatic disease is quite strong. The presence of TNF-α in PsA was first described in synovial explants [96] and subsequently in synovial fluid [55, 56] and synovial tissue [97] of PsA patients. TNF-α is primarily produced by macrophages. TNF-α displays a multitude of functions and plays a role in lymphocyte and neutrophil adhesion, increased vessel permeability, decreased haematopoesis, stimulation of collagenase and prostglandin E, and the production and stimulation of other cytokines. At the tissue level, TNF-α contributes to cartilage degradation, inhibition of bone formation, and bone resorption. TNF-α exerts its effect by binding to two distinct but structurally similar TNF receptors: the p55 and p75 receptor, which are present at the cell surface of almost every cell type. Binding of the trimeric TNF-α initiates the intracellular cell signalling. Binding to both receptors has overlapping but some distinct effects. Binding to the p55 receptor initiates mainly the inflammatory response while binding to the p75 receptor is important for TNF thymocyte proliferation, TNF-mediated skin necrosis, and apoptosis of activated mature lymphocytes. These receptors exist also in a soluble form and can act as natural TNF inhibitors. Levels of soluble p55 and p75 receptors are increased in PsA but to a lower extent than in RA [98]. The development of TNF blocking agents was based on the finding of naturally occurring soluble TNF receptors with blocking effect.

Clinical proof of the role of TNFα was demonstrated by the reduction of TNF-α expression after exposure to methotrexate [99]. Numerous studies have shown reduction of inflammatory infiltration and TNF-α after treatment with TNF-blocking agents.

RANK/RANKL

Receptor Activator of NFκ-B (RANK) is a transmembrane protein expressed by bone forming osteoblasts and is secreted upon cleavage or alternative splicing as a soluble protein. RANK interacts with Receptor Activator of NFκ-B ligand (RANKL), a transmembrane receptor on osteoclast precursor and dendritic cells. RANK/RANKL signalling is essential for osteoclastogenesis and osteoclast function in physiological bone remodelling but also in bone loss associated with inflammatory diseases. OPG functions as a decoy receptor for RANKL that prevents RANKL binding to its receptor RANK. As there is a prominent role for osteoclasts in the pathogenesis and development of bone erosions in PsA, the role of RANK/RANKL/OPG has been studied in PsA. Patients with psoriatic disease have increased serum levels of RANKL compared to controls and patients with PsA have increased levels of OPG compared to patients with only psoriasis [75]. The increased level of OPG may indicate ongoing bone formation in PsA. RANK is up-regulated in synovial tissue in PsA [100]. In patients with PsA the level of RANKL correlates with radiographic erosions, joint space narrowing, and osteolysis scores [77] but do not correlate with the degree of systemic bone loss in PsA.

Interleukin 17

IL-17 A is member of a large IL-17 family of cytokines and binds to IL-17 receptor expressed by a variety of cells such as monocytes, lymphocytes, lymphoid tissue inducer cells, synoviocytes, keratinocytes, epithelial cells, and fibroblasts. IL-17 acts as a homodimer or heterodimer with IL-17F and is produced by Th17 cells, a new subset of Th-cells. Il-17A is more potent than IL-17 F or the heterodimer in inducing inflammatory cytokine expression. IL-17-A act on a multitude of cells, including keratinocytes, in the skin and synovial like fibroblasts in the joint to increase the mediators sustaining the chronic inflammation. IL-17 A also acts on osteoblasts and OCPs to promote bone resorption. IL-17 is abundantly present in the circulation of PsA patients as well as in the synovial fluid [101]. The PsA joint, but not the RA joint, is enriched for IL-17+CD8+ T cells. Other cells, such as mast cells and neutrophils, can produce IL-17 and are also identified in psoriatic skin lesions and synovial tissue of PsA patients [102]. Moreover the levels of this T cell subset in the synovial fluid are correlated with disease activity measures and the radiographic erosion status after 2 years, suggesting a previously unrecognized contribution of these cells to the pathogenesis of PsA [103].

Interleukin 23

IL-23 is a heterodimeric cytokine composed of a p19 and a p40 subunit. It binds to the IL-23 receptor or to IL-12Rbeta-1. Both subunits are secreted by macrophages or dendritic cells. The IL 23R is expressed on a variety of cell types including TH17 cells, gamma delta T-cells, innate lymphoid cells, macrophages, dendritic cells, and monocytes. IL-23 is significantly increased in psoriasis lesions and increased synovial expression of the p19 unit of IL-23

is associated with disease activity in PsA. In animal models, IL-23 acts on resident T cells in the enthesis and promotes typical pathogenic changes with accompanying production of pro-inflammatory cytokines including IL-17 [29].

Conclusion

The pathogenesis of PsA and by extension psoriatic disease is complex. Although skin and joint involvement are linked, they can occur independently. While some immunological features occur in both manifestations there are some striking differences. In particular, the tissue response of the joints, cartilage and bone, is different from the skin response. New insights including a paradigm shift from PsA being an autoimmune disease towards a disease with an autoimmune but also an auto-inflammatory component will lead to a better understanding of the pathophysiology. It is clear that besides an important genetic component for the development and perpetuation of the inflammatory process, there are also important environmental factors involved, including trauma and the microbiome. An increased understanding of the pathophysiology must consequently lead to improved treatment strategies with better outcomes for the patient.

References

1. Braum LS, McGonagle D, Bruns A, et al. Characterisation of hand small joints arthropathy using high-resolution MRI–limited discrimination between osteoarthritis and psoriatic arthritis. Eur Radiol 2013;23(6):1686–93.
2. Zenz R, Ferl R, Kenner L, et al. Psoriasis-like skin disease and arthritis caused by inducible epidermal deletion of Jun proteins. Nature 2005;437:369–75.
3. McGonagle D, McDermott MF. A proposed classification of the immunological diseases. PLoS Med 2006;3(8):e297.
4. Karason A, Love TJ, Gudbjornsson B. A strong heritability of psoriatic arthritis over four generations – the Reykjavik Psoriatic Arthritis Study. Rheumatology (Oxford). 2009;48(11):1424–8.
5. O'Rielly DD, Rahman P. Genetics of psoriatic arthritis. Best Pract Res Clin Rheumatol 2014;28(5):673–85.
6. Bowes J, Loehr S, Budu-Aggrey A, et al. PTPN22 is associated with susceptibility to psoriatic arthritis but not psoriasis: evidence for a further PsA-specific risk locus. Ann Rheum Dis. 2015;74(10):1882–5.
7. Hüffmeier U, Uebe S, Ekici AB, et al. Common variants at TRAF3IP2 are associated with susceptibility to psoriatic arthritis and psoriasis. Nat Genet 2010;42(11):996–9.
8. Chandran V, Bull SB, Pellett FJ, et al. Human leukocyte antigen alleles and susceptibility to psoriatic arthritis. Hum Immunol. 2013;74(10):1333–8.
9. Winchester R, Minevich G, Steshenko V, et al. HLA associations reveal genetic heterogeneity in psoriatic arthritis and in the psoriasis phenotype. Arthritis Rheum 2012;64:1134–44.
10. Eder L, Chandran V, Pellet F, Shanmugarajah S, Rosen CF, Bull SB, Gladman DD. Human Leukocyte Antigen risk alleles for Psoriatic Arthritis among psoriasis patients. Ann Rheum Dis 2012;71:50–5.
11. Haroon M, Winchester R, Giles JT, Heffernan E, FitzGerald O. Certain class I HLA alleles and haplotypes implicated in susceptibility play a role in determining specific features of the psoriatic arthritis phenotype. Ann Rheum Dis. 2016;75(1):155–62.
12. Apel M, Uebe S, Bowes J, Giardina E, et al. Variants in RUNX3 contribute to susceptibility to psoriatic arthritis, exhibiting further common ground with ankylosing spondylitis. Arthritis Rheum. 2013;65(5):1224–31.
13. Zhu J, Qu H, Chen X, Wang H, Li J. Single nucleotide polymorphisms in the tumor necrosis factor-alpha gene promoter region alter the risk

of psoriasis vulgaris and psoriatic arthritis: a meta-analysis. PLoS One. 2013;23;8(5):e64376.

14. Moll JM, Wright V. Psoriatic arthritis. Semin Arthritis Rheum 1973;3(1):55–78.

15. Tinazzi I, McGonagle D, Biasi D, et al. Preliminary evidence that subclinical enthesopathy may predict psoriatic arthritis in patients with psoriasis. J Rheumatol. 2011;38(12):2691–2.

16. Simon D, Faustini F, Kleyer A, et al. Analysis of periarticular bone changes in patients with cutaneous psoriasis without associated psoriatic arthritis. Ann Rheum Dis. 2015;75(4):660–6.

17. Punzi L, Pianon M, Bertazzolo N, Fagiolo U, Rizzi E, Rossini P, Todesco S. Clinical, laboratory and immunogenetic aspects of post-traumatic psoriatic arthritis: a study of 25 patients. Clin Exp Rheumatol. 1998;16(3):277–81.

18. Pattison E, Harrison BJ, Griffiths CE, Silman AJ, Bruce IN. Environmental risk factors for the development of psoriatic arthritis: results from a case-control study. Ann Rheum Dis. 2008;67(5):672–6.

19. Eder L, Law T, Chandran V, Shanmugarajah S, et al. Association between environmental factors and onset of psoriatic arthritis in patients with psoriasis. Arthritis Care Res (Hoboken). 2011;63(8):1091–7.

20. Chandran V, Raychaudhuri SP. Geoepidemiology and environmental factors of psoriasis and psoriatic arthritis. J Autoimmun 2010;34:J314–21.

21. McGonagle D, Ash Z, Dickie L, McDermott M, Aydin SZ. The early phase of psoriatic arthritis. Ann Rheum Dis. 2011;70 Suppl 1:i71–6.

22. Poggenborg RP, Eshed I, Østergaard M, Sørensen IJ, Møller JM, Madsen OR, Pedersen SJ. Enthesitis in patients with psoriatic arthritis, axial spondyloarthritis and healthy subjects assessed by 'head-to-toe' whole-body MRI and clinical examination. Ann Rheum Dis. 2015;74(5):823–9.

23. Tan AL, Grainger AJ, Tanner SF, Emery P, McGonagle D. A high-resolution magnetic resonance imaging study of distal interphalangeal joint arthropathy in psoriatic arthritis and osteoarthritis: are they the same? Arthritis Rheum 2006;54(4):1328–33.

24. Kiuru MJ1, Niva M, Reponen A, Pihlajamäki HK. Bone stress injuries in asymptomatic elite recruits: a clinical and magnetic resonance imaging study. Am J Sports Med. 2005;33(2):272–6.

25. Aydin SZ, Bas E, Basci O, Filippucci E, et al. Validation of ultrasound imaging for Achilles entheseal fibrocartilage in bovines and description of changes in humans with spondyloarthritis. Ann Rheum Dis. 2010;69(12):2165–8.

26. Ng J, Tan AL, McGonagle D. Unifocal psoriatic arthritis development in identical twins following site specific injury: evidence supporting biomechanical triggering events in genetically susceptible hosts. Ann Rheum Dis. 2015;74(5):948–9.

27. Armaka M, Apostolaki M, Jacques P, Kontoyiannis DL, Elewaut D, Kollias G. Mesenchymal cell targeting by TNF as a common pathogenic principle in chronic inflammatory joint and intestinal diseases. J Exp Med. 200818;205(2):331–7.

28. Jacques P, Lambrecht S, Verheugen E, et al. Proof of concept: enthesitis and new bone formation in spondyloarthritis are driven by mechanical strain and stromal cells. Ann Rheum Dis 2014;73(2):437–45.

29. Sherlock JP, Joyce-Shaikh B, Turner SP, et al. IL-23 induces spondyloarthropathy by acting on ROR-γt+ CD3+CD4-CD8-entheseal resident T cells. Nat Med. 2012;18(7):1069–76.

30. Vasey FB, Deitz C, Fenske NA, Germain BF, Espinoza LR. Possible involvement of group A streptococci in the pathogenesis of psoriatic arthritis. J Rheumatol. 1982;9(5):719–22.

31. Wang Q, Vasey FB, Mahfood JP, et al. V2 regions of 16S ribosomal RNA used as a molecular marker for the species identification of streptococci in peripheral blood and synovial fluid from patients with psoriatic arthritis. Arthritis Rheum. 1999;42(10):2055–9.

32. Thomssen H, Hoffmann B, Schank M, et al. There is no disease-specific role for streptococci-responsive synovial T lymphocytes in the pathogenesis of psoriatic arthritis. Med Microbiol Immunol. 2000;188(4):203–7.

33. Palazzi C, Olivieri I, D'Amico E, et al. Hepatitis C virus infection in psoriatic arthritis. Arthritis Rheum. 2005;53(2):223–5.

34. Taglione E, Vatteroni ML, Martini P, et al. Hepatitis C virus infection: prevalence in psoriasis and psoriatic arthritis. J Rheumatol. 1999;26(2):370–2.

35. Njobvu P, McGill P. Psoriatic arthritis and human immunodeficiency virus infection in Zambia. J Rheumatol. 2000;27(7):1699–702.

36. Ouédraogo DD, Meyer O. Psoriatic arthritis in Sub-Saharan Africa. Joint Bone Spine. 2012;79(1):17–19.

37. Naik S, Bouladoux N, Wilhelm C, et al. Compartmentalized control of skin immunity by resident commensals. Science 2012;337(6098):1115–9.

38. Gao Z1, Tseng CH, Strober BE, Pei Z, Blaser MJ. Substantial alterations of the cutaneous bacterial biota in psoriatic lesions. PLoS One. 2008;3(7):e2719.

39. Fahlén A, Engstrand L, Baker BS, Powles A, Fry L. Comparison of bacterial microbiota in skin biopsies from normal and psoriatic skin. Arch Dermatol Res. 2012;304(1):15–22.

40. Castelino M, Eyre S, Upton M, Ho P, Barton A. The bacterial skin microbiome in psoriatic arthritis, an unexplored link in pathogenesis: challenges and opportunities offered by recent technological advances. Rheumatology (Oxford). 2014;53(5):777–84.

41. Scher JU, Ubeda C, Artacho A, et al. Decreased bacterial diversity characterizes the altered gut microbiota in patients with psoriatic arthritis, resembling dysbiosis in inflammatory bowel disease. Arthritis Rheumatol. 2015;67(1):128–39.

42. Curran SA, FitzGerald OM, Costello PJ, et al. Nucleotide sequencing of psoriatic arthritis tissue before and during methotrexate administration reveals a complex inflammatory T cell infiltrate with very few clones exhibiting features that suggest they drive the inflammatory process by recognizing autoantigens. J Immunol 2004;172(3):1935–44.

43. Fearon U, Reece R, Smith J, Emery P, Veale DJ. Synovial cytokine and growth factor regulation of MMPs/TIMPs: implications for erosions and angiogenesis in early rheumatoid and psoriatic arthritis patients. Ann N Y Acad Sci. 1999;878:619–21.

44. Kuroda K, Sapadin A, Shoji T, Fleischmajer R, Lebwohl M. Altered expression of angiopoietins and Tie2 endothelium receptor in psoriasis. J Invest Dermatol. 2001;116(5):713–20.

45. Kruithof E, Baeten D, De Rycke L, et al. Synovial histopathology of psoriatic arthritis, both oligo- and polyarticular, resembles spondyloarthropathy more than it does rheumatoid arthritis. Arthritis Res Ther. 2005;7(3):R569–80.

46. Gudbjörnsson B, Christofferson R, Larsson A. Synovial concentrations of the angiogenic peptides bFGF and VEGF do not discriminate rheumatoid arthritis from other forms of inflammatory arthritis. Scand J Clin Lab Invest. 2004;64(1):9–15.

47. Fearon U, Griosios K, Fraser A, et al. Angiopoietins, growth factors, and vascular morphology in early arthritis. J Rheumatol. 2003;30(2):260–8.

48. Biniecka M, Connolly M, Gao W, et al. Redox-mediated angiogenesis in the hypoxic joint of inflammatory arthritis. Arthritis Rheumatol. 2014;66(12):3300–10.

49. Veale D, Yanni G, Rogers S, Barnes L, Bresnihan B, Fitzgerald O. Reduced synovial membrane ELAM-1 expression, macrophage numbers and lining layer hyperplasia in psoriatic arthritis as compared with rheumatoid arthritis. Arthritis Rheum 1993;36:893–900.

50. Salvador G, Sanmarti R, Garcia-Peiró A, Rodríguez-Cros JR, Muñoz-Gómez J, Cañete JD. p53 expression in rheumatoid and psoriatic arthritis synovial tissue and association with joint damage. Ann Rheum Dis. 2005;64(2):183–7.

51. Cañete JD, Santiago B, Cantaert T, et al. Ectopic lymphoid neogenesis in psoriatic arthritis. Ann Rheum Dis. 2007;66(6):720–6.

52. Costello PJ, Winchester RJ, Curran SA. Psoriatic arthritis joint fluids are characterized by CD8 and CD4 T cell clonal expansions appear antigen driven. J Immunol. 2001;166(4):2878–86.

53. Costello P, Bresnihan B, O'Farrelly C, Fitzgerald O. Predominance of CD8+ T lymphocytes in psoriatic arthritis. J Rheumatol 1999;26:1117–24.

54. Goldstein I, Simon AJ, Ben Horin S, et al. Synovial VLA-1+ T cells display an oligoclonal and partly distinct repertoire in rheumatoid and psoriatic arthritis. Clin Immunol. 2008;128(1):75–84.

55. Partsch G, Steiner G, Leeb FB, Dunky A, Broll H, Smolen JS. Highly increased levels of tumor necrosis factor-α and other proinflammatory cytokines in psoriatic arthritis synovial fluid. J Rheumatol 1997;24:518–23.

56. Partsch G, Wagner E, Leeb BF, Dunky A, Steiner G, Smolen JS. Upregulation of cytokine receptors sTNF-R55, STNFR75, and sIL-2r in psoriatic arthritis synovial fluid. J Rheumatol 1998;25:105–10.

57. Mitra A, Raychaudhuri SK, Raychaudhuri SP. Functional role of IL-22 in psoriatic arthritis. Arthritis Res Ther 2012;article R65.

58. Wolk K, Witte E, Wallace E, et al. IL-22 regulates the expression of genes responsible for antimicrobial defense, cellular differentiation, and mobility in keratinocytes: a potential role in psoriasis. Eur J Immunol. 2006;36(5):1309–23.

59. Antonelli A, Fallahi P, Delle Sedie A, et al. High values of alpha (CXCL10) and beta (CCL2) circulating chemokines in patients with psoriatic arthritis, in presence or absence of autoimmune thyroiditis. Autoimmunity. 2008;41(7):537–42.

60. Flytlie HA, Hvid M, Lindgreen E, et al. Expression of MDC/CCL22 and its receptor CCR4 in rheumatoid arthritis, psoriatic arthritis and osteoarthritis. Cytokine. 2010;49(1):24–9.

61. Fraser A, Fearon U, Reece R, Emery P, Veale DJ. Matrix metalloproteinase 9, apoptosis, and vascular morphology in early arthritis. *Arthr Rheum*, 2001;44:2024–28.

62. Giannelli G1, Erriquez R, Iannone F, Marinosci F, Lapadula G, Antonaci S. MMP-2, MMP-9, TIMP-1 and TIMP-2 levels in patients with rheumatoid arthritis and psoriatic arthritis. Clin Exp Rheumatol. 2004;22(3):335–8.

63. McGonagle D, Lories RJ, Tan AL, Benjamin M. The concept of a 'synovio-entheseal complex' and its implications for understanding joint inflammation and damage in psoriatic arthritis and beyond. Arthritis Rheum. 2007;56(8):2482–91.

64. Emad Y, Ragab Y, Gheita T, et al. Knee enthesitis and synovitis on magnetic resonance imaging in patients with psoriasis without arthritic symptoms. J Rheumatol. 2012;39(10):1979–86.

65. Laloux L, Voisin MC, Allain J, et al. Immunohistological study of entheses in spondyloarthropathies: comparison in rheumatoid arthritis and osteoarthritis. Ann Rheum Dis. 2001;60(4):316–21.

66. McGonagle D, Marzo-Ortega H, O'Connor P, et al. Histological assessment of the early enthesitis lesion in spondyloarthropathy Ann Rheum Dis 2002;61:534–7.

67. McGonagle D, Gibbon W, O'Connor P, et al. Characteristic magnetic resonance imaging entheseal changes of knee synovitis in spondylarthropathy. Arthritis Rheum. 1998;41(4):694–700.

68. Jevtic V, Watt I, Rozman B, Kos-Golja M, Demsar F, Jarh O. Distinctive radiological features of small hand joints in rheumatoid arthritis and seronegative spondyloarthritis demonstrated by contrast-enhanced (Gd-DTPA) magnetic resonance imaging. Skeletal Radiol. 1995;24(5):351–5.

69. Lories RJ, Matthys P, de Vlam K, Derese I, Luyten FP. Ankylosing enthesitis, dactylitis, and onychoperiostitis in male DBA/1 mice: a model of psoriatic arthritis. Ann Rheum Dis. 2004;63(5):595–8.

70. Finzel S, Kraus S, Schmidt S, et al. Bone anabolic changes progress in psoriatic arthritis patients despite treatment with methotrexate or tumour necrosis factor inhibitors. Ann Rheum Dis. 2013;72(7):1176–81.

71. Lories RJ, Luyten FP, de Vlam K. Progress in spondylarthritis. Mechanisms of new bone formation in spondyloarthritis. Arthritis Res Ther 2009;11(2):221.

72. Finzel S, Sahinbegovic E, Kocijan R, Engelke K, Englbrecht M, Schett G. Inflammatory bone spur formation in psoriatic arthritis is different from bone spur formation in hand osteoarthritis. Arthritis Rheumatol 2014;66(11):2968–75.

73. Franck H, Ittel T. Serum osteocalcin levels in patients with psoriatic arthritis: an extended report. Rheumatol Int 2000;19(5):161–4.

74. Szentpetery A, McKenna MJ, Murray BF, et al. Periarticular bone gain at proximal interphalangeal joints and changes in bone turnover markers in response to tumor necrosis factor inhibitors in rheumatoid and psoriatic arthritis. J Rheumatol. 2013;40(5):653–62.

75. Chandran V, Cook RJ, Edwin J, et al. Soluble biomarkers differentiate patients with psoriatic arthritis from those with psoriasis without arthritis. Rheumatology (Oxford). 2010;49(7):1399–405.

76. Grisar J, Bernecker PM, Aringer M, et al. Ankylosing spondylitis, psoriatic arthritis, and reactive arthritis show increased bone resorption, but differ with regard to bone formation. J Rheumatol. 2002;29(7):1430–6.

77. Dalbeth N, Pool B, Smith T, Callon KE, Lobo et al. Circulating mediators of bone remodeling in psoriatic arthritis: implications for disordered osteoclastogenesis and bone erosion. Arthritis Res Ther. 2010;12(4):R164.

78. Grcevic D, Jajic Z, Kovacic N, et al. Peripheral blood expression profiles of bone morphogenetic proteins, tumor necrosis factor-superfamily molecules, and transcription factor Runx2 could be used as markers of the form of arthritis, disease activity, and therapeutic responsiveness. J Rheumatol. 2010;37(2):246–56.

79. Tassiulas I, Duncan SR, Centola M, Theofilopoulos AN, Boumpas DT. Clonal characteristics of T cell infiltrates in skin and synovium of patients with psoriaticarthritis. Hum Immunol. 1999;60(6):479–91. 28.

80. Chang JC, Smith LR, Froning KJ, et al. CD8+ T-cells in psoriatic lesions preferentially use T-cell receptors V beta 3 and/or V beta 13.1 genes. Ann NY Acad Sci. 1995;756:370–81.

81. Veale DJ, Barnes L, Rogers S, FitzGerald O. Immunohistochemical markers for arthritis in psoriasis. Ann Rheum Dis 1994;53:450–4.

82. Lee E, Trepicchio WL, Oestreicher JL, et al. Increased expression of interleukin 23 p19 and p40 in lesional skin of patients with psoriasis vulgaris. J Exp Med. 2004;199(1):125–30.

83. Menon B, Gullick NJ, Walter GJ, et al. Interleukin-17+CD8+ T cells are enriched in the joints of patients with psoriatic arthritis and correlate with disease activity and joint damage progression. Arthritis Rheumatol. 2014;66(5):1272–81.

84. Benham H, Norris P, Goodall J, et al. Th17 and Th22 cells in psoriatic arthritis and psoriasis. Arthritis Res Ther. 2013;15(5):R136.

85. Lande R, Botti E, Jandus C, et al. The antimicrobial peptide LL37 is a T-cell autoantigen in psoriasis. Nat Commun. 2014;5:5621.

86. Diani M, Altomare G, Reali E. T cell responses in psoriasis and psoriatic arthritis. Autoimmun Rev. 2015;14(4):286–92.

87. Jongbloed SL, Lebre MC, Fraser AR. Enumeration and phenotypical analysis of distinct dendritic cell subsets in psoriatic arthritis and rheumatoid arthritis. Arthritis Res Ther. 2006;8(1):R15.

88. Lande R, Giacomini E, Serafini B, et al. Characterization and recruitment of plasmacytoid dendritic cells in synovial fluid and tissue of patients with chronic inflammatory arthritis. J Immunol. 2004;173(4):2815–24.

89. Aochi S, Tsuji K, Sakaguchi M, Huh N, et al. Markedly elevated serum levels of calcium-binding S100A8/A9 proteins in psoriatic arthritis are due to activated monocytes/macrophages. J Am Acad Dermatol. 2011;64(5):879–87.

90. Ritchlin CT, Haas-Smith SA, Li P, Hicks DG, Schwarz EM. Mechanisms of TNF-alpha- and RANKL-mediated osteoclastogenesis and bone resorption in psoriatic arthritis. J Clin Invest. 2003;111(6):821–31.

91. Colucci S, Brunetti G, Cantatore FP, et al. Lymphocytes and synovial fluid fibroblasts support osteoclastogenesis through RANKL, TNFalpha, and IL-7 in an in vitro model derived from human psoriatic arthritis. J Pathol. 2007;212(1):47–55.

92. Chiu YG, Shao T, Feng C, et al. CD16 (FcRgammaIII) as a potential marker of osteoclast precursors in psoriatic arthritis. Arthritis Res Ther. 2010;12(1):R14.

93. Chiu YG, Ritchlin CT Characterization of DC-STAMP+ cells in human bone marrow. J Bone Marrow Res. 2013;19;1. Pii.

94. Anandarajah AP, Schwarz EM, Totterman S, et al. The effect of etanercept on osteoclast precursor frequency and enhancing bone marrow oedema in patients with psoriatic arthritis. Ann Rheum Dis. 2008;67(3):296–301.

95. de Vlam K, Gottlieb AB, Mease PJ. Current concepts in psoriatic arthritis: pathogenesis and management. Acta Derm Venereol. 2014;94(6):627–34.

96. Ritchlin C1, Haas-Smith SA, Hicks D, Cappuccio J, Osterland CK, Looney RJ. Patterns of cytokine production in psoriatic synovium. J Rheumatol. 1998;25(8):1544–52.

97. Danning CL, Illei GG, Hitchon C, Greer MR, Boumpas DT, McInnes IB. Macrophage-derived cytokine and nuclear factor kappaB p65 expression in synovial membrane and skin of patients with psoriatic arthritis. Arthritis Rheum. 2000;43(6):1244–56.

98. Cope AP, Aderka D, Doherty M, et al. Increased levels of soluble tumor necrosis factor receptors in the sera and synovial fluid of patients with rheumatic diseases.Arthritis Rheum. 1992;35(10):1160–9.

99. Kane D, Gogarty M, O'Leary J, Silva I, Bermingham N, Bresnihan B, Fitzgerald O. Reduction of synovial sublining layer inflammation and proinflammatory cytokine expression in psoriatic arthritis treated with methotrexate. Arthritis Rheum 2004;50(10):3286–95.

100. Ritchlin CT, Haas-Smith SA, Li P, Hicks DG, Schwarz EM. Mechanisms of TNF-alpha- and RANKL-mediated osteoclastogenesis and bone resorption in psoriatic arthritis. J Clin Invest 2003;111(6):821–31.

101. Mrabet D, Laadhar L, Sahli H, Zouari B, Haouet S, Makni S, Sellami S. Synovial fluid and serum levels of IL-17, IL-23, and CCL-20 in rheumatoid arthritis and psoriatic arthritis: a Tunisian cross-sectional study. Rheumatol Int 2013;33(1):265–6.

102. Menon B, Gullick NJ, Walter GJ, et al. Interleukin-17+CD8+ T cells are enriched in the joints of patients with psoriatic arthritis and correlate with disease activity and joint damage progression. Arthritis Rheumatol. 2014;66(5):1272–81.

103. Noordenbos T, Yeremenko N, Gofita I, et al. Interleukin-17-positive mast cells contribute to synovial inflammation in spondylarthritis. Arthritis Rheum. 2012;64(1):99–109.

CHAPTER 5

Genetics of psoriasis

Philip E. Stuart, Lam C. Tsoi, Caely A. Hambro, and James T. Elder

Impact of psoriasis

Psoriasis is a common immunologically mediated inflammatory disease (IMID) characterized by skin inflammation, epidermal hyperplasia, and increased risk of arthritis, as well as cardiovascular morbidity [1]. Substantial evidence indicates that psoriasis is driven by abnormal interactions between cells of the innate and adaptive host defence systems, including keratinocytes, dendritic cells, and T-cells, resulting in both a dysregulated immune response and markedly increased epidermal proliferation [2]. As is the case for all IMIDs, the precise aetiology of psoriasis remains unknown.

The economic burden of psoriasis is very substantial, with estimated direct costs of over $50 billion in 2013 [3]. The majority of the 150,000 newly diagnosed US cases annually appear in individuals <30 years of age, with 10,000 of these individuals being less than10 years old [4]. The cutaneous manifestations of psoriasis are visible and often uncomfortable and unpleasant, with a highly negative impact on quality of life [5].

Genetic epidemiology of psoriasis

Psoriasis has been reported to affect from 0.1% to 6.5% of individuals, depending on ethnicity and geographical location, with a tendency towards higher prevalence with increasing latitude [6]. Most estimates of psoriasis prevalence vary from 2% to 3% in European-origin populations [7, 8], and the incidence of psoriasis has been estimated at 60 per 100,000 person-years [9]. Psoriatic arthritis (PsA) develops over time in psoriasis patients, with most patients developing signs of skin disease prior to arthritis. A recent longitudinal study of PsA development in patients with psoriasis found that PsA develops at a rate of 2.7 per 100 psoriasis patients per year [10]. While population-based studies generally produce lower estimates (6–11%) [11–13], clinic-based studies have estimated that up to 40% of psoriatics may develop PsA, which is severe and deforming in 5% of cases [14]. The sex ratio has consistently been found to be essentially even for both psoriasis and PsA [7, 8, 11, 13, 15].

In this chapter, we will utilize the term cutaneous-only psoriasis (PsC) to refer to individuals affected with psoriasis for 10 or more years without developing any signs of PsA, and the term psoriasis vulgaris (PsV) to include PsA, PsC, and psoriatic individuals for whom a diagnosis of PsA is either unavailable or uncertain. This definition has yielded several genetic differences between PsA and PsC [16].

Psoriasis has a strong genetic component, as initially assessed by epidemiologic studies involving twins and families, and more recently confirmed by linkage studies in families and genetic association studies in cases and controls [17]. We [18], and more recently others [19], have reviewed twin studies in psoriasis. All of these studies found a substantially (2–3.5-fold) higher concordance of psoriasis in monozygotic (MZ) compared to dizygotic (DZ) twins [15]. The only available twin study of PsA, based on the Danish Twin Study, found concordance for PsA in 1 of 10 MZ twins compared to 1 of 26 DZ twins [20]. Estimates of heritability (the proportion of variation in overall disease liability due to genetic factors) have ranged from 50% to 90% for psoriasis in populations of European descent [19, 21–25]. Recurrence risk (i.e. disease prevalence in relatives compared to the general population) ranges from 4-19 in siblings (λ_s) or first degree relatives (λ_1) of psoriatic individuals [26–28]. Even higher genetic effects have been reported for PsA, with estimates of 80–100% for heritability [26, 27] and values ranging from 30 to 49 for λ_s and λ_1 [26–29]. Additional aspects of the genetic epidemiology of psoriasis, including its mode of inheritance, penetrance, and possible parent-of-origin effects, have been considered elsewhere [17].

Historical aspects of psoriasis genetics

HLA association studies

The major histocompatibility complex (MHC) contains the genes encoding human leukocyte antigens (HLA), along with many other genes involved in host defence [30]. Over time, methods of HLA typing have evolved from serological to DNA-based, with the latter methods progressing from oligonucleotide-based [31] to imputation-based, involving typing of single nucleotide polymorphisms (SNPs) across the MHC region [32] to next-generation sequencing [33]. HLA association studies of psoriasis began with serologic studies over 40 years ago [34]. Subsequently, the MHC component of psoriasis was given the locus name *PSORS1* (Mendelian Inheritance in Man #142840).

As might be expected given that CD8+ T-cells recognize antigen in the context of MHC Class I, the strongest MHC associations in psoriasis have consistently mapped to the Class I region 1. PsV is strongly associated with *HLA-C*06* in Caucasian [35] and Chinese populations [36, 37], particularly in patients with early onset, guttate psoriasis, positive family history, and more severe disease [35]. PsA is also associated with *HLA-C*06*, particularly in PsA patients with early onset of skin disease [38–40]. However, *HLA-C*06* is significantly less frequent in PsA than in PsV [41–44]. *HLA-B*27* is also associated with PsA [42–49], but the strength of association is much lower than in ankylosing spondylitis (AS) [45, 50]. Another longstanding finding is the association of PsA with *HLA-B*38* and *HLA-B*39* [41, 42, 46, 47, 50–55], which are closely related to each other and have structural homologies with *HLA-B*27* [56].

Our early studies of familial psoriasis typed HLA alleles by serologic and/or DNA methods, revealing associations with *HLA-B*57*, *HLA-DRB1*07*, and *HLA-DQB1*09* in addition to *HLA-C*06* [57]. All of these alleles belong to the extended MHC haplotype EH57.1 [58]. Early studies localized the disease determinant to the Class I end of this haplotype [57, 59]. However, there are many genes in the MHC Class I region, and they are in strong linkage disequilibrium (LD). To address the challenge of identifying the 'real' *PSORS1* gene, we initially carried out a cluster analysis of MHC haplotypes, which mapped *PSORS1* to the proximal MHC Class I region [60]. In 2006, we published more detailed recombinant ancestral haplotype mapping of the region in 678 families, along with DNA sequencing of the critical interval in two disease and five normal chromosomes. This analysis strongly implicated *HLA-C* rather than any of ten other nearby genes, including the attractive skin-expressed candidate corneodesmosin (*CDSN*) [61]. These findings were confirmed in a collection of 163 Chinese Han families [37].

Several studies have documented a strong association between PsV and an MHC Class I haplotype that is common in Japan and Thailand, but rare in Caucasians (*HLA-A*02:07, -C*01, -B*46:01*) [62–66]. This haplotype was associated with PsV when found in *cis* to any of three HLA Class II haplotypes [63], suggesting that a psoriasis determinant other than *HLA-C*06* resides on the Class I end of these haplotypes. There is evidence that this determinant is associated with later-onset disease [63]. We compared this haplotype to *HLA-C*06*-bearing haplotypes at the genomic level, and found that this haplotype is unlikely to share a specific disease allele in common with *HLA-C*06*, based not only on differences in DNA sequence, but also on differences in disease phenotype, including lower risk of disease, greater nail involvement, and later age at onset in *HLA-C*01-B*46* carriers compared with *HLA-C*06* carriers [67]. This haplotype has been associated with other autoimmune diseases, including myasthenia gravis and Graves' disease [68]. More recent analyses of the MHC in psoriasis will be detailed below.

Linkage studies

Genetic linkage studies measure transmission of alleles through generations or sharing of alleles between affected family members. Utilizing linkage as well as family-based association strategies, we and others made important advances in the genetic dissection of HLA associations in psoriasis (see HLA association studies) [60, 61, 67, 69, 70]. Outside of the MHC, genetic linkage studies in families, sib pairs, and trios reported 17 additional susceptibility loci [71–73]. However, other than *PSORS2* (17q24-q25) spanning the *CARD14* gene [74], *PSORS4* in the epidermal differentiation complex [75], *PSORS7* on chromosome 1p spanning the *IL23R* locus [76], and *PSORS6* on chromosome 19p13 spanning the *TYK2* locus [77], most of these non-MHC loci have not been replicated by other linkage studies, or confirmed in subsequent association studies. Similar difficulties have been encountered using the linkage approach to study other complex genetic diseases. In retrospect, we now appreciate that this is due to low penetrance of non-MHC genetic signals compared to those found in the MHC, leading to a high

frequency of unaffected carriers that markedly reduces the power of linkage analysis.

Psoriasis genetics in the 21st century

Two relatively recent technologies, high-throughput DNA sequencing and microarray-based analysis of SNPs, have revolutionized genetics in this century, with corresponding advances in the identification of psoriasis susceptibility loci. While the bulk of genetic discoveries in psoriasis have involved microarray-based SNP genotyping (see below), we begin with those discoveries made by DNA sequencing, due to the insights provided by sequencing into the nature of rare yet highly penetrant disease alleles in psoriasis.

DNA sequencing

Over the past decade, sequencing of individual genes has been extended to targeted groups of genes, whole exomes, and whole genomes by the development of several massively parallel, next-generation sequencing techniques [78]. Both types of sequencing strategies have been fruitfully utilized when combined with linkage analysis to identify rare and highly penetrant 'mutations' (as opposed to more common, but less penetrant 'variations'). A prime example of such success has been the identification of *CARD14* as the causative gene at the *PSORS2* locus. Three linkage studies of large pedigrees suggested highly penetrant but rare mutations at *PSORS2* [74, 79, 80]. Seventeen years after reporting *PSORS2* [74], Bowcock and colleagues used high-throughput sequencing of genomic DNA libraries from two *PSORS2* pedigrees and a sporadic case of psoriasis to identify gain-of-function mutations in *CARD14* that enhanced NF-κB activation in keratinocytes [81]. Soon thereafter, others used a similar linkage-targeted resequencing strategy to identify *CARD14* mutations in four pedigrees with pityriasis rubra pilaris, a highly inflammatory papulosquamous dermatosis with clinical features similar to psoriasis [82]. Targeted and whole-exome DNA sequencing also played key roles in the identification of mutations in *AP1S3* (chr 2q23) [83] and *IL36RN* (chr 2q13) genes [84–86] in generalized pustular psoriasis (GPP), a highly inflammatory disorder characterized by systemic inflammation and a lack of typical psoriatic plaques. *AP1S3* encodes a subunit of a multiprotein complex that promotes vesicular trafficking between the trans-Golgi network and endosomes. Silencing of *AP1S3* disrupted the endosomal translocation of TLR3, blocking the induction of IFN-β [83]. Interestingly, IFN-β has anti-inflammatory activities involving the inhibition of IL-1 production [87]. *IL36RN* encodes IL36Ra, an antagonist of the IL1-like protein IL-36. The mutated form of the IL36Ra protein was expressed at lower levels in GPP patients, resulting in increased production of IL-8 and other proinflammatory cytokines by keratinocytes [86]. IL-1 drives the pathogenesis of many autoinflammatory conditions [88], and IL-1 blockade is emerging as an effective treatment for pustular psoriasis [89, 90]. Thus far, mutations in *IL36RN* and *AP1S3* have not been reported in patients with pustular outbreaks in the context of chronic plaque psoriasis, a finding that is consistent clinically with the highly inflammatory presentation of 'classical' GPP. Together, these results suggest two mechanisms for dysregulation of IL-1 family signalling in GPP, with major autoinflammatory consequences.

Microarray-based genotyping

With the advent of massively parallel, array-based genotyping technologies, we and others studying polygenic disorders pivoted from linkage studies performed in pedigrees, to a genome-wide association study (GWAS) strategy performed in cases and controls. This evolution occurred because association is much more powerful than linkage in the search for common susceptibility alleles, provided that dense genotyping is possible [91]. This strategy has proven to be very successful for psoriasis, as it has for many other complex genetic disorders [92]. Because GWAS entails the testing of hundreds of thousands to millions of markers, it was important to establish a conservative threshold for statistical significance. While many factors enter into setting this threshold for GWAS, a value of $P \leq 5\times10^{-8}$ has emerged for declaring a genome wide statistically significant result [93, 94].

As shown in Table 5.1, during the past 35 years, case–control studies have identified loci in 86 genomic regions that are associated with psoriasis at genome-wide significance. Before 2007, only loci within the MHC reached this level of significance. Early case–control studies had effective sample sizes of well under 1,000 (where effective sample size is defined as the total number of individuals with a 1:1 balanced case–control design that has statistical power equal to that of the actual case–control dataset). Only loci in the MHC had effect sizes for risk of disease large enough (odds ratio>3) to achieve genome-wide significance in these early studies. More recently, an explosion in the number of loci discovered has occurred due to increasingly large sample sizes and interrogation of large numbers of genetic variants. These more recent well-powered studies have focused on populations of either white European or Chinese ancestry, so currently all known psoriasis loci except those in the MHC have been firmly established for only these two populations. For the MHC, in addition to the studies of Chinese and European ancestry peoples cited in Table 5.1, genome-wide significant association has also been reported for Japanese [95], Korean [96], Thai [63], Pakistani [97, 98], and Indian [99–101] populations. Eleven of the 86 known psoriasis risk loci (*IFNLR1, IL23R, LCE, IFIH1, ERAP1, TNIP1, IL-12B*, MHC, *FOSL1, NFKBIA*, and *CARD14*) are shared by European and Chinese populations. Fifty-five loci have been established for Europeans only, and 20 loci for Chinese only.

Since 2007, effective sample sizes of the combined discovery and replication stages have ranged from the low thousands to nearly 40,000 individuals for the most recent meta-analyses of Chinese [102] and European [103] subjects. Originally, these GWAS microarrays were designed to tag all of the common (i.e. minor allele frequency, MAF>0.05) variation throughout the genome. These early GWAS studies were typically carried out in two stages——a high cost-per-sample discovery stage, in which a subset of the available sample was genotyped for a large, comprehensive marker set, followed by a lower cost-per-sample replication stage in which the most promising findings from the discovery stage are typed in the remainder of the sample. Thus, in the first few years of the GWAS era, discovery samples were usually much smaller than replication samples, limiting the power to detect new loci. More recently, specialized chips that target all exons (Exomechip [104]) or genomic regions previously implicated in immune-mediated polygenic diseases (Immunochip [105]) have become popular, largely because they are generally less expensive. This approach has led to the appearance of several studies since 2012 using discovery datasets with

an effective sample size of 20,000 or larger. However, a large proportion of the discovery stage samples for most of these bigger studies only featured targeted coverage of the genome (i.e. Exomechip and/or Immunochip). Only a few studies, all in Caucasians, have carried out truly large discovery GWAS, with effective sample sizes from ~10,000 [106, 107] to ~30,000 [103]. In contrast, the largest meta-GWAS of Chinese ancestry individuals to date has an effective sample size of ~3,800 [108], which is likely a contributing factor as to why fewer psoriasis loci have been discovered for Chinese vs European ancestry populations (31 vs 66, respectively).

Sixteen of the loci in Table 5.1 have also been firmly established as susceptibility loci for PsA, and 12 for PsC. Compared to studies of psoriasis, those of PsA and PsC are fewer in number and of generally lower power, hampering discovery of genetic loci for these two subphenotypes. The most powerful and comprehensive genetic comparison of these two psoriasis subphenotypes to date [16] found that the strength of association of PsA vs PsC was approximately equal for most known psoriasis loci. This study identified significant differences in relative strength of PsA and PsC association for variants near *TNFAIP3, IL23R, TNFRSF9,* and *LCE3C/B* [16]. This study also confirmed previously reported differential association for variants in the MHC [42, 109–114] and near *IL23R* [112, 115] and *PTPN22* [116]. However, it did not replicate prior reports of nominally significant differences in PsA vs PsC association for loci near *IL-12B* [112, 117], *FBXL19* [118], *ZNF816* [117], *CSF2* [115], *CCR2* [119], or *IL13* [120–123]. The *IL23R* and *TNFAIP3* regions are of particular interest, as they appear to display locus heterogeneity for psoriasis phenotypes, with each region containing a variant increasing risk specifically for PsA but not PsC, as well as one or more LD-independent variants posing risk for both subphenotypes (Figure 5.1). Conversely, the *LCE3C/3B* and *TNFRSF9* loci confer risk for PsC but not PsA (Figure 5.2). The skin selectivity of the *LCE3C/3B* signal may reflect the fact that this locus resides in the epidermal differentiation complex, where many genes of the LCE, SPRR, and filaggrin families, as well as loricrin and involucrin, are selectively expressed in the skin or other stratified epithelia, but not in the joints.

The existence of secondary psoriasis association signals independent of the primary reported variant have been reported for 11 of the 86 susceptibility regions presented in Table 5.1; these include the MHC [107, 108, 112, 114, 124–127], *IL-12B* [107, 108, 112, 127], *IL-23R* [16, 102, 112, 128], *TYK2* [107, 129, 130], *IFIH1* [107, 108, 130], *ERAP1* [107, 108], *NOS2* [16], *REL* [129], *TRAF3IP2* [129], *GJB2* [128], and *IFNGR2/SON* [102]. Of these 11 regions, only for the first seven in the list have any of the reported secondary signals achieved genome-wide significance in a logistic regression model containing all independent signals in the region. Secondary signals for PsA have been reported for the MHC [114, 115], *IL-12B* [16, 115], *IFIH1* [16, 115], and *NOS2* [115], while multiple independent signals for PsC have been reported for the MHC [114] and *IL-12B* [16]. Statistical epistasis (meaning that the effect of genetic variation at one locus depends upon genotype at another locus) has been observed between the primary psoriasis signal in the MHC (*HLA-C*06:02*) and psoriasis risk loci in the *LCE* gene cluster [107, 131–133], near *ERAP1* [16, 107, 126, 129], and near *IL-12B* [133]. Statistically significant interaction among PsA or PsC loci has not yet been demonstrated [16].

As a group, the 66 genome-wide significant European-origin psoriasis loci (see Microarray-based genotyping) can explain ~28%

Table 5.1 Psoriasis susceptibility loci. Listed loci achieve genome-wide significance of association ($P \leq 5 \times 10^{-8}$) with psoriasis in the cited references. For each locus, dots indicate whether association with psoriatic arthritis (PsA) or with cutaneous-only psoriasis (PsC) has also been established at genome-wide significance, as well as whether the association with psoriasis has been demonstrated in European (Eur) or Chinese (Chn) origin individuals. Please note that the 'Function' column does not cover every gene and contains assumptions as to which genes in any given region might be most likely to be involved.

Candidate gene(s)	Chrom. region	PsA	PsC	Eur	Chn	References	Function
SLC45A1, TNFRSF9	1p36.23		•	•		107; 16	*TNFRSF9*: Inhibits proliferation of activated T lymphocytes and induces programmed cell death.
MTHFR, NPPA	1p36.22				•	102	*MTHFR*: Required for homocysteine remethylation to methionine. Genetic variation influences susceptibility to occlusive vascular disease, neural tube defects, colon cancer and acute leukaemia.
IFNLR1	1p36.11	•		•	•	107; 191; 192; 16	Forms a receptor complex with IL-10 receptor beta. Interacts with interferon-lambda family members IL28A, IL28B, and IL29.
RUNX3	1p36.11	•		•		107; 193; 16	Transcription factor (TF) required for development of IFN-γ producing pathogenic Th17 cells through binding with T-bet [194].
ZNF683	1p36.11				•	102	TF expressed in quiescent and long-lived effector-type CD8(+) T cells. Its function in human T cells seems adapted to lifelong, periodic pathogen challenges [195].
IL23R, C1orf141	1p31.3	•	•	•	•	112; 107; 128; 115; 102; 16; 130	*IL23R*: Subunit of the IL-23 receptor that pairs with IL12Rβ1 to initiate IL23A signalling. Associates with JAK2, and binds to STAT3 in a ligand-dependent manner.
LRRC7	1p31.1			•		106	*LRRC7*: Brain-expressed leucine-rich repeat protein found in the postsynaptic density. Contains a PDZ domain near its C-terminus.
FUBP1	1p31.1			•		103, 196	*FUBP1*: Encodes a single stranded DNA-binding protein that binds to multiple DNA elements, and has 3'-5' helicase activity. Binding to viral RNA is thought to play a role in several viral diseases.
PTPN22	1p13.2	•				116	*PTPN22*: Encodes a lymphoid-specific intracellular phosphatase regulating CBL function in the TCR signalling pathway. Also associated with T1D, RA, SLE, vitiligo, and Graves' disease.
LCE3B, LCE3C, LCE3D, LCE3A, C1orf68, KPRP	1q21.3		•	•	•	131; 124; 129; 132; 107; 128; 102; 108; 16; 130	*LCE3*: Late cornified envelope genes are expressed in differentiated keratinocytes. Genes of the *LCE3* group show increased expression in psoriatic skin and are induced after skin injury, whereas other LCE group genes are down-regulated [197].
AIM2	1q23.1				•	102	Encodes a cytoplasmic sensor that recognizes dsDNA of microbial or host origin. Upon binding to DNA, AIM2 assembles inflammasomes, which cleave the pro-inflammatory cytokines pro-IL-1β and pro-IL-18a [198].
FASLG	1q24.3			•		103	Encodes Fas ligand (CD95), a transmembrane protein of the TNF family. Fas ligand/receptor interactions regulate inflammation via apoptosis and promotion of inflammatory responses in macrophages, DCs, and keratinocytes [199].
DENND1B	1q31.3			•		115; 130	Functions as a guanine nucleotide exchange factor for the endosomal small GTPase RAB35, linking RAB35 activation with the clathrin machinery.
IKBKE	1q32.1			•		103	Encodes IKKε; essential for regulation of antiviral signaling. Activated downstream of cytosolic RNA/DNA sensors, and mediates activation of TFs including IRF3, IRF7, and NF-κB [200].
REL, LINC01185	2p16.1	•		•		129; 201; 107; 108; 16; 130	*REL*: Encodes c-Rel. a member of the NF-κB family with an important role in B-cell survival and proliferation. Amplified or mutated in human B-cell lymphomas. Mice lacking both REL and RELA in KC develop a psoriasiform dermatitis [202].
B3GNT2	2p15			•		107; 16; 130	Encodes a member of the beta-1,3-N-acetylglucosaminyl transferase family. Deficiency results in hyperactivation of lymphocytes [203].

Table 5.1 Continued

Candidate gene(s)	Chrom. region	PsA	PsC	Eur	Chn	References	Function
IL1RL1	2q12.1				•	102	IL1RL1: Encodes a member of the IL1 receptor family induced by proinflammatory stimuli, and involved in helper T cell function. Associated with atopic dermatitis in Oriental populations.
IFIH1, KCNH7	2q24.2	•		•	•	129; 107; 204; 108; 16; 130	IFIH1: Encodes a DEAD box protein upregulated in response to treatment with IFN-β. Variation in IFIH1 is associated with Type 1 diabetes, vitiligo, SLE, and ulcerative colitis.
PLCL2	3p24.3		•			106; 130	Encodes a phospholipase C-like protein with a pleckstrin homology domain. Variation has been associated with primary biliary cirrhosis, multiple sclerosis, and rheumatoid arthritis.
NFKBIZ	3q12.3		•			106	NFKBIZ: Encodes IκB-zeta which is an Act1 (TRAF3IP2)-dependent IL-17 target gene in mice [205] and humans [107].
CASR	3q21.1				•	102	Encodes a GPCR expressed in the parathyroid gland, which senses calcium concentration and modifies PTH secretion. Plays a key role in mineral homeostasis and KC differentiation.
GPR160	3q26.2				•	102	Associated with stroke in the Japanese population.
TP63	3q28		•			108	Encodes a member of the p53 family of TFs. Essential for epidermal development in mice. Mutations associated with ectodermal dysplasia, cleft lip/palate, others. Epidermal overexpression results in an AD-like phenotype [206].
NFKB1	4q24				•	204	Encodes a 105 kDa Rel-specific transcription inhibitor that can be processed to a 50 kD DNA binding subunit of the NF-κB protein complex. Activated by cytokines, oxidants, UV light, and bacterial or viral products.
CARD6	5p13.1		•			106	Encodes a microtubule-associated protein that interacts with RIP kinases and modulates signalling pathways converging on NF-kB.
ZFYVE16	5q14.1				•	102	Encodes an endosomal protein that regulates membrane trafficking in the endosome. Functions as a scaffold protein in the TGF-β pathway.
ERAP1, LNPEP	5q15			•	•	143; 129; 107; 191; 128; 204; 16; 130	ERAP1: Encodes an endoplasmic reticulum aminopeptidase involved in trimming HLA class I-binding peptide precursors for antigen presentation. Acts as a monomer or as an ERAP1/2 heterodimer. Epistasis with HLA Class I genes in psoriasis, AS, and Behçet's disease.
CSF2, P4HA2	5q31.1	•		•		115	CSF2: Encodes cytokine that controls production, differentiation, and function of PMNs and macrophages. Maps to a cluster of related genes at 5q31 involved in AML, including IL4, IL5, IL13.
IL13, IL4	5q31.1		•	•		112; 107; 108; 16; 130	Cytokines with overlapping functions produced by Th2 cells. Involved in B-cell maturation, differentiation, and IgE isotype switching. Down-regulates macrophage activity. IL3, IL5, IL4, and CSF2 form a gene cluster on chr 5q.
TNIP1, ANXA6	5q33.1	•	•	•		112; 143; 201; 107; 117; 127; 115; 102; 108; 16	TNIP1: Encodes an A20-binding protein involved in autoimmunity and tissue homeostasis through regulation of NFκB activation. Associated with myasthenia gravis, systemic sclerosis and SLE.
IL-12B, ADRA1B, RNF145	5q33.3	•	•	•	•	207; 208; 112; 124; 209; 210; 129; 107; 203; 127; 115; 102; 108; 16; 130	IL-12B: Encodes the p40 a subunit of IL-12, a cytokine that acts on T and NK cells. Expressed by DCs and activated macrophages, IL-12 is an essential inducer of Th1 development that protects against intracellular pathogens. IL-12B variation is associated with MS, CD, UC, and AS.
PTTG1	5q33.3				•	143	PTTG1: Encodes an anaphase-promoting complex substrate involved in sister chromatid separation. The gene product is tumorigenic and highly expressed in various tumours.

(continued)

Table 5.1 Continued

Candidate gene(s)	Chrom. region	PsA	PsC	Eur	Chn	References	Function
EXOC2, IRF4	6p25.3			•		107	IRF4: Encodes a TF that regulates IL-17A promoter activity and Th17-mediated colitis in vivo. Stabilizes the Th17 phenotype through IL-21. Variation is associated with pigmentation, RA, lymphoma, leukaemia, and schizophrenia.
CDKAL1	6p22.3			•		16	CDKAL1: Encodes a member of the methylthiotransferase family of unknown function. Variation associated with T2D, BMI, CD.
HLA-C, HLA-B, HLA-A, HLA-DR	6p21.33	•	•	•	•	211; 212; 213; 45; 109; 42; 214; 59; 215; 216; 217; 218; 219; 110; 220; 221; 111; 222; 112; 124; 125; 209; 210; 129; 133; 160; 201; 223; 113; 126; 107; 224; 114; 127; 115; 16	HLA-B and HLA-C present antigens to CD8+ T-cells. HLA-C also serves as a ligand for killer immunoglobulin-like receptors (KIRs) on NK cells. Beyond HLA-C, conditional analysis demonstrates strong associations between PsV and multiple HLA loci, with amino acid 45 at HLA-B distinguishing between PsC and PsA [114].
TRAF3IP2	6q21	•	•	•		209; 210; 129; 113; 107; 115; 108; 16; 130	Interacts with TRAF proteins and I-kappaB kinase and MAP kinases to activate NF-κB transcription factors that mediate innate immunity.
TNFAIP3	6q23.3		•	•		112; 107; 108; 16; 130	Rapidly induced by TNF; encodes a ubiquitin-editing enzyme involved in cytokine-regulated immune/inflammatory responses, and inhibition of NF-κB activation and TNF-induced apoptosis.
TAGAP	6q25.3			•		107	Encodes a protein activating a Rho GTPase protein for T-cell activation. Mutations are associated with RA, coeliac disease, and MS.
CCDC129	7p14.3				•	102	Encodes coiled-coil domain containing protein [129] involved in receptor binding.
ELMO1	7p14.1			•		107	An engulfment and cell motility protein that promotes phagocytosis and cell migration. Associated with glioma cell invasion and diabetic nephropathy.
CSMD1	8p23.2				•	143	A postulated tumour suppressor of squamous cell carcinomas [225].
DDX58	9p21.1			•		107	Encodes a protein with a caspase recruitment domain and RNA helicase-DEAD box motif. Recognizes dsRNA, controls immune responses.
KLF4	9q31.2			•		107; 130	A transcription factor that regulates p53 in G1-to-S phase transition after DNA damage. Necessary for skin barrier function.
TNFSF15	9q32			•		130	Induced by TNF and IL1-α; encodes a cytokine that activates NF-κB and MAP kinases. Induces apoptosis; inhibits endothelial cell proliferation.
ZNF365	10q21.2			•		103	Zinc finger protein; mutations are associated with uric acid-induced nephrolithiasis.
CAMK2G	10q22.2			•		106; 16	Encodes the gamma chain of a serine/threonine, Ca(2+)/calmodulin-dependent protein kinase.
ZMIZ1	10q22.3			•		226; 16	Regulates transcription factors, such as the androgen receptor, Smad3/4, and p53. Gene translocation with the ABL1 locus on chr 9 is associated with acute lymphoblastic leukaemia.
PTEN, KLLN, SNORD74	10q23.31			•		103, 196	PTEN: Tumour suppressor that negatively regulates the AKT/PKB signaling pathway. KLLN: Nuclear protein that increases S phase arrest and apoptosis and is upregulated by p53.
CHUK	10q24.31			•		103	A serine/threonine protein kinase that activates NF-κB via degradation of its inhibitor IκBα.
ZNF143	11p15.4				•	102	Zinc finger protein transcriptional activator that initiates RNA polymerase activity.

Table 5.1 Continued

Candidate gene(s)	Chrom. region	PsA	PsC	Eur	Chn	References	Function
RPS6KA4, PRDX5	11q13.1			•		226; 16	RPS6KA4: Serine/threonine kinase that phosphorylates CREB1, ATF1, and histone H3 to regulate genes involved in inflammation. PRDX5: A protective antioxidant enzyme that interacts with peroxisome receptor 1.
AP5B1, CFL1, FIBP, FOSL1	11q13.1			•	•	102, 103	FOSL1: Regulates cell proliferation/differentiation via interactions with other AP-1 family members.
ZC3H12C	11q22.3			•		107; 16	Encodes a protein that inhibits TNF-induced endothelial cell activation.
ETS1	11q24.3			•		107	Transcription factor with activator and repressor activity. Plays a role in stem cell development, cell aging, and tumorigenesis.
CD27, LAG3	12p13.3				•	204	CD27 encodes a member of the TNF receptor superfamily required for T-cell immunity [227]. LAG3 encodes a ligand for MHC class II receptors and is structurally related to CD4.
KLRK1, KLRC4	12p13.2			•		103	Transmembrane receptors that can activate NK and T cells. Targeted in immune disorder and cancer treatment.
IL23A, STAT2	12q13.3	•	•	•		112; 107; 115; 108; 16; 130	IL23A: A subunit of the IL-23 heterodimer, which acts on memory CD4(+) T cells to induce STAT4 and IFN-γ. STAT2: Transcriptional activator that forms a complex with STAT1 in response to IFN.
BRAP, MAPKAPK5	12q24.12			•		103	BRAP: sequesters BRCA1 to the cytoplasm. MAPKAPK5: Tumour suppressor activated by MAPKs in response to cell stress and inflammatory cytokines; phosphorylates HSP27.
IL31	12q24.31			•		103	Produced by Th2 T-cells, and acts on keratinocyte and epithelial cell receptors. May regulate allergic skin disorders and other allergic diseases.
GJB2	13q12.11				•	143; 128	A gap junction protein, also known as a connexin. Mutations of this gene account for over half of pre-lingual, recessive deafness cases.
COG6	13q14.11			•		108	Encodes a subunit of the conserved oligomeric Golgi complex.
LINC00330	13q14.2			•		108	Long intergenic non-coding RNA 330; function unknown.
UBAC2, RN7SKP9	13q32.3			•		103	UBAC2: UBA domain-containing 2, Implicated in Behçet's disease [228].
NFKBIA, PSMA6	14q13.2	•	•	•	•	118; 129; 107; 192; 102; 108; 16; 130	NFKBIA: Moves between cytoplasm and nucleus to inhibit NF-κB. Mutations associated with ectodermal dysplasia with T-cell immunodeficiency. PSMA6: encodes a proteasomal subunit involved in cleavage of MHC class I peptides.
SYNE2	14q23.2				•	102	A nuclear outer membrane protein that binds cytoplasmic F-actin to secure the nucleus to the cytoskeleton and maintain its structural integrity.
RP11-61O1.1	14q32.2			•		103	Non-coding gene of unknown function.
KLF13	15q13.3			•		103	A transcription factor containing 3 zinc finger DNA-binding domains [229]. Regulates HPV life cycle in keratinocytes [230].
PRM3, SOCS1	16p13.13			•		107; 130	PRM3: A sperm protamine, which condenses sperm DNA into a compact, inactive complex. SOCS1: A cytokine-induced negative feedback inhibitor of STAT signalling.
FBXL19, PRSS53, HSD3B7	16p11.2	•				118; 107; 108; 16; 130	FBXL19: An E3 ubiquitin ligase that ubiquitinates IL1 receptor-like 1 for degradation. PRSS53 encodes a protein with serine-type endopeptidase activity. HSD3B7 encodes a membrane-associated ER enzyme involved in the synthesis of bile acids.
NOS2	17q11.2	•	•	•		118; 107; 108; 116; 16	Encodes an inducible nitric oxide synthase that is markedly overexpressed in psoriasis lesions.

(continued)

Table 5.1 Continued

Candidate gene(s)	Chrom. region	PsA	PsC	Eur	Chn	References	Function
IKZF3	17q12				•	204	Encodes a TF in the Ikaros family of zinc-finger proteins. Controls proliferation and differentiation of B-cells; functions in chromatin remodelling.
PTRF, STAT3, STAT5A/B	17q21.2			•		107	*PTRF:* Enables dissociation and replacement of transcription complexes on emerging rRNA transcripts. Thought to play a role in the creation of plasma membrane caveolae. *STAT3, STAT5A, STAT5B:* Transcription factors involved in cell growth, apoptosis, and immunoregulation.
TRIM47, TRIM65	17q25.1			•		103	*TRIM65:* Tripartite Motif Containing 65. Deactivates p53 through ubiquitination. Up-regulated in non-small cell lung carcinoma [231].
TMC6	17q25.3				•	102	An integral membrane protein of the endoplasmic reticulum. Known as one of two genes causing epidermodysplasia verruciformis, a disease with increased susceptibility to HPV and SCC.
CARD14	17q25.3			•	•	107, 128	A caspase recruitment domain-containing protein of the MAGUK family, members of which act as scaffold proteins in cell adhesion, cell polarity, and signal transduction. Interacts with BCL10 to activate NF-κB and promote apoptosis.
PTPN2	18p11.21			•		103	Encodes a protein tyrosine phosphatase with a highly conserved catalytic motif. EGFR and the Shc adaptor protein are supposed substrates. Serves as a signalling molecule to regulate cell growth, differentiation, mitosis, and oncogenesis.
POLI, STARD6, MBD2	18q21.2			•		107	*POLI:* DNA polymerase involved in DNA repair and in mutation of immunogloublin genes. *STARD6:* Homologous to STAR proteins involved in sterol transport [232]. *MBD2:* Methyl-CpG binding protein that can repress or activate transcription.
SERPINB8	18q22.1				•	143	Protease inhibitor-8, a member of the ov-serpin subfamily. Serpins play a role in complement activation, fibrinolysis, coagulation, migration, apoptosis, and tumour suppression.
TYK2	19p13.2	•		•		129; 107; 115; 16; 130	Belongs to the JAK family of tyrosine kinases that phosphorylate cytokine receptors to propagate inflammatory signals. Functions in IFN-mediated anti-viral immunity; gene mutation has been linked to hyper IgE syndrome.
ILF3,CARM1	19p13.2			•		107; 16	*ILF3:* A dsRNA binding protein that regulates gene expression via mRNA stabilization. Influences redistribution of nuclear mRNA to the cytoplasm in T-cells. *CARM1:* An arginine methyltransferase that acts on histones to regulate gene expression.
FUT2	19q13.33			•		103; 130	Encodes the galactoside 2-L-fucosyltransferase enzyme, a Golgi membrane protein involved in the production of the H antigen precursor for the ABO blood group glycoproteins.
ZNF816	19q13.41				•	143; 128	Encodes a zinc finger protein with TF activity. Binds sequence-specific DNA.
RNF114, SNAI1	20q13.13			•		233; 107; 16; 130	*RNF114:* Ubiquitin-protein ligase that degrades the inhibitor of CDKN1A to induce G1-to-S phase transition. *SNAI1:* Zinc finger transcriptional repressor involved in mesodermal development.
IFNGR2, SON	21q22.11				•	102	*IFNGR2:* Non-ligand-binding beta chain of IFN-g receptor. Mutations result in susceptibility to mycobacterial disease.
RUNX1	21q22.12			•		108	The alpha subunit of core binding factor, which plays a role in hematopoietic development. Leads to leukaemia via chromosomal translocation.
YDJC, UBE2L3	22q11.21			•		226; 107	*YDJC:* Deacetylates carbohydrates in the breakdown of oligosaccharides. *UBE2L3:* Ubiquitin-conjugating enzyme that ubiquitinates p53, c-FOS, and p105.

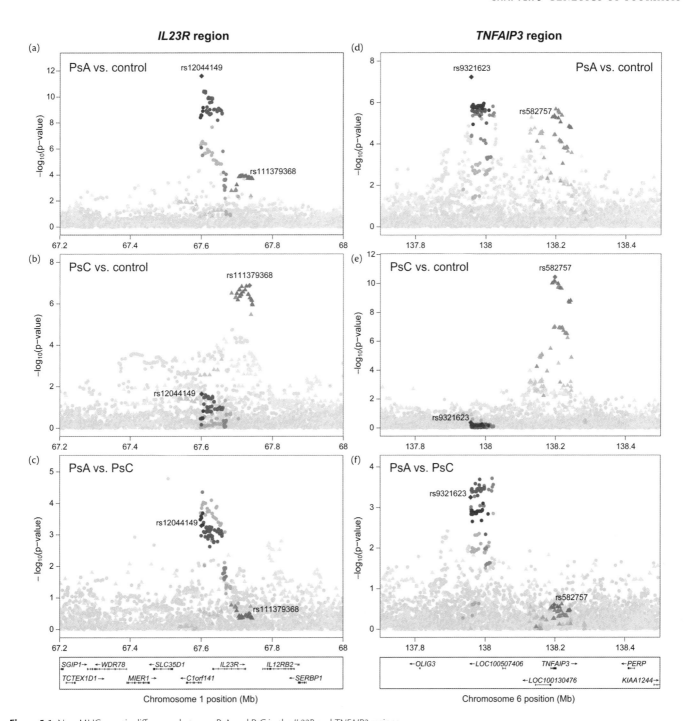

Figure 5.1 Non-MHC genetic differences between PsA and PsC in the *IL23R* and *TNFAIP3* regions.

Negative log10-transformed p-values from meta-analyses of association are shown for 800-kb regions encompassing genes *IL23R* (panels A-C) and *TNFAIP3* (panels D-F). For each region two reference SNPs with diamond symbols are labeled, denoting the variants that were most significantly associated for tests of PsA cases versus controls and PsC cases vs. controls. For all other plotted variants, the shape of the symbol denotes which index SNP the variant is in highest LD with (circles for the PsA index, triangles for the PsC index), and the grayscale intensity indicates the magnitude of the pairwise LD r² coefficient. Panels A and D show association results for PsA cases vs. controls, and panels B and E for PsC cases vs. controls. Panels C and F show results for a conservative parametric test of the difference in log(OR) values from the PsA vs. control and PsC vs. control comparisons. The bottom two panels give the physical positions of known genes in each region.

Reprinted from The American Journal of Human Genetics 97(6):816-836 Stuart P. et al. Genome-wide association analysis of psoriatic arthritis and cutaneous psoriasis reveals differences in their genetic architecture (2015) with permission from Elsevier.

of the genetic heritability [103], compared to the 22% of heritability that could be explained using only the 39 independent signals identified as of 2012 [107]. This relatively small increase reflects the fact that as sample sizes increase, the odds ratios of newly described signals tend to decrease. Moreover, these 66 loci generate a genetic risk score capable of discriminating cases and controls in our

sample with a predictive capacity (area under the receiver operating curve, or AUC) of ~0.75, a value that compares favourably to other complex genetic disorders [134]. However, higher predictive capacity is generally required to yield a clinically useful predictive test. Recently, several serum-derived biomarkers have been identified as tools for the prediction of PsA development in psoriatic patients,

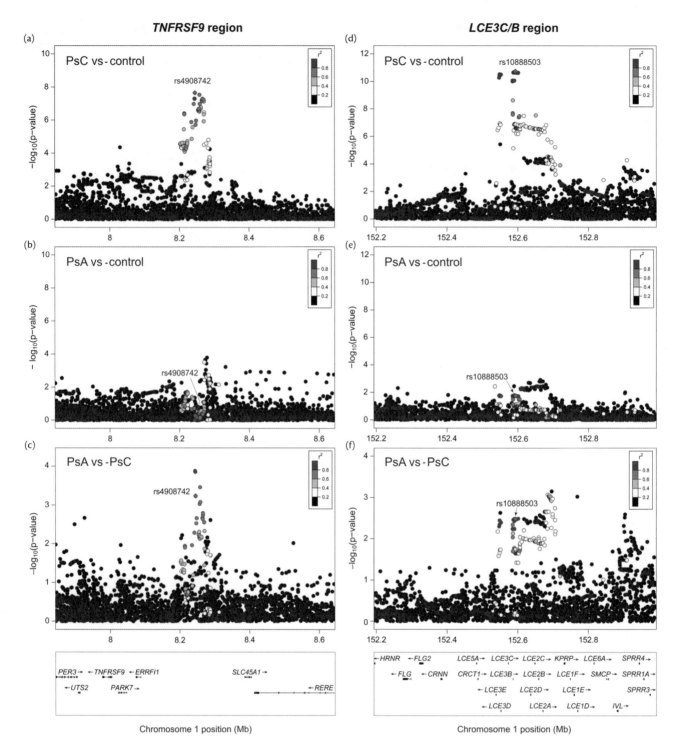

Figure 5.2 PsC-specific signals in the *TNFRSF9* and *LCE3* regions.

Negative log10-transformed p-values are shown for 800-kb regions encompassing genes *TNFRSF9* (panels A-C) and *LCE3C* and *LCE3B* (panels D-F). The most significantly-associated (index) SNP for the comparison of PsC cases with unaffected controls is shown for each region. The grayscale value of each symbol denotes the strength of LD (r^2 coefficient) with the index SNP. The comparison of PsA cases vs. controls is shown in panels A and C. The comparison of PsC cases vs. controls is shown in panels B and E. Panels C and F show the results of a parametric test of the difference in log(OR) values from the PsA vs. control and PsC vs. control comparisons. The physical positions of known genes in each region are shown in the bottom two panels.

Reprinted from The American Journal of Human Genetics 97(6):816-836 Stuart P. et al. Genome-wide association analysis of psoriatic arthritis and cutaneous psoriasis reveals differences in their genetic architecture (2015) with permission from Elsevier.

including proteins and microRNAs [135–137]. Because about one in four patients with PsC go on to develop PsA, by combining genetic results with other blood-derived biomarkers, development of a clinically useful tool for the prediction of PsA development in psoriatic patients is a feasible goal.

Unlike the high-penetrance, high-effect-size mutations emerging from the sequencing-based studies described earlier, the 'candidate genes' presented in Table 5.1 cannot simply be assumed to play a causal role underlying the observed associations. Indeed, identification of the biological processes responsible for these genetic signals is a major focus of current research in psoriasis and other complex genetic disorders [138]. Nevertheless, several lines of evidence point to the importance of host defence genes in the immunopathogenesis of psoriasis. Perhaps most evident is the fact that the magnitude and significance of psoriasis associations in the MHC dwarfs those of all other associated loci. To better assess the importance of defined biological processes and pathways across the entire genome, we developed an analysis tool called MEAGA (Minimum distance-based Enrichment Analysis for Genetic Association) which uses graphical algorithms to measure the overlap between observed genetic signals and annotated functions and pathways [139]. Using MEAGA, we identified 87 significantly enriched functions/pathways, many of which are immune-related functions such as lymphocyte differentiation/regulation, Type I interferon and pattern recognition, NF-κB signalling, and response to viruses/bacteria [103]. Because DNA accessibility in chromatin correlates well with gene activity [140], we also used a method similar to one described by others [141] to assess the overlap between psoriasis-associated genetic signals and open chromatin regions across a panel of different cell types. This analysis showed that the psoriasis signals are enriched in regulatory elements from different T-cell subsets (CD8+ T-cells and various CD4+ T-cell subsets including T_h0, T_h1, and T_h17) (Figure 5.3) [103]. Notably, ~70% of these either themselves harbour or are in high LD (r2≥0.8) with SNPs mapping to enhancers in these four cell types. This genetic evidence supporting the importance of immune and inflammatory host defence mechanisms in psoriasis is strongly supported by the increasing number of highly effective biological therapies for psoriasis, particularly those targeting TNF,

as well as the IL-23/Th17 pathway 2. These important advances are detailed elsewhere in this volume (see Chapter 26). As illustrated in Figure 5.4 and detailed in the figure legend and Table 5.1, many of the genetic signals uncovered by psoriasis GWAS can be viewed as participants in a "play in four acts", relating to (i) antigen presentation, (ii) activation of NF-κB, (iii) Th17 differentiation, and (iv) effects of IL-17 on cutaneous host defence [142].

HLA associations in psoriasis—what do they mean?

While the currently known European-origin signals explain 28% of the genetic heritability, genes in the MHC alone contribute 11.2% (i.e. ~40% of the heritability explained by the 66 known signals). However, deciphering the biological correlates of HLA association in psoriasis remains a challenging subject of research. One key facet of MHC function elucidated by genetics involves the importance of MHC Class I antigen processing and presentation. As noted earlier, *HLA-C*06* manifests epistasis (i.e. genetic interaction) with SNPs mapping to a region of chromosomal band 5q15 containing key genes involved in MHC Class I antigen processing (*ERAP1, ERAP2*, and *LNPEP*) [129, 143]. The *ERAP* genes encode endoplasmic reticulum-associated aminopeptidases that trim antigenic peptides to the optimal size for binding to MHC Class I molecules, which are 8–10 amino acids [144]. These enzymes act on peptides that are generated in the cytosol by proteasomal degradation and other proteolytic mechanisms, and subsequently transported to the endoplasmic reticulum by the products of MHC-encoded *TAP* genes. Epistasis involving the *ERAP* region has also been found in two other HLA Class I-associated diseases: *HLA-B*27* in ankylosing spondylitis [145], and *HLA-B*51* in Behçet's disease [146]. These observations provide genetic evidence for the importance of antigen presentation in the pathogenesis of psoriasis and other MHC Class I-associated diseases.

For many years, researchers have noted a strong association between psoriasis, *HLA-C*06*, and streptococcal infection [147, 148], as well as between ankylosing spondylitis, *HLA-B*27*, and Gram-negative bacterial infections of the gut [149], raising the question of whether 'molecular mimicry' might exist between microbial pathogens and host proteins, involving MHC Class I-mediated antigen presentation. *HLA-C*06* association is particularly strong for guttate psoriasis, an acute presentation of psoriasis that typically presents in childhood or early adolescence, often following the development of streptococcal pharyngitis [150]. Notably, skin-homing T-cell clones that are expanded in psoriatic skin lesions are also expanded in the tonsils of psoriatic patients [151]. Recent studies have shown that tonsillectomy improves psoriasis, both clinically and in terms of immune responses involving peptide antigens that cross-react between streptococcal M protein and 'hyperproliferative' keratins overexpressed in psoriatic skin [152]. Moreover, studies involving immunization of rabbits with heat-killed *Streptococcus pyogenes* identified antibodies reactive with the proteins ezrin, maspin, peroxiredoxin 2, heat shock protein 27 (hsp27), as well as the 'hyperproliferative' keratin K6. These same proteins also stimulated proliferation of CD8+ T-cells in psoriasis patients, particularly in *HLA-C*06*+ individuals [153].

These results provide genetic and biological support for a connection between psoriasis, HLA-C*06, and streptococcal pharyngitis involving cross-reactivity between streptococcal antigens and

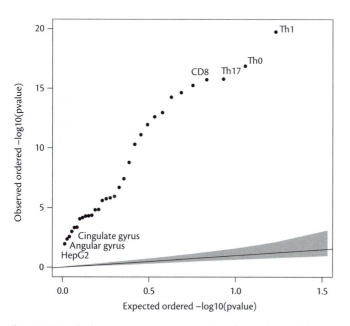

Figure 5.3 Overlap between psoriasis genetic signals and open chromatin in various cell types.

For various cell or tissue types with active enhancers predicted using the H3K27ac mark, we measured the enrichment of the enhancers among the psoriasis-associated loci. This quantile-quantile plot depicts the observed-ordered −log10 p values for enrichment of the number of regulatory elements overlapping with the psoriasis susceptibility loci shown in **Table 5.1** (y-axis) against the expected −log10 p values (x-axis). The grey-shaded area depicts the 95% interval for what would have been observed by chance. The cell types yielding the most significant p values are labeled; for illustration purposes, we also labeled cell or tissue types with the least significant p-values.

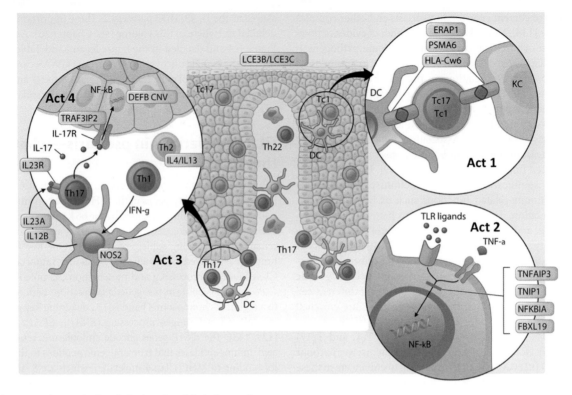

Figure 5.4 Immunopathogenesis of psoriasis, viewed as a 'play in four acts'.

Act 1—antigen presentation: Having been processed by proteasomes (*PSMA6* encodes a proteasomal subunit), followed by transport to the endoplasmic reticulum for further processing by ERAP1 in dendritic cells (DC), antigen in the binding pocket of HLA-C*06 interacts with a T-cell receptor, allowing activation and clonal expansion of antigen-specific CD8+ T-cell. This process may occur both in the dermis (activation of memory resident T-cell) and local lymph nodes (activation of naive T-cell). Subsequently, activated CD8+ T-cell migrate into the epidermis where they encounter HLA-C*06-Ag on the surface of the keratinocytes (or perhaps melanocytes). Activated CD8+ T-cell could also trigger the local release of soluble factors, including cytokines, chemokines, and/or innate immune mediators, which could further increase local inflammation and stimulate keratinocyte proliferation. **Act 2—NF-κB activation:** Multiple genes mapping to psoriasis susceptibility loci participate in the regulation of NF-κB in response to TNF, TLR ligands, and other innate immune mediators. **Act 3—Th17 expansion:** Th1 cell polarization is cross-regulated by IL-4 and/or IL-13 produced by Th2 cells. IFN-γ produced by Th1 cells activates DC, which produce iNOS (encoded by NOS2) and produce IL-23 (the p40 subunit of which is encoded by *IL-12B*). IL-23 interacts with IL-23 receptors (one subunit encoded by *IL23R*), leading to the survival and proliferation of Th17 cells. **Act 4—IL-17 responses:** IL-17 produced by Th17 cells binds to IL-17 receptors and activates downstream signalling via Act 1 (encoded by *TRAF3IP2*) on keratinocytes. In concert with TNF and/or other proinflammatory cytokines, IL-17 stimulates the production of defensins as well as chemokines, promoting host defense and leading to the infiltration of additional inflammatory cells into the lesion. The function of other candidate psoriasis genes in one or more of these 'acts' is provided in **Table 5.1**.

Adapted from Goldsmith et al. Fitzpatrick's Dermatology in General Medicine, 8th edition (2012) with permission from McGraw Hill, based on a figure from Nair et al. 'Psoriasis Bench to Bedside: Genetics meets Immunology' (2009) JAMA Dermatology 145(4) 462-464 Copyright©(2009) American Medical Association. All rights reserved.

keratin-related host proteins. However, newer data indicate that the role of HLA genes in psoriasis is likely to be even more complex, involving the genetic involvement of HLA-A, HLA-B, and HLA-DR in addition to HLA-C [114], an amino acid residue in HLA-B that discriminates between PsA and PsC [114], potentially altered regulation of *HLA-C*06* expression [154, 155], and presentation by HLA-C*06 of melanocyte-derived peptides not related to keratins or streptococci [155].

Participation of multiple HLA alleles

We used conditional logistic regression to control for the effects of *HLA-C*06* in a sample of 9,247 European-descent psoriatic patients (3,038 PsA and 3,098 PsC) and 13,589 controls, revealing evidence for multiple peaks of association within the MHC [114] (Figure 5.5). Similar observations have also been made in smaller samples [125, 126]. Using SNP data to impute HLA alleles, we found that multiple MHC Class I and Class II alleles are associated with psoriasis at genome-wide significance ($P<5.0\times10^{-8}$), including *HLA-C*06:02, HLA-C*12:03, HLA-B* amino acid positions 67 and 9, *HLA-A* amino acid position 95, and *HLA-DQα1* amino acid position 53 [114]. After accounting for all of these independent

associations, we found no evidence for additional risk conferred by variation in *MICA*, an HLA-like gene located in the MHC Class III region that has previously been associated with PsA [157, 158].

HLA-B amino acid 45 distinguishes PsA from PsC

As reviewed in 'HLA association studies' above, early HLA association studies identified differences between PsA and psoriasis in general (i.e. PsV), whereas more recent studies have defined PsC in such a way that the subject was documented not to have joint symptoms at the time of entry into the study [44, 159, 160]. Using the operational definition of PsC described earlier (i.e. skin psoriasis for at least 10 years without a history of joint complaints) in an effort to account for the delayed onset of PsA relative to skin psoriasis [10], we recently identified genetic associations that differ between PsC and PsA within the MHC [114]. We mapped differential HLA association of PsC vs PsA to amino acid 45 of HLA-B, with carriage of glutamic acid at this position increasing risk for PsA vs PsC far more than any classical HLA-B allele [114]. While Glu 45 is present in known PsA-associated *HLA-B* alleles, including *HLA-B*08, HLA-B*27, HLA-B*38,* and *HLA-B*39* [161], we found that the increased risk for PsA vs PsC persisted after controlling for

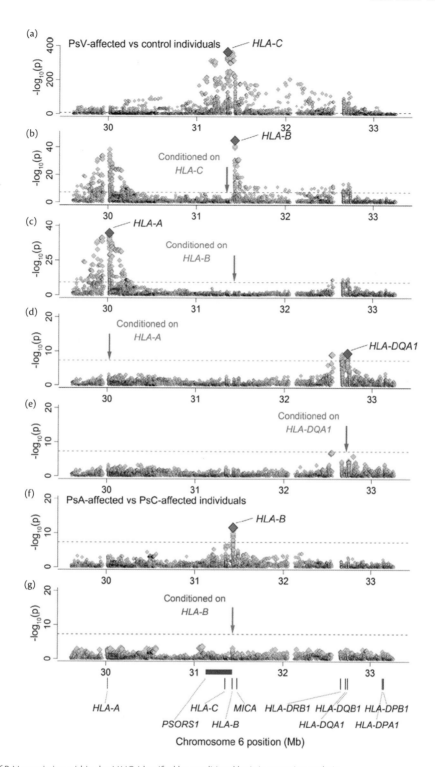

Figure 5.5 Multiple peaks of PsV association within the MHC, identified by conditional logistic regression analysis.

Association plots between MHC variants for PsV and its subphenotypes of PsA and PsC. Each diamond represents the $-\log_{10}(p)$ of the variants, including SNPs, classical HLA or MICA alleles, and amino acid polymorphisms encoded by the *HLA* genes or *MICA*. The dotted horizontal line represents the significance threshold of $p = 5 \times 10^{-8}$. The bottom panel shows the physical positions of the HLA genes, MICA, and *PSORS1* on chromosome 6 (UCSC Genome Browser hg18). We tested four binary phenotypes: (A) PsV-affected vs control individuals, (B) PsA-affected vs control individuals, (C) PsC-affected vs control individuals, and (D) PsA-affected versus PsC-affected individuals.

Reprinted from Okada et al., Fine mapping Major Histocompatibility Complex associations in psoriasis and its clinical subtypes (2014) *American Journal of Human Genetics* 95:162-72 (2014) under Creative Commons license CC BY 3.0.

these alleles, suggesting that Glu 45 in HLA-B exerts an important molecular effect [114]. Of note, amino acid residue 45 is located in the antigen-binding groove, in close proximity to residues 9 and 67, which themselves distinguish PsV from controls after controlling for *HLA-C*06* (Figure 5.6). The presence of Glu at residue 45 favours binding of arginine in the P2 position that interfaces with the B pocket of the HLA-B peptide-binding groove, whereas the presence of Lys at HLA-B residue 45, which confers decreased risk for PsA vs PsC in the context of the HLA-B*44 allele, favours binding of glutamic acid in the P2 position [161]. To date, however,

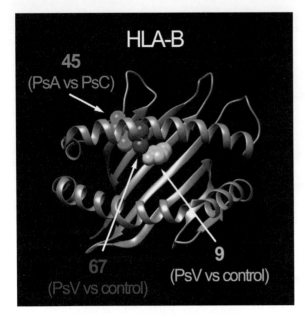

Figure 5.6 Proximity of disease-associated amino acid variants in HLA-B. HLA-B amino acid residues at positions 9 and 67 that are associated with overall PsV risk are highlighted. The residue at amino acid position 45 that is associated with different risks for PsA vs. PsC is indicated by the white arrow from position 45.
Reprinted from Okada et al., Fine mapping Major Histocompatibility Complex associations in psoriasis and its clinical subtypes (2014) American Journal of Human Genetics 95:162–72 (2014) under Creative Commons license CC BY 3.0.

no specific antigens have been identified for PsA [162]. Additional complexity arises because different clinical subtypes of PsA may have different HLA associations [161].

Altered regulation of HLA-C*06

Our recent MHC analysis [114] revealed that *HLA-C*06*, as an allele, yielded the most significant p value for PsV ($P=1.7\times10^{-364}$), with a larger effect size than any individual amino acid residue or combination of residues. This outcome differs from studies of psoriasis-associated HLA loci other than *HLA-C*06* [114], and from HLA associations in HIV elite controllers [163] and rheumatoid arthritis [164], all of which implicated specific amino acid residues as the most significant determinants of risk, rather than HLA alleles. As suggested by others [155], *HLA-C*06* might be associated with psoriasis due to distinctive regulatory features. Indeed, the 3′-untranslated region (UTR) of *HLA-C*06* contains a variant micro-RNA binding site for miR148a that results in loss of repression of *HLA-C*06* expression [154]. However, other *HLA-C* alleles also carry this variant, but are not psoriasis-associated. Thus, it remains possible that some unique feature of the combination of amino acid variants present in the antigen-binding groove of HLA-C*06 may be responsible for enhanced presentation of psoriasis-related antigens.

Presentation of other antigens by HLA-C*06

Recently, Prinz and colleagues reported that ADAMTS-like protein 5, a fibrillin-like, heparin-binding protein specifically expressed by melanocytes, stimulates HLA-C*06-restricted psoriatic T-cell responses in psoriatic individuals [156]. While it is somewhat surprising that a melanocyte antigen might be responsible for keratinocyte hyperplasia, the restricted localization of melanocytes

to the epidermis provides a plausible explanation for the skin-targeting of immune responses in psoriasis.

Future genetic studies of psoriasis: Challenges and opportunities

While providing remarkable insights into disease pathogenesis, genetic studies of psoriasis (and other IMIDs) present several challenges. In addition to the modest odds ratios associated with most IMID susceptibility loci, ~80–90% of these genetic signals do not appear to encode deleterious changes in protein structure [165–171]. While the discovery that many genetic variants exert their effects at the level of gene regulation is very exciting, the most elegant feature of genetic analysis—the ability to work with genomic DNA from blood or other sources—is replaced by a more complex scenario which requires analysis of disease-relevant cell types in physiologic context. Besides uncertainty as to which cell types are disease-relevant, these signals may be emanating from only a small fraction of the cell types present in diseased tissue, and the pathogenic cell types are often hard to access experimentally in humans. Thus, the translation of disease-associated genetic variation into biologic effects requires strategic re-tooling of available resources, from genetics to genomics and epigenetics [138]. To address these challenges, several unique resources are available. Besides GWAS studies, microarray and RNA-seq based transcriptomes of normal vs psoriatic skin have revealed many expression quantitative trait loci (eQTL) [172], critical transcriptional networks [173, 174], and hundreds of novel long non-coding RNAs with immune-related functions [175]. Transcriptome data is also available for several relevant component cell types [176–179], and advanced data-mining tools have been developed for elucidation of the nature of non-coding genetic variation [180], for allele-specific read analysis [181], for skin disease classification [182], and for cross-population analysis of genetic associations [183] and eQTLs [184].

Deleterious protein changes are rare among GWAS variants in psoriasis [16, 103, 107] as well as other autoimmune diseases [165–170]. This fact demands that psoriasis genetic signals need to be interpreted in the context of regulatory variation. Any such analysis should ideally be focused on biologically relevant cell types, and at the same time account for the topological complexity of chromatin, with enhancers and promoters often mapping many kilobases away from each other due to chromatin looping [185, 186]. While the epigenome is clearly influenced by cell physiology [187] and environmental factors [188], it also reflects the effects of genetic variation [141, 189]. Thus, if we are to understand the true nature of disease-associated genetic variation, it is essential to understand the chromatin landscape of relevant cells and tissues, and to integrate the landscapes of chromatin structure and gene regulation with respect to genetic variation. This approach is very promising, as eQTLs often co-localize with accessible chromatin [141, 189]. In the case of psoriasis, skin-homing T-cells and myeloid dendritic cells are attractive targets for analysis, as they can be obtained from blood, and appear to mediate many aspects of psoriasis pathogenesis. ATAC-seq (Assay of Transposase-Accessible Chromatin combined with sequencing) is a recently-developed tool for probing chromatin structure [190]. While a number of different assays for open chromatin are available [78], ATAC-seq is particularly well-suited for this purpose because it can be performed on as few as 50,000 cells per sample, which is in the range of skin-homing CD4+

and CD8+ T-cells that can be obtained from ~100 ml of blood. By carrying out ATAC-seq on these cell types in 100–200 individuals, while assessing the transcriptomes in parallel using RNA-seq, it should be possible to assess how psoriasis-associated genetic variations affect chromatin structure for most common variants (i.e. MAF >5%).

Summary

In this chapter, we have presented a large body of information on psoriasis genetics. The major conclusion is that psoriasis is an immune-mediated disease in which innate and adaptive host defence responses are modified by genetic factors that not only modulate the overall risk of psoriasis, but also dictate whether the disease affects the skin and/or the joints. We apologize that it has not been possible to cite all of the many excellent studies that have contributed to this vibrant field.

References

1. Gudjonsson JE, Elder JT. Psoriasis. In: Goldsmith L, Katz SI, Gilchrest BA, Paller AS, Woolf K, Leffell DJ, editors. Dermatology in General Medicine. 1. 8th ed. New York: McGraw-Hill; 2012. p. 197–231.

2. Kim J, Krueger JG. The immunopathogenesis of psoriasis. Dermatologic clinics. 2015;33(1):13–23. PubMed PMID: 25412780.

3. Brezinski EA, Dhillon JS, Armstrong AW. Economic burden of psoriasis in the United States: A Systematic Review. JAMA Dermatol. 2015;151(6):651–8. PubMed PMID: 25565304.

4. Krueger GG, Bergstresser PR, Lowe NJ, Voorhees JJ, Weinstein GD. Psoriasis. J Am Acad Dermatol. 1984;11(5 Pt 2):937–47.

5. Gupta MA, Schork NJ, Gupta AK, Kirkby S, Ellis CN. Suicidal ideation in psoriasis. Int J Dermatol. 1993;32(3):188–90.

6. Raychaudhuri SP, Farber EM. The prevalence of psoriasis in the world. J Eur Acad Dermatol Venereol. 2001;15(1):16–7. PubMed PMID: 11451313.

7. Schafer T. Epidemiology of psoriasis. Review and the German perspective. Dermatology. 2006;212(4):327–37. PubMed PMID: 16707882.

8. Naldi L. Epidemiology of psoriasis. Curr Drug Targets Inflamm Allergy. 2004;3(2):121–8. PubMed PMID: 15180464.

9. Bell LM, Sedlack R, Beard CM, Perry HO, Michet CJ, Kurland LT. Incidence of psoriasis in Rochester, Minn, 1980–3. Arch Dermatol. 1991;127(8):1184–7. PubMed PMID: 1863076.

10. Eder L, Haddad A, Rosen CF, et al. The incidence and risk factors for psoriatic arthritis in patients with psoriasis—a prospective cohort study. Arthritis Rheumatol. 2015 Nov 10. PubMed PMID: 26555117.

11. Ogdie A, Langan S, Love T, Haynes K, Shin D, Seminara N, et al. Prevalence and treatment patterns of psoriatic arthritis in the UK. Rheumatology (Oxford). 2013;52(3):568–75. PubMed PMID: 23221331. Pubmed Central PMCID: PMC3573270.

12. Gelfand JM, Gladman DD, Mease PJ, Smith N, Margolis DJ, Nijsten T, et al. Epidemiology of psoriatic arthritis in the population of the United States. J Am Acad Dermatol. 2005;53(4):573. PubMed PMID: 16198775.

13. Asgari MM, Wu JJ, Gelfand JM, Salman C, Curtis JR, Harrold LR, et al. Validity of diagnostic codes and prevalence of psoriasis and psoriatic arthritis in a managed care population, 1996–2009. Pharmacoepidemiol Drug Saf. 2013;22(8):842–9. PubMed PMID: 23637091. Pubmed Central PMCID: PMC3720770.

14. Gladman DD. Natural history of psoriatic arthritis. Baillieres Clin Rheumatol. 1994;8(2):379–94.

15. Lonnberg AS, Skov L, Duffy DL, et al. Genetic factors explain variation in the age at onset of psoriasis: A population-based twin study. Acta Derm Venereol. 2015; 96(1):35-8. PubMed PMID: 26073043.

16. Stuart PE, Nair RP, Tsoi LC, et al. Genome-wide association analysis of psoriatic arthritis and cutaneous psoriasis reveals differences in their genetic architecture. Am J Hum Genet. 2015;97(6):816–36. PubMed PMID: 26626624.

17. Rahman P, Elder JT. Genetic epidemiology of psoriasis and psoriatic arthritis. Ann Rheum Dis. 2005;64 Suppl 2:ii37–9; discussion ii40–1. PubMed PMID: 15708933.

18. Elder JT, Nair RP, Guo SW, Henseler T, Christophers E, Voorhees JJ. The genetics of psoriasis. Arch Dermatol. 1994;130(2):216–24.

19. Lonnberg AS, Skov L, Skytthe A, Kyvik KO, Pedersen OB, Thomsen SF. Heritability of psoriasis in a large twin sample. Br J Dermatol. 2013;169(2):412–6. PubMed PMID: 23574549.

20. Pedersen OB, Svendsen AJ, Ejstrup L, Skytthe A, Junker P. On the heritability of psoriatic arthritis. Disease concordance among monozygotic and dizygotic twins. Ann Rheum Dis. 2008;67(10):1417–21. PubMed PMID: 18218666.

21. Ananthakrishnan R, Eckes L, Walter H. On the genetics of psoriasis. An analysis of Hellgren's data for a model of multifactorial inheritance. Arch Dermatol Forsch. 1973;247(1):53–8.

22. Ananthakrishnan R, Eckes L, Walter H. On the genetics of psoriasis: An analysis of Lomholt's data from Faroe Islands for a multifactorial mode of inheritance. J Genet (Orissa). 1974;61:142–50.

23. Brandrup F, Green A, Holm N. [Occurrence of psoriasis in Denmark]. Ugeskr Laeger. 1982 Nov 22;144(47):3538–41. PubMed PMID: 7168048. Praevalensen af psoriasis i Danmark.

24. Duffy DL, Spelman LS, Martin NG. Psoriasis in Australian twins. J Am Acad Dermatol. 1993;29(3):428–34.

25. Grjibovski AM, Olsen AO, Magnus P, Harris JR. Psoriasis in Norwegian twins: contribution of genetic and environmental effects. J Eur Acad Dermatol Venereol. 2007;21(10):1337–43. PubMed PMID: 17958839.

26. Moll JM, Wright V, O'Neill T, Silman AJ. Familial occurrence of psoriatic arthritis. Ann Rheum Dis. 1973;32(3):181–201.

27. Myers A, Kay LJ, Lynch SA, Walker DJ. Recurrence risk for psoriasis and psoriatic arthritis within sibships. Rheumatology (Oxford). 2005;44(6):773–6. PubMed PMID: 15757963.

28. Chandran V, Schentag CT, Brockbank JE, Pellett FJ, Shanmugarajah S, Toloza SM, et al. Familial aggregation of psoriatic arthritis. Ann Rheum Dis. 2009;68(5):664–7. PubMed PMID: 18524791.

29. Karason A, Love TJ, Gudbjornsson B. A strong heritability of psoriatic arthritis over four generations--the Reykjavik Psoriatic Arthritis Study. Rheumatology (Oxford). 2009;48(11):1424–8. PubMed PMID: 19741010.

30. Trowsdale J, Knight JC. Major histocompatibility complex genomics and human disease. Annu Rev Genomics Hum Genet. 2013;14:301–23. PubMed PMID: 23875801.

31. Erlich HA, Opelz G, Hansen J. HLA DNA typing and transplantation. Immunity. 2001;14(4):347–56. PubMed PMID: 11336680.

32. de Bakker PI, Raychaudhuri S. Interrogating the major histocompatibility complex with high-throughput genomics. Hum Mol Genet. 2012;21(R1):R29–36. PubMed PMID: 22976473. Pubmed Central PMCID: PMC3459647.

33. Hosomichi K, Shiina T, Tajima A, Inoue I. The impact of next-generation sequencing technologies on HLA research. J Hum Genet. 2015;60(11):665–73. PubMed PMID: 26311539. Pubmed Central PMCID: PMC4660052.

34. Russell TJ, Schultes LM, Kuban DJ. Histocompatibility (HL-A) antigens associated with psoriasis. N Engl J Med. 1972;287(15):738–40.

35. Henseler T, Christophers E. Psoriasis of early and late onset: characterization of two types of psoriasis vulgaris. J Am Acad Dermatol. 1985;13(3):450–6.

36. Fan X, Yang S, Sun LD, et al. Comparison of clinical features of HLA-Cw*0602-positive and -negative psoriasis patients in a Han Chinese population. Acta Derm Venereol. 2007;87(4):335–40. PubMed PMID: 17598037.

37. Fan X, Yang S, Huang W, et al. Fine mapping of the psoriasis susceptibility locus PSORS1 supports HLA-C as the susceptibility

gene in the Han Chinese population. PLoS Genet. 2008;4(3):e1000038. PubMed PMID: 18369457.

38. Gladman DD, Cheung C, Ng CM, Wade JA. HLA-C locus alleles in patients with psoriatic arthritis (PsA). Hum Immunol. 1999;60(3):259–61.

39. Al-Heresh AM, Proctor J, Jones SM, et al. Tumour necrosis factor-alpha polymorphism and the HLA-Cw*0602 allele in psoriatic arthritis. Rheumatology (Oxford). 2002;41(5):525–30.

40. Ho PY, Barton A, Worthington J, Thomson W, Silman AJ, Bruce IN. HLA-Cw6 and HLA-DRB1*07 together are associated with less severe joint disease in psoriatic arthritis. Ann Rheum Dis. 2007;66(6):807–11. PubMed PMID: 17223660.

41. Murray C, Mann DL, Gerber LN, et al. Histocompatibility alloantigens in psoriasis and psoriatic arthritis. Evidence for the influence of multiple genes in the major histocompatibility complex. J Clin Invest. 1980;66(4):670–5.

42. Gladman DD, Anhorn KA, Schachter RK, Mervart H. HLA antigens in psoriatic arthritis. J Rheumatol. 1986;13(3):586–92.

43. Winchester R, Minevich G, Steshenko V, et al. HLA associations reveal genetic heterogeneity in psoriatic arthritis and in the psoriasis phenotype. Arthritis and rheumatism. 2011 Oct 17. PubMed PMID: 22006066.

44. Eder L, Chandran V, Pellet F, et al. Human leucocyte antigen risk alleles for psoriatic arthritis among patients with psoriasis. Ann Rheum Dis. 2011;71(1):50–5 PubMed PMID: 21900282.

45. Armstrong RD, Panayi GS, Welsh KI. Histocompatibility antigens in psoriasis, psoriatic arthropathy, and ankylosing spondylitis. Ann Rheum Dis. 1983;42(2):142–6.

46. Beaulieu AD, Roy R, Mathon G, et al. Psoriatic arthritis: risk factors for patients with psoriasis—a study based on histocompatibility antigen frequencies. J Rheumatol. 1983;10(4):633–6.

47. McHugh NJ, Laurent MR, Treadwell BL, Tweed JM, Dagger J. Psoriatic arthritis: clinical subgroups and histocompatibility antigens. Ann Rheum Dis. 1987;46(3):184–8.

48. Muto M, Nagai K, Mogami S, Nakano J, Sasazuki T, Asagami C. HLA antigens in Japanese patients with psoriatic arthritis. Tissue Antigens. 1995;45(5):362–4.

49. Queiro R, Torre JC, Gonzalez S, et al. HLA antigens may influence the age of onset of psoriasis and psoriatic arthritis. J Rheumatol. 2003;30(3):505–7.

50. Espinoza LR, Vasey FB, Gaylord SW, et al. Histocompatibility typing in the seronegative spondyloarthropathies: a survey. Semin Arthritis Rheum. 1982;11(3):375–81.

51. Crivellato E, Zacchi T. HLA-B39 and the axial type of psoriatic arthritis. Acta Derm Venereol. 1987;67(3):249–50.

52. Trabace S, Cappellacci S, Ciccarone P, Liaskos S, Polito R, Zorzin L. Psoriatic arthritis: a clinical, radiological and genetic study of 58 Italian patients. Acta Derm Venereol Suppl (Stockh). 1994;186:69–70.

53. Hohler T, Weinmann A, Schneider PM, et al. TAP-polymorphisms in juvenile onset psoriasis and psoriatic arthritis. Hum Immunol. 1996;51(1):49–54.

54. Gonzalez S, Brautbar C, Martinez-Borra J, et al. Polymorphism in MICA rather than HLA-B/C genes is associated with psoriatic arthritis in the Jewish population. Hum Immunol. 2001;62(6):632–8.

55. Gonzalez S, Martinez-Borra J, Lopez-Vazquez A, Garcia-Fernandez S, Torre-Alonso JC, Lopez-Larrea C. MICA rather than MICB, TNFA, or HLA-DRB1 is associated with susceptibility to psoriatic arthritis. J Rheumatol. 2002;29(5):973–8.

56. Bravo MJ, Colmenero Jde D, Alonso A, Caballero A. HLA-B*39 allele confers susceptibility to osteoarticular complications in human brucellosis. J Rheumatol. 2003;30(5):1051–3.

57. Jenisch S, Henseler T, Nair RP, et al. Linkage analysis of HLA markers in familial psoriasis: strong disequilibrium effects provide evidence for a major determinant in the HLA-B/ -C region. American journal of human genetics. 1998;63(1):191–9.

58. Degli-Esposti MA, Leaver AL, Christiansen FT, Witt CS, Abraham LJ, Dawkins RL. Ancestral haplotypes: conserved population MHC haplotypes. Hum Immunol. 1992;34(4):242–52.

59. Schmitt-Egenolf M, Eiermann TH, Boehncke WH, Ständer M, Sterry W. Familial juvenile onset psoriasis is associated with the human leukocyte antigen (HLA) class I side of the extended haplotype Cw6- B57-DRB1*0701-DQA1*0201-DQB1*0303: a population- and family-based study. J Invest Dermatol. 1996;106(4):711–4.

60. Nair RP, Stuart P, Henseler T, et al. Localization of psoriasis-susceptibility locus PSORS1 to a 60-kb interval telomeric to HLA-C. Am J Hum Genet. 2000;66(6):1833–44. PubMed PMID: 10801386. Pubmed Central PMCID: 1378062.

61. Nair RP, Stuart PE, Nistor I, et al. Sequence and haplotype analysis supports HLA-C as the psoriasis susceptibility 1 gene. Am J Hum Genet. 2006;78(5):827–51. PubMed PMID: 16642438. Pubmed Central PMCID: 1474031.

62. Vejbaesya S, Eiermann TH, Suthipinititharm P, et al. Serological and molecular analysis of HLA class I and II alleles in Thai patients with psoriasis vulgaris. Tissue Antigens. 1998;52(4):389–92.

63. Choonhakarn C, Romphruk A, Puapairoj C, Jirarattanapochai K, Leelayuwat C. Haplotype associations of the major histocompatibility complex with psoriasis in Northeastern Thais. Int J Dermatol. 2002;41(6):330–4.

64. Nakagawa H, Asahina A, Akazaki S, et al. Association of Cw11 in Japanese patients with psoriasis vulgaris. Tissue Antigens. 1990;36(5):241–2.

65. Koizumi H, Fukaya T, Tsukinaga I, Ohkawara A, Wakisaka A, Aizawa M. HLA antigens in psoriasis vulgaris. Acta Dermatol Kyoto. 1988;83:483–8.

66. Ozawa A, Miyahara M, Sugai J, Iizuka M, Kawakubo Y, et al. HLA class I and II alleles and susceptibility to generalized pustular psoriasis: significant associations with HLA-Cw1 and HLA-DQB1*0303. J Dermatol. 1998;25(9):573–81.

67. Stuart PE, Nair RP, Hiremagalore R, Kullavanijaya P, Tejasvi T, et al. Comparison of MHC class I risk haplotypes in Thai and Caucasian psoriatics shows locus heterogeneity at PSORS1. Tissue Antigens. 2010;76(5):387–97. PubMed PMID: 20604894. Pubmed Central PMCID: PMC2970686.

68. Barber LD, Percival L, Valiante NM, et al. The inter-locus recombinant HLA-B*4601 has high selectivity in peptide binding and functions characteristic of HLA-C. J Exp Med. 1996;184(2):735–40.

69. Trembath RC, Clough RL, Rosbotham JL, et al. Identification of a major susceptibility locus on chromosome 6p and evidence for further disease loci revealed by a two stage genome-wide search in psoriasis. Hum Mol Genet. 1997;6(5):813–20.

70. Veal CD, Capon F, Allen MH, et al. Family-based analysis using a dense single-nucleotide polymorphism-based map defines genetic variation at PSORS1, the major psoriasis-susceptibility locus. Am J Hum Genet. 2002;71(3):554–64.

71. Sagoo GS, Tazi-Ahnini R, Barker JW, et al. Meta-analysis of genome-wide studies of psoriasis susceptibility reveals linkage to chromosomes 6p21 and 4q28-q31 in Caucasian and Chinese Hans population. J Invest Dermatol. 2004;122(6):1401–5.

72. Sagoo GS, Cork MJ, Patel R, Tazi-Ahnini R. Genome-wide studies of psoriasis susceptibility loci: a review. J Dermatol Sci. 2004;35(3):171–9. PubMed PMID: 15381238.

73. Karason A, Gudjonsson JE, Jonsson HH, et al. Genetics of psoriasis in Iceland: evidence for linkage of subphenotypes to distinct Loci. J Invest Dermatol. 2005;124(6):1177–85. PubMed PMID: 15955092.

74. Tomfohrde J, Silverman A, Barnes R, Fernandez-Vina MA, et al. Gene for familial psoriasis susceptibility mapped to the distal end of human chromosome 17q. Science. 1994;264(5162):1141–5. PubMed PMID: 8178173.

75. Capon F, Semprini S, Dallapiccola B, Novelli G. Evidence for interaction between psoriasis-susceptibility loci on chromosomes 6p21 and 1q21 [letter]. Am J Hum Genet. 1999;65(6):1798–800.

76. Veal CD, Clough RL, Barber RC, et al. Identification of a novel psoriasis susceptibility locus at 1p and evidence of epistasis between PSORS1 and candidate loci. J Med Genet. 2001;38(1):7–13.

77. Lee YA, Ruschendorf F, Windemuth C, et al. Genomewide scan in german families reveals evidence for a novel psoriasis-susceptibility locus on chromosome 19p13. Am J Hum Genet. 2000;67(4):1020–4.

78. Shendure J, Lieberman Aiden E. The expanding scope of DNA sequencing. Nat Biotechnol. 2012;30(11):1084–94. PubMed PMID: 23138308. Pubmed Central PMCID: PMC4149750.

79. Hwu WL, Yang CF, Fann CS, et al. Mapping of psoriasis to 17q terminus. J Med Genet. 2005;42(2):152–8. PubMed PMID: 15689454.

80. Birnbaum RY, Zvulunov A, Hallel-Halevy D, et al. Seborrhea-like dermatitis with psoriasiform elements caused by a mutation in ZNF750, encoding a putative C2H2 zinc finger protein. Nat Genet. 2006;38(7):749–51. PubMed PMID: 16751772.

81. Jordan CT, Cao L, Roberson ED, et al. PSORS2 is due to mutations in CARD14. Am J Hum Genet. 2012 May 4;90(5):784–95. PubMed PMID: 22521418. Pubmed Central PMCID: PMC3376640.

82. Fuchs-Telem D, Sarig O, van Steensel MA, et al. Familial pityriasis rubra pilaris is caused by mutations in CARD14. Am J Hum Genet. 2012 Jul 13;91(1):163–70. PubMed PMID: 22703878. Pubmed Central PMCID: 3397268.

83. Setta-Kaffetzi N, Simpson MA, Navarini AA, et al. AP1S3 mutations are associated with pustular psoriasis and impaired Toll-like receptor 3 trafficking. Am J Hum Genet. 20141;94(5):790–7. PubMed PMID: 24791904. Pubmed Central PMCID: 4067562.

84. Marrakchi S, Guigue P, Renshaw BR, et al. Interleukin-36-receptor antagonist deficiency and generalized pustular psoriasis. N Engl J Med. 2011;365(7):620–8. PubMed PMID: 21848462.

85. Onoufriadis A, Simpson MA, Pink AE, et al. Mutations in IL36RN/IL1F5 Are Associated with the severe episodic inflammatory skin disease known as generalized pustular psoriasis. Am J Hum Genet. 2011;89(3):432–7. PubMed PMID: 21839423.

86. Setta-Kaffetzi N, Navarini AA, Patel VM, et al. Rare pathogenic variants in IL36RN underlie a spectrum of psoriasis-associated pustular phenotypes. J Invest Dermatol. 2013;133(5):1366–9. PubMed PMID: 23303454.

87. Gonzalez-Navajas JM, Lee J, David M, Raz E. Immunomodulatory functions of type I interferons. Nat Rev Immunol. 2012;12(2):125–35. PubMed PMID: 22222875. Pubmed Central PMCID: PMC3727154.

88. Aksentijevich I, Kastner DL. Genetics of monogenic autoinflammatory diseases: past successes, future challenges. Nat Rev Rheumatol. 2011;7(8):469–78. PubMed PMID: 21727933.

89. Viguier M, Guigue P, Pages C, Smahi A, Bachelez H. Successful treatment of generalized pustular psoriasis with the interleukin-1-receptor antagonist Anakinra: lack of correlation with IL1RN mutations. Ann Intern Med. 2010;153(1):66–7. PubMed PMID: 20621920.

90. Huffmeier U, Watzold M, Mohr J, Schon MP, Mossner R. Successful therapy with anakinra in a patient with generalized pustular psoriasis carrying IL36RN mutations. Br J Dermatol. 2014;170(1):202–4. PubMed PMID: 23909475.

91. Risch N, Merikangas K. The future of genetic studies of complex human diseases. Science. 1996;273(5281):1516–7.

92. Welter D, MacArthur J, Morales J, et al. The NHGRI GWAS Catalog, a curated resource of SNP-trait associations. Nucleic Acids Res. 2014;42(Database issue):D1001–6. PubMed PMID: 24316577. Pubmed Central PMCID: 3965119.

93. Jannot AS, Ehret G, Perneger T. P < 5 x 10–8 has emerged as a standard of statistical significance for genome-wide association studies. J Clin Epidemiol. 2015;68(4):460–5. PubMed PMID: 25666886.

94. Sham PC, Purcell SM. Statistical power and significance testing in large-scale genetic studies. Nat Rev Genet. 2014;15(5):335–46. PubMed PMID: 24739678.

95. Ozawa A, Ohkido M, Inoko H, Ando A, Tsuji K. Specific restriction fragment length polymorphism on the HLA-C region and susceptibility to psoriasis vulgaris. J Invest Dermatol. 1988;90(3):402–5.

96. Kim TG, Lee HJ, Youn JI, Kim TY, Han H. The association of psoriasis with human leukocyte antigens in Korean population and the influence of age of onset and sex. J Invest Dermatol. 2000;114(2):309–13.

97. Shaiq PA, Stuart PE, Latif A, Schmotzer C, Kazmi AH, Khan MS, et al. Genetic associations of psoriasis in a Pakistani population. Br J Dermatol. 2013;169(2):406–11. PubMed PMID: 23495851. Pubmed Central PMCID: 3731395.

98. Munir S, ber Rahman S, Rehman S, et al. Association analysis of GWAS and candidate gene loci in a Pakistani population with psoriasis. Mol Immunol. 2015;64(1):190–4. PubMed PMID: 25481369.

99. Umapathy S, Pawar A, Mitra R, et al. Hla-a and Hla-B alleles associated in psoriasis patients from Mumbai, Western India. Indian J Dermatol. 2011;56(5):497–500. PubMed PMID: 22121262. Pubmed Central PMCID: 3221207.

100. Indhumathi S, Rajappa M, Chandrashekar L, Ananthanarayanan PH, Thappa DM, Negi VS. The HLA-C*06 allele as a possible genetic predisposing factor to psoriasis in South Indian Tamils. Archives of dermatological research. 2016;308(3):193–9. PubMed PMID: 26796545.

101. Chandra A, Lahiri A, Senapati S, et al. Increased risk of psoriasis due to combined effect of HLA-Cw6 and LCE3 risk alleles in Indian population. Scientific Reports. 2016;6:24059. PubMed PMID: 27048876.

102. Zuo X, Sun L, Yin X, et al. Whole-exome SNP array identifies 15 new susceptibility loci for psoriasis. Nat Commun. 2015;6:6793. PubMed PMID: 25854761. Pubmed Central PMCID: PMC4403312.

103. Tsoi LC, Stuart PE, Tian C, et al. Large scale meta-analysis characterizes genetic architecture for common psoriasis associated variants. Nat Commun. 2017 May 24;8:15382. PubMed PMID: 28537254. Pubmed Central PMCID: PMC5458077.

104. Huyghe JR, Jackson AU, Fogarty MP, et al. Exome array analysis identifies new loci and low-frequency variants influencing insulin processing and secretion. Nat Genet. 2013;45(2):197–201. PubMed PMID: 23263489. Pubmed Central PMCID: 3727235.

105. Cortes A, Brown MA. Promise and pitfalls of the Immunochip. Arthritis Res Ther. 2011 Feb 1;13(1):101. PubMed PMID: 21345260.

106. Tsoi LC, Spain SL, Ellinghaus E, et al. Enhanced meta-analysis and replication studies identify five new psoriasis susceptibility loci. Nat Commun. 2015;6:7001. PubMed PMID: 25939698. Pubmed Central PMCID: 4422106.

107. Tsoi LC, Spain SL, Knight J, et al. Identification of 15 new psoriasis susceptibility loci highlights the role of innate immunity. Nat Genet. 2012 Nov 11;44(12):1341–8. PubMed PMID: 23143594. Pubmed Central PMCID: PMC3510312.

108. Yin X, Low HQ, Wang L, Li Y, et al. Genome-wide meta-analysis identifies multiple novel associations and ethnic heterogeneity of psoriasis susceptibility. Nat Commun. 2015;6:6916. PubMed PMID: 25903422.

109. Woodrow JC, Ilchysyn A. HLA antigens in psoriasis and psoriatic arthritis. Journal of medical genetics. 1985;22(6):492–5. PubMed PMID: 3866077. Pubmed Central PMCID: 1049511.

110. Lascorz J, Burkhardt H, Huffmeier U, et al. Lack of genetic association of the three more common polymorphisms of CARD15 with psoriatic arthritis and psoriasis in a German cohort. Ann Rheum Dis. 2005;64(6):951–4. PubMed PMID: 15539411.

111. Ho PY, Barton A, Worthington J, et al. Investigating the role of the HLA-Cw*06 and HLA-DRB1 genes in susceptibility to psoriatic arthritis: comparison with psoriasis and undifferentiated inflammatory arthritis. Ann Rheum Dis. 2008;67(5):677–82. PubMed PMID: 17728335. Pubmed Central PMCID: 2563264.

112. Nair RP, Duffin KC, Helms C, et al. Genome-wide scan reveals association of psoriasis with IL-23 and NF-kappaB pathways. Nat Genet. 2009;41(2):199–204. PubMed PMID: 19169254. Pubmed Central PMCID: PMC2745122.

113. Julia A, Tortosa R, Hernanz JM, et al. Risk variants for psoriasis vulgaris in a large case-control collection and association with clinical subphenotypes. Hum Mol Genet. 2012 Oct 15;21(20):4549–57. PubMed PMID: 22814393.

114. Okada Y, Han B, Tsoi LC, et al. Fine mapping major histocompatibility complex associations in psoriasis and its clinical subtypes. Am J Hum Genet. 2014;95(2):162–72. PubMed PMID: 25087609. Pubmed Central PMCID: 4129407.

115. Bowes J, Budu-Aggrey A, Huffmeier U, et al. Dense genotyping of immune-related susceptibility loci reveals new insights into the genetics of psoriatic arthritis. Nat Commun. 2015;6:6046. PubMed PMID: 25651891. Pubmed Central PMCID: 4327416.

116. Bowes J, Loehr S, Budu-Aggrey A, et al. PTPN22 is associated with susceptibility to psoriatic arthritis but not psoriasis: evidence for a further PsA-specific risk locus. Ann Rheum Dis. 2015;74(10):1882–5. PubMed PMID: 25923216. Pubmed Central PMCID: PMC4602265.

117. Yang Q, Liu H, Qu L, et al. Investigation of 20 non-HLA (human leucocyte antigen) psoriasis susceptibility loci in Chinese patients with psoriatic arthritis and psoriasis vulgaris. Br J Dermatol. 2013;168(5):1060–5. PubMed PMID: 23252691.

118. Stuart PE, Nair RP, Ellinghaus E, et al. Genome-wide association analysis identifies three psoriasis susceptibility loci. Nat Genet. 2010;42(11):1000–4. PubMed PMID: 20953189. Pubmed Central PMCID: PMC2965799.

119. Soto-Sanchez J, Santos-Juanes J, Coto-Segura P, et al. Genetic variation at the CCR5/CCR2 gene cluster and risk of psoriasis and psoriatic arthritis. Cytokine. 2010;50(2):114–6. PubMed PMID: 20153665.

120. Callis Duffin K, Freeny IC, Schrodi SJ, et al. Association between IL13 polymorphisms and psoriatic arthritis is modified by smoking. J Invest Dermatol. 2009;129(12):2777–83. PubMed PMID: 19554022.

121. Bowes J, Eyre S, Flynn E, et al. Evidence to support IL-13 as a risk locus for psoriatic arthritis but not psoriasis vulgaris. Ann Rheum Dis. 2011;70(6):1016–9. PubMed PMID: 21349879. Pubmed Central PMCID: 3086035.

122. Eder L, Chandran V, Pellett F, et al. IL13 gene polymorphism is a marker for psoriatic arthritis among psoriasis patients. Ann Rheum Dis. 2011;70(9):1594–8. PubMed PMID: 21613309.

123. Chang YT, Chou CT, Yu CW, et al. Cytokine gene polymorphisms in Chinese patients with psoriasis. Br J Dermatol. 2007;156(5):899–905. PubMed PMID: 17388919.

124. Zhang XJ, Huang W, Yang S, et al. Psoriasis genome-wide association study identifies susceptibility variants within LCE gene cluster at 1q21. Nat Genet. 2009;41(2):205–10. PubMed PMID: 19169255.

125. Feng BJ, Sun LD, Soltani-Arabshahi R, et al. Multiple loci within the major histocompatibility complex confer risk of psoriasis. PLoS Genet. 2009;5(8):e1000606. PubMed PMID: 19680446. Pubmed Central PMCID: PMC2718700.

126. Knight J, Spain SL, Capon F, Hayday A, et al. Conditional analysis identifies three novel major histocompatibility complex loci associated with psoriasis. Hum Mol Genet. 2012 Dec 1;21(23):5185–92. PubMed PMID: 22914738. Pubmed Central PMCID: 3490509.

127. Das S, Stuart PE, Ding J, et al. Fine mapping of eight psoriasis susceptibility loci. Eur J Hum Genet. 2015;23(6):844–53. PubMed PMID: 25182136.

128. Tang H, Jin X, Li Y, Jiang H, et al. A large-scale screen for coding variants predisposing to psoriasis. Nat Genet. 2014;46(1):45–50. PubMed PMID: 24212883.

129. Strange A, Capon F, Spencer CC, et al. A genome-wide association study identifies new psoriasis susceptibility loci and an interaction between HLA-C and ERAP1. Nat Genet. 2010;42(11):985–90. PubMed PMID: 20953190.

130. Dand N, Mucha S, Tsoi LC, et al. Exome-wide association study reveals novel psoriasis susceptibility locus at TNFSF15 and rare protective alleles in genes contributing to type I IFN signalling. Hum Mol Genet. 2017;26(21):4301–13. PubMed PMID: 28973304.

131. de Cid R, Riveira-Munoz E, Zeeuwen PL, et al. Deletion of the late cornified envelope LCE3B and LCE3C genes as a susceptibility factor for psoriasis. Nat Genet. 2009;41(2):211–5. PubMed PMID: 19169253.

132. Riveira-Munoz E, He SM, Escaramis G, et al. Meta-analysis confirms the LCE3C_LCE3B deletion as a risk factor for psoriasis in several ethnic groups and finds interaction with HLA-Cw6. J Invest Dermatol. 2011 Nov 25. PubMed PMID: 21107349.

133. Zheng HF, Zuo XB, Lu WS et al. Variants in MHC, LCE and IL12B have epistatic effects on psoriasis risk in Chinese population. J Dermatol Sci 2011;61(2):124–8. PubMed PMID: 21208785.

134. Jostins L, Barrett JC. Genetic risk prediction in complex disease. Hum Mol Genet. 2011 Oct 15;20(R2):R182–8. PubMed PMID: 21873261.

135. Cretu D, Liang K, Saraon P, Batruch I, Diamandis EP, Chandran V. Quantitative tandem mass-spectrometry of skin tissue reveals putative psoriatic arthritis biomarkers. Clin Proteomics. 2015;12(1):1. PubMed PMID: 25678896. Pubmed Central PMCID: PMC4304122.

136. Cretu D, Prassas I, Saraon P, Batruch I, et al. Identification of psoriatic arthritis mediators in synovial fluid by quantitative mass spectrometry. Clin Proteomics. 2014;11(1):27. PubMed PMID: 25097465. Pubmed Central PMCID: PMC4108225.

137. Paek SY, Han L, Weiland M, et al. Emerging biomarkers in psoriatic arthritis. IUBMB Life. 2015;67(12):923–7. PubMed PMID: 26602058.

138. Edwards SL, Beesley J, French JD, Dunning AM. Beyond GWASs: illuminating the dark road from association to function. Am J Hum Genet. 2013 Nov 7;93(5):779–97. PubMed PMID: 24210251. Pubmed Central PMCID: 3824120.

139. Tsoi LC, Elder JT, Abecasis GR. Graphical algorithm for integration of genetic and biological data: proof of principle using psoriasis as a model. Bioinformatics. 2014; 31(8):1243-9. PubMed PMID: 25480373.

140. Weintraub H, Groudine M. Chromosomal subunits in active genes have an altered conformation. Science. 1976;193(4256):848–56.

141. Farh KK, Marson A, Zhu J, Kleinewietfeld M, Housley WJ, Beik S, et al. Genetic and epigenetic fine mapping of causal autoimmune disease variants. Nature. 2015;518(7539):337–43. PubMed PMID: 25363779. Pubmed Central PMCID: 4336207.

142. Nair RP, Ding J, Duffin KC, et al. Psoriasis bench to bedside: genetics meets immunology. Arch Dermatol. 2009;145(4):462–4. PubMed PMID: 19380669. Pubmed Central PMCID: PMC2739283.

143. Sun LD, Cheng H, Wang ZX, et al. Association analyses identify six new psoriasis susceptibility loci in the Chinese population. Nat Genet. 2010;42(11):1005–9. PubMed PMID: 20953187.

144. Shastri N, Cardinaud S, Schwab SR, Serwold T, Kunisawa J. All the peptides that fit: the beginning, the middle, and the end of the MHC class I antigen-processing pathway. Immunol Rev. 2005;207:31–41. PubMed PMID: 16181325.

145. Evans DM, Spencer CC, Pointon JJ, et al. Interaction between ERAP1 and HLA-B27 in ankylosing spondylitis implicates peptide handling in the mechanism for HLA-B27 in disease susceptibility. Nat Genet. 2011;43(8):761–7. PubMed PMID: 21743469.

146. Kirino Y, Bertsias G, Ishigatsubo Y, et al. Genome-wide association analysis identifies new susceptibility loci for Behcet's disease and epistasis between HLA-B*51 and ERAP1. Nat Genet. 2013;45(2):202–7. PubMed PMID: 23291587. Pubmed Central PMCID: PMC3810947.

147. Gudjonsson JE, Karason A, Antonsdottir AA, et al. HLA-Cw6-positive and HLA-Cw6-negative patients with Psoriasis vulgaris have distinct clinical features. J Invest Dermatol. 2002;118(2):362–5. PubMed PMID: 11841557.

148. Gudjonsson JE, Thorarinsson AM, Sigurgeirsson B, Kristinsson KG, Valdimarsson H. Streptococcal throat infections and exacerbation of chronic plaque psoriasis: a prospective study. Br J Dermatol. 2003;149(3):530–4. PubMed PMID: 14510985.

149. Calin A, Fries JF. An 'experimental' epidemic of Reiter's syndrome revisited. Follow-up evidence on genetic and environmental factors. Ann Intern Med. 1976;84(5):564–6.

150. Mallon E, Bunce M, Savoie H, et al. HLA-C and guttate psoriasis. Br J Dermatol. 2000;143(6):1177–82.

151. Diluvio L, Vollmer S, Besgen P, Ellwart JW, Chimenti S, Prinz JC. Identical TCR beta-chain rearrangements in streptococcal angina and skin lesions of patients with psoriasis vulgaris. J Immunol. 2006 Jun 1;176(11):7104–11. PubMed PMID: 16709873.

152. Thorleifsdottir RH, Sigurdardottir SL, Sigurgeirsson B, et al. Improvement of psoriasis after tonsillectomy is associated with a decrease in the frequency of circulating T cells that recognize streptococcal determinants and homologous skin determinants. J Immunol. 2012;188(10):5160–5. PubMed PMID: 22491250.

153. Besgen P, Trommler P, Vollmer S, Prinz JC. Ezrin, maspin, peroxiredoxin 2, and heat shock protein 27: potential targets of a streptococcal-induced autoimmune response in psoriasis. J Immunol. 2010;184(9):5392–402. PubMed PMID: 20363977.

154. Kulkarni S, Savan R, Qi Y, Gao X, Yuki Y, Bass SE, et al. Differential microRNA regulation of HLA-C expression and its association with HIV control. Nature. 2011;472(7344):495–8. PubMed PMID: 21499264. Pubmed Central PMCID: PMC3084326.

155. Clop A, Bertoni A, Spain SL, Simpson MA, Pullabhatla V, Tonda R, et al. An in-depth characterization of the major psoriasis susceptibility locus identifies candidate susceptibility alleles within an HLA-C enhancer element. PLoS One. 2013;8(8):e71690. PubMed PMID: 23990973. Pubmed Central PMCID: 3747202.

156. Arakawa A, Siewert K, Stohr J, Besgen P, Kim SM, Ruhl G, et al. Melanocyte antigen triggers autoimmunity in human psoriasis. J Exp Med. 2015;212(13):2203–12. PubMed PMID: 26621454.

157. Pollock R, Chandran V, Barrett J, et al. Differential major histocompatibility complex class I chain-related A allele associations with skin and joint manifestations of psoriatic disease. Tissue Antigens. 2011;77(6):554–61. PubMed PMID: 21457151.

158. Pollock RA, Chandran V, Pellett FJ, et al. The functional MICA-129 polymorphism is associated with skin but not joint manifestations of psoriatic disease independently of HLA-B and HLA-C. Tissue Antigens. 2013;82(1):43–7. PubMed PMID: 23611695.

159. Pollock RA, Pellett FJ, Chandran V, Gladman DD. Expression patterns of natural killer receptor genes in inflamed joints and peripheral blood of patients with psoriatic arthritis. Tissue Antigens. 2011;78(5):345–7. PubMed PMID: 21883096.

160. Winchester R, Minevich G, Steshenko V, et al. HLA associations reveal genetic heterogeneity in psoriatic arthritis and in the psoriasis phenotype. Arthritis Rheum. 2012;64(4):1134–44. PubMed PMID: 22006066.

161. FitzGerald O, Haroon M, Giles JT, Winchester R. Concepts of pathogenesis in psoriatic arthritis: genotype determines clinical phenotype. Arthritis Res Ther. 2015;17:115. PubMed PMID: 25948071. Pubmed Central PMCID: PMC4422545.

162. Barnas JL, Ritchlin CT. Etiology and pathogenesis of psoriatic arthritis. Rheum Dis Clin North Am. 2015;41(4):643–63. PubMed PMID: 26476224.

163. International_HIV_Controllers_Study, Pereyra F, Jia X, McLaren PJ, et al. The major genetic determinants of HIV-1 control affect HLA class I peptide presentation. Science. 2010;330(6010):1551–7. PubMed PMID: 21051598.

164. Raychaudhuri S, Sandor C, Stahl EA, et al. Five amino acids in three HLA proteins explain most of the association between MHC and seropositive rheumatoid arthritis. Nat Genet. 2012;44(3):291–6. PubMed PMID: 22286218. Pubmed Central PMCID: PMC3288335.

165. Okada Y, Wu D, Trynka G, et al. Genetics of rheumatoid arthritis contributes to biology and drug discovery. Nature. 2013;506(7488):376–81. PubMed PMID: 24390342.

166. International Multiple Sclerosis Genetics C, Beecham AH, Patsopoulos NA, Xifara DK, et al. Analysis of immune-related loci identifies 48 new susceptibility variants for multiple sclerosis. Nat Genet. 2013;45(11):1353–60. PubMed PMID: 24076602. Pubmed Central PMCID: 3832895.

167. Parkes M, Cortes A, van Heel DA, Brown MA. Genetic insights into common pathways and complex relationships among immune-mediated diseases. Nat Rev Genet. 2013;14(9):661–73. PubMed PMID: 23917628.

168. Trynka G, Hunt KA, Bockett NA, et al. Dense genotyping identifies and localizes multiple common and rare variant association signals in celiac disease. Nat Genet. 2011;43(12):1193–201. PubMed PMID: 22057235. Pubmed Central PMCID: PMC3242065.

169. Manku H, Langefeld CD, Guerra SG, et al. Trans-ancestral studies fine map the SLE-susceptibility locus TNFSF4. PLoS Genet. 2013;9(7):e1003554. PubMed PMID: 23874208. Pubmed Central PMCID: 3715547.

170. Liu JZ, Almarri MA, Gaffney DJ, et al. Dense fine-mapping study identifies new susceptibility loci for primary biliary cirrhosis. Nat Genet. 2012;44(10):1137–41. PubMed PMID: 22961000.

171. [No authors listed] Little boxes. Nat Genet. 2014 Jun 26;46(7):659. PubMed PMID: 24965724.

172. Ding J, Gudjonsson JE, Liang L, et al. Gene expression in skin and lymphoblastoid cells: Refined statistical method reveals extensive overlap in cis-eQTL signals. Am J Hum Genet. 2010;87(6):779–89. PubMed PMID: 21129726. Pubmed Central PMCID: PMC2997368.

173. Li B, Tsoi LC, Swindell WR, et al. Transcriptome analysis of psoriasis in a large case-control Sample: RNA-Seq rovides insights into disease mechanisms. J Invest Dermatol. 2014;134(7):1828–38. PubMed PMID: 24441097. Pubmed Central PMCID: 4057954.

174. Swindell WR, Johnston A, Xing X, Voorhees JJ, Elder JT, Gudjonsson JE. Modulation of epidermal transcription circuits in psoriasis: new links between inflammation and hyperproliferation. PLoS One. 2013;8(11):e79253. PubMed PMID: 24260178. Pubmed Central PMCID: 3829857.

175. Tsoi LC, Iyer MK, Stuart PE, et al. Analysis of long non-coding RNAs highlights tissue-specific expression patterns and epigenetic profiles in normal and psoriatic skin. Genome Biol. 2015;16:24. PubMed PMID: 25723451. Pubmed Central PMCID: 4311508.

176. Swindell WR, Johnston A, Voorhees JJ, Elder JT, Gudjonsson JE. Dissecting the psoriasis transcriptome: inflammatory- and cytokine-driven gene expression in lesions from 163 patients. BMC Genomics. 2013;14:527. PubMed PMID: 23915137. Pubmed Central PMCID: 3751090.

177. Swindell WR, Xing X, Stuart PE, et al. Heterogeneity of inflammatory and cytokine networks in chronic plaque psoriasis. PLoS One. 2012;7(3):e34594. PubMed PMID: 22479649. Pubmed Central PMCID: PMC3315545.

178. Swindell WR, Stuart PE, Sarkar MK, et al. Cellular dissection of psoriasis for transcriptome analyses and the post-GWAS era. BMC Med Genomics. 2014;7:27. PubMed PMID: 24885462. Pubmed Central PMCID: 4060870.

179. Swindell WR, Xing X, Voorhees JJ, Elder JT, Johnston A, Gudjonsson JE. Integrative RNA-seq and microarray data analysis reveals GC content and gene length biases in the psoriasis transcriptome. Physiol Genomics. 2014;46(15):533–46. PubMed PMID: 24844236. Pubmed Central PMCID: 4121624.

180. Flutre T, Wen X, Pritchard J, Stephens M. A statistical framework for joint eQTL analysis in multiple tissues. PLoS Genet. 2013;9(5):e1003486. PubMed PMID: 23671422. Pubmed Central PMCID: 3649995.

181. Harvey CT, Moyerbrailean GA, Davis GO, Wen X, Luca F, Pique-Regi R. QuASAR: quantitative allele-specific analysis of reads. Bioinformatics. 2014 Dec 4. PubMed PMID: 25480375.

182. Inkeles MS, Scumpia PO, Swindell WR, et al. Comparison of molecular signatures from multiple skin diseases identifies mechanisms of immunopathogenesis. J Invest Dermatol. 2015;135(1):151–9. PubMed PMID: 25111617. Pubmed Central PMCID: 4268388.

183. Wang C, Zhan X, Bragg-Gresham J, Kang HM, et al. Ancestry estimation and control of population stratification for sequence-based association studies. Nat Genet. 2014;46(4):409–15. PubMed PMID: 24633160. Pubmed Central PMCID: 4084909.

184. Wen X, Luca F, Pique-Regi R. Cross-population joint analysis of eQTLs: Fine mapping and functional annotation. PLoS Genet. 2015; 11(4):e1005176. PubMed PMID: 25906321. PMCID: PMC4408026.

185. Simonis M, Klous P, Splinter E, et al. Nuclear organization of active and inactive chromatin domains uncovered by chromosome conformation capture-on-chip (4C). Nat Genet. 2006;38(11):1348–54. PubMed PMID: 17033623.

186. Ghavi-Helm Y, Klein FA, Pakozdi T, et al. Enhancer loops appear stable during development and are associated with

paused polymerase. Nature. 2014; 512(7512):96–100. PubMed PMID: 25043061.

187. Chen Y, Mistry DS, Sen GL. Highly rapid and efficient conversion of human fibroblasts to keratinocyte-like cells. J Invest Dermatol. 2014;134(2):335–44. PubMed PMID: 23921950. Pubmed Central PMCID: 3875612.

188. Groudine M, Weintraub H. Propagation of globin DNAase I-hypersensitive sites in absence of factors required for induction: a possible mechanism for determination. Cell. 1982;30(1):131–9.

189. Degner JF, Pai AA, Pique-Regi R, et al. DNase I sensitivity QTLs are a major determinant of human expression variation. Nature. 2012;482(7385):390–4. PubMed PMID: 22307276. Pubmed Central PMCID: 3501342.

190. Buenrostro JD, Giresi PG, Zaba LC, Chang HY, Greenleaf WJ. Transposition of native chromatin for fast and sensitive epigenomic profiling of open chromatin, DNA-binding proteins and nucleosome position. Nat Methods. 2013;10(12):1213–8. PubMed PMID: 24097267. Pubmed Central PMCID: 3959825.

191. Cheng H, Li Y, Zuo XB, Tang HY, et al. Identification of a missense variant in LNPEP that confers psoriasis risk. J Invest Dermatol. 2014;134(2):359–65. PubMed PMID: 23897274.

192. Li Y, Cheng H, Zuo XB, et al. Association analyses identifying two common susceptibility loci shared by psoriasis and systemic lupus erythematosus in the Chinese Han population. J Med Genet. 2013;50(12):812–8. PubMed PMID: 24070858.

193. Apel M, Uebe S, Bowes J, Giardina E, et al. Variants in RUNX3 contribute to susceptibility to psoriatic arthritis, exhibiting further common ground with ankylosing spondylitis. Arthritis Rheum. 2013;65(5):1224–31. PubMed PMID: 23401011.

194. Wang CQ, Suarez-Farinas M, Nograles KE, et al. IL-17 induces inflammation-associated gene products in blood monocytes and treatment with ixekizumab reduces their expression in psoriasis patient blood. J Invest Dermatol. 2014;134(12):2990–3 PubMed PMID: 24999591.

195. Braun J, Frentsch M, Thiel A. Hobit and human effector T-cell differentiation: The beginning of a long journey. Eur J Immunol. 2015;45(10):2762–5. PubMed PMID: 26440905.

196. Tsoi LC, Stuart PE, Tian C, et al. Large-scale meta-analysis characterizes genetic architecture for common psoriasis-associated variants. Nat Commun. 2017;8:15382. PubMed PMID: 28537254.

197. Niehues H, van Vlijmen-Willems IM, Bergboer JG, et al. Late cornified envelope (LCE) proteins: Distinct expression patterns of LCE2 and LCE3 members suggest nonredundant roles in human epidermis and other epithelia. Br J Dermatol 2015; 174(4):795–802. PubMed PMID: 26556599.

198. Man SM, Karki R, Kanneganti TD. AIM2 inflammasome in infection, cancer and autoimmunity: role in DNA sensing, inflammation and innate immunity. Eur J Immunol. 2015;46(2):269–80. PubMed PMID: 26626159.

199. Cullen SP, Martin SJ. Fas and TRAIL 'death receptors' as initiators of inflammation: Implications for cancer. Semin Cell Dev Biol. 2015;39:26–34. PubMed PMID: 25655947.

200. Fitzgerald KA, McWhirter SM, Faia KL, et al. IKKepsilon and TBK1 are essential components of the IRF3 signaling pathway. Nat Immunol. 2003;4(5):491–6. PubMed PMID: 12692549.

201. Ellinghaus E, Stuart PE, Ellinghaus D, et al. Genome-wide meta-analysis of psoriatic arthritis identifies susceptibility locus at REL. J Invest Dermatol 2012;132(4):1133–40. PubMed PMID: 22170493. Pubmed Central PMCID: 3305829.

202. Grinberg-Bleyer Y, Dainichi T, Oh H, et al. Cutting edge: NF-kappaB p65 and c-Rel control epidermal development and immune homeostasis in the skin. J Immunol. 2015;194(6):2472–6. PubMed PMID: 25681334. Pubmed Central PMCID: PMC4355158.

203. Togayachi A, Kozono Y, Kuno A, et al. Beta3GnT2 (B3GNT2), a major polylactosamine synthase: analysis of B3GNT2-deficient mice. Methods Enzymol. 2010;479:185–204. PubMed PMID: 20816167.

204. Sheng Y, Jin X, Xu J, Gao J, et al. Sequencing-based approach identified three new susceptibility loci for psoriasis. Nat Commun. 2014;5:4331. PubMed PMID: 25006012.

205. Sonder SU, Saret S, Tang W, Sturdevant DE, Porcella SF, Siebenlist U. IL-17-induced NF-kappaB activation via CIKS/Act1: physiologic significance and signaling mechanisms. J Biol Chem. 2012;286(15):12881–90. PubMed PMID: 21335551. Pubmed Central PMCID: PMC3075635.

206. Rizzo JM, Oyelakin A, Min S, et al. DeltaNp63 regulates IL-33 and IL-31 signaling in atopic dermatitis. Cell Death Differ. 2016; 23(6):1073–85. PubMed PMID: 26768665.

207. Cargill M, Schrodi SJ, Chang M, et al. A large-scale genetic association study confirms IL12B and leads to the identification of IL23R as psoriasis-risk genes. Am J Hum Genet. 2007;80(2):273–90. PubMed PMID: 17236132.

208. Nair RP, Ruether A, Stuart PE, Jenisch S, et al. Polymorphisms of the IL12B and IL23R genes are associated with psoriasis. J Invest Dermatol. 2008;128(7):1653–61. PubMed PMID: 18219280. Pubmed Central PMCID: PMC2739284.

209. Huffmeier U, Uebe S, Ekici AB, et al. Common variants at TRAF3IP2 are associated with susceptibility to psoriatic arthritis and psoriasis. Nat Genet. 2010;42(11):996–9. PubMed PMID: 20953186. Pubmed Central PMCID: PMC2981079.

210. Ellinghaus E, Ellinghaus D, Stuart PE, et al. Genome-wide association study identifies a psoriasis susceptibility locus at TRAF3IP2. Nat Genet. 2010;42(11):991–5. PubMed PMID: 20953188.

211. Brenner W, Gschnait F, Mayr WR. HLA B13, B17, B37 and Cw6 in psoriasis vulgaris: association with the age of onset. Arch Dermatol Res 1978;28;262(3):337–9. PubMed PMID: 718258.

212. Gunn I, Leheny W, Lakshmipathi T, Lamont MA, Faed M. HLA antigens in a Scottish psoriatic population. Tissue Antigens. 1979;14(2):157–64.

213. Tiilikainen A, Lassus A, Karvonen J, Vartiainen P, Julin M. Psoriasis and HLA-Cw6. Br J Dermatol. 1980;102(2):179–84.

214. Ikaheimo I, Silvennoinen-Kassinen S, Karvonen J, Tiilikainen A. Alanine at position 73 of HLA-C is associated with psoriasis vulgaris in Finland. Br J Dermatol. 1994;131(2):257–9.

215. Enerback C, Martinsson T, Inerot A, et al. Evidence that HLA-Cw6 determines early onset of psoriasis, obtained using sequence-specific primers (PCR-SSP). Acta Derm Venereol. 1997;77(4):273–6.

216. Jenisch S, Henseler T, Nair RP, et al. Linkage analysis of human leukocyte antigen (HLA) markers in familial psoriasis: strong disequilibrium effects provide evidence for a major determinant in the HLA-B/-C region. Am J Hum Genet. 1998;63(1):191–9. PubMed PMID: 9634500.

217. Gonzalez S, Martinez-Borra J, Torre-Alonso JC, et al. The MICA-A9 triplet repeat polymorphism in the transmembrane region confers additional susceptibility to the development of psoriatic arthritis and is independent of the association of Cw*0602 in psoriasis. Arthritis Rheum. 1999;42(5):1010–6.

218. Luszczek W, Kubicka W, Cislo M, et al. Strong association of HLA-Cw6 allele with juvenile psoriasis in Polish patients. Immunol Lett. 2003;85(1):59–64.

219. Chang YT, Tsai SF, Lee DD, et al. A study of candidate genes for psoriasis near HLA-C in Chinese patients with psoriasis. Br J Dermatol. 2003;148(3):418–23.

220. Queiro R, Gonzalez S, Lopez-Larrea C, et al. HLA-C locus alleles may modulate the clinical expression of psoriatic arthritis. Arthritis Res Ther. 2006;8(6):R185. PubMed PMID: 17166285.

221. Reich K, Huffmeier U, Konig IR, et al. TNF polymorphisms in psoriasis: association of psoriatic arthritis with the promoter polymorphism TNF*-857 independent of the PSORS1 risk allele. Arthritis Rheum. 2007;56(6):2056–64. PubMed PMID: 17530646.

222. Liu Y, Helms C, Liao W, et al. A genome-wide association study of psoriasis and psoriatic arthritis identifies new disease loci. PLoS Genet. 2008;4(3):e1000041. PubMed PMID: 18369459.

223. Eder L, Chandran V, Pellett F, et al. Differential human leucocyte allele association between psoriasis and psoriatic arthritis: a family-based association study. Ann Rheum Dis. 2012;71(8):1361–5. PubMed PMID: 22586163.

224. Chandran V, Bull SB, Pellett FJ, Ayearst R, Rahman P, Gladman DD. Human leukocyte antigen alleles and susceptibility to psoriatic arthritis. Hum Immunol 2013;74(10):1333–8. PubMed PMID: 23916976.

225. Lau WL, Scholnick SB. Identification of two new members of the CSMD gene family. Genomics. 2003;82(3):412–5. PubMed PMID: 12906867.

226. Ellinghaus D, Ellinghaus E, Nair RP, et al. Combined analysis of genome-wide association studies for Crohn disease and psoriasis identifies seven shared susceptibility loci. Am J Hum Genet. 2012 Apr 6;90(4):636–47. PubMed PMID: 22482804. Pubmed Central PMCID: 3322238.

227. Hendriks J, Gravestein LA, Tesselaar K, van Lier RA, Schumacher TN, Borst J. CD27 is required for generation and long-term maintenance of T cell immunity. Nature Immunol 2000;1(5):433–40. PubMed PMID: 11062504.

228. Sawalha AH, Hughes T, Nadig A, et al. A putative functional variant within the UBAC2 gene is associated with increased risk of Behcet's disease. Arthritis and rheumatism. 2011;63(11):3607–12. PubMed PMID: 21918955. Pubmed Central PMCID: PMC3205238.

229. Scohy S, Gabant P, Van Reeth T, et al. Identification of KLF13 and KLF14 (SP6), novel members of the SP/XKLF transcription factor family. Genomics. 2000 Nov 15;70(1):93–101. PubMed PMID: 11087666.

230. Zhang W, Hong S, Maniar KP, Cheng S, et al. KLF13 regulates the differentiation-dependent human papillomavirus life cycle in keratinocytes through STAT5 and IL-8. Oncogene. 2016;35(42):5565–75. PubMed PMID: 27041562.

231. Li Y, Ma C, Zhou T, Liu Y, Sun L, Yu Z. TRIM65 negatively regulates p53 through ubiquitination. Biochem Biophys Res Commun. 2016;22:473(1):278–82. PubMed PMID: 27012201.

232. Soccio RE, Adams RM, Romanowski MJ, Sehayek E, Burley SK, Breslow JL. The cholesterol-regulated StarD4 gene encodes a StAR-related lipid transfer protein with two closely related homologues, StarD5 and StarD6. Proc Natl Acad Sci U S A. 2002 May 14;99(10):6943–8. PubMed PMID: 12011452. Pubmed Central PMCID: PMC124508.

233. Capon F, Bijlmakers MJ, Wolf N, et al. Identification of ZNF313/RNF114 as a novel psoriasis susceptibility gene. Hum Mol Genet. 2008;17(13):1938–45. PubMed PMID: 18364390.

CHAPTER 6

Genetics of psoriatic arthritis

Robert Winchester, Darren D. O'Rielly,
and Proton Rahman

Introduction

The overall psoriasis phenotype is clinically heterogeneous, consisting of the two major subtypes: cutaneous psoriasis (PsV) and psoriatic arthritis (PsA). Moreover, the clinical phenotype of PsA is itself heterogeneous, and some of the musculoskeletal phenotypic features of PsA are found in other spondyloarthritis diseases. This heterogeneity raises the question of whether it has a determinative genetic basis or is simply the product of chance differences. Genetic epidemiology studies have consistently demonstrated that PsA is characterized by a strong genetic component. We will articulate how these genetic studies give strong support to considering the psoriasis phenotype as genetically heterogeneous, and that PsA is genetically different from PsV without musculoskeletal involvement.

The pathogenesis of PsA embodies a complex interplay between genetic, immunological, and environmental factors. Accordingly, we will review the current genetic knowledge with respect to PsA pathogenesis. This will include the significant contribution from the major histocompatibility complex (MHC) region, which accounts for approximately one-third of the genetic contribution, as well as the more numerous newly discovered non-MHC loci identified from large international genome-wide association studies (GWAS) based on single-nucleotide polymorphisms (SNPs). These have revealed genes specific for PsA susceptibility as well as genes that encode proteins which share pathways with other closely related diseases, such as psoriasis. We will detail how the candidate genes achieving genome-wide significance in GWAS can be grouped into barrier integrity genes, innate immune response genes, and adaptive immune response genes, involving CD8 T-lymphocytes and Th-17 lymphocyte signalling. In particular, the prominent emerging role of the Th-17 signalling pathway in PsA pathogenesis will be highlighted.

Significant individual variability in drug efficacy and adverse events is well recognized and continues to be an ongoing challenge in managing patients with psoriatic disease; accordingly, we will discuss how the emergence of therapeutic agents that target specific molecular pathways has heightened the interest in identifying pharmacogenetic targets that will lead to personalized medicine. The delineation of this heterogeneity will likely have a major impact on the design of clinical trials and will be highly relevant to a personalized medicine approach to the patient with PsA, including more effective screening strategies and therapy.

The remarkable accumulation of knowledge gained in recent years from studies of PsA and its allied diseases is fundamentally changing our concept of the overall psoriasis phenotype and the spondylitis group of diseases in general, as well as our understanding of the genetics of PsA in particular. This knowledge includes: identification of many genes that contribute to the predisposition to develop PsA, especially using newer molecular genomic methods; the details of how these genes operate to cause inflammation; the relationship between genotype and the resulting clinical phenotype; the discovery of new therapeutic agents that more effectively act on the inflammatory processes, and how genetic variation can affect response to treatment in PsA; and advances in imaging technology to assess the extent and consequences of inflammation. Underlying these advances is the fundamental genetic paradigm: that the genes associated with susceptibility to develop PsA, not only serve to mark those who are likely to develop the disease, but that the particular product encoded by the susceptibility allele is importantly involved in the molecular mechanisms that result in the disease, and further that they contribute to the specific clinical phenotype the disease takes in that individual.

Although much knowledge has been gleaned from recent large-scale studies investigating the genetics of PsA, challenges still remain. Despite the number of genes identified in PsA, only a small fraction of the heritability is explained coining the term 'missing heritability'. We will discuss sources that are likely responsible for this phenomenon and provide a roadmap for future genetic investigations in PsA.

Genetic epidemiology of PsA

Population- and family-based studies demonstrate a strong familial basis to psoriatic disease, in keeping with clinical experience that PsV and PsA clearly segregate in families. From a clinician's perspective, it may appear that the more prevalent PsV is more heritable than PsA, but population-based genetic epidemiological studies demonstrate the opposite effect [1]. The strength of the genetic contribution, termed the recurrence rate, is estimated by calculating the relative proportion of disease in siblings (or other relatives) as compared with the prevalence of disease in the general population. The recurrence ratio was first reported in 1973, where prevalence of PsA in first degree relatives (i.e. 5.5%) vs the prevalence of PsA in a UK general population (i.e. 0.1%) [2], yielded a recurrence ratio of 55 as compared with a sibling recurrence ratio in PsV of 4 to 10. More recently, a Canadian study reported a PsA sibling recurrence risk of 30.8 [3] and an Icelandic reported a heritability of 39 [4]. Collectively, these studies consistently report a greater heritability for PsA compared with PsV.

Twin studies are an alternative, robust method to estimate heritability of a complex disease since higher concordance of psoriatic disease among monozygotic twins compared to dizygotic twins strongly implicates genetic factors. The only published and relatively small twin study in PsA reported a proband-wise concordance rate of 6/11 (i.e. 55%) in monozygotic twins and 6/28 (i.e. 21%) in dizygotic twins, consistent with the strong genetic contribution of PsA [5].

There is an excess of paternal transmission in PsA: the proportion of probands with an affected father (i.e. 0.65) was significantly greater than the expected proportion (i.e. 0.5) assuming no influence of sex on transmission [6]. This was confirmed in a larger study of 849 PsA probands where 57% of fathers and 43% of mothers were affected [7]. This suggests that PsA is characterized by genomic imprinting, an epigenetic effect that causes differential gene expression depending on the sex of the transmitting parent.

Genetics of PsA

The identification of the genes responsible for the increased heritability of PsA has been a lengthy preoccupation of many investigators. Progress was limited by the concept of the biologic nature of the disease, available technologies for gene determination, prevailing diagnostic criteria for PsA, and the size of the study population. Chapter 5 will review the detailed genetics of PsV; however, since the two diseases are interrelated clinically, and share similar immunopathology; we will compare the genetics of PsV and PsA. We will first focus on the genetics surrounding the major histocompatibility complex (MHC) and then the non-MHC genetics as they relate to PsA disease pathogenesis.

MHC genetics

With emerging evidence suggesting PsA might be an immune-mediated disease, the first candidate susceptibility genes to be examined were the highly polymorphic *HLA* genes that critically regulate the adaptive immune response through the binding and presentation of peptides to T cells. The studies of the association of PsA with certain *HLA* alleles began with Brewerton's identification in 1974 of a significantly increased frequency of *HLA-B*27* in individuals with PsA, especially in those with axial involvement [8]. Then HLA diversity was determined using serologic typing methods, which were arduous and much less precise than the current DNA-based methods. At about the same time, the dominant HLA allele associated with susceptibility to psoriasis was identified as *HLA-C*06:02*, as it is now designated, although in the period of serologic studies it was termed 'HLA-Cw6'. *HLA-C*06:02* is found in approximately 60% of PsV cases, see Chapter 5. As anticipated from the presence of psoriasis in PsA, PsA is also associated with *HLA-Cw6* as first reported by Murray et al. [9], where HLA-Cw6 was identified in 34.6% of PsA, 50% of PsV and 13.5% of controls.

However, in later studies the proportion of serologically defined *HLA-C*06:02* varied from 60% to 15–20%, the latter levels similar to its frequency in healthy controls; see [10] for a more detailed summary and analysis of the divergent results among these earlier reports. These pioneering studies on HLA were limited by imprecision of the serologic method of determining HLA alleles, the use of control populations not carefully ethnically matched to the patient population, and reliance on incompletely validated case definitions for PsA diagnosis.

Genetic heterogeneity within the overall psoriasis or psoriatic disease phenotype

The development of improved disease classification criteria and the newer methodology to directly determine the MHC allele by detailed sequence-based DNA typing, or by sequence-specific probe techniques allowed several groups to address the fundamental question of the homogeneity of the overall psoriatic disease phenotype and specifically the genetic relationship between PsV and PsA with very similar results [11, 12]. One such study based on the determination of HLA alleles by sequence-based DNA typing methods involved the assembly of a PsV cohort of patients with psoriasis presenting to a dermatology clinic, who were determined to be without features of arthritis, spondylitis, or enthesitis through examination by a rheumatologist. This cohort was compared with a PsA cohort, ascertained by CASPAR criteria, from the same relatively homogeneous Caucasian population presenting to a rheumatology clinic, in effect comparing the dermatologist's perspective of psoriasis to the rheumatologist's, and asking whether the two perspectives were equivalent in terms of their HLA alleles determined by sequence-based DNA typing methods [12]. *HLA-C*06:02*, the major susceptibility gene associated with PsV, was found in was 57.5% of the PsV cohort, but was only 28.7% in the PsA cohort ($P=9.94\times10^{-12}$). Consequently, the hypothesis of genetic homogeneity of the psoriasis phenotype and psoriatic disease was rejected. This implied that despite the overall similarity of the appearance of psoriasis in both PsA and PsV, these two major psoriatic disease subtypes, cutaneous psoriasis and PsA, do not entirely arise from the action of the same HLA genes. Although, since the control frequency of *HLA-C*06:02* is 19.7%, the frequency of this allele, 28.7% in PsA, is significantly increased OR=1.8(1.3–2.5) indicating that in this subset of PsA patients, susceptibility to the disease was associated with *HLA-C*06:02*, paralleling the association with PsV.

Genetic heterogeneity of psoriatic arthritis

The next challenge was to focus on PsA and determine whether there were other HLA alleles involved in determining PsA susceptibility. Four alleles of the *HLA-B* locus, *HLA-B*27:05:02*, 15.6% OR=2.6 (1.7–4.2); *HLA-B*39:01:01*, 6.4% OR=3.5(1.6-7.6); *HLA-B*38:01:01* and *HLA-B*08:01*, OR=1.6 (1.2–2.0) were each also significantly associated with PsA susceptibility compared with both controls and PsV, Table 6.1. Highly similar results were obtained by Eder et al. [11]. Intriguingly, the *HLA-B*39.06* allele, which differs by only a few amino acids from *HLA-B*39:01*, but has an ancestral haplotype containing a different *HLA-C* allele was not associated with PsA susceptibility, emphasizing the relatively precise molecular basis for susceptibility [5]. Unlike *HLA-C*06:02*, these alleles do not carry an elevated risk for PsV in the absence of arthritis, and in the case of *HLA-B*08:01*, it is significantly decreased in frequency in cutaneous psoriasis, suggesting a possible protective role in PsV development. Reflecting the genetic heterogeneity of PsA, the five different MHC alleles that denote individuals at risk for PsA each encode molecules with considerably different properties and are not associated with genes in common elsewhere on their haplotypes, other than the sharing of *HLA-C*12:03* by *HLA-B*39:01:01* and *HLA-B*38:01:01*.

These five PsA susceptibility alleles are almost exclusively present in seven classic ancestral haplotypes in individuals of Northern European ancestry (*HLA-B*08:01-C*07:01*, *HLA-B*27:05-C*02:02*, *HLA-B*27:05-C*01:02*, *HLA-B*37:01-C*06:02*, *HLA-B*57:01-C*06:02*, *HLA-B*39:01-C*12:03* and *HLA-B*38:01-C*12:03*), Table 6.1. Apart from *HLA-C*06:02*, mainly found on two ancestral haplotypes (*HLA-B*37:01-C*06:02* and *HLA-B*57:01-C*06:02*), none of the other *HLA-B* alleles were associated with *HLA-C*06:02*.

Table 6.1 Risk of developing psoriatic arthritis and MHC class I alleles or haplotypes

In populations of Northern European ancestry the development of psoriatic arthritis predominantly occurs in individuals who inherit one or more of the following MHC class I alleles or haplotypes:

Alleles	Haplotypes
HLA-B*08:01	HLA-B*08:01 – C*07:01
HLA-B*27:05:02	HLA-B*27:05:02 – C*01:02
	HLA-B*27:05:02 – C*02:02
HLA-B*38:01	HLA-B*38:01 – C*12:01
HLA-B*39:01	HLA-B*39:01 – C*12:01
HLA-C*06:02	HLA-B*37:01 – C*06:02
	HLA-B*57:01 – C*06:02

Psoriatic arthritis is significantly less likely to develop in those with the following alleles or haplotypes:

HLA-B*44:02:01	HLA-B*44:02 – C*05:02
HLA-B*44:03:02	HLA-B*44:03 – C*16:01

It is very highly likely these five susceptibility alleles act to confer susceptibility, but because of the strong linkage disequilibrium in these haplotypes, it is likely that other genes on the haplotypes participate in the process.

Architecture and function of HLA molecules encoded by susceptibility alleles

Intriguingly, several other *HLA* alleles are disproportionally decreased in frequency in PsA, for example, *HLA-B*44:02*, is present in 24.6% of controls, but only 14.8% of PsA patients, OR=0.53(0.36–0.80), and *HLA-B*44:03* is similarly reduced OR=0.47(0.24–0.92) [12]. The structure of the *HLA-B*44:02* and *HLA-B*44:03* molecules and their peptide binding properties contrasts with that of the two HLA-B molecules encoded by *HLA-B*27:05:02* and *HLA-B*39:01:01* alleles in terms of the charge of a peptide binding pocket and the charge of the amino they preferably bind, as described previously [12]. *HLA-B*27:05:02* and *HLA-B*39:01:01* molecules have negatively charged glutamic acid in the B pocket at position 45 that preferentially binds a positively charged second amino acid side chain (P2) of a peptide, e.g. Arginine or Lysine. *HLA-B*08:01* and *HLA-B*38:01* molecules have analogous negatively charged pockets, while the two molecules associated with decreased susceptibility have exactly the opposite charge and peptide binding properties, Table 6.2.

This finding provides additional support to the concept that particular peptides preferably bound by HLA molecules encoded by the PsA susceptibility alleles play an important role in influencing the development, either positively or negatively, of the immune response underlying PsA. This interpretation was supported by the recent study from Okada and colleagues in a large cohort of PsA patients using imputed HLA typing of *HLA-B* alleles from SNPs [13]. Imputation from SNP analysis is technically much easier than determining the allele sequence, allowing large number of patients to be studied, but is less precise because relatively few regions of the allele are determined in the SNP analysis, preventing accurate allele assignment. The finding that

Table 6.2 The amino acid charge in the HLA-B molecule P2 peptide binding pocket determines the type of amino acid at P2 in the peptide preferentially bound by the HLA-B molecule and influences whether the allele confers increased or decreased susceptibility to psoriatic arthritis

HLA-B Molecule	P2 Pocket Amino acid at position 45 or 67 in HLA-B molecule		Binding Peptide P2 amino acid preference	Risk estimate of allele encoding HLA-B molecule
	45	67		Odds ratio
B*27:05:02	Glu	Cys	Arg	3.18
B*38:01:01	Glu	Cys	Arg	1.73
B*39:01:01	Glu	Cys	Arg	3.74
B*44:02:01	Lys	Ser	Glu	0.53
B*44:03:02	Lys	Ser	Glu	0.47

resistance and susceptibility allomorphic molecules for PsA susceptibility encode molecules of contrasting charge, Table 6.2, is similar to the molecular architecture underlying the shared epitope hypothesis in rheumatoid arthritis susceptibility, where, the allomorphs associated with susceptibility in the P4 pocket of the class II HLA-DR molecule have a positively charged lysine or arginine, while those alleles such as encoded by *HLA-DRB1*04:03* associated with greatly decreased susceptibility have a negatively charged amino acid in the pocket [14]. Why allomorphs with the ability to bind charged peptides seem implicated in susceptibility to several different autoimmune diseases is intriguing, and could relate to greater degeneracy of the binding pockets or the property of charged amino acid side chains to be post-translationally modified.

Interval between the onset of psoriasis and the development of PsA

The standard teaching is that PsA follows the onset of PsV by 10–15 years. However, one of the first clues that the genes implicated in PsA susceptibility were acting in divergent ways was that the interval between the onset of psoriasis and the development of PsA was influenced by the patient's HLA type. In patients with *HLA-B*27:05:02* or *HLA-B*39:01:01*, arthritis develops much closer to, the appearance of psoriasis. Indeed nearly a third of *HLA-B*27:05:02* patients had the onset of skin disease after the onset of musculoskeletal disease (i.e. psoriatic arthritis sine psoriasis) [12]. Conversely in *HLA-C*06:02* patients, the interval between skin disease and musculoskeletal disease was the expected lag of over a decade This suggested susceptibility genes determine the time interval between the clinical appearance of the skin and musculoskeletal phenotypes of PsA as a quantitative trait. Thus the genetic effect of *HLA-B*27:05:02* results in similar penetrance and roughly contemporaneous appearance of both musculoskeletal and skin disease, while *HLA-C*06:02* specifies highly penetrant severe cutaneous disease and delayed milder musculoskeletal disease with greatly reduced penetrance.

Relationship of PsA allelic heterogeneity to PsA phenotypic heterogeneity

In addition to the finding that several different *HLA-B* or *HLA-C* genes are implicated in susceptibility recently emerging findings show that these alleles or their haplotypes are differentially and often additively associated with different clinical features of PsA. Precedent for an effect of susceptibility alleles on disease phenotype has been present since the initial study by Brewerton et al. [8], where *HLA-B*27* was proposed as being linked to the presence of axial disease in PsA. However, in subsequent studies this association has been inconsistent [15, 16–19]. Analogously, *HLA-C*06:02* has been reported to be associated with fewer involved or damaged joints [20].

Axial involvement in psoriatic arthritis is more strongly associated with HLA-B*08 rather than HLA-B*27

McEwen described that while ankylosing spondylitis is characterized by predominantly symmetrical sacroiliitis and uniform ascending axial involvement, PsA sacroiliitis is more likely to be asymmetric and axial involvement much less uniform [21]. In a recent study [22], sacroiliitis was found in 25% of PsA patients by X-Ray, where the radiologist was blinded to the clinical and HLA genotype of the patient, with 18% having asymmetric sacroiliitis and 6.4% symmetric sacroiliitis. PsA spondylitis was significantly associated with both *HLA-B*27:05:02* and *HLA-B*08:01*. Among the one quarter of PsA cases with symmetrical sacroiliitis, 61% had *HLA-B*27:05:02*, P<0.000, OR=10.6 (3.8–29), while only 16.1% had *HLA-B*08:01*, P=0.32, Table 6.3. Moreover, symmetrical sacroiliitis and *HLA-B*27:05* was male preponderant (OR=11.91), resembling ankylosing spondylitis, and were consistent with the classic report by Brewerton et al. of *HLA-B*27* and axial disease in PsA [8]. A recent study additionally supports this concept [23].

Unexpectedly and in marked contrast, the asymmetric involvement found in three quarters of the psoriatic arthritis patients with sacroiliitis was not significantly associated with *HLA-B*27:05:02*, P=0.19, but rather 62% of asymmetric sacroiliitis patients were *HLA-B*08:01*, P<0.000, OR=3.7 (1.9–6.9). This later finding provides a genetic explanation for the distinctive predominant pattern of asymmetric axial involvement described by McEwen several decades ago [21], and clearly indicates the fact that the predominant form of axial spondyloarthritis in PsA differs from that of ankylosing spondylitis both genetically and phenotypically.

Table 6.3 Genotype determines phenotype: The frequency of *HLA-B*27:05:02* is significantly increased in those with symmetrical sacroiliitis, while the frequency of *HLA-B*08:01* is increased in those with asymmetric sacroiliitis

Susceptibility allele	Susceptibility allele frequency in 282 patients with:		
	Any sacroiliitis	Symmetric sacroiliitis	Asymmetric sacroiliitis
HLA-B*27:05:02	23%	**61.1%**	9.8%
	P = 0.059	**P < 0.000**	P = 0.185
	OR = 1.92	**OR = 10.63**	OR = 0.52
	(0.97–3.79)	**(3.9–29.3)**	(0.19–1.39)
HLA-B*08:01	**50.7%**	16.7%	**62.7%**
	P = 0.006	P = 0.07	**P <0.000**
	OR = 2.15	OR = 0.32	**OR=3.8**
	(1.06–1.77)	(0.91–1.14)	**(1.9–7.0)**

Genotypic associations of other clinical features of the heterogeneous PsA phenotype

Some other elements of the heterogeneous PsA phenotype are also differently associated with the various HLA susceptibility alleles, as discussed in greater detail, see [22, 25] For example, enthesitis and dactylitis, are both significantly positively associated with *HLA-B*27:05*, while these traits are negatively associated with *HLA-B*44:02* and *HLA-B*44:03*. In enthesitis, the pattern of the strong association differed slightly from that of symmetric sacroiliitis, appearing predominantly driven by the *HLA-B*27:05:02-C*01:02:01* haplotype, and less so by *HLA-B*27:05:02* itself. Joint deformity and ankylosis, in contrast, was associated with *HLA-B*08:01*, but not *HLA-B*27:05*, and here also *HLA-B*44:02* and *HLA-B*44:03* are negatively associated with these more synovial features of PsA.

The *HLA-C*06:02:01* allele and *HLA-B*57:01:01-C*06:02:01* haplotype that are the primary susceptibility elements of PsV susceptibility were not positively associated with any of these axial, entheseal, or articular features and were significantly negatively associated with asymmetric sacroiliitis. However, there was evidence that the presence of *HLA-B*37:01* on the *HLA-B*37:01-C*06:02* haplotype exerts an epistatic effect on the subphenotype conferred by *HLA-C*06:02:01*, since the presence of this haplotype was positively associated with joint fusion, and an increased severity index in propensity analyses [22].

Genotypic contributions to phenotype assessed by propensity analysis

In these univariate associations between phenotypic traits and HLA alleles and haplotypes on one chromosome, each gene associated with susceptibility appeared to define a particular subphenotype. This action was often modified by the presence of additional HLA susceptibility alleles found on the ancestral haplotype containing the susceptibility allele [22]. However, genes in trans also contribute, as shown by the positive and negative associations of phenotypic traits with different alleles at the same locus, e.g. *HLA-B*27* and *HLA-B*44* alleles. To explore further the potential genotypic effects of pairwise combinations of different *HLA-B* and *HLA-C* alleles/haplotypes inherited from each parent, one can create allele/haplotype risk scores for the combination of two haplotypes by combining single alleles/haplotypes separately associated with being in the highest PsA severity propensity tertile based on the features studied by univariate analysis. This approach provided evidence that the character and severity of PsA phenotype is determined at the genotype level with genes of both chromosomes contributing additively to the composite phenotype [22]. The highest propensity score for severe PsA was with *HLA-B*27:05:02-C*02:02:02*, *HLA-B*08:01:01-C*07:01:01*, and *HLA-B*37:01:01-C*06:02:01*, but not the *HLA-B*27:05:02-C*01:01:01*, or *HLA-B*57:01:01-C*06:02:01* haplotypes[22]. In contrast, HLA-B*44 haplotypes were associated with presence of milder disease.

A more severe or a milder disease phenotype occurs in an apparent additive manner according to the presence of various combinations of these haplotypes. Accordingly, HLA typing may prove helpful in assessing the potential for more or less intense disease and the choice of a therapeutic agent. It is also clear that much more remains to be described about genotype–phenotype relations, including the need for validation studies, especially in ethnic groups where one can sort out relative contributions of certain alleles in the haplotype.

Limitations and future directions

The extreme linkage disequilibrium among the alleles comprising ancestral haplotypes implicated in PsA susceptibility and phenotype, in relatively ethnically homogeneous populations is an advantage in initial studies because the lower variance increases the power of the analysis and the pitfall of ethnic stratification between the different cohorts and subsets is greatly diminished. However, this advantage is a detriment in the next stage of analysis where one seeks to dissect the contribution of a given allele on the haplotype and identify its epistatic interactions. Moreover, these initial studies leave unanswered the question of the contribution of different HLA alleles to susceptibility in other than Northern Europe origin populations. This necessitates validation studies in different subsets of the European population and extension to other populations with psoriatic arthritis that lack major susceptibility ancestral haplotypes such as *HLA-B*08:01-C*07:01*, *HLA-B*27:05-C*02:02*, *HLA-B*27:05-C*01:02*, and *HLA-B*57:01-C*06:02*.

Implication of genetic and phenotypic heterogeneity on personalized medicine

Further extensions of the relationship between HLA susceptibility genes and features that define the PsA phenotype of a given patient should lead to predicting at the onset of psoriatic disease whether the disease is more likely to exhibit a more severe musculoskeletal phenotype, as for example, exhibited by combinations of *HLA-B*27:05:02* haplotypes with *HLA-B*08:01*; a more milder musculoskeletal phenotypes as seen in those with combinations of *HLA-C*06:02*, *HLA-B*44:02*, and *HLA-B*44:03* haplotypes; or manifest itself with primarily cutaneous involvement. This would allow suggesting use of more powerful biologics early on in one individual, and a much more symptomatic use of mild agents in another.

The PsA genotypic heterogeneity introduces further genetic heterogeneity into the axial spondyloarthritis group. How to include these *HLA-B*08* patients in the current axial spondyloarthritis classification is not resolved, since they lack the *HLA-B*27* criterion [24]. Moreover, it remains undetermined whether the *HLA-B*08* patients with axial disease respond similarly or differently to therapies.

There remain large gaps in understanding mechanisms underlying the effect of the above-described HLA class I alleles that results in the development of phenotypically heterogeneous forms of psoriatic disease. We presume the different peptide binding properties of the molecules encoded by these alleles determine immune systems with different T cell recognition specificities for various peptides likely derived from different self-molecules. The details of the overall mechanisms of inflammation triggered by the response to these different self-peptides may be an additional level of functional heterogeneity cause by the differing HLA susceptibility alleles, but at this time these potentially different inflammatory pathways remain hypothetical and represent paradigms for future genotype–phenotype–pharmacogenetic relationships implicit in the idea of personalized medicine.

Potential impact of genotypic and phenotypic heterogeneity on psoriatic arthritis classification, diagnosis criteria, and therapeutic trials

Some of the phenotypic traits used in certain diagnostic criteria, such as enthesitis, dactylitis, axial disease, are influenced by the combination of susceptibility alleles comprising the patient's genotype. In theory, since the current diagnostic criteria use these genotypically controlled phenotypic features, it might be possible that PsV individuals who are *HLA-B*57:01-C*06:02* and lack the PsA alleles associated with these distinctive PsA phenotypic traits, would be less likely to be affirmed as having PsA.

Accordingly, delineating the genotype of patients in clinical trials of PsA may become more widespread. This would assure biologically comparable treatment groups, especially because the different genotypes associated with PsA may themselves be associated with different predominant inflammatory pathways that respond differently to therapeutic agents.

Non-MHC genetics

The identification of additional genes that contribute to PsA susceptibility was a major challenge first approached by identifying alleles throughout the genome shared between PsA cases. In the only reported PsA genome-wide linkage study, analysis on a large Icelandic cohort reported a LOD (logarithm of odds) score of 2.17 on chromosome 16q21, and when conditioned on paternal transmission, the LOD score increased to a statistically significant 4.19, suggesting PsA cases share genes in this region [4]. This showed the promise of genome-wide interrogation, but was constrained by limited power and technical challenges and has been largely replaced by the second genome-wide approach, a case–control format of identification of genes associated with PsA.

GWAS are a powerful method of studying the genetics associated with complex psoriatic diseases and have greatly accelerated the identification of genetic variants. The first-generation of GWAS in PsA has already been performed in multiple cohorts and has yielded consistent results [26–30] (Table 6.4). PsA genes identified include those located in the MHC region as expected, *HLA-B*, *HLA-C*, and those located outside the MHC including *IL-12B*, *IL-23R*, *STAT2*, *TNIP1*, *TRAF3IP2*, *TYK2*, *FBXL19*, and *REL*. The majority of these genes have also been identified in PsV, emphasizing potential shared pathways. However, these first-generation studies have included relatively small numbers of PsA patients and, in view of the greater clinical and HLA heterogeneity of PsA compared with PsV, it is evident that considerably larger cohorts will be required to more completely delineate PsA genetics. Results from GWAS have highlighted pathways that contribute to disease pathogenesis, strongly suggesting that the pathophysiology underpinning PsA may reflect an integrated model involving the disruption of distinct signalling pathways comprised of barrier integrity, innate immune response, antigen presentation, and adaptive immune response particularly those mediated by Th-17 signalling (Tables 6.4 & 6.5).

Barrier integrity

Although no genetic loci involved in barrier integrity have reached a genome-wide level of significance in PsA, several candidate gene studies have been performed. The most notable association was with the *LCE3* gene cluster, which encodes stratum corneum proteins critical for epidermal differentiation [31]. The association between *LCE3C_LCE3B-del* and PsA has produced conflicting results in different studies [32–34]. A meta-analysis comprised 7,758 control subjects and 2,325 patients with PsA, including three previous studies in six different populations, demonstrated a significant

Table 6.4 Non-MHC genetic loci associated with PsA identified from genome-wide association studies

Chr.	Gene	Ethnicity	Immune response	Shared risk allele with psoriasis (Yes/No)
19p13.2	TYK2	European	Innate immunity (Interferon and NFkB signalling) Adaptive immunity (Th-17 differentiation)	Yes
12q13.3	STAT2	European	Innate immunity (Interferon signalling)	Yes
5q32-q33.1	TNIP1	European	Innate immunity (NFkB signalling)	Yes
2p13-p12	REL	European	Innate immunity (NFkB signalling)	Yes
16p11.2	FBXL19	European	Innate immunity (NFkB signalling)	Yes
5q31.1-33.1	IL-12B	European	Adaptive immunity (Th-17 differentiation)	Yes
1p31.3	IL-23R	European	Adaptive immunity (Th-17 differentiation)	Yes
6q21	TRAF3IP2	European	Adaptive immunity (Th-17 effector signalling)	Yes

association between PsA and the *LCE3C_LCE3B-del* tag SNP in Italian and Spanish cohorts [35].

Innate immunity

Activation of the innate immune response could be the initial trigger, which sets in motion an inflammatory cascade initiating

Table 6.5 Non-MHC genetic loci associated with PsA that failed to reach a genome-wide level of significance

Chr.	Gene	Ethnicity	Immune response	Shared risk allele with psoriasis (Yes/No)
1q21.3	LCE3C_ LCE3B-del	European	Barrier integrity	Yes
6p21.3	TNFα	European	Innate immunity (TNFα signalling)	Yes
12q13.3	IL-23A	European	Adaptive immunity (Th-17 differentiation)	Yes
17q21.31	STAT3	European	Adaptive immunity (Th-17 differentiation)	Yes
3p14.3	IL-17RD	European	Adaptive immunity (Th-17 effector signalling)	Unknown

PsA pathogenesis. The resultant inflammatory milieu and related downstream cellular signalling tips the immune balance towards autoimmunity. Interferons and tumour necrosis factor-α (TNFα) appear to represent the predominant cytokines involved as evidenced by their release from dendritic cells in damaged skin and synovial fluid, respectively [36, 37].

Interferon signalling

Interferon (INF) is a key early mediator of inflammation through interactions with innate immune receptors producing proinflammatory cytokines such as TNFα and interleukin (IL)-1 [38]. Two genetic loci involved in INF signalling, *TYK2* and *STAT2*, have reached genome-wide significance in PsA [26–30]. *TYK2* encodes a tyrosine kinase involved in the initiation of IFNα signalling and NFkB activation [39]. *STAT2* is an essential transcription factor in INF-mediated anti-proliferative signalling whose function is regulated by tyrosine phosphorylation, which is the trigger for STAT-dimerization, subsequent nuclear translocation, and transcriptional activation of IFN-stimulated genes [40]. Variations within genes encoding proteins crucial for INF signalling have been identified in PsV GWAS including *ELMO1, TYK2, SOCS1, IFIH1, RNF114, IRF4, DDX58*, and *IFNLR1* [27, 29, 30, 41–47].

TNFα signalling

TNFα induces the production of inflammatory chemokines resulting in the accumulation of proinflammatory leukocytes, including neutrophils, monocytes, and activated T cells [48]. Of relevance to PsA, TNFα stimulates bone loss by mobilizing osteoclast precursors from the bone marrow and inhibits osteoblast differentiation and function [49, 50]. Alterations in TNFα signalling by genetic alteration may initiate transcription of numerous target genes contributing to PsV or PsA pathogenesis. Although GWAS failed to detect any association signals for TNFα genetic variants, a meta-analysis with 2,159 PsV and 2,360 PsA patients revealed a significant association between *TNFα* -238A/G and -857T/C polymorphism and PsA susceptibility [51]. In contrast, the variant genotypes and alleles of *TNFα* -308A/G were protective against PsV.

NFκB signalling

The NFκB complex is activated upon liberation from inhibitor of kappa B kinase (IκB), secondary to cytokine stimulation, most notably, TNFα and IL-17. The importance of NFκB signalling is supported by the presence of altered NFκB activity in psoriatic disease [52]. Several genetic loci involved in NFκB signalling, *TNIP1, REL, FBXL19*, and *TYK2*, have reached genome-wide significance in PsA [26–30]. The product of *TNIP1* (TNFAIP3-interacting protein 1) interacts with TNFAIP3 to inhibit TNF-induced NFκB-dependent gene expression [53]. *REL* genes encode a subunit of the NFκB complex that is essential for proper signalling [54] and the product of *FBXL19* reversibly inhibits NFκB signalling [42]. *TYK2* encodes a tyrosine kinase involved in the initiation of IFN signalling and NFκB activation [55]. Genetic variations encoding proteins crucial for NFκB signalling have also been identified in PsV GWAS including *TNFAIP3, TNIP1, TYK2, REL, NFKBIA, CARD14, CARM1, NOS2, UBE2L3*, and *FBXL19* [27, 29, 30, 41–47]. Collectively, these data strongly support an important role of INF, TNFα and NFkB signalling in PsA and PsV pathogenesis.

Antigen presentation

Antigen presentation to the adaptive immune system by the innate immune system is a critical event in evoking psoriatic disease and disruption of antigen presentation and alteration of CD8 T cell signalling can result in inappropriate targeting and destruction of cells thereby contributing to PsA pathogenesis. Variations within *HLA-B* and *HLA-C* identified in GWAS reflect the contribution of the MHC. With respect to PsV, variations within genes encoding proteins crucial for antigen presentation have been identified in GWAS investigating susceptibility to PsV including *HLA-B*, *HLA-C*, *ERAP1*, *ERAP2*, and *MICA* [27, 29, 30, 41–47]. Collectively, these genes encode proteins that are involved in proper antigen presentation and may underlie PsA pathogenesis.

Adaptive immunity

Recent studies have proposed that Th-17 cells play a pivotal role in PsA pathology given that TNF-α, INF-γ, INF-α, and IL-1β all induce the secretion of IL-23 by myeloid dendritic cells which cause the differentiation of Th-17 cells [56]. Moreover, the Th-17 pathway, through its intermediaries, forms complex interactions with TNFα and NFκB, and consequently, plays an important role in both the innate immune response as well as bone remodelling [57]. These findings suggest that both IL-23 and IL-17 influence the activation of the NFκB pathway. Indeed, the discovery of IL-17 and the Th-17 subset has substantially changed our understanding of disease pathogenesis. In this section, we will focus on the genetics involved in both Th-17 differentiation and downstream Th-17 mediated signalling.

Th-17 differentiation

IL-17-promoting cytokines (e.g. TGF-β, IL-6, IL-1β, and IL-23) and their signalling pathways induce Th-17 cell differentiation, which contributes to the psoriatic phenotype. With the exception of IL-23, very limited information exists regarding the molecular pathology of these cytokines. As a result, only IL-23 will be covered in this section. IL-23 is a heterodimeric cytokine that binds IL-23R and IL-12Rβ1, promotes the expansion and survival of Th-17 cells, and acts as a pro-inflammatory mediator [58, 59]. PsA GWAS have only identified two genetic variations located within *IL-12β* and *IL-23R* [26–30]. Results from candidate gene studies have revealed an association of *IL-23A* and *STAT3* [60, 61]. IL-12 and IL-23 share the p40 subunit encoded by *IL-12B*, *IL-23A* encodes the p19 subunit of IL-23, and *IL-23R* encodes a subunit of the IL-23 receptor. STAT3 encodes for Stat3, which is required for the differentiation of Th-17 cells through the induction of RORγ [62, 63]. GWAS in PsV have revealed that variations located within *IL-12β*, *IL-23A*, *IL-23R*, *TYK2*, *STAT3*, *SOCS1*, and *ETS1* [27, 29, 30, 41–47]. These studies support a prominent role of IL-23 in the pathogenesis of both PsA and PsV.

Th-17 effector signalling

Th-17 effector signalling, which is comprised of IL-17, IL-21, and IL-22, produces autoimmunity, setting the stage for the development of PsA. Given the limited amount of genetic data available for IL-21 and IL-22, only IL-17 will be covered in this section. The relevance of the IL-17 in PsA is supported by the elevation of IL-17/IL-17R in synovial fluid from PsA patients [64, 65]. A single genetic variation located within *TRAF3IP2* has been discovered by PsA GWAS [26–30]. *TRAF3IP2* encodes TRAF3 interacting protein 2, which is essential for Th-17 cell mediated inflammatory responses and its dysregulation may affect both IL-17 and NFκB signalling [66]. A study of the *TRAF3IP2* variant associated with PsA revealed near complete loss of ability of the protein to interact with TRAF6 [29], therefore, TRAF3IP2 represents a key bridge between innate immunity and IL-17 mediated adaptive immunity. Although GWAS have not identified a direct association of IL-17 with either PsA or PsV, a family-based PsV association study in a Tunisian family revealed an association between *IL-17RD* (rs12495640), which is a member of the IL-17 receptor (IL-17R) family [67]. However, in PsA patients of northern Italian origin, *IL-17A* and *IL-17RA* allelic variants were not associated with disease susceptibility [68]. The net effect of such genetic variants is altered expression of Th-17 cells and subsequent production of IL-17, which induces additional proinflammatory cytokines and angiogenic factors, thereby contributing to PsA disease pathogenesis. It is expected that additional genetic loci involved in Th-17 signalling reaching genome-wide level of significance will be discovered in PsA, similar to that in PsV.

The search for PsA-weighted or -specific genes continues

The majority of genes associated with PsA are also associated with PsV. This finding is not surprising as PsA is a distinct entity within PsV and both diseases exhibit significant clinical, immunological, and therapeutic overlap. PsA and PsV also share multiple genes with other immune-mediated inflammatory disorders such as Crohn's disease (CD), rheumatoid arthritis (RA), systemic lupus erythematosus (SLE), and ankylosing spondylitis (AS). Examples of shared genes are: *TNFAIP3* (CD, RA, SLE), *IL-23R* (AS, CD), *ERAP-1* (AS, CD), *IL-12B* (CD), *REL* (RA), and *PTPN22* (RA) [69]. However, the specific variants or haplotypes of these genes may differ between the autoimmune diseases.

Regarding the non-MHC genes, variants appear to be either specific to or at least more weighted towards PsA (Table 6.6). Dense genotyping of immune-mediated susceptibility loci in approximately 2,000 PsA patients and over 8,000 controls, reported a distinct PsA risk variant at IL-23R that was independent of any psoriasis associated *IL-23R* SNP [26] The same study identified a SNP within the 5q31 susceptibility locus specifically associated with PsA; an association independent of an *IL-13* SNP that was also previously identified in PsA within this region. Finally, a large targeted case–control study in PsA demonstrated a genome-wide level of significant for an association of the *PTPN22* variant (rs2476601) in PsA [70]. Importantly, no association with this SNP was noted in a large PsV cohort. Notably, this *PTPN22* SNP is also associated with RA, particularly those that carry the anti-citrullinated protein antibody, as well other autoimmune diseases.

For PsA-weighted genes, the effect size of a *TRAF3IP2* variant appears to be more prevalent in PsA compared with PsV [27]. *TRAF3IP2* encodes Act1, an adapter protein essential for Th17-mediated inflammatory responses and thus is of great interest in the pathogenesis of PsA. A similar trend has been noted for *FBXL19*, where the allele frequency for PsA is greater than PsV. This gene encodes a member of the Skp1-Cullin-F-box family of E3 ubiquitin ligases and reversibly inhibits NFκB signalling [44]. Identification of these PsA-specific genes is a further testament to our conviction that PsA and PsV are genetically distinct entities that co-exist with many shared elements.

Although GWAS has contributed greatly to our understanding of psoriatic disease pathogenesis, much of the genetic burden of

Table 6.6 Non-MHC genetic loci that have been reported as either PsA-specific or heavily weighted toward PsA

Chr.	Gene	Ethnicity	Immune response	Shared risk variant with psoriasis (Yes/No)
PsA-specific genetic loci				
1p13.2	PTPN22 (rs2476601)	European	Innate immunity (Interferon signalling) Adaptive immunity (Th-17 effector signalling)	No
5q31	Unknown (rs715285)	European	Unknown	No
1p31.3	IL-23R (rs12044149)	European	Adaptive immunity (Th-17 differentiation)	No
PsA-weighted genetic loci				
6q21	TRAF3IP2 (rs33980500)	European	Adaptive immunity (Th-17 effector signalling)	Yes
16p11.2	FBXL19	European	Innate immunity (NFκB signalling)	Yes

psoriatic disease remains unexplained, hence the term 'missing heritability'

GWAS have generated countless new candidate genes that were not suspected prior to initiating those studies. Although most of these candidates are not likely to be causal variants, its relevance is magnified by the occurrence of selected genes in major pathways suspected of causing psoriatic disease. Despite the number of genes identified in psoriatic disease by GWAS, only a small fraction of the heritability is explained. There is certainly the opportunity to identify more genetic variants in PsA by deploying larger datasets of patients, denser SNP coverage, and meta-analyses coupled with strategic imputation. The unexplained heritability of PsA is attributed, at least, in part, to inherent technology limitations, as GWAS is particularly suited to capture common variants. Consequently, violation of the common disease–common variant model may lead to 'missing heritability' [71]. However, searching solely for common variants in common disease will identify a fraction of the entire genetic burden as evidenced with large GWAS in CD where identification of recent genes have made very marginal differences to the total heritability [72]. Many sources have been proposed to account for this missing heritability including imperfect SNP-tagging (producing weak GWAS signals), rare variants, structural variations (CNVs), epigenetics (e.g. methylation analysis), epistatic interactions, gene–environment interactions, parent-of-origin effects, and phenotype misclassification [73, 74].

Exome sequencing holds great promise for rare variant discovery particularly in familial studies. As genomic technologies improve, detection of associations with variants of lower frequency is increasingly becoming possible. As large-scale parallel-sequencing studies of many thousands of individuals become commonplace, then sufficient power is likely to be gained, allowing both rare and common variants to be discovered to a greater extent. A unique gain-of-function mutation that segregated with psoriasis was identified using exome sequencing, which altered splicing within CARD14 [75]. This study illustrates that rare variants with large effect size can be identified through technological advancements like massive parallel sequencing.

Structural variations have been largely overlooked with respect to the heritability of psoriatic disease. Searching for different types of genetic variants such as CNVs has also led to the identification of several genes for psoriatic disease. For example, a genome-wide investigation targeting CNVs identified a significant association between the LCE3C_LCE3B deletion and increased susceptibility to psoriasis in several populations [31]. Therefore, it appears that quantitative variation in gene dosage may also contribute to susceptibility to PsA, but further investigation in larger cohorts is warranted.

In addition to genetic predisposition factors, epigenetic factors may play a role in the onset and progression of psoriatic disease. DNA methylation is an epigenetic silencing mechanism, which occurs at the 5′-carbon of cytosine residue within the CpG dinucleotides by DNA methyltransferases [76]. Although studies of genome-wide DNA methylation in PsA patients are lacking, numerous genome-wide DNA methylation studies have been performed in psoriasis. For example, MeDIP-Seq has revealed much higher number of hypermethylated regions in the affected skin of psoriatic patients, including in genes enriched for the immune system, cell cycle regulation, and apoptotic mechanisms [77].

Incorporation of gene/gene and gene/environment interactions in patient care may improve the ability to predict which individuals will develop psoriatic disease and identify patients who are more likely to rapidly progress. Complex diseases have complex genetic and epigenetic interactions that remain to be fully elucidated. Careful evaluation of gene–gene and gene–environment interactions should be performed secondary to identification of genetic variants. Interactions between two genetic variants has already been reported in PsV, where SNPs tagging HLA-Cw*0602 demonstrated a statistical interaction with ERAP-1 [46], as well as the LCE3C_LCE3B-del variant [78]. Gene–environment interactions are even more complex to evaluate as quantitating the exposure is quite challenging. For example, cigarette smoking appears to modulate certain autoimmune disorders in a subset of patients with genetic alternations. In PsA, two separate cohorts have reported a statistical interaction between cigarette smoking and IL-13; however, its biological explanation and clinical significance remains unclear [79, 80]. Models incorporating multiple genes may need to be developed if genetic variants are to be used as a predictive tool similar to the cumulative weighted genotype relative risk score developed by Chen et al. [81].

In addition to disease susceptibility and progression, responses to targeted biologics that are prescribed to treat PsA are also affected by genetic variation. Although this field is still in its infancy, as adequately powered studies for biologic agents are still lacking for psoriatic disease, there are limited reports that speak to the possible broad applicability of this approach towards personalized medicine. For example, TNFα inhibitors are strikingly effective in PsA; however, 30–40% of patients exhibit no therapeutic response. A number of studies designed to address this dichotomous response to TNFi has demonstrated that genetic variants are correlated with the presence or absence of a response [82–85]. For example, better therapeutic response to TNFα inhibition was noted for those carrying the *TNFα-308* GG genotype compared with those carrying the AA or AG genotypes [85]. PsA patients being treated with etanercept demonstrated a trend toward a better response when carrying the *TNFα-489A* allele [83]. The TNF receptor 1A (*TNFR1A*) variant (AA genotype of SNP rs767455) was associated with a better EULAR response at 3 months for PsA patients treated with infliximab [82]. PsA patients receiving six months of infliximab reported higher EULAR responses in the presence of the TNF-related apoptosis inducing ligand receptor 1 (*TRAIL-R1*) variant (CC genotype of SNP rs20575) [82]. These candidate gene studies suggest genetic variation does contribute to pharmacokinetics and pharmacodynamics of targeted biologic therapy in PsA patients.

Better understanding how genetics underscores disease susceptibility, severity, progression, and response to targeted therapy is of paramount importance in order for the concept of personalized medicine to become a reality for PsA patients. PsA is a very heterogeneous disease making genetic investigation more challenging compared with PsV, and this heterogeneity partially accounts for the greater amount of unexplained heritability in PsA. Fine mapping of the MHC region and GWAS studies have illuminated new candidate genes that were not suspected prior to initiating those studies and have contributed greatly to our understanding of PsA pathogenesis. Employing recent technological advancements, like whole-exome sequencing, transcriptome and methylome analyses, in combination with functional studies will likely result in the identification of new genetic variants in PsA. It is expected that identification of rare variants, structural variations (CNVs), epigenetics, epistatic interactions, and gene-environment interactions will help account for the 'missing heritability' in PsA. Importantly, incorporation of genetic variants along with gene/gene and gene/environment interactions in risk assessment modelling may improve the ability to predict which individuals will develop psoriatic disease, identify PsA patients who are more likely to rapidly progress, and identify patients who will response to targeted biologic therapy.

References

1. Rahman P, Elde, JT. Genetic epidemiology of psoriasis and psoriatic arthritis. Ann Rheum Dis, 2005; 64: Suppl 2:ii37–9; discussion ii40–1.
2. Moll JM, Wright V. Familial occurrence of psoriatic arthritis. Ann Rheum Dis, 1973; 32(3): 181–201.
3. Chandran V, Schentag CT, Brockbank JE, et al. Familial aggregation of psoriatic arthritis. Ann Rheum Dis, 2009; 68(5): 664–7.
4. Karason A, Love TJ. Gudbjornsson B. A strong heritability of psoriatic arthritis over four generations--the Reykjavik Psoriatic Arthritis Study. Rheumatology (Oxford), 2009;48(11):1424–8.
5. Pedersen OB, Svendsen AJ, Ejstrup L, Skytthe A, Junker P. On the heritability of psoriatic arthritis. Disease concordance among monozygotic and dizygotic twins. Ann Rheum Dis, 2008; 67(10):1417–21.
6. Rahman P, Gladman DD, Schentag CT, Petronis A. Excessive paternal transmission in psoriatic arthritis. Arthritis Rheum, 1999. 42(6):1228–31.
7. Pollock RA, Thavaneswaran A, Pellett F, et al. Further evidence supporting a parent-of-origin effect in psoriatic disease. Arthritis Care Res (Hoboken), 2015; 67(11):1586–90.
8. Brewerton DA, Caffrey M, Nicholls A, Walters D, James DC. HL-A 27 and arthropathies associated with ulcerative colitis and psoriasis. Lancet, 1974;956–8.
9. Murray C, Caffrey M, Nicholls A, Walters D, James DC. Histocompatibility alloantigens in psoriasis and psoriatic arthritis. Evidence for the influence of multiple genes in the major histocompatibility complex. J Clin Invest, 1980;66(4):670–5.
10. Winchester R, Genetics of Psoriasis and Psoriatic Arthritis, in Psoriatic and Reactive Arthritis—A Companion to Rheumatology, C.T. Ritchlin and O. FitzGerald, Editors. 2007, Elsevier: Amsterdam, pp.65–80.
11. Eder L, Chandran V, Pellet F, et al. Human leucocyte antigen risk alleles for psoriatic arthritis among patients with psoriasis. Ann Rheum Dis, 2012; 71(1):50–5.
12. Winchester R., Minevich G, Steshenko V, et al. HLA associations reveal genetic heterogeneity in psoriatic arthritis and in the psoriasis phenotype. Arthritis Rheum, 2012; 64(4):1134–44.
13. Okada Y, Han B, Tsoi EL, et al. Fine mapping major histocompatibility complex associations in psoriasis and its clinical subtypes. Am J Hum Genet, 2014. 95(2):162–72.
14. Gregersen PK, Silver J, Winchester RJ. The shared epitope hypothesis. An approach to understanding the molecular genetics of susceptibility to rheumatoid arthritis. Arthritis Rheum, 1987;30(11):1205–13.
15. Queiro, R., Sarasqueta C, Belzunegui J, Gonzalez C, Figueroa M, Torre-Alonso JC. Psoriatic spondyloarthropathy: a comparative study between HLA-B27 positive and HLA-B27 negative disease. Sem Arthritis Rheum 2002; 31(6):413–8.
16. Gladman D, Anhorn KA, Schachter RK, Mervart H. HLA antigens in psoriatic arthritis. J. Rheumatol 1986:13:586.
17. Gladman DD, Farwell, VT. The role of HLA antigens as indicators of disease progression in psoriatic arthritis. Multivariate relative risk model. Arthritis Rheum 1995; 38(6):845–50.
18. Queiro-Silva R, Torre-Alonso JC, Tinturé-Eguren T, López-Lagunas I. The effect of HLA-DR antigens on the susceptibility to, and clinical expression of psoriatic arthritis. Scand J Rrheumatol 2004;33(5):318–22.
19. Grubić Z, Perić P, Cecuk-Jelicić E, Zunec R, Curković B, Kerhin-Brkljacić V. The distribution of HLA alleles class I and class II among patientes with psoriatic arthritis in Croatia. Reumatizam, 2004. 51(1):5–11.
20. Ho PY, Barton A, Worthington J, Thomson W, Silman AJ, Bruce IN. HLA-Cw6 and HLA-DRB1*07 together are associated with less severe joint disease in psoriatic arthritis. Ann Rheum Dis, 2007; 66(6):807–11.
21. McEwen C, McEwen C, DiTata D, Lingg C, Porini A, Good A, Rankin T. Ankylosing spondylitis and spondylitis accompanying ulcerative colitis, regional enteritis, psoriasis and Reiter's disease. A comparative study. Arthritis Rheum, 1971;14(3):291–318.
22. Haroon M, Winchester R, Giles JT, Heffernan E, FitzGerald O. Certain class I HLA alleles and haplotypes implicated in susceptibility play a role in determining specific features of the psoriatic arthritis phenotype. Ann Rheum Dis 2014;73(8):1487–94.
23. Castillo-Gallego C, Aydin SZ, Emery P, McGonagle DG, Marzo-Ortega H. Magnetic resonance imaging assessment of axial psoriatic arthritis: extent of disease relates to HLA-B27. Arthritis Rheum, 2013; 65(9):2274–8.
24. Rudwaleit M. New approaches to diagnosis and classification of axial and peripheral spondyloarthritis. Curr Opin Rheumatol, 2010;22(4):375–80.
25. FitzGerald O, Haroon M, Giles JT, Winchester R. Concepts of pathogenesis in psoriatic arthritis: genotype determines clinical phenotype. Arthritis Res Ther, 2015;17(1):115.
26. Bowes J, Budu-Aggrey A, Huffmeier U et al. Dense genotyping of immune-related susceptibility loci reveals new insights into the genetics of psoriatic arthritis. Nat Commun, 2015;6:6046.
27. Ellinghaus E. Ellinghaus D, Stuart PE, et al. Genome-wide association study identifies a psoriasis susceptibility locus at TRAF3IP2. Nat Genet, 2010;42(11):991–5.
28. Ellinghaus E, Stuart PE, Ellinghaus D, et al. Genome-wide meta-analysis of psoriatic arthritis identifies susceptibility locus at REL. J Invest Dermatol, 2012;132(4):1133–40.
29. Huffmeier U, Uebe S, Ekici AB, et al. Common variants at TRAF3IP2 are associated with susceptibility to psoriatic arthritis and psoriasis. Nat Genet, 2010; 42(11):996–9.

30. Liu, Y., et al. A genome-wide association study of psoriasis and psoriatic arthritis identifies new disease loci. PLoS Genet, 2008. 4(3):e1000041.

31. de Cid R, Riveira-Munoz E, Zeeuwen PL et al. Deletion of the late cornified envelope LCE3B and LCE3C genes as a susceptibility factor for psoriasis. Nat Genet, 2009;41(2):211–5.

32. Bowes J, Flynn E, Ho P, et al. Variants in linkage disequilibrium with the late cornified envelope gene cluster deletion are associated with susceptibility to psoriatic arthritis. Ann Rheum Dis, 2010; 69(12):2199–203.

33. Chiraz BS, Myriam A, Ines Z, et al. Deletion of late cornified envelope genes, LCE3C_LCE3B-del, is not associated with psoriatic arthritis in Tunisian patients. Mol Biol Rep, 2014; 41(6):4141–6.

34. Huffmeier U, Estivill X, Riveira-Munoz E, et al. Deletion of LCE3C and LCE3B genes at PSORS4 does not contribute to susceptibility to psoriatic arthritis in German patients. Ann Rheum Dis, 2010;69(5):876–8.

35. Docampo E, Giardina E, Riveira-Muñoz E, et al. Deletion of LCE3C and LCE3B is a susceptibility factor for psoriatic arthritis: a study in Spanish and Italian populations and meta-analysis. Arthritis Rheum, 2011; 63(7):1860–5.

36. Ganguly D, Chamilos G, Lande R, et al. Self-RNA-antimicrobial peptide complexes activate human dendritic cells through TLR7 and TLR8. J Exp Med, 2009;206(9):1983–94.

37. Lories RJ, de Vlam K. Is psoriatic arthritis a result of abnormalities in acquired or innate immunity? Curr Rheumatol Rep, 2012;14(4):375–82.

38. Hertzog P, Forster S, Samarajiwa S. Systems biology of interferon responses. J Interferon Cytokine Res, 2011; 31(1):5–11.

39. Li Y, Ohms SJ, Sun C, Fan J. NF-kappaB controls Il2 and Csf2 expression during T cell development and activation process. Mol Biol Rep, 2013; 40(2):1685–92.

40. Steen HC, Gamero AM. STAT2 phosphorylation and signaling. JAKSTAT, 2013; 2(4):e25790.

41. Ellinghaus D, Ellinghaus E, Nair RP et al. Combined analysis of genome-wide association studies for Crohn disease and psoriasis identifies seven shared susceptibility loci. Am J Hum Genet, 2012;90(4):636–47.

42. Genetic Analysis of Psoriasis Consortium, the Wellcome Trust Case Control Consortium 21, Strange A, et al. A genome-wide association study identifies new psoriasis susceptibility loci and an interaction between HLA-C and ERAP1. Nat Genet, 2010;42(11):985–90.

43. Nair RP, Duffin KC, Helms C, et al. Genome-wide scan reveals association of psoriasis with IL-23 and NF-kappaB pathways. Nat Genet, 2009. 41(2):199–204.

44. Stuart P, Nair RP, Ellinghaus E, et al. Genome-wide association analysis identifies three psoriasis susceptibility loci. Nat Genet, 2010;42(11):1000–4.

45. Sun LD, Cheng H, Wang ZX, et al. Association analyses identify six new psoriasis susceptibility loci in the Chinese population. Nat Genet, 2010;2(11):1005–9.

46. Tsoi LC, Spain SL, Knight J, et al. Identification of 15 new psoriasis susceptibility loci highlights the role of innate immunity. Nat Genet, 2012;44(12):1341–8.

47. Zhang XJ, Huang W, Yang S, et al. Psoriasis genome-wide association study identifies susceptibility variants within LCE gene cluster at 1q21. Nat Genet, 2009;41(2):205–10.

48. Koch AE. Chemokines and their receptors in rheumatoid arthritis: future targets? Arthritis Rheum, 2005. 52(3):710–21.

49. Gilbert L, He X, Farmer P, et al. Inhibition of osteoblast differentiation by tumor necrosis factor-alpha. Endocrinology, 2000. 141(11):3956–64.

50. Li P, Schwarz EM, O'Keefe RJ, Ma L, Boyce BF, Xing L. RANK signaling is not required for TNFalpha-mediated increase in CD11(hi) osteoclast precursors but is essential for mature osteoclast formation in TNFalpha-mediated inflammatory arthritis. J Bone Miner Res, 2004;19(2):207–13.

51. Zhu J, Qu H, Chen X, Wang H, Li J. Single nucleotide polymorphisms in the tumor necrosis factor-alpha gene promoter region alter the risk of psoriasis vulgaris and psoriatic arthritis: a meta-analysis. PLoS One, 2013; 8(5):e64376.

52. Abdou AG, Hanout HM. Evaluation of survivin and NF-kappaB in psoriasis, an immunohistochemical study. J Cutan Pathol, 2008; 35(5):445–51.

53. Verstrepen L, Garpentier I, Verhelst K, Beyaert R. ABINs: A20 binding inhibitors of NF-kappa B and apoptosis signaling. Biochem Pharmacol, 2009;78(2):105–14.

54. De Molfetta GA, Lucíola Zanette D, Alexandre Panepucci R, et al. Role of NFKB2 on the early myeloid differentiation of CD34+ hematopoietic stem/progenitor cells. Differentiation, 2010; 80(4-5):195–203.

55. Lu, T., Jackson MW, Wang B, et al. Regulation of NF-kappaB by NSD1/FBXL11-dependent reversible lysine methylation of p65. Proc Natl Acad Sci U S A, 2010;107(1):46–51.

56. Ryan C, Abramson A, Patel M, Menter A. Current investigational drugs in psoriasis. Expert Opin Investig Drugs, 2012;21(4):473–87.

57. Bulek K, Liu C, Swaidani S, et al. The inducible kinase IKKi is required for IL-17-dependent signaling associated with neutrophilia and pulmonary inflammation. Nat Immunol, 2011;12(9):844–52.

58. Oppmann B, Lesley R, Blom B, et al. Novel p19 protein engages IL-12p40 to form a cytokine, IL-23, with biological activities similar as well as distinct from IL-12. Immunity, 2000;13(5):715–25.

59. Pappu R, Ramirez-Carrozzi V, Sambandam A. The interleukin-17 cytokine family: critical players in host defence and inflammatory diseases. Immunology, 2011. 134(1):8–16.

60. Bowes J, Orozco G, Flynn E, et al. Confirmation of TNIP1 and IL23A as susceptibility loci for psoriatic arthritis. Ann Rheum Dis, 2011; 70(9):1641–4.

61. Cenit MC, Ortego-Centeno N, Raya E, et al. Influence of the STAT3 genetic variants in the susceptibility to psoriatic arthritis and Behcet's disease. Hum Immunol, 2013; 74(2):230–3.

62. Harris TJ, Grosso JF, Yen HR, et al. Cutting edge: An in vivo requirement for STAT3 signaling in TH17 development and TH17-dependent autoimmunity. J Immunol 2007;179(7):4313–7.

63. Ivanov, II, McKenzie BS, Zhou L, et al. The orphan nuclear receptor RORgammat directs the differentiation program of proinflammatory IL-17+ T helper cells. Cell, 2006; 126(6):1121–33.

64. Mrabet D, Laadhar L, Sahli H, et al. Synovial fluid and serum levels of IL-17, IL-23, and CCL-20 in rheumatoid arthritis and psoriatic arthritis: a Tunisian cross-sectional study. Rheumatol Int, 2013;33(1):265–6.

65. Raychaudhuri SP, Raychaudhuri SK, Genovese MC. IL-17 receptor and its functional significance in psoriatic arthritis. Mol Cell Biochem, 2012;359(1–2):419–29.

66. Sonder SU, Saret S, Tang W, et al. IL-17-induced NF-kappaB activation via CIKS/Act1: physiologic significance and signaling mechanisms. J Biol Chem, 2011; 286(15):12881–90.

67. Ammar M, Bouchlaka-Souissi C, Zaraa I et al. Family-based association study in Tunisian familial psoriasis. Int J Dermatol, 2012;51(11):1329–34.

68. Catanoso MG, Boiardi L, Macchioni P, et al. IL-23A, IL-23R, IL-17A and IL-17R polymorphisms in different psoriatic arthritis clinical manifestations in the northern Italian population. Rheumatol Int, 2013; 33(5):1165–76.

69. O'Rielly DD, Rahman P. Genetics of susceptibility and treatment response in psoriatic arthritis. Nat Rev Rheumatol, 2011; 7(12):718–32.

70. Bowes J, Loehr S, Budu-Aggrey A et al. PTPN22 is associated with susceptibility to psoriatic arthritis but not psoriasis: evidence for a further PsA-specific risk locus. Ann Rheum Dis, 2015; 74(10):1882–5.

71. McClellan J. King MC. Genetic heterogeneity in human disease. Cell, 2010;141(2):210–7.

72. Liu JZ, Sommeren S, Huang H, et al. Association analyses identify 38 susceptibility loci for inflammatory bowel disease and highlight shared genetic risk across populations. Nat Genet, 2015; 47(9):979–86.

73. Eichler EE, Flint J, Gibson G, et al. Missing heritability and strategies for finding the underlying causes of complex disease. Nat Rev Genet, 2010;11(6):446–50.

74. Manolio TA, Collins FS, Cox NJ, et al. Finding the missing heritability of complex diseases. Nature, 2009. 461(7265):747–53.

75. Jordan CT, Cao L, Roberson ED, et al. PSORS2 is due to mutations in CARD14. Am J Hum Genet, 2012; 90(5):784–95.

76. Chatterjee R, Vinson C. CpG methylation recruits sequence specific transcription factors essential for tissue specific gene expression. Biochim Biophys Acta, 2012;1819(7):763–70.

77. Zhang, P., et al. Whole-genome DNA methylation in skin lesions from patients with psoriasis vulgaris. J Autoimmun, 2013;41:17–24.

78. Riveira-Munoz E, Zhao M, Liang G, et al. Meta-analysis confirms the LCE3C_LCE3B deletion as a risk factor for psoriasis in several ethnic groups and finds interaction with HLA-Cw6. J Invest Dermatol, 2011;131(5):1105–9.

79. Duffin KC, Freeny IC, Schrodi SJ, et al. Association between IL13 polymorphisms and psoriatic arthritis is modified by smoking. J Invest Dermatol, 2009;129(12):2777–83.

80. Eder L, Chandran V, Pellett F, et al. IL13 gene polymorphism is a marker for psoriatic arthritis among psoriasis patients. Ann Rheum Dis, 2011;70(9):1594–8.

81. Chen H, Poon A, Yeung C, et al. A genetic risk score combining ten psoriasis risk loci improves disease prediction. PLoS One, 2011;6(4):e19454.

82. Morales-Lara MJ, Cañete JD, Torres-Moreno D, et al. Effects of polymorphisms in TRAILR1 and TNFR1A on the response to anti-TNF therapies in patients with rheumatoid and psoriatic arthritis. Joint Bone Spine, 2012;79(6):591–6.

83. Murdaca G, Gulli R, Spanò F, et al. TNF-alpha gene polymorphisms: association with disease susceptibility and response to anti-TNF-alpha treatment in psoriatic arthritis. J Invest Dermatol, 2014;134(10):2503–9.

84. Ramirez J, Fernández-Sueiro JL, López-Mejías R, et al. FCGR2A/CD32A and FCGR3A/CD16A variants and EULAR response to tumor necrosis factor-alpha blockers in psoriatic arthritis: a longitudinal study with 6 months of followup. J Rheumatol, 2012;39(5):1035–41.

85. Seitz M, Wirthmüller U, Möller B, Villiger PM. The -308 tumour necrosis factor-alpha gene polymorphism predicts therapeutic response to TNFalpha-blockers in rheumatoid arthritis and spondyloarthritis patients. Rheumatology (Oxford), 2007;. 46(1):93–6.

CHAPTER 7

Immunology and cytokine pathways

Bruce Kirkham

Introduction

This chapter will review our knowledge of the immunological processes thought to underpin the pathogenesis of psoriatic arthritis (PsA). It will review the increasing knowledge of cytokine pathways, in particular the interleukin 17/interleukin 23 pathway increasingly thought to play a central role in both PsA and psoriasis (PsO). Linking new knowledge of genetics, cytokines, and their cellular sources has led to major changes in current thought concerning the immunopathogenesis of these conditions.

As has been well described in preceding chapters, PsA is now differentiated from rheumatoid arthritis (RA), the most common inflammatory arthritis, initially by clinical characteristics and more recently by striking genetic differences [1]. PsA clearly belongs to the spondyloarthritis group of inflammatory arthritides. The most clear differentiating factors from RA have come from genetic studies which show no role for Class II MHC genes, but relationships to Class I MHC similar to other spondylarthropathies (SpA) [2]. Also similar to psoriasis and SpAs, PsA has relationships to cytokine genes, mainly in the interleukin-17 (IL-17)/23 pathways [3]. The specific association of PsA with Runx3 polymorphisms indicate a key role for CD8 cell mediated pathology and IL-17 responsiveness [4].

Cytokine networks

Cytokines form a large group of proteins, made by immune and sometimes non-immune cells that influence the response of both immune and non-immune cells, usually by interacting with a specific cell surface receptor. They can have pro- or anti-inflammatory properties and influence cells locally or systemically. Cytokines are often grouped into families by structure, and many cytokines have multiple effects [5]. An important role of cytokines is to coordinate immune and bystander non-immune cell activity in response to a stimulus, often infectious in nature. Many cytokines are found at sites of inflammation such as an inflamed joint. It is difficult to discern if a particular cytokine plays a key role in a particular arthropathy. Cytokine-targeted therapies have given us important information on this question, well reviewed by Schett et al. [6]. They have suggested that key cytokine 'nodes' play a pivotal role in different inflammatory conditions. Disease-specific responses to targeted cytokine inhibition relate not just to the cytokine, but to its influence on often non-immune cells, e.g. fibroblasts in the joint and keratinocytes in the skin. The key cytokine in PsA to date is tumour necrosis factor alpha (TNF-α). TNF inhibition has profound disease suppressive effects on almost all aspects of PsA disease including axial involvement and joint damage progression. Many other therapies that are successful in RA, such as B cell depletion and anti-interleukin (IL)-6 receptor blocking, have little effect in PsA. IL-17A inhibition has recently been found to have similar effects to TNF inhibition [7, 8]. IL-17 is an example of the complexity of cytokine families, with IL-17A to F now identified as structurally related family members, with differing properties, interacting with a family of receptors called IL-17R, now with five members, IL-17R A to F, which function as homo- or heterodimers, just to add to the complexity (Figure 7.1) [9]. Of potentially great importance in pathogenesis, IL-17 shows significant synergy with TNF-α in both inflammation and joint damage [6].

Cellular composition of PsA synovial pathology

Synovial tissue in normal joints and tendon sheaths consists of a thin intimal lining layer made up of fibroblast-like synoviocytes and intimal lining layer macrophages, resting on a subsynovial layer of loose connective tissue, containing blood vessels, nerve endings, fibroblasts, and adipocytes [10]. Normal synovial tissue contains a few immune cells including mast cells and macrophages in this subsynovial layer [10]. Inflamed joints are characterised by increased synovial lining cell numbers which causes it to be thicker, increased sublining vascularity and numbers of subsynovial cells, including T and B lymphocytes, macrophages, dendritic cells, fibroblasts, neutrophils and mast cells [11, 12], with a 10-fold increase in cellularity compared to non-inflamed joints [13].

Simple histology of synovial biopsies is similar for all types of inflammatory arthritis. Over the last 30 years, more detailed immunohistochemical studies have described the cellular composition of the synovial infiltrate to elucidate the immunopathogenesis of PsA [14]. Subsequent studies of cytokine and inflammatory mediator production give more detail of synovial cells function [15]. Recently high throughput techniques using gene expression and proteomic approaches have investigated the totality of cellular function in different arthritides.

Several studies compared the synovial cell types in PsA with the most common inflammatory arthritis, rheumatoid arthritis (RA) [16–19]. These studies generally report differences between PsA and

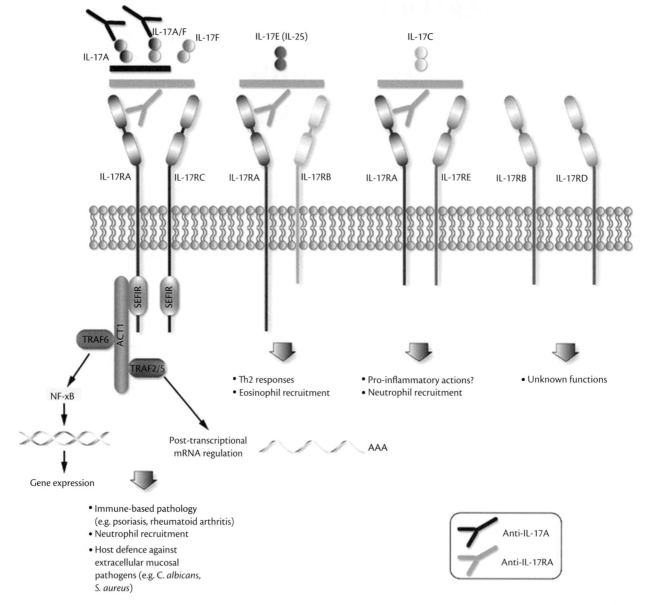

Figure 7.1 Interleukin-17 (IL-17) and IL-17 receptor family members and their biological roles. Intracellular signalling pathways of IL-17R and targets of IL-17 pathway inhibitors. Bars (according to shade) define cytokine functional inhibition by antibody.

Reprinted from Kirkham B, Kavanaugh A., and Reich K 'Interleukin-17A: a unique pathway in immune-mediated diseases: psoriasis, psoriatic arthritis, and rheumatoid arthritis' (2014) Immunology 141(2):1330142 with permission from John Wiley & Sons Ltd.

RA in cellularity and lining layer thickness. However, many patient groups were not matched for disease duration and therapy, key factors which might influence cellular composition. Danning and colleagues compared synovial membrane (SM) cellular and cytokine immunostaining in 25 subjects with PsA [20] with skin biopsies and 20 with RA, matched for disease duration, DMARD use, and erosive status [18]. More people with RA received glucocorticoids. PsA SM had thinner lining layer but increased lining layer CD68 macrophages, and interleukin (IL) -1beta (IL-1β) and TNF-α staining. Sublining vascularity and overall cellularity and cytokine staining were similar, but PsA synovium had reduced CD3 T cell numbers. More recently van Kuijk and colleagues investigated synovial pathology in patients with RA and PsA, matched for disease duration and therapy [19]. The numbers of fibroblast-like synoviocytes and macrophages were similar, but synovial CD3+T cell numbers were

considerably lower in PsA, and plasma cell numbers trended lower in patients with PsA. Staining for TNF-α, IL-lβ, IL-6, and IL-18 was similar in PsA and RA, as was matrix metalloproteinases, adhesion molecule, and vascular marker expression.

PsA is one of the spondyloarthridities along with ankylosing spondylitis (AS), reactive arthritis, inflammatory bowel disease (Crohn's disease and ulcerative colitis), related arthritis, and a less well-defined group called undifferentiated SpA (uSpA). Smaller studies suggested SM immunopathology of the different SpA subtypes was very similar. Baeten and colleagues reported one of the largest studies to date [20]. Synovial biopsies obtained from 99 SpA and 86 RA patients with active knee synovitis were analysed for 15 histological and immunohistochemical markers (Table 7.1).

The first group of 82 SpA patients was made up of 19 AS, 33 PsA, 24 USpA, 4 SpA associated with inflammatory bowel disease, and

Table 7.1 Histopathological features and scoring systems used to evaluate synovial inflammation.

Assessed by histology	
Lining-layer hyperplasia	Semiquantitative
Degree of vascularity	Semiquantitative
Inflammatory infiltration	Semiquantitative
Lymphoid aggregates	Present or absent
Plasma cells	Semiquantitative
Polymorphonuclear leukocytes	Semiquantitative
Assessed by immunohistochemistry	
CD1a	Present or absent
CD3	Semiquantitative
CD20	Semiquantitative
CD68 lining layer	Semiquantitative
CD68 sublining layer	Semiquantitative
CD163 lining layer	Semiquantitative
CD163 sublining layer	Semiquantitative
Intracellular citrullinated peptides	Present or absent
MHC class II–HC gp39 peptide complex, recognized by mAb 12A	Present or absent

Reprinted from Baeten et al. Infiltration of the synovial membrane with macrophage subsets and polymorphonuclear cells reflects global disease activity in spondyloarthropathy. Arthritis Res Ther 2005, 7:R359–R369, under CC by 2.0.

2 with reactive arthritis. A validation group consisted of 4 patients with AS, 5 with PsA and 8 with USpA. They reported no differences between the SpA subgroups using the study parameters

They then assessed the differences in SpA synovial histopathological features compared to RA. The two groups were matched for disease duration with high erythrocyte sedimentation rate (ESR),/ C-reactive protein(CRP) levels; more people with RA received disease modifying antirheumatic drugs (DMARDs) (41% vs 28% PsA) and glucocorticoids (30% vs 0%). SpA synovitis had higher vascularity and more CD163+ macrophages and polymorphonuclear leukocytes (PMN), and less lining-layer hyperplasia, and fewer lymphoid aggregates, CD1a+ cells, intracellular citrullinated proteins, and MHC–HC gp39 complexes compared to RA synovitis. A recent study by this group shows changes in lining layer macrophage cell markers, suggesting more IL-10 related changes in PsA compared to RA [21].

Despite the differences in cell composition of PsA and RA SM, studies of cytokine expression show few differences. Ritchlin and colleagues studied tissue mRNA expression by multi-gene assay, and cytokine levels in explant supernatants at day 10, comparing PsA, RA, and osteoarthritis (OA), and psoriatic skin [22]. Synovial tissues were scored histologically by a pathologist blind to the clinical diagnosis. PsA explants released elevated levels of IL-1β, IL-2, IL-10, interferon-gamma (IFNγ), and TNF-α, but not IL-4 or IL-5, with similar gene mRNA expression in whole synovial tissue. Cytokine levels were greater in PsA than RA, despite higher histopathologic scores in RA. Production of IL-1β, IFNγ, and IL-10 were strongly correlated. Levels of IFNγ, IL-1β, and

IL-10 were higher in psoriatic synovium than psoriatic dermal plaques.

More recently, Yeremenko and colleagues compared synovial molecular and cellular processes [23], identifying differentially expressed genes by pan-genomic microarray, confirmed by quantitative polymerase chain reaction and immunohistochemical analyses of synovial biopsy samples from patients with SpA (n=63), RA (n=28), and gout (n=9). Microarray analysis identified 64 up-regulated transcripts in SpA synovitis compared to RA. Pathway analysis revealed a myogene signature specific for SpA, which was independent of disease duration, treatment, and SpA subtype (non-psoriatic vs psoriatic). Synovial tissue staining identified the myogene-expressing cells as vimentin-positive, prolyl4-hydroxylase–positive, CD90+, CD146+ mesenchymal cells in the intimal lining layer and sublining areas. A small number of patients tested before and after TNF-α inhibitor therapy showed no change in the SpA specific myogene signature.

B lymphocytes are consistently found in PsA synovium, in contrast to few found in PsO skin [11, 24]. Organized lymphoid structures similar to follicles seen in lymphoid organs such as lymph nodes or spleen, and formed by ectopic lymphoid neogenesis, are also seen [25]. These are found in patients with RA, and have been related to rheumatoid factor (RF) and cyclic citrullinated peptide antibody status. In PsA, similar structures are reported, although the size and organization of these ectopic lymphoid structures is probably less than in RA [11]. Synovial gene expression relating to these structures by quantitative PCR for 21 cytokines (CCR7, IFN-γ, IL-1β, IL-2, IL-6, IL-7, IL-8, IL-10, IL-12A, IL-13, IL-15, IL-17A, IL-18, IL-21, IL-22, IL-23A, IL-28, IL-33, transforming growth factor beta (TGF-β1), TNF-α, and lymphotoxin (LTβ)), was explored in synovial fluid (SF) and SM samples from 46 patients with PsA, which clinically was often mild (median swollen and tender joint count 1, IQR 1:2) [26]. Most cytokines were expressed in most patients, although some were expressed in fewer than 50% [IL-13(24%), IL-17A (33%), IL-21 (43%), IL-22 (15%), and IL- 28A (43%)]. SF cytokine protein levels were less frequently positive and not correlated to SM mRNA expression; IL-12 and IL-28A were not detected and 11 cytokines detected in less than half of SF samples. IL-6, IL-15, and CC chemokine-ligand 20 (CCL20) were detected in either SM or SF in more than 80% of patients. Although 43% of patients demonstrated lymphoid neogenesis, cytokine expression was only different for two cytokines: IL-23A mRNA was increased and TGF-β1 was lower in patients with lymphoid neogenesis, with IL-15 expression trending higher. IL-23 mRNA levels correlated with disease activity measures and SF levels of IL-6 and CCL20 correlated with CRP.

A detailed study of SM and SF B lymphocytes in 13 patients with RA and 15 patients with PsA showed B cells in PsA had subtly different surface markers of activation from RA [27]. Increased CD86, HLA-DR, and HLA-DQ expression was found in patients with both RA and PsA. HLA-DP was significantly lower in PsA. CD40 expression was increased in SF B cells from PsA, but not RA. Extending this study, Cantaert and colleagues, explored if innate-like CD5 positive B cells, originally described in mouse models of colitis, with putative regulatory functions, were present in SpA [28]. They studied peripheral blood samples from 40 patients with SpA (9 PsA, 29 AS, 1 uSpA), 26 matched healthy controls and 23 patients with RA, and SM samples from 7 patients with RA and 6 with SpA. CD5 B cells were found in SpA SM naive, marginal zone-like, and memory B cell compartments, but not in RA. Similar to their murine counterparts, CD5 B cells from patients with SpA showed low levels of somatic hypermutation, slightly increased HLA–DR, but low CD80 and CD86 costimulatory molecule surface expression. Functionally, *in vitro* activation did not up-regulate these costimulatory molecules but induced significant production of IL-10 and IL-6 production, suggesting these cells have immunoregulatory capacity.

The functional meaning of SM B cells in PsA is unclear as auto-antibody levels are infrequent and of low titre. Recent interest in newly identified antibodies against citrullinated protein antibodies (ACPA) and carbamylated proteins (anti-CarP) are of great interest in RA [29]. Shi and colleagues assessed serum antibody levels in 2,086 patients seen at the Leiden Early Arthritis Clinic [30]. Of the 969 patients (47%) diagnosed with RA, 54% had ACPA, 59% IgM RF, and 44% anti-CarP antibodies. A low proportion of patient with PsA were positive for ACPA 6%, RF 10%, and anti-CarP 9%, similar to peripheral SpA 8%, 4%, and 15%, and OA 7%, 20%, and 11%, respectively. Healthy controls had 2% anti-CarP antibody positivity. A recent report from Chimenti and colleagues of 30 people with PsA (known to be ACPA negative) compared to 40 healthy controls, showed very low levels in controls with subsequent low cut-off levels for positivity, with 16/30 PsA patients with levels more than 64.4 units [31].

Recent reports using high through put transcriptome analysis add new information. Dolcino and colleagues identified specific gene signatures in paired peripheral blood cells (PBC) and synovial biopsies from 10 patients with PsA using Affymetrix arrays, validated by Q-PCR, FACS analysis and detection of soluble mediators [32]. Synovial biopsies of patients showed a modulation of approximately 200 genes compared to healthy donor blood. Among the differentially expressed genes, upregulation of Th17 related genes and type I interferon inducible genes were noted and FACS analysis confirmed the Th17 polarization. The synovial transcriptome showed gene clusters (bone remodelling, angiogenesis, and inflammation), with 90 genes modulated in both compartments (PBC and synovium) suggesting pathways in PBC mirror the inflamed synovium. The osteoactivin gene was highly upregulated in both PBC and synovial biopsies and high levels of osteoactivin protein was found in PsA sera, but not in serum from other inflammatory arthritides. The authors suggest the co-activation of IFN and Th17 pathways is typical of autoimmunity, and that osteoactivin may be a possible disease biomarker.

In contrast, Pollock and colleagues compared whole blood gene expression between patients with active PsA (n=20), cutaneous psoriasis (PsO) (n=20) and healthy controls (n=12) using Human Oligo microarrays [33]. PsA and PsO patients were matched for psoriasis area severity index and psoriasis duration, and controls were matched for age, sex, and ethnicity. At an adjusted false discovery rate q<0.05, 1,125 genes were differentially expressed between patients with PsA and healthy controls (56% upregulated and 44% downregulated), and 494 genes were differentially expressed between patients with PsA compared to PsO (24% upregulated and 76% downregulated). Differentially expressed genes in blood were lower in PsO patients, so not significantly different to controls. Genes upregulated in PsA compared with PsO were enriched in patterns relating to membrane, cell proliferation, cytokine activity, ribonucleoprotein, and tumour necrosis factor, and genes downregulated in PsA related to chromatin modification, nuclear

lumen, RNA splicing, and DNA/RNA helicase activity. The 'top hits' were involved in processes such as Toll-like receptor signalling (*LY96, ABCA1, TICAM1*), NK cell activation (*CD58, CLEC2B*), gene expression regulation by NF-κB (*BCL2A1*), osteoclastogenesis (*TGFBR3, NOTCH2NL*), epidermal development (*CSTA*), cell–cell recognition, signalling, and movement (*MSN, EZR*), and chromatin modification (*SETD2, SMARCA4*). More detailed exploration of the NFκB pathway using quantitative PCR arrays identified additional differentially expressed genes between PsA and PsO patients. Thirteen of 18 genes tested were significant in a replication cohort, with four (*NOTCH2NL, CXCL10, HAT1*, and *SETD2*) having fold changes concordant with the discovery cohort. The authors conclude their results suggest innate immunity may be important, via Toll-like receptor signalling, NF-κB, and various chromatin remodelling complexes, consistent with evidence implicating environmental triggers of the innate immune system, such as infections or tissue damage (the 'deep' Kobner phenomenon) in the development of PsA in PsO patients [34]. Variability of results from this work also shows that attention must be paid to clinical variables when selecting patients.

One of the most informative reports studied gene array of skin and synovial samples taken on the same day from 12 individuals with both PsA and psoriasis, confirmed by PCR, immunohistology, and cell immunofluorescence [35]. Gene expression in PsA synovium was more closely related to gene expression in PsA skin than to synovium in other forms of arthritis. However, gene expression patterns in psoriatic skin and synovium differed with a stronger IL-17 signature in skin than synovium, while TNF and IFN-γ gene signatures were more similar.

These studies confirm and extend earlier studies showing significant differences in the cellular composition of synovitis in SpA and RA. They suggest less B cell activity and more non-adaptive cellular immune and mesenchymal pathway dependent immune activation in PsA.

Enthesitis in spondyloarthritis

The spondyloarthropathies are characterized clinically by inflammation of the enthesis. Sub-clinical and intra-articular enthesitis detected by MRI, prompted McConagle and colleagues to suggest this might be a site of early inflammation in PsA, and with Benjamin, they coined the term 'synovio-entheseal complex', to emphasize the organized anatomy of these structures, with close proximity to synovial tissue [36]. This theory was given a major stimulus by an animal model of continuous high level IL-23 delivered by minicircle DNA in the context of a passive transfer model of collagen-antibody-induced arthritis, where enthesitis was an early lesion [37]. The entheseal cells that responded to IL-23, were CD3+CD4–CD8–IL-23R+ROR-γt+ T lymphoid cells, which produced IL-17 and 22, suggesting a role of innate immune cells and enthesitis in early PsA [38]. This hypothesis is the subject of a lively debate [2], but emphasizes the potential role of IL-23 in SpA. In normal human entheseal tissue, cadaveric studies (mean age 84 years [range 49–101]), showed degenerative changes and infiltrates of small numbers of inflammatory cells, mainly lymphoid cells (typically 10), with venous dilatation in 73% of sites [39]. Macrophage-like cells were sometimes seen, neutrophils were scarce, and synovial tissue, present at many sites, contained inflammatory infiltrates. Laloux and colleagues compared entheseal cellular immunopathology in pre-specified sites from surgical samples in eight subjects with AS, four with RA, most of whom were taking glucocorticoids, and three with OA [40]. Cellular infiltrates, most commonly in the bone marrow site of the enthesitis, showed significantly higher CD3, CD4 and particularly CD8 cells in patients with AS, compared to RA and OA. Access to human entheseal tissue in early arthritis is difficult. Ultrasound guided needle biopsy in five subjects with early enthesitis, confirmed by MRI and ultrasonography, was compared to control tissue obtained from two subjects at spinal surgery [41]. The SpA group showed increased vascularity and cellular infiltration compared with normal subjects. The most common infiltrating cells were CD68+ macrophages, with a few lymphocytes. Enthesis is a site of high mechanical stress which may trigger an auto-inflammatory response. A recent study, where mice that had their hind legs suspended to reduce mechanical stress, showed significantly less entheseal infiltrates compare to normally mobile control mice [42].

Serum markers of immune activity

Serum changes can sometimes give insights into important pathways of activity. Three areas of interest will be summarized here: levels of S100 calcium binding proteins (including calprotectin), adipokines, and bone-related immune active proteins.

S100A8/S100A9 (calprotectin) and S100A12 are major calcium-binding proteins highly expressed in granulocytes and early differentiation stages of monocytes. The human S100A8 protein is also known as myeloid-related protein 8, and S100A9 protein is also known as MRP-14. S100A12 is also known as extracellular newly identified receptor for advanced glycation end product–binding protein (EN-RAGE) [43]. In PsA SM, these proteins are mainly detected in perivascular areas of the sublining layer, very different to RA where they are found in the lining layer and sublining aggregates [44]. As S100A12 plays a key role in endothelial cell activation this pattern may have functional consequences. Serum levels are elevated both in PsA and RA, with reduced levels after methotrexate and TNF-inhibitor therapy [45]. Turina and colleagues found serum levels of calprotectin, hs-CRP, pentraxin-3, VEGF (all $P < 0.001$), and MMP-3 ($P = 0.062$), but not IL-6 and alpha-2-macroglobulin, were increased in SpA (n=18) vs healthy controls (n=20) [46]. Treatment with infliximab, but not placebo, significantly decreased calprotectin and hs-CRP levels, with a trend for MMP-3. Hansson and colleagues noted patients suffering polyarthritic patterns of PsA (n=33) had significantly higher levels of S-calprotectin compared with controls (n=31) and patients with mono-/oligoarthritis PsA (n=32). Serum levels of S-calprotectin correlated with hs-CRP, swollen joint count, and CXCL10 [47].

Patients with PsA have increased rates of obesity compared to healthy controls and also to people with PsO [48]. Adipose tissue is mainly composed of adipocytes, with a stromal–vascular fraction, which includes macrophages [49]. Adipocytes secrete adipokines which play diverse physiologic roles, including insulin resistance, but can also interact with immune cells. It is proposed that leptin, visfatin, and resistin have pro-inflammatory activities. In contrast, the most frequently measured adipokine, adiponectin (particularly the low molecular weight isoform) is believed to have anti-inflammatory effects. Adipose tissue can also produce pro-inflammatory cytokines such as TNFα, IL-6, and IL-8, and chemokines such as monocyte chemoattractant protein-1 (MCP-1).

Eder and colleagues found the prevalence of metabolic syndrome trended higher in PsA patients (n=203) compared to PsO (n=155) (36.5% vs 27.1%, P=0.056). Significant increases in prevalence of insulin resistance, and levels of adiponectin and in women, leptin, were noted [50]. Xue and colleagues compared adipokines in 41 people with PsA and 24 healthy controls [51]. Patients with PsA had higher leptin and omentin levels, but lower adiponectin and chemerin levels, and also higher TNF-α, RANKL, and osteoclast numbers assessed by TRAP staining. Serum levels of TNF-α, RANKL, leptin, and omentin positively correlated with osteoclast numbers. Continuing the exploration of bone active serum markers, Dalbeth and colleagues found patients with PsA (n=38) compared to those with psoriasis (n=10) and healthy controls (n=12) had higher circulating concentrations of Dikkopf-1 (Dkk-1), a bone anabolic protein, and M-CSF, but not RANKL [52]. In PsA, M-CSF and RANKL positively correlated with radiographic erosion, joint space narrowing, and osteolysis scores. Peripheral blood CD14+/CD11b+ cells, osteoclast-like cell numbers and resorptive pits after culture with RANKL and M-CSF, correlated with radiographic damage scores, and M-CSF concentrations correlated with the percentage of peripheral blood CD14+/CD11b+ cells.

These studies illustrate that systemic inflammatory mediators and cells, adipokines and bone active molecules are a feature of the immunological and pathogenic landscape of PsA which differentiates it from the more skin based pathology of PsO.

New concepts of pathogenesis

New knowledge is producing a major transformation in understanding of the immuno-pathogenesis of PsO [53] and PsA [54]. Initially PsO was thought to be a disorder of abnormal keratinocyte function. Then as psoriatic skin was infiltrated by cells of the acquired or adaptive immune system, psoriasis was considered an 'auto-immune' condition. However the epidemiology and more recently genetic basis of psoriasis has led to changes in this view [53, 55]. Environmental factors related to psoriasis include trauma (the well-known but poorly understood Koebner phenomenon], infections (streptococcal, viral including HIV], hypocalcaemia in generalized pustular psoriasis, psychogenic stress, and some drugs. This epidemiology, with genetic relationships relating to non-immune pathways, has produced the current view that psoriasis could be a dysregulated inflammatory response to multiple environmental stimuli [23, 53]. Similarly concepts of the pathogenesis of PsA, previously considered a T-lymphocyte-driven autoimmune condition are also under discussion [54, 56]. Recent genome-wide association studies in PsA identify variants of the *TRAF3IP2* gene, encoding Act-1 (NF-κB activator 1), a key mediator of IL-17 signalling [57, 58], and the *RUNX3* gene [59], a transcription factor that promotes CD8+ T-cell development in the thymus, as risk factors for disease development. In addition, there has been renewed interest in the role of mechanical stress and inflammation at the enthesis [60]. These new concepts have been supported by new information relating to the role and type of cells producing IL-17 and the related IL-23 pathway [37]. Many of these cells are part of the innate immune system, a vital system for rapid responses to many environmental and infectious stimuli, which interact with the adaptive immune system, which is generally slower to respond to an initial stimulus, but has memory [37].

The innate immune system

Innate immunity plays a key role in the early response to pathological insults especially infections [61]. Cells of the innate immune system can respond immediately to signals from pathogens or cellular damage, with cytokine and cell-to-cell responses. This provides early defence and also interacts with the acquired immune system to stimulate and direct this system's initial response [62]. The skin, as the primary interface with the external environment, provides the first line of host defence against injury and infection [63]. Similar to the lung and gut mucosal barrier, the skin is equipped with a diverse set of immune cells which can react to different insults, but also have the potential to cause abnormal responses and disease. Many are innate immune system cells, including several lymphoid cell subsets, polymorphonuclear neutrophils, dendritic cells, and tissue Langerhans cells [64, 65].

Natural killer (NK) cells, gamma delta (γδ) T-cells and innate lymphoid cells (ILCs) are important lymphocyte subsets able both to produce cytokines including IL-17 and to kill cellular targets [66]. NK cells are large granular lymphocytes, defined by their expression of CD56 and the lack of a T-cell receptor (TCR)–CD3 complex, whose functions include killing cells that are expressing stress-induced molecules. NK cells are part of a group of cells called innate lymphoid cells which do not have rearranged T-cell receptors (TCR). They react to cytokines and cellular ligands, produced in tissues after infection or injury, as well as to pathogen-associated molecular patterns [67]. NK cells have receptors that recognize and respond to human leucocyte antigen (HLA), including the killer immunoglobulin-like receptors (KIRs). Some KIRs can recognize different forms of HLA-B27 and this pathway has been implicated in spondyloarthritis pathogenesis [68]. HLA-B27 genotype is highly expressed in the PsA subset presenting with axial (spinal) components of the disease, so a similar pathogenic mechanism may be involved in this group [2].

ILCs are lymphoid cells that do not express the usual markers of T and B cells [69]. Three groups are described in humans, relating to their dependence on the transcriptional repressor Inhibitor of DNA binding 2 (Id2) and on the IL-2Rγ chain. The ILC3 subset, which also includes lymphoid tissue inducer cells, is dependent on the transcription factor RORγT, as well as expression of the IL-7Rα chain, and can produce IL-17A and/or IL-22 upon stimulation [70]. In humans, ILC3 can be subdivided on the basis of the expression of the natural cytotoxicity receptors—NKp44, NKp46, and NKp30—which identifies those cells that can produce IL-22 and / or IL-17A.

γδ cells are a population of CD3 T-cells that express a TCR comprising, γ and δ chains, related but distinct from the usual T cell αβTCR [64]. γδ T-cells are enriched in epithelial and mucosal tissues [71]. Similar to NK cells, γδ T cells are involved in non-MHC-restricted cytotoxicity in cell-mediated immune responses. The γδ TCR does not engage MHC-antigen complexes like αβ T cells but acts more like a pattern recognition receptor, recognizing factors produced by bacterial metabolic pathways, cell damage, and inflammatory cytokines produced by macrophages or dendritic cells responding to infectious signals [66]. Most human γδ T cells are either the Vδ1+ (peripheral blood) or Vδ2+ subclasses (epithelial sites).

Recently, it has become clear that cytokine patterns generating functional phenotypes initially seen in adaptive immune lymphocytes, such as Th1 and Th2 subsets, are replicated in innate lymphocytes. These data are summarized in a recent review suggesting that both innate and adaptive immune responses can be divided into three groups, Type 1 (IFNγ dependent), Type 2 (IL-4 etc), and Type 3 (IL-17 pathway) [72].

Innate and adaptive immune cells in psoriatic arthritis

γδ T cells

Spadero and colleagues investigated γδ TCR antigen and NK surface marker positive cells by flow cytometry in PB and SF lymphocytes from people with PsA (n=17), RA (n=16), and healthy controls [73]. Both PsA and RA patients had reduced peripheral blood γδ T cells compared to healthy controls (percentages and absolute numbers), with similar levels in SF and PB. In contrast, PB levels of NK and NK-T lymphocytes were similar in all groups; however, SF levels were lower than PB in both PsA and RA. There were no significant correlations of the different cell subsets with clinical or serological measures. Kenna et al. studied PB IL-23R+T cells in 17 patients with active AS, 8 with PsA, 9 with RA, and 20 healthy subjects [74]. The proportion of PB IL-23R+T cells was two-fold higher in patients with AS compared to healthy controls, due to a three-fold increase in IL-23R+ γδ T cells. In vitro stimulation with IL-23 and/or anti-CD3/CD28 enhanced IL-17 secretion by IL-23R+γδ T cells, but not IL-23R– γδ T cells in AS patients. Since IL-23 is a maturation and growth factor for IL-17–producing cells, increased IL-23R expression may regulate the function of this putative pathogenic γδ T cell population.

γδ T cells mediate rapid tissue responses in murine skin and participate in cutaneous immune regulation including protection against cancer [75], but little is known about the role of human γδ cells in cutaneous disease. Laggner and colleagues showed that human blood contains a subset of pro-inflammatory cutaneous lymphocyte antigen (a marker of cells that traffic to the skin) and C-C chemokine receptor 6 positive Vγ9Vδ2 T cells, which is rapidly recruited into abnormal human skin [76]. Patients with psoriasis had increased Vγ9Vδ2 T cells in psoriatic skin, with lower peripheral blood levels, compared to healthy controls and patients with atopic dermatitis, which normalized after successful treatment of skin psoriasis. These cells produced pro-inflammatory mediators including IL-17A and activated keratinocytes in a TNF-α and IFN-γ dependent process.

NK cells

Dalbeth and Callan reported on NK cell frequency in paired samples of peripheral blood and SF from 22 patients with inflammatory arthritis, 5 of whom had SpA (3 PsA, 2 AS) [77]. PB and SF cell numbers were similar, but SF cells showed a different distribution of NK cell phenotypes, most expressing high levels of CD56. Most SF NK cells did not express CD16 or KIR/KAR, but expressed high levels of CD94 and an NK receptor called natural killer group 2 member A (NKG2A). Synovial NK cells responded to a combination of IL-12 and IL-15 by rapidly secreting IFNγ. It was suggested that this subset may be recruited from the periphery and further activated by cytokines in the joint. Tang et al. had previously reported that IL-15 is capable of arming CD8 effector T cells to kill independently of their TCR via NKG2D in a cytosolic phospholipase A2 (cPLA2)-dependent process [78]. As NK cells also express NKG2D, they investigated if resting NK cells could be primed to the effector phase by IL-15, and studied a possible role for this pathway in PsA. They reported PsA patients had upregulated IL-15 and major histocompatibility complex class I chain-related A (MICA) in synovial tissues. This environment enabled NK cell activation and killing via NKG2D and cPLA2, and incubating blood NK cells with IL-15 reproduced the joint NK cell phenotype. These findings, similar to those of Dalbeth and Callan [77], suggest a possible pathogenic role for NK cells, activated by environmental stress signals and primed by IL-15.

Lower peripheral blood NK cell numbers were confirmed by Conigliara and colleagues who found RA (n=82) and PsA (n=32) patients had reduced peripheral blood NK and B cell numbers compared to healthy controls [79]. NK and B cell numbers increased to normal levels in both groups after etanercept therapy, with NK cell increases associated with clinical responses in both RA and PsA.

NK cells are rare in healthy skin. In patients with psoriasis the frequency of cells expressing NK receptors, such as CD56, is significantly increased in lesional skin, with decreased peripheral blood levels compared to healthy controls [80, 81]. Their pathological relevance is unclear, but injecting peripheral blood NK cells from subjects with psoriasis into human skin grafts in mice can form psoriasiform-like changes [82].

Innate lymphoid cells

ILCs were characterized in the peripheral blood (PB) of healthy controls, patients with PsO and PsA, and SF of patients with PsA and RA [83]. Fewer CCR6+ ILCs were found in PsA PB than in healthy control PB. In PsA SF, ILCs were four-fold more abundant than PsA PB, and enriched for CCR6+ ILCs compared to PsA PB and RA SF. Natural cytotoxicity receptor NKp44+ group 3 ILCs were rare in PB and RA SF, but abundant in PsA SF. Increased numbers of IL-17A-producing ILCs, positive for surface CCR6, NKp44, and melanoma cell adhesion molecule (MCAM) were present in PsA SF compared to RA SF. Blood NKp44+, CCR6+, MCAM+ ILC numbers inversely correlated with PsA disease activity.

In PsO, a substantial proportion of IL-17A and IL-22 producing cells in skin and blood of normal individuals and psoriasis patients are CD3 negative innate lymphocytes [84]. In contrast to the PsA report above, circulating NKp44+ ILC3 in blood of psoriasis patients was increased compared to healthy individuals or atopic dermatitis patients, with more than 50% of circulating NKp44+ ILC3 expressing the cutaneous lymphocyte-associated antigen indicating their potential for skin homing. Psoriasis skin had an increased frequency of total ILC compared to blood, and NKp44+ ILC3 were also increased in non-lesional psoriatic skin compared to normal skin. Teunissen and colleagues [85] confirmed these findings and showed NKp44+ ILC3 cells from skin and blood of psoriasis patients produced IL-22, suggesting they may participate in psoriasis pathology.

MAIT cells

Mucosa-associated invariant T (MAIT) cells are innate T cells that are abundant in humans, which possess an evolutionarily conserved invariant T cell receptor α chain restricted by the nonpolymorphic class Ib major histocompatibility (MHC) molecule, MHC class I-related protein (MR1). MAIT cells are activated by a MR1-bound riboflavin (vitamin B$_2$) metabolite [86]. As animals cannot synthesize riboflavin, riboflavin derivatives act as signals for the immune system to a broad range of microbial pathogens. MAIT cells produce cytokines such as IFN-γ, TNF, and IL-17A [86]. Recent reports have suggested that the majority of IL-17A+ CD8+ T cells in the blood are MAIT cells. MAIT cells are found in psoriatic skin; however, they are not increased in abundance [87]. The majority of IL-17A+CD8+ T cells in psoriasis skin plaques are devoid of MAIT cell characteristics [88, 89]. In our study of SF in patients with PsA, IL-17+ SF cells showed no increase in MAIT cells compared to peripheral blood [90].

Dendritic cells

Dendritic cells (DCs) play a key role in accumulating and processing antigens and presenting them to the immune system with cytokines such as IL-12 and IL-23 which have profound effects on the type of adaptive lymphoid response. Initially their immuno-stimulatory roles were recognized, but recently key immunoregulatory roles have also been suggested [91]. Jongbloed and colleagues characterized the immunophenotype and functional characteristics of myeloid DCs (mDCs) and plasmacytoid DCs (pDCs) in patients with PsA and RA [92]. Peripheral blood pDC numbers were significantly reduced in both PsA and RA, with an immature phenotype compared to healthy controls, with decreased CD62L expression on both subsets. mDCs and pDCs were present in PsA and RA synovial fluid with the mDC:pDC ratio significantly exceeding that in PB. Synovial fluid pDCs displayed an immature phenotype comparable with PB pDCs. In contrast, RA and PsA synovial fluid mDCs displayed a more mature phenotype (increased CD80, CD83, and CD86 expression) compared to PB mDCs. Both SF subsets matured following Toll-like receptor (TLR) stimulation. pDCs from PB and SF produced INF-γ and TNFα on TLR9 stimulation, but only SF pDCs produced IL-10. Similarly, mDCs from PB and SF produced similar TNFα levels in response to TLR2, but SF mDCs produced more IL-10 than PB controls. These data show the potential for these cells to play a role both in a pro and anti-inflammatory role [93].

Lande and colleagues examined the presence and phenotype of SF pDCs in patients with RA, PsA, and OA [94]. pDC cells were 4- to 5-fold higher in RA SF and PsA SF than OA SF, and similar to above were in an immature state, but matured when exposed ex vivo to viral agents or unmethylated DNA. CXCR3 and CXCR4 were expressed by both blood and SF pDCs and the chemokines, CXCL-10, CXCL-11, and CXCL-12, present in RA and PsA SF could stimulate chemotaxis of blood-derived pDCs. These findings suggest that chemokines drive recruitment of pDCs from blood to the inflamed synovium in both PsA and RA.

Recently Wenink and colleagues tested the hypothesis that an impaired response by DCs might compromise the clearance of bacteria and predispose to chronic inflammation, by studying cytokine production by DC from healthy controls and patients with RA, PsA, and PsO in response to mycobacterial, other bacterial, and TLR ligands [95]. Proinflammatory cytokine secretion by PsA DCs was impaired after in vitro challenge with mycobacterial and TLR-2 ligands. This impairment was associated with elevated serum levels of CRP. Expression of TLR-2 and other receptors known to mediate mycobacterial recognition was stable, but intracellular TLR inhibitors were higher in DCs from PsA patients. The authors suggest their findings indicate that DCs from PsA patients have a disordered immune response toward some species of (myco)bacteria.

Impaired clearance of bacteria may generate chronic inflammation of joints, entheses, skin, and the gut.

Human skin studies have focused on the role of immunostimulatory DCs during skin inflammation [96]. In human skin, myeloid DCs that reside in the dermis represent a major subset of dermal DCs during tissue homeostasis. Recently, Chu and colleagues, showed that CD141+ dermal DCs are a major IL-10–producing skin-resident DC subset [97]. These cells induced T cell hyporesponsiveness and CD25hi regulatory T cells that suppress skin inflammation. Vitamin D3 (VitD3)-induced CD141+ cells generated from blood DCs shared phenotypic and functional features of skin-resident CD141+ dermal DCs. They regulate alloimmunity functions, and the authors suggest they may have similar role *in vivo*.

CD4 cells

CD25+CD4+ regulatory T cells participate in the regulation of immune responses and have been shown to be present in RA joints [98]. Cao and colleagues investigated the presence and regulatory function of these cells in SF and PB samples obtained during relapse from 36 patients with spondyloarthropathies, 21 adults with juvenile idiopathic arthritis and 135 patients with RA [99]. Of 192 patients, 182 demonstrated a higher frequency of CD25bright CD4+ T cells in SF than in peripheral blood. Interestingly compared to healthy subjects, patients had significantly fewer CD25brightCD4+ T cells in PB. Functional studies in eight patients showed CD25brightCD4+ T SF cells suppressed the production of both type 1 and 2 cytokines including IL-7, and proliferation, independent of diagnosis. This and other studies mainly in RA, show regulatory T cells are present in most inflammatory arthritides, with functions that could potentially regulate immune activation, but the effectiveness of their regulatory role *in vivo* is unclear.

Expression of the adhesion molecule, CD146/MCAM/MelCAM, on T cells has been associated with recent activation, memory subsets, and Th17 effector function, and is elevated in inflammatory arthritis. Wu and colleagues compared the expression of CD146 on PB and SF CD4+ T cells from healthy donors and patients with RA, AS or PsA [100]. CD146+CD4+ and IL-17+CD4+ T cell frequencies were increased in PB cells from PsA patients, compared with healthy donors, and in SF compared with PB. CD146+CD4+ T cells were enriched for secretion of IL-17 (alone or with IL-22 or IFN-γ) and putative Th17-associated surface markers (CD161 and CCR6), but not others (CD26 and IL-23 receptor). CD4+ T cells producing IL-22 or IFN-γ, without IL-17, were less commonly present in the CD146+ subset. However, the majority of cells secreting these cytokines lacked CD146. These data suggest CD146 is not a sensitive or specific marker of Th17 cells.

CD8 cells

An early finding of immune cells that differentiated PsA from RA was that in PsA, SF CD8+T cells were enriched compared to CD4+T cells, reversing the CD4:CD8 ratio [101]. This difference was greatest in patients with oligoarticular PsA, but not significantly different from PsA patients with polyarticular disease. The authors suggested CD8 T cells may play an important role in the pathogenesis in PsA, a HLA class I mediated disease

This group went on to use TCR beta-chain nucleotide sequencing to determine whether the oligoclonal expansions previously reported in PsA [102], represent extreme determinant spreading among driving clones that recognize autoantigens or were non-antigen-driven, inflammation-related expansions [103]. They hypothesized that clones persisting after methotrexate treatment, which reduced but did not eliminate disease activity, may drive inflammation. Seventy-six percent of the T cell clones in active tissue were polyclonal and unexpanded, accounting for 31% of transcripts, and were reduced by methotrexate therapy. Most expanded clones in the inflamed joint did not persist during methotrexate treatment, were found only in inflammatory sites, exhibited no structural homology to one another, and were either CD4 or CD8 in lineage, suggesting they were non-autoantigen-driven, inflammation-related expansions. The 12% of the expanded clones which could be grouped into clonal sets suggesting antigen drive, were exclusively CD8 lineage, persisted during methotrexate administration, and were present in both SF and blood. However, a major set of these putative driver CD8 clones exhibited a previously described EBV-specific beta-chain motif, emphasizing that the dominant feature of the disease was activation of multiple clones apparently lacking specificity for an inciting autoantigen. The authors suggested that alternative routes of CD8 T cell activation such as the killer immunoglobulin receptor might have an important role. This hypothesis remains central to the B27-induced unfolded protein response for AS [68], as discussed under 'The innate immune system'.

Immunohistochemical studies of IL-17 expression in psoriasis skin show neutrophils and mast cells are the most frequently stained cells [104]. Neutrophils had originally been shown to produce IL-17 mRNA in studies of lung pathology [105]. Neutrophil staining for IL-17A was almost completely lost within 2 weeks of beginning treatment with an anti-IL-17A monoclonal antibody, secukinumab, at a time when skin changes are first noted. In contrast, mononuclear cells including lymphocytes and mast cells remained positive up to 12 weeks [106]. These findings in skin were replicated in earlier studies of SM, where mast cells are the most numerous cells staining for IL-17A in both PsA and RA [107–109]. A recent study of spinal facet joints from patients with AS compared to OA, demonstrated significant bone marrow immune cell infiltrates, with IL-17-secreting cells detected at a higher frequency in AS than OA [110]. The majority of IL-17+ cells were indicative of neutrophils, while CD3+ T cells and AA-1+ mast cells were less often IL-17-positive. The issue of whether mast cells produce IL-17, i.e. contain detectable IL-17mRNA for IL-17, or absorb IL-17 via IL-17 receptors is as yet unclear.

These immunohistochemical findings led some observers to hypothesize that IL-17+ T lymphocytes may not play a role in PsA or PsO [111, 112]. However, when skin cells from patients with PsO, were investigated by biopsy tissue digestion and preparation of mononuclear cells, followed by short *in vitro* stimulation and flow cytometry, it was clear that IL-17+ T lymphocytes were present [113]. Res and colleagues, noted that in psoriatic plaques, both CD4+IL-17+ and CD8+IL-17+ lymphocytes were detected [114], with the frequency of CD8+IL-17+ cells related to the psoriasis severity. CD8+ IL-17+ cells, previously detected in response to bacterial infections had been termed 'Tc17' cells to differentiate them from the well-known Th17 cells [115]. They have less cytotoxic capacity compared to the usual CD8+ IFNγ+ cytotoxic T cell, and probably have an immune activating role [115]. Preliminary studies of naive CD8 T cells show they follow a similar differentiation pathway to Th17 cells, utilizing IL-1β, IL-6 and TGF- β, with a secondary critical role for IL-23 in stabilizing the cell type and triggering Il-17 production [116]. A recent report suggests skin mast cells are positive for IL-17A mRNA, but that most IL-17A is produced by skin CD8+ lymphocytes, with mast cells producing more IL-22 [117].

Our group recently reported for the first time, that the PsA joint, but not the RA joint, is enriched for IL-17+CD8+ T cells [90]. Mononuclear cells from paired samples of SF and PB from 21 patients with PsA or RA (n=14) were stimulated *ex vivo*, and T cells examined by flow cytometry. In PsA, both IL-17+CD4- (predominantly CD8+, i.e. Tc17 cells) and IL-17+CD4+T cells (Th17 cells) were significantly enhanced in SF compared to PB. In contrast, in RA, only IL-17+CD4+T cells were increased in the SF. The Tc17 cells in PsA SF positively correlated with multiple disease activity measures, including CRP level, ESR, Disease Activity Score in 28 joints and power Doppler ultrasound score, and were increased in PsA patients with erosive disease compared to those with non-erosive disease, while SF Th17 cell levels did not significantly correlate with any measures. CD107a, perforin, and granzyme B were attenuated in IL-17+CD8+ T cells compared to IFNγ+CD8+T cells, indicating these IL-17+CD8+ T cells are not prototypical cytotoxic cells. These findings suggest a similarity in immunopathologic characteristics of PsA and PsO, and emphasize the difference to RA. They also provide a mechanism for the long-suggested potential pathogenic role for CD8+ T cells in PsA [101]. In addition, we found no increase in γδ cells or MAIT cells in SF compared to PB, and did not detect differences in the frequencies of PB IL-17+ T cells from patients with PsA, RA, or age matched healthy controls, similar to some previous reports [74, 110].

van Baarsen and colleagues recently reported very different results to previous immunohistochemical studies. They studied SM biopsies from 15 patients with PsA, 11 RA, 10 inflammatory OA and 7 controls from non-inflamed knee joints [118]. Frozen sections stained for IL-17A, IL-17F, and the IL-17 receptors, IL-17RA and IL-17RC, were evaluated by digital image analysis, and confocal microscopy and double-staining with CD4, CD8, CD15, CD68, CD163, CD31, von Willebrand factor, peripheral lymph node addressin, lymphatic vessel endothelial hyaluronan receptor 1, mast cell tryptase, and retinoic acid receptor–related orphan receptor γt (RORγt) to determine which synovial cells expressed IL-17A and IL-17F. In contrast to previous studies, they found IL-17A, IL-17F, IL-17RA, and IL-17RC were abundantly expressed in synovial tissues of all patient groups. IL-17RA was mainly present in the sublining layer and IL-17RC in the intimal lining layer. Quantitative digital image analysis demonstrated only IL-17A was significantly more highly expressed in arthritis patients compared to non-inflamed control patients. The expression of IL-17A, IL-17F, and their receptors was similar in different patient groups, but highly variable between individual patients. CD4+ and CD8+ cells coexpressed IL-17A, and few cells coexpressed IL-17F. IL-17A and IL-17F were not detected in CD15+ neutrophils, and mast cells were infrequently positive for IL-17A or IL-17F. Many cells were positive for the transcription factor RORγt, and colocalization of RORγt and IL-17A/IL-17F suggested those cell are producing IL-17. The authors suggest heterogeneous expression levels may explain non-response to anti-IL-17 therapy in some patients.

The synovium is characterized by abundant fibroblast cells, which may have a key role in mediating inflammatory pathways and have been extensively studied in RA [6]. Few studies in PsA

are reported but a recent study of the effects of Janus kinase inhibition on fibroblast function suggested PsA fibroblasts are activated similar to RA [119]. PsA fibroblasts showed functions of invasion, network formation, and migration, with spontaneous secretion of IL-6, IL-8, MCP-1, MMP9/MMP2, MMP3, IP-10, and IL-10. A recent immunohistochemical study showed RANKL was expressed by fibroblast-like synoviocytes as well as sublining T lymphocytes [120]. RANK-positive osteoclast precursors but no mature TRAP-positive osteoclasts were detected. Interestingly despite different rates and patterns of joint damage, the results were not different between nonpsoriatic SpA, psoriatic SpA or RA groups. Only a subset of patients with the best systemic response to TNF inhibition had decreased intimal lining layer RANKL expression. PsA synovium has more (non-degranulated) mast cells compared to RA synovium [11]. A study of IL-33 and its receptor ST2, which have a potential role of stimulating mast cells, showed heterogenous synovial biopsy mRNA levels and staining of IL-33 in endothelial cells and sometimes fibroblasts, that were not different between patients with PsA, RA, or OA. IL-33 was undetectable in serum and SF in PsA, and serum ST2 levels only higher in RA [121].

Conclusion

Increased knowledge of innate immunity and the important role of IL-17/23 biology in both psoriasis and psoriatic arthritis, have led to new theories of immunopathogenesis in both conditions [122]. Many innate immune cells reside in skin, which could directly translate environmental signals into a chronic adaptive immune response. The joint has fewer resident innate immune cells and is less well researched. The new information summarized here will provide important hypotheses for investigation of pathogenic pathways. Differences in non-immune cell function may also be critical mediators of response [6], e.g. production of IL-12 or IL-23 by dendritic cells. Keratinocytes in skin [123] and fibroblasts in joints may be critical in mediating cytokine production and effector function.

References

1. Eder L, Chandran V, Gladman DD. What have we learned about genetic susceptibility in psoriasis and psoriatic arthritis? Curr Opin Rheumatol 2015;27:91–8. Review.
2. FitzGerald O, Haroon M, Giles JT, Winchester R. Concepts of pathogenesis in psoriatic arthritis: genotype determines clinical phenotype. Arthritis Res Ther 2015;17(1):115.
3. Nair RP, Duffin KC, Helms C, et al. Genome-wide scan reveals association of PsO with IL-23 and NF-κB pathways. Nat Genet 2009;41:199–204.
4. Veale D. Psoriatic arthritis: recent progress in Pathophysiology and drug development. Arthritis Res Ther 2013;15: 224 10.1186/ar4414
5. Dinarello CA, Cannon JG, Wolff SM, et al. Tumor necrosis factor (cachectin) is an endogenous pyrogen and induces production of interleukin 1. J Exp Med 1986;163(6):1433–50.
6. Schett G, Elewaut D, McInnes IB, Dayer JM, Neurath MF. How cytokine networks fuel inflammation: toward a cytokine-based disease taxonomy. Nat Med 2013;19:822–4.
7. McInnes IB, Mease PJ, Kirkham B, et al. Secukinumab, a human anti-interleukin-17A monoclonal antibody, in patients with psoriatic arthritis (FUTURE 2): a randomised, double-blind, placebo - controlled, phase 3 trial. Lancet. 2015;386: 1137–46.
8. Mease PJ, McInnes IB, Kirkham B, et al. Secukinumab nhibition of interleukin-17A in patients with psoriatic arthritis. N Engl J Med 2015;373:1329–39.

9. Gaffen SL, Jain R, Garg AV, Cua DJ. IL-23-IL-17 immune axis: Discovery, mechanistic understanding, and clinical testing. Nat Rev Immunol 2014;14:585–600.

10. Smith MD, Barg E, Weedon H, et al. Microarchitecture and protective mechanisms in synovial tissue from clinically and arthroscopically normal knee joints. Ann Rheum Dis 2003;62:303–7.

11. van de Sande MG, Baeten DL. Immunopathology of synovitis: from histology to molecular pathways. Rheumatology (Oxford) 2015; pii: kev330. Review.

12. van Kuijk AW, Tak PP. Synovitis in psoriatic arthritis: immunohistochemistry, comparisons with rheumatoid arthritis, and effects of therapy. Curr Rheumatol Rep 2011;13:353–9.

13. Van Landuyt KB, Jones E A, McGonagle D, Luyten F P, Lories R J. Flow cytometric characterization of freshly isolated and culture expanded human synovial cell populations in patients with chronic arthritis. Arthritis Res Ther 2010;12:R15.

14. Codullo V, McInnes IB. Synovial tissue response to treatment in psoriatic arthritis. Open Rheumatol J 2011;5:133–7. doi: 10.2174/1874312901105010133.

15. Baeten D, Van Damme N, Van den Bosch F et al. Impaired Th1 cytokine production in spondyloarthropathy is restored by anti-TNFalpha. Ann Rheum Dis 2001;60:750–5.

16. Kruithof E, Baeten D, De RL, Vandooren B, et al. Synovial histo-pathology of psoriatic arthritis, both oligo- and polyarticular, resembles spondyloarthropathy more than it does rheumatoid arthritis. Arthritis Res Ther 2005;7:R569–80.

17. Veale D, Yanni G, Rogers S, Barnes L, Bresnihan B, Fitzgerald O. Reduced synovial membrane macrophage numbers, ELAM-1 expression, and lining layer hyperplasia in psoriatic arthritis as compared with rheumatoid arthritis. Arthritis Rheum. 1993;36:893–900.

18. Danning CL, Illei GG, Hitchon C, Greer MR, Boumpas DT, McInnes IB. Macrophage-derived cytokine and nuclear factor kappaB p65 expression in synovial membrane and skin of patients with psoriatic arthritis. Arthritis Rheum. 2000;43(6):1244–56.

19. van Kuijk AWR, Reinders-Blankert P, Smeets TJM, Dijkmans BAC, Tak PP. Detailed analysis of the cell infiltrate and the expression of mediators of synovial inflammation and joint destruction in the synovium of patients with psoriatic arthritis: implications for treatment. Ann Rheum Dis 2006;65:1551–1557.

20. Baeten D, Kruithof E, De Rycke L, et al. Infiltration of the synovial membrane with macrophage subsets and polymorphonuclear cells reflects global disease activity in spondyloarthropathy. Arthritis Res Ther 2005; 7:R359–69.

21. Ambarus CA, Noordenbos T, de Hair MJ, Tak PP, Baeten DL. Intimal lining layer macrophages but not synovial sublining macrophages display an IL-10 polarized-like phenotype in chronic synovitis. Arthritis Res Ther 2012;14:R74.

22. Ritchlin C, Haas-Smith SA, Hicks D, Cappuccio J, Osterland CK, Looney RJ. Patterns of cytokine production in psoriatic synovium. J Rheumatol 1998;25:1544–52.

23. Yeremenko N, Noordenbos T, Cantaert T, et al. Disease-specific and inflammation-independent stromal alterations in spondylarthritis synovitis. Arthritis Rheum. 2013; 65: 174–85.

24. Mak RKH, Hundhausen C, Nestle FO, Progress in understanding the immunopathogenesis of psoriasis. Clinical subtypes, histological features and associated comorbidities. Actas Dermosifiliogr. 2009;100 (Suppl 2):2–13.

25. Veale DJ, Barnes L, Rogers S, FitzGerald O Immunohistochemical markers for arthritis in psoriasis. Ann Rheum Dis 1994;53:450–4.

26. Celis R, Planell N, Fernández-Sueiro JL et al. Synovial cytokine expression in psoriatic arthritis and associations with lymphoid neogenesis and clinical features. Arthritis ResTher 2012;14:R93.

27. Armas-González E, Díaz-Martín A, Domínguez-Luis MJ, et al. Differential antigen-presenting b cell phenotypes from synovial microenvironment of patients with rheumatoid and psoriatic arthritis. J Rheumatol 2015;42:1825–34.

28. Cantaert T, Doorenspleet ME, FrancoSalinas G, et al. Increased numbers of CD5_B lymphocytes with a regulatory phenotype in spondylarthritis. Arthritis Rheum 2012;64:1859–68.

29. Jiang X, Trouw LA, van Wesemael TJ, Shi J, et al. Anti-CarP antibodies in two large cohorts of patients with rheumatoid arthritis and their relationship to genetic risk factors, cigarette smoking and other autoantibodies. Ann Rheum Dis 2014;73:1761–8.

30. Jing Shi J, van Steenbergen HW, van Nies JAB, et al. The specificity of anti-carbamylated protein antibodies for rheumatoid arthritis in a setting of early arthritis. Arth Res Ther 2015;17:339.

31. Chimenti MS, Triggianese P, Nuccetelli M, et al. Auto-reactions, autoimmunity and psoriatic arthritis. Autoimmun Rev 2015;14:1142–6.

32. Dolcino M, Ottria A, Barbieri A, et al. Gene expression profiling in peripheral blood cells and synovial membranes of patients with psoriatic arthritis. PLoS ONE 2015; 10(6):e0128262.

33. Pollock RA, Abji F, Liang K, et al. Gene expression differences between psoriasis patients with and without inflammatory arthritis. J Invest Dermatol 2015;135:620–3.

34. Riol-Blanco L, Ordovas-Montanes J, Perro M, et al. Nociceptive sensory neurons drive interleukin-23 mediated psoriasiform skin inflammation. Nature 2014;510:157–61.

35. Belasco J, Louie JS, Gulati N, et al. Comparative genomic profiling of synovium versus skin lesions in psoriatic arthritis. Arth Rheumatol 2015;67:934–44.

36. Benjamin M, Mcgonagle D. Histopathologic changes at 'synovio-enthesal complexes' suggesting a novel mechanism for synovitis in osteoarthritis and spondylarthritis. Arthritis Rheum 2007;56:3601–9.

37. Sherlock JP, Joyce-Shaikh B, Turner SP, et al. IL-23 induces spondyloarthropathy by acting on ROR-γt+ CD3+ CD4– CD8– entheseal resident T cells. Nat Med 2012; 18: 1069–76.

38. Cua DJ, Tato CM. Innate IL-17-producing cells: the sentinels of the immune system. Nat Rev Immunol 2010;10:479–89.

39. Benjamin M, Mcgonagle D, The anatomical basis for disease localisation in seronegative spondyloarthropathy at entheses and related sites. J Anat 2001;199:503–26.

40. Laloux L, Voisin MC, Allain J, et al. Immunohistological study of entheses in spondyloarthropathies: comparison in rheumatoid arthritis and osteoarthritis. Ann Rheum Dis 2001;60:316–21.

41. McGonagle D, Marzo-Ortega H, O'Connor P, et al. Histological assessment of the early enthesitis lesion in spondyloarthropathy. Ann Rheum Dis 2002;61:534–7.

42. Vieira-Sousa E, van Duivenvoorde LM, Fonseca JE, Lories RJ, Baeten DL. Review: animal models as a tool to dissect pivotal pathways driving spondyloarthritis. Arthritis Rheumatol 2015;67:2813–27.

43. Foell D, Roth J. Proinflammatory S100 proteins in arthritis and autoimmune disease. Arthritis Rheum 2004;50:3762–71. Review.

44. Foell D, Kane D, Bresnihan B, et al. Expression of the pro-inflammatory protein S100A12 (EN-RAGE) in rheumatoid and psoriatic arthritis. Rheumatology 2003;2:1383–9.

45. Aochi S, Tsuji K, Sakaguchi M et al. Markedly elevated serum levels of calcium-binding S100A8/A9 proteins in psoriatic arthritis are due to activated monocytes/macrophages. J Amer Acad Derm 2011;64:879–87.

46. Turina MC, Yeremenko N, Paramarta JE, De Rycke L, Baeten D. Calprotectin (S100A8/9) as serum biomarker for clinical response in proof-of-concept trials in axial and peripheral spondyloarthritis. Arthritis Res Ther 2014;16:413.

47. Hansson C, Eriksson C, Alenius G-M. S-Calprotectin (S100A8/S100A9): A Potential Marker of Inflammation in Patients with Psoriatic Arthritis. J Immunol Res. 2014, Article ID 696415.

48. Canete JD, Mease P. The link between obesity and psoriatic arthritis. Ann Rheum Dis 2012;71:1265–6.

49. Toussirot E, Aubin F, Dumoulin G. Relationships between adipose tissue and psoriasis, with or without arthritis. Frontiers Immunol 2014;12:5, 368. doi: 10.3389/fimmu.2014.00368

50. Eder L, Jayakar J, Pollock R, et al. Serum adipokines in patients with psoriatic arthritis and psoriasis alone and their correlation with disease activity. Ann Rheum Dis 2013;72:1956–61.

51. Xue Y, Jiang L, Cheng Q, et al. Adipokines in psoriatic arthritis patients: the correlations with osteoclast precursors and bone erosions. PLoS ONE 2012;7:e46740.

52. Dalbeth N, Pool B, Smith T, et al. Circulating mediators of bone remodeling in psoriatic arthritis: implications for disordered osteoclastogenesis and bone erosion. Arthritis Res Ther 2010; 12: R164.

53. Lowes MA, Suárez-Fariñas M, Krueger JG. Immunology of psoriasis. Annu Rev Immunol 2014;32:227–55.

54. Ambarus C, Yeremenko N, Tak PP, Baeten D. Pathogenesis of spondyloarthritis: autoimmune or autoinflammatory? Curr Opin Rheumatol 2012;24:351–8.

55. Boehncke WH, Schön MP. Psoriasis. Lancet 2015;386(9997):983–94.

56. Smith JA, Colbert RA. The IL-23/IL-17 Axis in spondyloarthritis pathogenesis: Th17 and beyond arthritis rheumatol. 2014; 66: 231–41.

57. Huffmeier U, Uebe S, Ekici AB, et al. Common variants at TRAF3IP2 are associated with susceptibility to psoriatic arthritis and psoriasis. Nat Genet 2010;42:996–9.

58. Doyle MS, Collins ES, FitzGerald OM, Pennington SR. New insight into the functions of the interleukin-17 receptor adaptor protein Act1 in psoriatic arthritis. Arth Res Ther 2012;14:226.

59. Apel M, Uebe S, Bowes J, et al. Variants in RUNX3 contribute to susceptibility to psoriatic arthritis, exhibiting further common ground with ankylosing spondylitis. Arthritis Rheum 2013;65:1224–31.

60. McGonagle D, Benjamin M, Tan AL. The pathogenesis of psoriatic arthritis and associated nail disease: not autoimmune after all? Curr Opin Rheumatol. 2009;21:340–7.

61. R. Medzhitov, C. Janeway Jr., Innate immunity. N Engl J Med 2000;343:338–44.

62. Isailovic N, Daigo K, Mantovani A, Selmi C. Interleukin-17 and innate immunity in infections and chronic inflammation. J Autoimmun. 2015; 60:1–11.

63. Diani M, Altomare G, Reali E. T cell responses in psoriasis and psoriatic arthritis. Autoimmun Rev. 2015;14:286–92.

64. Al-Mossawi MH, Ridley A, Kiedel S, Bowness P. The role of natural killer cells, gamma delta T-cells and other innate immune cells in spondyloarthritis. Curr Opin Rheumatol 2013;25:434–9.

65. Koyasu S, Moro K. Role of innate lymphocytes in infection and inflammation. Front Immunol. 2012;3:101.

66. Sutton CE, Mielke LA, Mills KHG. IL-17-producing γδ T cells and innate lymphoid cells. Eur. J. Immunol. 2012;42:2221–31.

67. Spits H, Cupedo T. Innate lymphoid cells: emerging insights in development, lineage relationships, and function. Annu Rev Immunol 2012;30:647–75.

68. Bowness P, Ridley A, Shaw J, et al. Th17 cells expressing KIR3DL2þ and responsive to HLA-B27 homodimers are increased in ankylosing spondylitis. J Immunol 2011;186:2672–80.

69. McKenzie AN, Spits H, Eberl G. Innate lymphoid cells in inflammation and immunity. Immunity 2014;41:366–74.

70. Montaldo E, Juelke K, Romagnani C. Group 3 innate lymphoid cells (ILC3s): origin, differentiation, and plasticity in humans and mice. Eur J Immunol 2015;45(8):2171–82. doi: 10.1002/eji.201545598.

71. Gray EE, Suzuki K, Cyster JG. Cutting edge: identification of a motile IL-17-producing gammadelta T cell population in the dermis. J Immunol 2011;186:6091–5.

72. Annunziato F, Romagnani C, Romagnani S. The 3 major types of innate and adaptive cell-mediated effector immunity. J Allergy Clin Immunol 2015;135:626–35.

73. Spadaro A, Scrivo R, Moretti T, et al. Natural killer cells and gamma/delta T cells in synovial fluid and in peripheral blood of patients with psoriatic arthritis. Clin Exp Rheumatol 2004;22:389–94.

74. Kenna TJ, Davidson SI, Duan R, et al. Enrichment of circulating interleukin-17–secreting interleukin-23 receptor–positive γδt cells in patients with active ankylosing spondylitis. Arthritis Rheum 2012;64:1420–9.

75. Sumaria N, Roediger B, Ng LG, et al. Cutaneous immunosurveillance by self-renewing dermal gammadelta T cells. J Exp Med 2011;208:505–18.

76. Laggner U, Di Meglio P, Perera GK, et al. Identification of a novel pro-inflammatory human skin-homing Vγ9Vδ2 T cell subset with a potential role in psoriasis. J Immunol 2011;187:2783–93.

77. Dalbeth N, Callan MFC. A Subset of natural killer cells is greatly expanded within inflamed joints. Arthritis Rheum 2002;46:1763–72.

78. Tang F, Sally B, Ciszewski C, et al. Interleukin 15 primes natural killer cells to kill via nkg2d and cpla2 and this pathway is active in psoriatic arthritis. PLoS ONE 2013;8(9):e76292.

79. Conigliaro P, Triggianese P, Perricone C, et al. Restoration of peripheral blood natural killer and B cell levels inpatients affected by rheumatoid and psoriatic arthritis during etanercept treatment. Clin Exp Immunol 2014;177:234–43.

80. Ottaviani C, Nasorri F, Bedini C et al. CD56 (bright) CD16(-) NK cells accumulate in psoriatic skin in response to CXCL10 and CCL5 and exacerbate skin inflammation. Eur J Immunol 2006;36:118–28.

81. Luci C, Gaudy-Marqueste C, Rouzaire P, et al. Peripheral natural killer cells exhibit qualitative and quantitative changes in patients with psoriasis and atopic dermatitis. Br J Dermatol 2012;166:789–96.

82. Gilhar A, Ullmann Y, Kerner H et al. Psoriasis is mediated by a cutaneous defect triggered by activated immunocytes: induction of psoriasis by cells with natural killer receptors. J Invest Dermatol 2002; 119:384–91.

83. Leijten EF, van Kempen TS, Boes M, et al. Brief report: enrichment of activated group 3 innate lymphoid cells in psoriatic arthritis synovial fluid. Arthritis Rheumatol, 2015;XX:2222.

84. Villanova F, Flutter B, Tosi I, et al. Characterization of innate lymphoid cells (ILC) in human skin and blood demonstrates increase of NKp44+ ILC3 in psoriasis. J Invest Dermatol 2014;134:984–91.

85. Teunissen MBM, Munneke JM, Bernink JH, et al. Composition of innate lymphoid cell subsets in the human skin: enrichment of ncr+ ilc3 in lesional skin and blood of psoriasis patients. J Invest Dermatol 2014;134(9):2351–60.

86. Cowley SC, MAIT cells and pathogen defence. Cell Mol Life Sci 2014;71:4831–40.

87. Dusseaux M, Martin E, Serriari N, et al. Human MAIT cells are xenobiotic-resistant, tissue-targeted,CD161hi IL-17-secreting T cells. Blood 2011;117:1250–9.

88. Johnston A, Gudjonsson JE, Psoriasis and the MAITing game: a role for IL-17A+ invariant TCR CD8+ T cells in psoriasis? J Invest Dermatol 2014;134:2864–6.

89. Teunissen MBM, Yeremenko NG, Baeten DLP, et al. The IL-17A-producing CD8+ T-cell population in psoriatic lesional skin comprises mucosa-associated invariant T cells and conventional T cells. J Invest Dermatol 2014;134(12):2898–907. doi: 10.1038/jid.2014.261.

90. Menon B, Gullick NJ, Walter GJ, et al. Interleukin-17+CD8+T cells are enriched in the joints of patients with psoriatic arthritis and correlate with disease activity and joint damage progression. Arthritis Rheum 2014;66:1272–81.

91. Merad M, and Manz, MG. Dendritic cell homeostasis. Blood.2009; 113:3418–27.

92. Jongbloed SL, Lebre MC, Fraser AR, et al. Enumeration and phenotypical analysis of distinct dendritic cell subsets in psoriatic arthritis and rheumatoid arthritis. Arthritis Res Ther 2006;8:R15.

93. Gaston JS, Jarvis LB, Zhang L, Goodall JC. Dendritic cell: T-cell interactions in spondyloarthritis. Adv Exp Med Biol 2009;649:263–76.

94. Lande R, Giacomini E, Serafini B, et al. Characterization and recruitment of plasmacytoid dendritic cells in synovial fluid and tissue of patients with chronic inflammatory arthritis. J Immunol 2004;173:2815–24.

95. Wenink MH, Santegoets KC, Butcher J, et al. Impaired dendritic cell proinflammatory cytokine production in psoriatic arthritis. Arthritis Rheum 2011;63:3313–22.

96. Nestle FO, Di Meglio P, Qin J-Z, Nickoloff BJ. Skin immune sentinels in health and disease, Nat Rev Immunol 2009;9:679–691.

97. Chu C-C, Ali N, Karagiannis P, et al. Resident CD141 (BDCA3)+ dendritic cells in human skin produce IL-10 and induce regulatory T cells that suppress skin inflammation. J Exp Med 2012;209:935–94.

98. Walter GJ, Evans HG, Menon B, et al. Interaction with activated monocytes enhances cytokine expression and suppressive activity of human CD4+CD45ro+CD25+CD127(low) regulatory T cells. Arthritis Rheum 2013;65:627–38.

99. Cao D, van Vollenhoven R, Klareskog L, Trollmo C, Malmström V. CD25brightCD4+ regulatory T cells are enriched in inflamed joints of patients with chronic rheumatic disease. Arthritis Res Ther 2004;6:R335–R346.

100. Wu C, Goodall JC, Busch R, Gaston JSH. Relationship of CD146 expression to secretion of interleukin (IL)-17, IL-22 and interferon-γ by CD4+ T cells in patients with inflammatory arthritis. Clin Exp Immunology 2014;179:378–91.

101. Costello P, Bresnihan B, O'Farrelly C, FitzGerald O. Predominance of CD8+ T lymphocytes in psoriatic arthritis. J Rheumatol 1999;26:1117–24.

102. Tassiulas I, Duncan SR, Centola M, Theofilopoulos AN, Boumpas DT. Clonal characteristics of T cell infiltrates in skin and synovium of patients with psoriatic arthritis. Hum Immunol 1999;60:479–91.

103. Curran SA, FitzGerald OM, Costello PJ, et al. Nucleotide sequencing of psoriatic arthritis tissue before and during methotrexate administration reveals a complex inflammatory T cell infiltrate with very few clones exhibiting features that suggest they drive the inflammatory process by recognizing autoantigens. J Immunol 2004;172:1935–44.

104. Lin AM, Rubin CJ, Khandpur R, et al. Mast cells and neutrophils release IL-17 through extracellular trap formation in psoriasis. J Immunol 2011;187(1):490–500.

105. Ferretti S, Bonneau O, Dubois GR, Jones CE, Trifilieff A. IL-17, produced by lymphocytes and neutrophils, is necessary for lipopolysaccharide-induced airway neutrophilia: IL-15 as a possible trigger. J Immunol 2003;170(4):2106–12.

106. Reich K, Papp KA, Matheson RT, et al. Evidence that a neutrophil-keratinocyte crosstalk is an early target of IL-17A inhibition in psoriasis. Exp Dermatol 2015;24(7):529–35.

107. Hueber AJ, Asquith DL, Miller AM, et al. Mast cells express IL-17A in rheumatoid arthritis synovium. J Immunol 2010;184:3336–40.

108. Noordenbos T, Yeremenko N, Gofita I, et al. Interleukin-17–positive mast cells contribute to synovial inflammation in spondylarthritis. Arthritis Rheum 2012;64:99–109.

109. Moran EM, Heydrich R, Ng CT, et al. IL-17A expression is localised to both mononuclear and polymorphonuclear synovial cell infiltrates. PLoS One 2011;6:e24048.

110. Appel H, Maier R, Wu P, et al. Analysis of IL-17+ cells in facet joints of patients with spondyloarthritis suggests that the innate immune pathway might be of greater relevance than the Th17-mediated adaptive immune response. Arthritis Res & Ther 2011;13: R95.

111. Yeremenko N, Baeten D. IL-17 in spondyloarthritis: is the T-party over? Arthritis Res Ther 2011;13:115.

112. Kryczek I, Bruce AT, Gudjonsson JE, et al. Induction of IL-17+T cell trafficking and development by IFN-γ: mechanism and pathological relevance in psoriasis. J Immunol 2008;181:4733–41.

113. Ortega C, Fernandez AS, Carrillo JM, et al. IL-17-producing CD8 T lymphocytes from psoriasis skin plaques are cytotoxic effector cells that secrete Th17-related cytokines. J Leukoc Biol 2009;86:435–43.

114. Res PC, Piskin G, de Boer OJ, et al. Overrepresentation of IL-17A and IL-22 producing CD8 T cells in lesional skin suggests their involvement in the pathogenesis of psoriasis. PLoS One 2010;5:e14108.

115. Andersson J, Samarina A, Fink J, Rahman S, Grundstrom S. Impaired expression of perforin and granulysin in CD8+T cells at the site of infection in human chronic pulmonary tuberculosis. Infect Immun 2007;75:5210–22.

116. Huber M, Heink S, Grothe H, et al. A Th17-like developmental process leads to CD8(+) Tc17 cells with reduced cytotoxic activity. Eur J Immunol 2009;39:1716–25.

117. Mashiko S, Bouguermouh S, Rubio M, Baba N, Bissonnette R, Sarfati M. Human mast cells are major IL-22 producers in patients with psoriasis and atopic dermatitis. J Allergy Clin Immunol 2015; pii: S0091–6749(15)00175-X.

118. van Baarsen LGM, Lebre MC, van der Coelen D, et al. Heterogeneous expression pattern of interleukin 17A (IL-17A), IL-17F and their receptors in synovium of rheumatoid arthritis, psoriatic arthritis and osteoarthritis: possible explanation for nonresponse to anti-IL-17 therapy? Arthr Res Ther 2014;16:426.

119. Gao W, McGarry T, Orr C, McCormick J, Veale DJ, Fearon U. Tofacitinib regulates synovial inflammation in psoriatic arthritis, inhibiting STAT activation and induction of negative feedback inhibitors. Ann Rheum Dis 2016;75:311–5.

120. Vandooren B, Cantaert T, Noordenbos T, Tak PP, Baeten D. The abundant synovial expression of the RANK/RANKL/Osteoprotegerin system in peripheral spondylarthritis is partially disconnected from inflammation. Arthritis Rheum 2008;58:718–29.

121. Talabot-Ayer D, McKee T, Gindre P, et al. Distinct serum and synovial fluid interleukin (IL)-33 levels in rheumatoid arthritis, psoriatic arthritis and osteoarthritis. Joint Bone Spine. 2012;79:32–7.

122. Kirkham BW, Kavanaugh A, Reich K. Interleukin-17A: a unique pathway in immune mediated diseases: Psoriasis, psoriatic arthritis, and rheumatoid arthritis. Immunology 2014;141:133–42.

123. Chiricozzi A, Guttman-Yassky E, Suarez-Farinas M, et al. Integrative responses to IL-17 and TNF-α in human keratinocytes account for key inflammatory pathogenic circuits in psoriasis. J Invest Dermatol 2011;131:677–87.

CHAPTER 8

Mechanisms of bone destruction and proliferation in psoriatic arthritis

Rik Lories

Introduction

Structural damage to the skeletal tissues is a feared complication of chronic inflammatory and degenerative joint disease [1]. Together with inflammation, structural damage contributes to the pain, the loss of function and the resulting disability associated with these common and debilitating disorders. The contribution of joint damage towards the morbidity of patients with chronic arthritis increases as disease duration extends [1, 2]. In many patients with long-standing joint disease in whom inflammation may be adequately controlled with currently available treatment strategies, structural damage is the main culprit for persistent clinical problems.

For psoriatic arthritis (PsA) patients, potential structural damage to the joint is a major concern [2, 3]. Strikingly, in PsA and in typical contrast to other chronic joint diseases, damage to the different structures of the joint, in particular the bone, the cartilage but also the synovium and joint-associated ligaments, is often unpredictable and may vary between different joints both within individuals as well as among different patients. Joint destruction characterized by the development of erosions in bone often associated with or leading to loss of articular cartilage, as well as joint remodelling with extensive new bone formation potentially leading to joint ankylosis can both be recognized [1] and can occur in distinct ways in different joints from an individual patient (Figure 8.1).

The heterogeneity in clinical disease presentation that includes mono-, oligo-, and polyarthritis, dominant peripheral as well as dominant axial disease, as well as in severity of disease, both from the clinical and from the structural perspective, illustrate the difficult challenge in developing a comprehensive and unifying perspective on structural damage in PsA [1]. It is therefore important to know that careful epidemiological observations have refuted the old concept that PsA is a relative benign disease in most patients. Effectively, in the Toronto cohort study as well as in the Dublin early PsA cohort, the risk of erosions and the risk of subsequent disability has been clearly recognized [2, 4] and should fundamentally influence the way we consider structural damage and try to prevent it in this important disease. Effectively, individual joint inflammation is clearly associated with subsequent damage [5].

From the patient perspective, the recognition of PsA as a potentially severe and debilitating disease highlights the importance and impact of structural damage and has direct clinical consequences: a holistic approach towards PsA therapy should include drug or non-pharmacological strategies aiming at preventing or minimizing structural damage. The development and implementation of such strategies requires good knowledge of the underlying mechanisms at the tissue, cellular, and molecular level. This is not an easy challenge as direct access to the tissues of interest in patients and healthy individuals is by default limited, and there is no animal model that completely mimics the human disease. In this chapter, current insights into mechanisms of structural damage to the joint in PsA are discussed and put into a clinical perspective in particular with regards to current and future therapeutic interventions.

Basics of bone development, growth, and homeostasis

Understanding the mechanisms underlying structural damage including eventual repair or remodelling efforts within the skeletal tissues requires some insights into the basic signalling cascades and cells that play a key role in bone development, growth, and homeostasis. It is important to also recognize the differences between these physiological processes and the different processes that contribute to joint destruction in patients with PsA: loss of articular cartilage, the development of bone erosions, and osteolysis, as well as new bone formation potentially leading to joint ankylosis.

From a semantic point of view, bone modelling refers to the shaping and growth of the skeleton within predetermined boundaries. Skeletal development is executed following a strict plan and, like most developmental processes, is based on gradients of morphogens and growth factors influencing the differentiation of distinct progenitor populations [6, 7]. Most of the skeletal elements are formed through a process of endochondral bone formation. The key steps are the proliferation and condensation of progenitor cells at the site of the future bone, with increased cell–cell interaction resulting in chondrogenic differentiation and the formation of a cartilage template (Figure 8.2). Cells within this template undergo progressive differentiation steps going through different stages (proliferating chondrocytes, prehypertrophic chondrocytes, hypertrophic chondrocytes) (Figure 8.3). The latter population is considered the terminal differentiation status of the chondrocyte. Whereas the extracellular matrix surrounding the early differentiation status chondrocytes is rich in type II collagen and not-calcified, hypertrophic chondrocytes produce a matrix rich in type

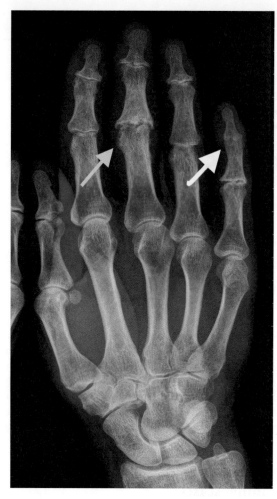

Figure 8.1 Radiographic image of structural damage in the hand of a patient with psoriatic arthritis. Different joints show signs of cartilage loss, erosive lesions and remodeling. The grey arrow indicates a bone erosion, the white arrow shows a joint that is partially ankylosed.

Endochondral bone formation is a tightly regulated process to which different developmental cascades contribute [6]. Bone morphogenetic proteins are a family of growth factors with strong chondro- and osteogenic properties [8]. They were initially discovered as a protein fraction from demineralized bone capable of inducing the cascade of endochondral bone formation ectopically and *in vivo*, e.g. upon injection of purified bone extract into the muscle of rodents [9]. Other key pathways include the Wnt and Hedgehog cascades. Wnt signalling determines cell fate in different types of tissue and organs. Wnt signalling is very complex with different intracellular cascades activated by the distinct ligand and receptor interactions from the Wnt family [10]. During endochondral bone formation, Wnt signalling has a negative effect on very early phases of chondrogenesis but appears to stimulate further differentiation once the process has been triggered and also stimulates direct differentiation of bone-forming osteoblasts from osteoprogenitor cells [10] (Figures 8.2, 3 and 4). Hedgehog signalling is another pathway with a key role in chondrogenic differentiation [11]. These three cascades have also been associated with new bone formation and joint damage in patients with PsA and related disorders, in particular spondyloarthritis (see below).

Endochondral bone formation is not the only process responsible for building the elements of the skeleton. The process described above leads to the formation of the primary ossification centres [6]. At the same time, a bony collar is formed through a process of direct ossification, in which osteoblast progenitor cells directly differentiate into osteoblasts (Figure 8.4). Upon the initial development of the bone, the process of endochondral bone formation is further organized in the growth plates, going through the same molecular cascades.

Bone is a very dynamic tissue and physiological remodelling of bone is a constant feature [12, 13]. Cycles of bone breakdown and build-up provide the body with a means to constantly adapt the skeleton to the strain imposed. These bone remodelling cycles are maintained by three different cell types: osteoblasts as anabolic cells, osteoclasts as catabolic cells, and osteocytes as orchestrating mechanosensitive cells (Figure 8.5). The osteoblasts belong to the mesenchymal lineage and produce the characteristic extracellular matrix of bone that becomes calcified and gives the bone its unique strength. Osteocytes are terminally differentiated osteoblasts that become trapped in the calcified extracellular matrix. Osteoclasts are multinucleated giant cells originating from the fusion of

X collagen and this is calcified. This matrix is subsequently invaded by vessels and bone progenitor cells, resulting in apoptosis of the chondrocytes, breakdown of the original extra-cellular matrix, and replacement of the cartilage template by bone (Figure 8.4).

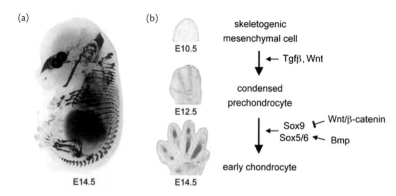

Figure 8.2 Chondrocyte early differentiation and development of cartilage. A. Alcian blue staining of a mouse embryo at E14.5 demonstrates that chondrocyte differentiation of skeletogenic cells leads to the formation of a primary skeleton that is entirely cartilaginous. B. Sections through the developing paws of mouse embryos illustrate the major steps of early chondrogenesis. At E10.5, the limb bud is filled with skeletogenic cells. By E12.5, some of these cells have formed precartilaginous condensations that prefigure the future digits. By E14.5, condensed prechondrocytes have undergone chondrocyte early differentiation. The sections are stained with Alcian blue and nuclear fast red. Reprinted from Lefebvre V, Bhattaram P. Vertebrate skeletogenesis. Curr Top Dev Biol. 2010;90:291-317 with permission from Elsevier.

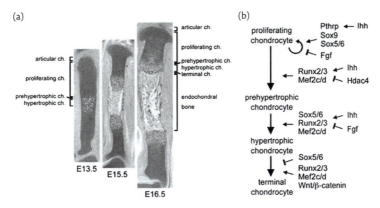

Figure 8.3 Chondrocyte maturation and development of cartilage growth plates. A. Sections through a mouse embryo tibia illustrate the development of growth plates and endochondral bone. At E13.5, early chondrocytes in the center of cartilage primordia undergo prehypertrophic and hypertrophic maturation. They reach terminal maturation and are replaced by endochondral bone by E15.5. Later on, growth plates maintain themselves and elongate developing bones. Chondrocytes keep proliferating and give rise, layer by layer, to maturing chondrocytes. These cells which eventually die and are replaced by bone. The sections are stained with Alcian blue and nuclear fast red. B. Schematic of the molecular control of growth plate chondrocytes Reprinted from Lefebvre V, Bhattaram P. Vertebrate skeletogenesis. Curr Top Dev Biol. 2010;90:291-317 with permission from Elsevier.

differentiating osteoclast precursor cells that are derived from the monocytic lineage [14]. The key molecules that orchestrate the differentiation, maturation, and activation of osteoclasts have been well defined: monocyte-colony stimulating factor (MCSF) and Receptor of NFkappa B ligand (RANKL). RANKL can be produced by different cells types including osteocytes and osteoblasts, but also activated T cells and synoviocytes [15], and binds to the RANK receptor on osteoclast precursor cells. The interaction between

RANK and RANKL is further regulated by osteoprotegerin that can act as a decoy receptor for RANKL and thereby inhibits osteoclast differentiation and activation.

Structural damage in psoriatic arthritis

As explained in the Introduction, both clinical and radiographic manifestations of PsA are characterized by surprising variability

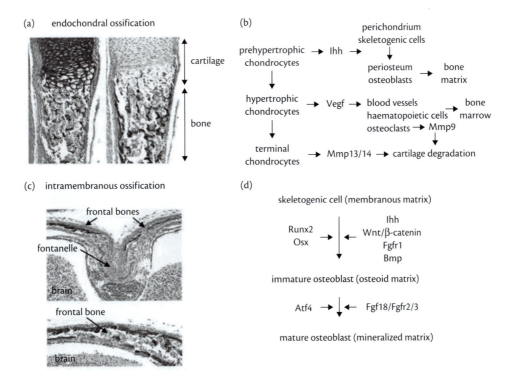

Figure 8.4 Osteoblast differentiation and intramembranous and endochondral ossification. A. Sections through an endochondral bone in a newborn mouse show the replacement of cartilage by bone. The left section is stained with Alcian blue and the right one with the von Kossa reagent, which leaves a brown precipitate on the mineralized bone matrix. B. Schematic showing how growth plate chondrocytes and bone-forming cells interact with each other to achieve endochondral ossification. C. Coronal sections of a newborn mouse head. In the suture linking the two frontal bones (top panel), osteoblast precursors are surrounded by an abundant collagenous matrix. Further away (bottom panel), osteoblasts mature and deposit a mineralized bone matrix. This matrix is stained with the von Kossa reagent. D. Schematic of the molecular control of osteoblast differentiation Reprinted from Lefebvre V, Bhattaram P. Vertebrate skeletogenesis. Curr Top Dev Biol. 2010;90:291-317 with permission from Elsevier.

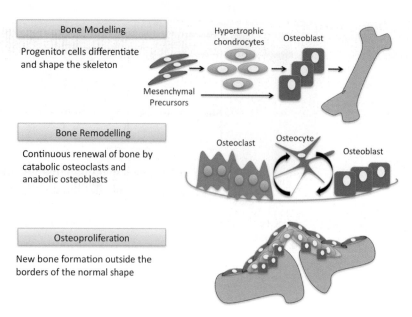

Figure 8.5 Concepts of bone formation. Bone modeling is a developmental process that determines the shape and structure of the skeleton. In this well-orchestrated process, progenitors differentiate by endochondral or direct bone formation. Bone remodeling refers to the continuous renewal of the skeleton by bone resorbing osteoclasts (multinucleated cells) and bone-forming osteoblasts. The osteocytes are mechanosensitive cells and orchestrate the bone remodeling cycle. Bone modeling in SpA is a disease-associated process, in which new bone formation is occurring outside the original borders of the skeleton. Reprinted from Lories RJ, Schett G. Pathophysiology of new bone formation and ankylosis in spondyloarthritis. Rheum Dis Clin North Am. 2012;38(3):555–67 with permission from Elsevier.

and unpredictability. In the 1970s, outstanding clinical observation and recording allowed Moll and Wright to propose different subforms of PsA based on clinical and radiographic manifestations [16]. These subforms include polyarticular disease, oligo-articular disease, distal interphalangeal joint predominant arthritis, arthritis mutilans, and spondyloarthritic PsA.

Polyarticular disease may be very similar in its clinical manifestation to that seen in patients with rheumatoid arthritis. Suggestions that this disease is actually PsA are based on the presence of the skin disorder in patients or their closest blood relatives; on the absence of rheumatoid arthritis associated auto-antibodies, such as rheumatoid factor and anti-citrullinated protein antibodies; or on the co-involvement of distal interphalangeal joints that are typically not affected in rheumatoid arthritis patients. Radiographic evidence suggesting that these patients have psoriatic rather than rheumatoid arthritis may be based on differences in appearances of erosions and signs of joint remodelling such as enthesophytes and osteophytes (Figure 8.1) the latter characteristically absent in patients with rheumatoid arthritis. Nevertheless, the clinical overlap between these patients and those with rheumatoid arthritis can be a challenge. Current data clearly support the view that polyarticular PsA is more related to other forms of PsA than to rheumatoid arthritis [17, 18].

Oligoarticular disease typically involves large joints in the lower limb. The radiographic manifestations are again variable. Both erosion (loss of articular cartilage) and formation of osteophytes or enthesophytes are seen (Figure 8.6). The overall impact of the structural damage, in particular of damage to the bone, is again variable. In large joints, such as the knee, the articular cartilage loss and damage to the ligaments may be more important in determining the long-term outcome than the presence of juxta-articular erosions or osteophytes.

Spondyloarthritic PsA shares most features, including the typical presence of inflammatory back pain, with radiographic and non-radiographic axial spondyloarthritis. Some differences, however, are striking. Back pain, as such, may be less common in patients with radiographic signs of disease in axial PsA than in axial spondyloarthritis. Psoriatic spondylitis often only shows unilateral sacroiliac disease and cervical spine involvement, and the syndesmophytes in the PsA patients are typically larger and plumper [20, 21]. The latter observation suggests that some of the genetic susceptibility underlying psoriatic disease and axial spondyloarthritis may influence the radiographic outcome of disease or that common symptoms may only identify a partial overlap in underlying disease mechanisms [22].

Isolated but mostly polyarticular distal interphalangeal joint arthritis is a challenging form of PsA in terms of both correct diagnosis and treatment. This subform of PsA is commonly

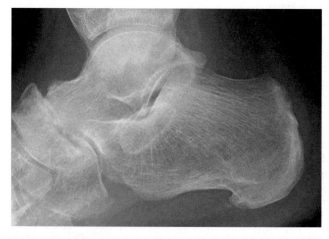

Figure 8.6 Damage to the ankle joint in a patient with oligoarticular psoriatic arthritis. There is cartilage loss and decreased joint space width in the talonavicular joint and an enthesophyte at the insertion of the fascia plantaris.

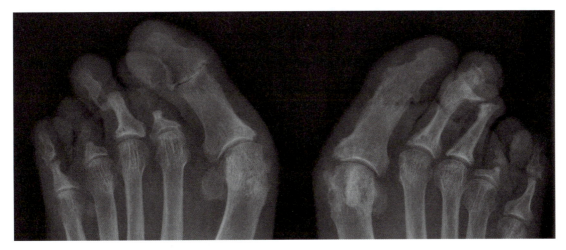

Figure 8.7 Arthritis mutilans in the feet of a patient with psoriatic arthritis. The osteodestruction even results in the virtual disappearance of some phalanges.

associated with the presence of nail disease, a feature that can help in establishing the correct diagnosis. Radiographic damage includes both erosive, bone-destructive disease, and loss of cartilage, as well as features of joint remodelling. In the absence of nail disease, the distinction between this form of PsA and erosive osteoarthritis of the hands can be a considerable challenge. However, differentiating these diseases is important as therapeutic strategies are different. The observation that the small ligaments and their entheses appear involved in both PsA and erosive hand osteoarthritis has suggested the existence of common mechanisms of disease and underpins a novel hypothesis that there is no sharp dividing line between the two entities with biomechanical factors contributing to the onset of both [23, 24]

Arthritis mutilans is a relatively rare but very severe subform of PsA [25] (Figure 8.7). It is characterized by extreme and rapid joint destruction with extensive osteolysis and flail joints. The consequences for joint function are typically severe. The excessive destruction appears to be a relatively unique feature for this disease.

The anatomic basis of bone destruction and remodelling in psoriatic arthritis

The enigmatic and unpredictable combination of bone catabolic and anabolic features of radiographic damage in these patients has been very difficult to understand from a cellular and tissue perspective. PsA has traditionally been included within the spondyloarthritis concept. This disease definition encompassed a number of related clinical entities that share genetic, pathophysiologic, and radiographic characteristics [26]. The spondyloarthritis concept includes, in addition to PsA, ankylosing spondylitis, reactive arthritis, inflammatory bowel disease associated arthritis, juvenile and undifferentiated forms. More recent revisiting of the concept introduced a distinction between predominant axial spondyloarthritis, including ankylosing spondylitis and non-radiographic axial spondyloarthritis, and predominant peripheral spondyloarthritis. The introduction of nuclear magnetic resonance imaging in the rheumatology field was useful to better define most forms of spondyloarthritis as enthesitis-related arthritis, thereby corroborating the earlier conceptual link between spondyloarthritis and enthesitis based on pathology and radiographic studies [27, 28]. In this context, it is important to note that the enthesitis concept is

defined at the tissue level and not the clinical presentation. Primary enthesitis within an articular joint may lead to synovitis and osteitis, and therefore clinically present as arthritis and synovitis.

The concept of enthesitis as unifying or primary disease localization has been criticized and challenged as any of the diseases within the spondyloarthritis concept can clinically and imaging-wise present as enthesitis, synovitis, or osteitis [29]. Nevertheless this concept is useful to better understand not only the pathophysiology of disease but also joint destruction and joint remodelling including progressive ankylosis. For PsA in particular, the co-occurrence of enthesitis, synovitis, and osteitis has led to the definition of the synovio-entheseal complex as key localization of disease [30]. Whereas the enthesis is a pauci-cellular and extra-cellular matrix rich tissue that appears relatively resistant to cell influx, the synovium and underlying bone marrow are highly vascularized tissues with enormous potential for inflammatory cell accrual suggesting that danger or chemotactic signals originating from the enthesitis can easily lead to synovitis or osteitis.

The enthesis is by default a site exposed to biomechanical stress. The hypothesis that biomechanical stress can be a triggering or perpetuating factor in the development of PsA has been supported by experimental and clinical evidence [31, 32]. Genetically modified mice that lack a regulatory element in the tumour necrosis factor gene, a strategy that results in endogenous TNF overexpression, develop enthesitis, arthritis, and inflammatory bowel disease [32]. However, tail suspension and unloading of the hind-paws reduces inflammation in this model. In addition, in a model of joint remodelling tail suspension also reduces new bone formation. Of particular interest, a specific immune cell population responsive to interleukin 23 has been discovered in the mouse enthesis suggesting that sentinel cells populate these tissues, most likely to detect microdamage [33, 34]. In addition, clinical epidemiological data have demonstrated that new bone formation, similar to that seen in patients with PsA, also develops in patients with skin disease only albeit without the typical signs and symptoms of inflammation [35].

All these observations may be useful to understand some of the pivotal differences in structural damage as seen in patients with PsA compared to those with rheumatoid arthritis. As the stabilizing and biomechanically challenged tissues of the joint are involved in onset and development of disease in PsA, the initiating events may not only result in inflammation typically associated with tissue destruction but also rapid loss of joint stability. In rheumatoid arthritis, inflammation develops in the synovium but may be the consequence of a more distantly originating immune reaction. In contrast in PsA, the intimate link between the development of inflammation and damage to the biomechanically challenged tissues that include both the enthesis and the synovium may trigger a stabilizing and remodelling tissue response. This two-faced aspect of the disease therefore results in both joint destruction driven by inflammation as well as joint remodelling to with both inflammation-driven damage and endogenous repair responses contribute.

The molecular basis of tissue destruction and remodelling in psoriatic arthritis

Joint destruction

Osteoclasts have key roles in joint destruction [1, 36]. As outlined above (see 'Basics of bone development, growth, and homeostasis'), these cells belong to the monocytic lineage and differentiate under control of cytokines M-CSF and RANKL [37] (Figure 8.8). Their unique properties include their attachment to the calcified surfaces of the bone and their ability to create a highly acidic microenvironment at this surface. In this way, the osteoclasts are the only cell type in the body that is capable of effectively breaking down the calcified bone matrix by specific enzymes within this acidic microenvironment.

Bone remodelling with continuous cycles of bone breakdown and synthesis is a carefully orchestrated and well-controlled process under physiological circumstances (Figure 8.5). However, this mechanism appears deregulated in diseases such as PsA and rheumatoid arthritis. Within the joints and under chronic inflammatory conditions, the amount of RANKL and the net balance between RANKL and its decoy receptor OPG can be shifted as different proinflammatory cytokines appear to increase RANKL expression. In physiological bone remodelling osteocytes appear to be the main source of RANKL [14, 38]. However, in inflammatory joint diseases other cells, including activated T cells and activated synovial fibroblasts, can produce RANKL and these cells are increased within the joint environment [1, 15, 36]. These factors lead to abnormal osteoclast activation at the sites of inflammation and the development of bone erosions in the joint.

Destructive lesions in some patients with PsA can be remarkable, a feature that remains unexplained. Ritchlin et al., demonstrated increased amount of osteoclast precursor cells in patients with PsA, a positive correlation with joint erosions, and a high sensitivity to TNF-induced activation [39], but this does not really explain the local effects, in particular the osteolysis seen in patients with arthritis mutilans. Osteoclast-activating effects of auto-antibodies, in particular of anti-citrullinated protein antibodies, have been demonstrated in patients with rheumatoid arthritis [40], but there is no evidence for the presence of similar or other antibodies in PsA that would have a similar effect. Other factors that could play a role in joint destruction include genetic variation in some cytokines, e.g. interleukin-4 [41].

In contrast to the large number of studies on the activation and phenotype of synovial fibroblasts in rheumatoid arthritis [42], relatively little is known about the specific activation of these cells in PsA. It seems likely, however, that the activation of these cells by the presence of proinflammatory cytokines results in upregulation of enzymes that can breakdown the cartilage matrix, e.g. matrix metalloproteinases and ADAMTS enzymes, and that this mechanism contributes to joint destruction.

New bone formation and ankylosis

The direct study of joint tissues involved in PsA is difficult. Synovial fluid and synovial tissue are best studied but even gaining access to these is an invasive procedure. Samples of entheseal tissue and areas of new bone formation are a far bigger challenge to obtain. The phenotypical overlap with other forms of spondyloarthritis does allow some insights into the molecular and cellular mechanisms involved. The limited amount of histology data available from patients suggest that both endochondral and membranous bone formation contribute to new bone formation and ankylosis [43–48]. The current hypothesis states that skeletal progenitor populations commit towards differentiation into either chondrocytes or osteoblasts during new bone formation in PsA. At the molecular level, data from mouse models suggest that new bone formation is directed by growth factors that also play a role in skeletal development including bone morphogenetic proteins (BMPs), Wnt proteins, hedgehog proteins, and fibroblast growth factors.

BMPs are potent growth factors that not only play important roles in skeletal development but also in body patterning and in the development of other organ systems. BMPs are part of a large family of ligands related to transforming growth factor beta. The different ligands and promiscuous receptor associations lead to the activation of distinct signalling cascades, thereby allowing distinct BMPs to have wide-ranging effects on specific cell types. Regulatory mechanisms include the expression of endogenous extracellular and intracellular antagonists and the complex

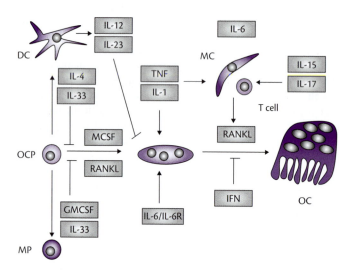

Figure 8.8 Osteoclast precursors (OCP) differentiate and fuse to mature osteoclasts (OC). This process is governed by macrophage colony stimulating factors (MCSF) and receptor activator of NF-κB ligand (RANKL). Tumour necrosis factor (TNF) and interleukins (IL)- 6, -15 and -17 support this process. Dendritic cell (DC) derived cytokines IL-12 and IL-23 suppress this process as well as IL-4 and IL-33, which initiate DC rather than OC differentiation. Also granulocyte/macrophage CSF supporting macrophage differentiation inhibit the process of osteoclast differentiation. MC: mesenchymal cells. Reprinted from Schett G. Effects of inflammatory and anti-inflammatory cytokines on the bone. Eur J Clin Invest. 2011;41(12):1361-6 with permission from Wiley.

interactions of co-activator and co-repressors at the level of transcription. Such interactions are essential for the fine-tuning of this signalling system [8]. In skeletal development, BMPs play an essential role in the early phases of chondrogenesis by stimulating chondrogenic differentiation including the late hypertrophic stages of chondrogenesis [6]. Different BMPs have also direct positive effects on osteoblast differentiation.

The role of the BMP pathway in new bone formation in the joints was studied in animal models of PsA and spondyloarthritis [49–51].The spontaneous arthritis model in aging male DBA/1 mice is a model characterized by a short phase of acute inflammation and by impressive bone remodelling starting from the entheses that may lead to joint ankylosis [52]. Histology of the model shows endochondral bone formation with consecutive phases of chondrocyte proliferation, condensation, differentiation, and hypertrophy, and ultimately replacement of the cartilage template by bone. Different BMPs are demonstrated by immunohistochemistry in this mouse model and activation of intracellular BMP Smad signalling molecules is associated with the early phases of the disease [50]. When noggin (an endogenous BMP antagonist that interferes with ligand-receptor binding) is overexpressed, ankylosis could be inhibited in both preventive and therapeutic experiments [50].

Wnt proteins have also been associated with joint remodelling [53, 54]. The Wnt family mediates its effects by using complex ligand–receptor interactions as well as activation of different intracellular signalling cascades. Canonical Wnt signalling primarily involves translocation of intracellular β-catenin molecule to the nucleus. In skeletal development and biology, Wnts stimulate bone formation and their expression appears regulated by the mechanosensing osteocytes. Wnts stimulate new bone formation by direct effects on osteoblasts [6, 10]. Moreover, Wnt proteins tightly regulate articular cartilage homeostasis and shifts in the balance between Wnt ligands and endogenous antagonists appear important in osteoarthritis [10].

The link between Wnt signalling and ankylosis in arthritis was originally demonstrated in the human TNF transgenic mouse model of arthritis [53, 54]. This model is commonly used as a mouse model of rheumatoid arthritis and characterized by extensive joint destruction. However, induction of Wnt signalling by neutralization of the Wnt antagonist dickkopf-1 (DKK1), previously linked to systemic bone loss, resulted in osteoproliferation and ankylosis in peripheral and axial joints. This local phenomenon was accompanied by a systemic gain of bone mass indicating that enhancing Wnt signalling in this model also affects bone remodelling in addition to bone modelling. DKK1 is a factor induced by proinflammatory cytokines such as TNF [53].

Hedgehog proteins also have key roles in skeletal development and are the mediators of an essential feedback loop that controls bone growth [6, 11]. This feedback loop is established with parathyroid hormone related protein. Indian hedgehog (IHH) defines the rate of chondrocyte proliferation and hypertrophy. IHH binds to the Smoothened and Patched receptor complex and leads to an activation of the GLI transcription factors. GLI1 and GLI2 are considered transcriptional activators, while GLI3 acts as a transcriptional repressor. A small compound that inhibits hedghog signalling by directly interfering with Smoothened, limits osteoproliferation in a model of inflammatory arthritis [55].

Clinical relevance of joint destruction and remodelling

Overall, the clinical impact of tissue destruction and remodelling in PsA has been studied less extensively than in rheumatoid arthritis. However, limited disease-oriented data strongly support the concept that both in the short as well as the long term, tissue damage is key determinant of function and quality of life [2, 56]. This is obviously directly clear in patients with arthritis mutilans in whom the often rapid and complete destruction of joints results in severe loss of function [25] but is often underestimated in patients that differ from those with the most severe forms. In addition the importance of damage to the articular cartilage—often less obvious—on classical X-rays is underestimated.

Scoring systems and their applications in clinical trials focused mostly on the destructive aspects of disease [57]. For remodelling of the spine different scoring systems exist that evaluate progression of ankylosis and a specific method has been proposed for patients with PsA [58]. Like axial spondyloarthritis, it is clear that axial PsA can lead to severe symptoms and disability [59]. Of note, only a few scoring systems that are not very commonly used also assess the impact of joint remodelling in peripheral joints [60, 61].

Therapeutic strategies

Historically therapeutic trials in PsA have been relatively rare. This has changed with the introduction of cytokine-targeted therapeutic strategies, in particular anti-tumour necrosis factor drugs. The clinical success of etanercept, infliximab, adalimumab, golimumab, and certolizumab pegol has also translated in effective inhibition of radiographic progression characterized by joint destruction with the soluble receptor as well as the monoclonal antibodies showing similar effects [62–74]. More recently similar data have been obtained with a new drug targeting IL-12 and IL-23 (ustekinumab) [75, 76]. Joint destruction appears clearly driven by inflammation [77].

Within these clinical trials, however, the remodelling features that characterize joint destruction in patients with PsA have not been studied in a similar way. It is therefore unclear how these drugs will affect these processes. Earlier data from the spondyloarthritis field have suggested that for axial disease and progressive ankylosis current strategies have a limited effect that may only become apparent after many years of treatment [78–80]. These observations suggested that non-inflammatory factors likely influence joint remodelling. Taking into account the perspective that some of the remodelling may be triggered by loss of joint stability, this perspective would predict that the effects of successful therapy would result in different outcomes when treatment is started early (before damage or instability) as compared to the outcome seen when therapy is started when the joint is already affected. Of note, some patients with PsA have shown impressive signs of joint repair after successful treatment with anti-TNF drugs [81].

Conclusion

Joint destruction and new bone formation potentially leading to ankylosis are important features of PsA. These different forms of damage can all contribute to the impact of disease, in particular to loss of function and disability. The increased attention towards the impact and severity of PsA in the last decades has underlined the importance of preventing any type of structural damage. Current therapeutic interventions targeting inflammation appear successful at limiting joint destruction. The impact of therapy on preventing ankylosis appears limited. Our knowledge of the cells and molecules involved in these processes is largely based on mouse models. Nevertheless, these insights could form the basis for further development of strategies. This will likely require more insights into the factors that trigger the different types of joint destruction and into those that determine the outcome in the different joints of an individual patient.

References

1. Schett G, Coates LC, Ash ZR, Finzel S, Conaghan PG. Structural damage in rheumatoid arthritis, psoriatic arthritis, and ankylosing spondylitis: traditional views, novel insights gained from TNF blockade, and concepts for the future. Arthritis Res Ther. 2011;13 Suppl 1:S4.

2. Gladman DD, Stafford-Brady F, Chang CH, Lewandowski K, Russell ML. Longitudinal study of clinical and radiological progression in psoriatic arthritis. J Rheumatol. 1990;17(6):809–12.

3. Sokoll KB, Helliwell PS. Comparison of disability and quality of life in rheumatoid and psoriatic arthritis. J Rheumatol. 2001;28(8):1842–6.

4. Kane D, Stafford L, Bresnihan B, FitzGerald O. A prospective, clinical and radiological study of early psoriatic arthritis: an early synovitis clinic experience. Rheumatology (Oxford). 2003;42(12):1460–8.

5. Cresswell L, Chandran V, Farewell VT, Gladman DD. Inflammation in an individual joint predicts damage to that joint in psoriatic arthritis. Ann Rheum Dis. 2011;70(2):305–8.

6. Lefebvre V, Bhattaram P. Vertebrate skeletogenesis. Curr Top Dev Biol. 2010;90:291–317.

7. Bianco P, Robey PG. Skeletal stem cells. Development. 2015;142(6):1023–7.

8. Lories RJ, Luyten FP. Bone morphogenetic protein signaling and arthritis. Cytokine Growth Factor Rev. 2009;20(5-6):467–73.

9. Urist MR. Bone: formation by autoinduction. Science. 1965;150(3698):893–9.

10. Lories RJ, Corr M, Lane NE. To Wnt or not to Wnt: the bone and joint health dilemma. Nat Rev Rheumatol. 2013;9(6):328–39.

11. Alman BA. The role of hedgehog signalling in skeletal health and disease. Nat Rev Rheumatol. 2015.

12. Farr JN, Khosla S. Skeletal changes through the lifespan–from growth to senescence. Nat Rev Endocrinol. 2015.

13. Bellido T. Osteocyte-driven bone remodeling. Calcif Tissue Int. 2014;94(1):25–34.

14. Nakashima T, Takayanagi H. New regulation mechanisms of osteoclast differentiation. Ann N Y Acad Sci. 2011;1240:E13–8.

15. Schett G, Gravallese E. Bone erosion in rheumatoid arthritis: mechanisms, diagnosis and treatment. Nat Rev Rheumatol. 2012;8(11):656–64.

16. Moll JM, Wright V. Psoriatic arthritis. Semin Arthritis Rheum. 1973;3(1):55–78.

17. Helliwell PS, Porter G, Taylor WJ, Group CS. Polyarticular psoriatic arthritis is more like oligoarticular psoriatic arthritis, than rheumatoid arthritis. Ann Rheum Dis. 2007;66(1):113–7.

18. Kruithof E, Baeten D, De Rycke L, et al. Synovial histopathology of psoriatic arthritis, both oligo- and polyarticular, resembles spondyloarthropathy more than it does rheumatoid arthritis. Arthritis Res Ther. 2005;7(3):R569–80.

19. Dougados M. Psoriatic arthritis: is it for real? Joint Bone Spine. 2007;74(4):311–2.

20. Helliwell PS, Hickling P, Wright V. Do the radiological changes of classic ankylosing spondylitis differ from the changes found in the spondylitis associated with inflammatory bowel disease, psoriasis, and reactive arthritis? Ann Rheum Dis. 1998;57(3):135–40.

21. Jeannou J, Goupille P, Avimadje MA, Zerkak D, Valat JP, Fouquet B. Cervical spine involvement in psoriatic arthritis. Rev Rhum Engl Ed. 1999;66(12):695–700.

22. Haroon M, Winchester R, Giles JT, Heffernan E, FitzGerald O. Certain class I HLA alleles and haplotypes implicated in susceptibility play a role in determining specific features of the psoriatic arthritis phenotype. Ann Rheum Dis. 2016;75(1):155–62.

23. McGonagle D, Hermann KG, Tan AL. Differentiation between osteoarthritis and psoriatic arthritis: implications for pathogenesis and treatment in the biologic therapy era. Rheumatology (Oxford). 2015;54(1):29–38.

24. McGonagle D, Tan AL, Grainger AJ, Benjamin M. Heberden's nodes and what Heberden could not see: the pivotal role of ligaments in the pathogenesis of early nodal osteoarthritis and beyond. Rheumatology (Oxford). 2008;47(9):1278–85.

25. Jadon DR, Shaddick G, Tillett W, et al. Psoriatic arthritis mutilans: characteristics and natural radiographic history. J Rheumatol. 2015;42(7):1169–76.

26. Dougados M, Baeten D. Spondyloarthritis. Lancet. 2011;377(9783): 2127–37.

27. Ball J. The enthesopathy of ankylosing spondylitis. Br J Rheumatol. 1983;22(4 Suppl 2):25–8.

28. McGonagle D, Gibbon W, Emery P. Classification of inflammatory arthritis by enthesitis. Lancet. 1998;352(9134):1137–40.

29. Paramarta JE, van der Leij C, Gofita I, et al. Peripheral joint inflammation in early onset spondyloarthritis is not specifically related to enthesitis. Ann Rheum Dis. 2014;73(4):735–40.

30. McGonagle D, Lories RJ, Tan AL, Benjamin M. The concept of a 'synovio-entheseal complex' and its implications for understanding joint inflammation and damage in psoriatic arthritis and beyond. Arthritis Rheum. 2007;56(8):2482–91.

31. McGonagle D, Thomas RC, Schett G. Spondyloarthritis: may the force be with you? Ann Rheum Dis. 2014;73(2):321–3.

32. Jacques P, Lambrecht S, Verheugen E, et al. Proof of concept: enthesitis and new bone formation in spondyloarthritis are driven by mechanical strain and stromal cells. Ann Rheum Dis. 2014;73(2):437–45.

33. Sherlock JP, Joyce-Shaikh B, Turner SP, et al. IL-23 induces spondyloarthropathy by acting on ROR-gammat+ CD3+CD4-CD8- entheseal resident T cells. Nat Med. 2012;18(7):1069–76.

34. Lories RJ, McInnes IB. Primed for inflammation: enthesis-resident T cells. Nat Med. 2012;18(7):1018–9.

35. Simon D, Faustini F, Kleyer A, et al. Analysis of periarticular bone changes in patients with cutaneous psoriasis without associated psoriatic arthritis. Ann Rheum Dis. 2015;75(4):660–6.

36. Schett G, David JP. The multiple faces of autoimmune-mediated bone loss. Nat Rev Endocrinol. 2010;6(12):698–706.

37. Schett G. Effects of inflammatory and anti-inflammatory cytokines on the bone. Eur J Clin Invest. 2011;41(12):1361–6.

38. Nakashima T, Hayashi M, Fukunaga T, Kurata K, Oh-Hora M, Feng JQ, et al. Evidence for osteocyte regulation of bone homeostasis through RANKL expression. Nat Med. 2011;17(10):1231–4.

39. Ritchlin CT, Haas-Smith SA, Li P, Hicks DG, Schwarz EM. Mechanisms of TNF-alpha- and RANKL-mediated osteoclastogenesis and bone resorption in psoriatic arthritis. J Clin Invest. 2003;111(6):821–31.

40. Harre U, Georgess D, Bang H, Bozec A, Axmann R, Ossipova E, et al. Induction of osteoclastogenesis and bone loss by human autoantibodies against citrullinated vimentin. J Clin Invest. 2012;122(5):1791–802.

41. Rahman P, Snelgrove T, Peddle L, Siannis F, Farewell V, Schentag C, et al. A variant of the IL4 I50V single-nucleotide polymorphism is associated with erosive joint disease in psoriatic arthritis. Arthritis Rheum. 2008;58(7):2207–8.

42. Karouzakis E, Neidhart M, Gay RE, Gay S. Molecular and cellular basis of rheumatoid joint destruction. Immunol Lett. 2006;106(1):8–13.

43. Appel H, Kuhne M, Spiekermann S, Ebhardt H, Grozdanovic Z, Kohler D, et al. Immunohistologic analysis of zygapophyseal joints in patients with ankylosing spondylitis. Arthritis Rheum. 2006;54(9):2845–51.

44. Appel H, Kuhne M, Spiekermann S, Kohler D, Zacher J, Stein H, et al. Immunohistochemical analysis of hip arthritis in ankylosing spondylitis: evaluation of the bone-cartilage interface and subchondral bone marrow. Arthritis Rheum. 2006;54(6):1805–13.

45. Appel H, Loddenkemper C, Grozdanovic Z, Ebhardt H, Dreimann M, Hempfing A, et al. Correlation of histopathological findings and magnetic resonance imaging in the spine of patients with ankylosing spondylitis. Arthritis Res Ther. 2006;8(5):R143.

46. Appel H, Maier R, Loddenkemper C, Kayser R, Meier O, Hempfing A, et al. Immunohistochemical analysis of osteoblasts in zygapophyseal joints of patients with ankylosing spondylitis reveal repair mechanisms similar to osteoarthritis. J Rheumatol. 2010;37(4):823–8.

47. Francois RJ. Some pathological features of ankylosing spondylitis as revealed by microradiography and tetracycline labelling. Clin Rheumatol. 1982;1(1):23–9.

48. Francois RJ, Gardner DL, Degrave EJ, Bywaters EG. Histopathologic evidence that sacroiliitis in ankylosing spondylitis is not merely enthesitis. Arthritis Rheum. 2000;43(9):2011–24.

49. Lories RJ, Daans M, Derese I, Matthys P, Kasran A, Tylzanowski P, et al. Noggin haploinsufficiency differentially affects tissue responses in destructive and remodeling arthritis. Arthritis Rheum. 2006;54(6):1736–46.

50. Lories RJ, Derese I, Luyten FP. Modulation of bone morphogenetic protein signaling inhibits the onset and progression of ankylosing enthesitis. J Clin Invest. 2005;115(6):1571–9.

51. Lories RJ, Haroon N. Bone formation in axial spondyloarthritis. Best Pract Res Clin Rheumatol. 2014;28(5):765–77.

52. Lories RJ, Matthys P, de Vlam K, Derese I, Luyten FP. Ankylosing enthesitis, dactylitis, and onychoperiostitis in male DBA/1 mice: a model of psoriatic arthritis. Ann Rheum Dis. 2004;63(5):595–8.

53. Diarra D, Stolina M, Polzer K, Zwerina J, Ominsky MS, Dwyer D, et al. Dickkopf-1 is a master regulator of joint remodeling. Nat Med. 2007;13(2):156–63.

54. Uderhardt S, Diarra D, Katzenbeisser J, David JP, Zwerina J, Richards W, et al. Blockade of Dickkopf (DKK)-1 induces fusion of sacroiliac joints. Ann Rheum Dis. 2010;69(3):592–7.

55. Ruiz-Heiland G, Horn A, Zerr P, Hofstetter W, Baum W, Stock M, et al. Blockade of the hedgehog pathway inhibits osteophyte formation in arthritis. Ann Rheum Dis. 2012;71(3):400–7.

56. Husted JA, Tom BD, Farewell VT, Schentag CT, Gladman DD. Description and prediction of physical functional disability in psoriatic arthritis: a longitudinal analysis using a Markov model approach. Arthritis Rheum. 2005;53(3):404–9.

57. van der Heijde D, Sharp J, Wassenberg S, Gladman DD. Psoriatic arthritis imaging: a review of scoring methods. Ann Rheum Dis. 2005;64 Suppl 2:ii61–4.

58. Lubrano E, Marchesoni A, Olivieri I, D'Angelo S, Spadaro A, Parsons WJ, et al. Psoriatic arthritis spondylitis radiology index: a modified index for radiologic assessment of axial involvement in psoriatic arthritis. J Rheumatol. 2009;36(5):1006–11.

59. Chandran V, Barrett J, Schentag CT, Farewell VT, Gladman DD. Axial psoriatic arthritis: update on a longterm prospective study. J Rheumatol. 2009;36(12):2744–50.

60. Wassenberg S, Fischer-Kahle V, Herborn G, Rau R. A method to score radiographic change in psoriatic arthritis. Z Rheumatol. 2001;60(3):156–66.

61. Tillett W, Jadon D, Shaddick G, Robinson G, Sengupta R, Korendowych E, et al. Feasibility, reliability, and sensitivity to change of four radiographic scoring methods in patients with psoriatic arthritis. Arthritis Care Res (Hoboken). 2014;66(2):311–7.

62. Antoni CE, Kavanaugh A, van der Heijde D, et al. Two-year efficacy and safety of infliximab treatment in patients with active psoriatic arthritis: findings of the Infliximab Multinational Psoriatic Arthritis Controlled Trial (IMPACT). J Rheumatol. 2008;35(5):869–76.

63. Eder L, Thavaneswaran A, Chandran V, Gladman DD. Tumour necrosis factor alpha blockers are more effective than methotrexate in the inhibition of radiographic joint damage progression among patients with psoriatic arthritis. Ann Rheum Dis. 2014;73(6):1007–11.

64. Gladman DD, Mease PJ, Ritchlin CT, et al. Adalimumab for long-term treatment of psoriatic arthritis: forty-eight week data from the adalimumab effectiveness in psoriatic arthritis trial. Arthritis Rheum. 2007;56(2):476–88.

65. Goulabchand R, Mouterde G, Barnetche T, Lukas C, Morel J, Combe B. Effect of tumour necrosis factor blockers on radiographic progression of psoriatic arthritis: a systematic review and meta-analysis of randomised controlled trials. Ann Rheum Dis. 2014;73(2):414–9.

66. Kavanaugh A, Antoni CE, Gladman D, et al. The Infliximab Multinational Psoriatic Arthritis Controlled Trial (IMPACT): results of radiographic analyses after 1 year. Ann Rheum Dis. 2006;65(8):1038–43.

67. Kavanaugh A, McInnes IB, Mease P, et al. Clinical efficacy, radiographic and safety findings through 5 years of subcutaneous golimumab treatment in patients with active psoriatic arthritis: results from a long-term extension of a randomised, placebo-controlled trial (the GO-REVEAL study). Ann Rheum Dis. 2014;73(9):1689–94.

68. Kavanaugh A, McInnes IB, Mease PJ, et al. Clinical efficacy, radiographic and safety findings through 2 years of golimumab treatment in patients with active psoriatic arthritis: results from a long-term extension of the randomised, placebo-controlled GO-REVEAL study. Ann Rheum Dis. 2013;72(11):1777–85.

69. Kavanaugh A, van der Heijde D, Beutler A, et al. Patients with psoriatic arthritis who achieve minimal disease activity in response to golimumab therapy demonstrate less radiographic progression: Results through 5 years of the randomized, placebo-controlled, GO-REVEAL study. Arthritis Care Res (Hoboken). 2016;68(2):267–74.

70. Kavanaugh A, van der Heijde D, McInnes IB, et al. Golimumab in psoriatic arthritis: one-year clinical efficacy, radiographic, and safety results from a phase III, randomized, placebo-controlled trial. Arthritis Rheum. 2012;64(8):2504–17.

71. van der Heijde D, Kavanaugh A, Gladman DD, et al. Infliximab inhibits progression of radiographic damage in patients with active psoriatic arthritis through one year of treatment: Results from the induction and maintenance psoriatic arthritis clinical trial 2. Arthritis Rheum. 2007;56(8):2698–707.

72. Mease PJ, Kivitz AJ, Burch FX, et al. Continued inhibition of radiographic progression in patients with psoriatic arthritis following 2 years of treatment with etanercept. J Rheumatol. 2006;33(4):712–21.

73. Mease PJ, Kivitz AJ, Burch FX, et al. Etanercept treatment of psoriatic arthritis: safety, efficacy, and effect on disease progression. Arthritis Rheum. 2004;50(7):2264–72.

74. Mease PJ, Ory P, Sharp JT, et al. Adalimumab for long-term treatment of psoriatic arthritis: 2-year data from the Adalimumab Effectiveness in Psoriatic Arthritis Trial (ADEPT). Ann Rheum Dis. 2009;68(5):702–9.

75. Kavanaugh A, Puig L, Gottlieb AB, et al. Maintenance of clinical efficacy and radiographic benefit through 2 years of ustekinumab therapy in patients with active psoriatic arthritis: Results from the PSUMMIT 1 trial. Arthritis Care Res (Hoboken). 2015;67(12):1739–49.

76. Kavanaugh A, Ritchlin C, Rahman P, et al. Ustekinumab, an anti-IL-12/23 p40 monoclonal antibody, inhibits radiographic progression in patients with active psoriatic arthritis: results of an integrated analysis of radiographic data from the phase 3, multicentre, randomised, double-blind, placebo-controlled PSUMMIT-1 and PSUMMIT-2 trials. Ann Rheum Dis. 2014;73(6):1000–6.

77. Gladman DD, Mease PJ, Choy EH, Ritchlin CT, Perdok RJ, Sasso EH. Risk factors for radiographic progression in psoriatic arthritis: subanalysis of the randomized controlled trial ADEPT. Arthritis Res Ther. 2010;12(3):R113.

78. Baraliakos X, Haibel H, Listing J, Sieper J, Braun J. Continuous long-term anti-TNF therapy does not lead to an increase in the rate of new bone formation over 8 years in patients with ankylosing spondylitis. Ann Rheum Dis. 2014;73(4):710–5.

79. Braun J, Baraliakos X, Hermann KG, et al. The effect of two golimumab doses on radiographic progression in ankylosing spondylitis: results through 4 years of the GO-RAISE trial. Ann Rheum Dis. 2014;73(6):1107–13.

80. van der Heijde D, Landewe R, Baraliakos X, et al. Radiographic findings following two years of infliximab therapy in patients with ankylosing spondylitis. Arthritis Rheum. 2008;58(10):3063–70.

81. Eder L, Chandran V, Gladman DD. Repair of radiographic joint damage following treatment with etanercept in psoriatic arthritis is demonstrable by 3 radiographic methods. J Rheumatol. 2011;38(6):1066–70.

Clinical features

CHAPTER 9

Psoriasis: skin and nails

Cheryl F. Rosen and Brian Kirby

Clinical features

Chronic plaque psoriasis is characterized by well-demarcated erythematous, scaly plaques. The scalp is commonly affected. Psoriasis may affect any part of the skin. It is estimated that 20% of patients have severe disease with more than 10% of the body surface area affected [1].

Guttate psoriasis presents generally with multiple erythematous scaly papules and plaques. This flare occurs commonly as a sequela to streptococcal infection, usually pharyngitis. The eruption usually occurs 10 days to 2 weeks after the infection [2]. Patients may have no disease between guttate flares or have residual chronic plaque psoriasis.

Erythrodermic psoriasis is a rare variant, occurring in less than 10% of patients with the disease [2]. Erythroderma is defined as generalized erythema and scale, with >90% of the body surface area affected. There is a differential diagnosis of erythroderma, and if there is no past history of psoriasis, a biopsy may be required to establish the diagnosis, ruling out cutaneous T cell lymphoma, a drug-induced eruption, and severe atopic dermatitis. Patients may be systemically unwell with a risk of cutaneously derived systemic infection such as staphylococcal septicaemia, due to disruption of the epidermal barrier. Temperature dysregulation may occur. High output cardiac failure is a rare complication.

Generalized pustular psoriasis is another rare variant of psoriasis [3]. Patients experience a sudden onset of generalized macular erythema with multiple pustules scattered over the skin surface. Many patients with generalized pustular psoriasis have no cutaneous findings between pustular episodes. When accompanied by fever and malaise, the disease may be referred to as von Zumbusch pustular psoriasis. Generalized pustular psoriasis may be precipitated by systemic illness or the abrupt withdrawal of systemic steroids. Less commonly, the discontinuation of the widespread use of potent topical steroids can lead to a generalized pustular flare. The use of oral steroids in patients with moderate to severe psoriasis should thus be undertaken with caution. A slow gradual tapering of the systemic steroid is recommended to minimize the risk of a rebound flare of chronic plaque psoriasis or, less commonly generalized pustular disease.

Inverse psoriasis

Intertriginous or inverse psoriasis is the psoriasis phenotype where the predominant locations of involvement are in the folds, such as the intergluteal cleft, axillae, and inguinal folds [4]. In a study that examined the incidence of psoriasis phenotypes in three large databases, inverse psoriasis was found to occur in 24–30% of patients with psoriasis. The affected areas are erythematous but are generally not scaly, due to the increased moisture in these areas. Inverse psoriasis may be itchy and painful and very distressing for the patient. Separate scoring systems have been developed to account for this flexural involvement. Involvement of the intergluteal cleft has been found to be associated with an increased risk of developing psoriatic arthritis [5].

Sebopsoriasis

This is a facial phenotype with psoriatic plaques appearing in a seborrheic pattern, with involvement of the nasolabial folds, the eyebrows, and the glabella.

Palmoplantar psoriasis and Palmoplantar pustulosis

Palmoplantar psoriasis affects the plantar aspect of the feet and palms of the hands and may affect 12–16% of patients with psoriasis [4]. Palmoplantar pustulosis is a distinct condition characterized by the development of pustules on a background of well-demarcated erythema. Yellow to white pustules appear on a background of erythema. As the individual pustules resolve, they may leave a brown dried crust. The pustules and the erythema may be itchy and painful, particularly if fissures develop. Walking may become very difficult and palmar involvement can interfere with the ability to perform the activities of daily living.

It remains unclear whether palmoplantar pustulosis is a variant of psoriasis or is a distinct condition associated with psoriasis [6]. The genetics of palmoplantar pustulosis may be distinct from psoriasis [7]. Palmoplantar pustulosis has been reported to occur predominantly in women and may be more strongly associated with cigarette smoking than chronic plaque psoriasis [8]. However, the percentage of people with palmoplantar pustulosis who have psoriasis on other parts of their skin has been found to be as high as 73% [9]. A study that compared the clinical and epidemiological data of patients affected by palmoplantar plaque psoriasis and palmoplantar pustulosis showed that 90% of patients with palmoplantar pustulosis had palmoplantar plaque psoriasis at the time of initial assessment or later on in their course [10]. There was no statistical difference between palmoplantar plaque psoriasis and palmoplantar pustulosis with respect to age of onset and duration of disease, family history of psoriasis, concomitant arthritis, or smoking habits [10]. Acrodermatitis continua of Hallopeau is a rare severe variant of palmoplantar pustulosis with addition painful pustular involvement of the nails and often bone resorption of the affected digits.

Nail psoriasis

Psoriasis can affect the nails in up to 25% of patients [4]. The presence of nail involvement is a risk factor for the development of psoriatic arthritis with a relative risk of 2.5 [5, 11]. Prevalence estimates of nail involvement in psoriatic arthritis suggest that approximately 50% of patients have nail psoriasis. Nail pitting is the most common feature. It is due to retention of nuclei in nail matrix keratinocytes (known as parakeratosis) with subsequent cell loss in the nail plate. Pitting is asymptomatic. Onycholysis is the separation of the nail plate from the underlying nail bed. Trauma can accelerate this process. Inflammation of the nail bed can lead to a yellow-brown discolouration of the distal nail plate called 'oil on water spots'. Subungual debris, with hyperkeratosis of the distal nail bed appears to be secondary to increased proliferation of the nail matrix. Psoriatic dystrophic nails may occasionally develop onychomycosis, particularly of the toenails. If this is suspected, nail clippings for fungal microscopy and culture should be done, because treatment of the nail fungus may improve the appearance and function of the nails.

Nail involvement can cause pain and significant functional impairment, resulting in the restriction of daily activities. Quality of life can be greatly impacted by nail psoriasis [12].

The treatment of nail psoriasis is unsatisfactory. Topical therapies are ineffective. Intralesional injection of triamcinolone acetonide into the nail matrix under local anaesthesia may be effective, but the pain from the injections limits its use. It may cause bone resorption. Systemic therapies have variable efficacy in nail psoriasis with the best results reported for cyclosporine (5mg/kg per day). The use of immunosuppressive medications may be justified for treating isolated nail psoriasis, if the nail disease is severe and has great impact on the quality of life. In a systematic review of treatment of nail psoriasis, infliximab and golimumab were found to cause significant nail improvement [13]. Cyclosporine, methotrexate, and ustekinumab were not found to be superior to their respective comparators: etretinate, cyclosporine, and placebo [13].

Ethnicity

Psoriasis appears to be more common in countries that are further from the equator and in Caucasians. It is rare in indigenous North Americans and one study actually found 0% prevalence in South American Indians [1].

There are two peak ages of incidence of chronic plaque psoriasis, the first occurring between 16 and 22 years and the second between 57 and 62 years of age. This has led to the concept of type I psoriasis and type II psoriasis [14]. This bimodal pattern of early and late onset psoriasis was also found in a more recent study [15].

Gender

Psoriasis vulgaris affects females and males equally although there may be an earlier age of onset in females. Clinical trials of therapies for moderate to severe psoriasis suggest that men are twice as likely to be enrolled in such trials. This may be due to men having more severe cutaneous disease but may be due to a bias in enrolling patients [16]. However, clinical trials in psoriatic arthritis suggest that there is an equal distribution of psoriatic arthritis between the sexes.

Pathophysiology

Psoriasis is characterized by hyperproliferation of the epidermis. In normal skin, basal cells proliferate and migrate outward through the layers of the epidermis as they differentiate. In the stratum corneum, the outer layer of the skin, keratinocytes die, become anucleated, having accumulated keratins and certain lipids, and provide the barrier function of the skin. With time, these cells are shed. This process normally takes 30–35 days. In psoriatic involved skin, this process is accelerated, with turnover of the epidermis occurring every 4–4.5 days. This results in a lack of normal keratinocyte differentiation with the formation of an abnormal stratum corneum that clinically manifests as scale [17].

There is a marked influx of immunocytes into the dermis and epidermis in psoriasis. These include cells of the innate and adaptive immune systems. Dendritic cells in the epidermis and upper dermis become activated [17]. This activation may be antigen driven.

A recent paper suggests that a protein expressed on the surface of melanocytes (ADAMTS-like protein 5) may act as an autoantigen in psoriasis [18]. The pathophysiology/aetiology of psoriasis is discussed in Chapters 4 to 8.

Early plaque formation is associated with an influx of neutrophils, mast cells, macrophages, and T cells into the dermis. This is followed by infiltration of the epidermis by neutrophils and T lymphocytes. Collections of neutrophils are seen with in the epidermis, called spongiform pustules of Kogoj and Munro's microabscesses. Numerous cytokines are produced which activate epidermal hyperproliferation. These cytokines include tumour necrosis factor alpha, interleukin (IL)-23, IL-17, and IL-22. There appears to be an autoinflammatory loop in the involved skin of psoriasis patients [17].

The overexpression of cytokines produced by Th1 and Th17 cells characterizes psoriasis plaques but cells of the innate immune system such as neutrophils may also produce IL-17 [19].

Psoriatic plaques are noted to have an increased number of blood vessels in the dermis [20], with the formation of new blood vessels in the papillary dermis. There is overexpression of angiogenic factors such as vascular endothelial growth factor (VEGF) in the plaques of psoriasis. VEGF may act as a chemoattractant and further enhance the inflammatory processes in the skin. This increased vascularity is seen on histology and becomes apparent clinically, when the scale of a psoriatic plaque is lifted off revealing multiple bleeding points (Auspitz sign).

There is considerable evidence for the role of neuroinflammation in psoriasis. Cutaneous nerve fibres are seen in abundance in involved skin. These fibres appear to be in close proximity with mast cells in the papillary dermis. They overexpress nerve growth factor, substance p, and calcitonin gene related peptide, neurotransmitters that can act as chemokines. These neurotransmitters can therefore further enhance cutaneous inflammation and epidermal hyperproliferation [21].

Genetics of psoriasis

There is an increased risk of developing psoriasis in family members of people with psoriasis. Please see Chapter 5.

Environmental factors

Psoriasis is associated with several environmental and lifestyle factors. Both guttate and chronic plaque psoriasis may be triggered and exacerbated by infection [22]. Streptococcal tonsillitis is strongly associated with a flare of guttate psoriasis. This is especially true in younger patients and those who carry the HLA-Cw6 allele. Molecular mimicry may play a role in this phenomenon. There is strong homology between the streptococcal M protein and keratin 17 that is overexpressed in involved psoriasis skin. It is proposed that streptococcal infection leads to an expansion of T cell clones which cross react with keratin 17 in the skin [23]. This concept is supported by studies demonstrating that an oligoclonal expansion of T cells occurs in the tonsils of psoriasis patients whose disease is exacerbated by streptococcal infection [24]. The same T cell clones are also found in increased numbers in the skin and blood of these patients. Treatment with antibiotics is not effective in guttate psoriasis [25]. This may be due to intracellular location of streptococci in the tonsils making the streptococci resistant to penicillin. However, tonsillectomy may result in remission of cutaneous psoriasis in up to 50% of patients whose disease is exacerbated by streptococcal tonsillitis [26]. Streptococcal infection and tonsillectomy do not affect psoriatic arthritis.

Human immunodeficiency virus infection

Human immunodeficiency virus (HIV)infection is associated with both the onset and exacerbation of psoriasis and psoriatic arthritis, particularly in patients with the HLA-Cw6 allele. This psoriatic paradox is not understood but it has been suggested that immune alterations induced by HIV infection lead to the inflammatory response in psoriasis and psoriatic arthritis. This supports the importance of CD8+ T cells in psoriasis pathogenesis, as with depletion of CD4+ cells the CD8+ cells can act unimpeded. Treatment with highly active antiretroviral therapy (HAART) is effective in controlling the psoriasis exacerbated by HIV infection in the majority of patients [27].

Medications

Several medications have been reported to exacerbate psoriasis, primarily as case reports [28]. However, there seems to be little doubt that lithium may exacerbate psoriasis and may make the disease more resistant to therapy. The mechanism underlying this effect of lithium is unknown.

The antimalarial medications, hydroxychloroquine and chloroquine, may exacerbate psoriasis. This is uncommon but these drugs should be avoided if possible in patients with moderate to severe psoriasis. Exacerbation of psoriasis with beta-blockers appears to be a rare event. Psoriasis should not be a contraindication to the use of beta-blockers, if needed for the treatment of co-morbidities such as hypertension or angina.

The abrupt withdrawal of systemic steroids can result in an exacerbation of psoriasis. If oral steroids are required to treat other conditions in people with moderate to severe psoriasis, a gradual tapering of the dose over several weeks is strongly recommended.

Anti-TNF biologics

New onset psoriasis, known as paradoxical psoriasis, has been reported to develop in people on anti-TNF agents [29]. Many of these patients are being treated with anti-TNF biologics for diseases other than psoriasis or psoriatic arthritis, such as Crohn's disease or ankylosing spondylitis [30, 31]. Palmoplantar and pustular forms of psoriasis are predominantly reported. Many patients can remain on TNF inhibitors and the paradoxical psoriasis can be managed by topical therapy or phototherapy. However, some patients will require a change in biologic therapy.

Psychological distress

Moderate to severe psoriasis is associated with psychological distress and impaired quality of life [32]. The presence of psoriatic arthritis increases both distress and quality of life impairment [32, 33]. Patients with moderate to severe psoriasis are more likely to suffer from depression than controls and to require treatment with antidepressant medication. Rates of depression have been reported in up to 23% of patients. Depression appears to be independent risk factor for psoriasis [32]. Increased rates of stigmatization, suicidal ideation, anxiety, and suicide have been reported in patients with psoriasis. Psychological distress may exacerbate psoriasis [32]. Psychological interventions have been reported to be effective in reducing psychological distress and the physical disease but these reports have been inconsistent. Screening for anxiety and depression in patients with moderate to severe disease is recommended.

Ultraviolet radiation/sunlight

Many patients report improvement in psoriasis with sunlight exposure, which has led to the therapeutic use of artificial sources of ultraviolet radiation, particularly narrow band ultraviolet B radiation. However, a minority have photoexacerbated psoriasis, noting worsening of their disease with sun exposure [34].

Physical trauma

Up to 25% of patients report that skin injury can flare their disease. This is known as the Koebner phenomenon [35]. It has been suggested that lifting heavy loads and injury may induce psoriatic arthritis in patients with psoriasis [36].

Cigarette smoking

Cigarette smoking is associated with an increased risk of developing psoriasis [37], as has been noted in rheumatoid arthritis. This is true for chronic plaque psoriasis but the association is stronger for palmoplantar pustulosis. The mechanism that links smoking and psoriasis is unknown but it is well established that smoking does have profound effects on immune function [38].

Alcohol misuse

Chronic plaque psoriasis is associated with alcohol misuse [39]. It is not clear whether psoriasis patients drink more alcohol due to the psychological distress associated with psoriasis or whether alcohol excess itself exacerbates psoriasis. It may be that both are correct. A Finnish study reported greatly increased rates of alcohol-related mortality in patients with psoriasis compared to controls [40]. Alcohol misuse was reported in up to 32% of patients with moderate to severe disease in an Irish population [41]. Alcohol misuse was linked to higher levels of anxiety and depression in an English cohort of psoriasis patients [42]. Psoriasis may be the only autoimmune disease where such a strong link with alcohol exists. The mechanism underlying the relationship between psoriasis and alcohol excess is not known.

Obesity and metabolic syndrome

Patients with moderate to severe psoriasis are more likely to be obese and have metabolic syndrome than control populations [43]. In a large American epidemiological study, the Nurses' Health Study, increasing obesity appeared to precede psoriasis [44]. In a smaller study of patients with psoriasis being treated with phototherapy, increasing body mass index was associated with more severe psoriasis as measured by PASI [45]. Adipocytes produce cytokines such as TNF-α that may contribute to worsening psoriasis. Decreasing body mass index by diet or bariatric surgery may reduce psoriasis severity [46].

Cardiovascular disease

Moderate to severe psoriasis is associated with an increased risk of cardiovascular disease and mortality [47]. This risk is higher among younger patients but the excess risk persists throughout life. Psoriasis patients also have an increased incidence of traditional cardiovascular risk factors including higher rates of cigarette smoking, hypertension, dyslipidaemia, type II diabetes, obesity, and excessive alcohol intake. Studies that have controlled for these traditional risk factors have demonstrated that both psoriasis and psoriatic arthritis are independent risk factors for premature cardiovascular disease [48].

Systemic inflammation is known to cause premature cardiovascular injury and may play a role in the increased risk of cardiovascular events in patients with severe psoriasis. However, the relative contribution of systemic inflammation compared to traditional risk factors is unknown. Patients with moderate to severe psoriasis should be screened for hypertension, dyslipidaemia, and type II diabetes as these people are at higher risk than the general population. Several studies suggest that systemic treatment of moderate to severe psoriasis may reduce the risk of cardiovascular disease, although this has not been fully established [49–52].

Measurement of psoriasis severity and outcome measures

The Psoriasis Area and Severity Index (PASI) remains the most widely used method for assessing psoriasis severity in clinical trials and clinical practice [53]. The PASI assesses psoriasis severity by giving a score for erythema, induration, and scale of an average plaque for each of the following areas: the arms, lower limbs including the buttocks, trunk, and head. The score for each part of the body is then multiplied by a number representing the extent of involvement in that part. A composite score is then calculated. The PASI may range from 0 to 72 but PASI values over 40 are rare. A PASI of >10 is indicative of moderate to severe psoriasis.

The PASI was originally developed to assess changes in psoriasis severity for a clinical trial of etretinate [53]. It has been adopted by regulatory agencies as the standard for assessing psoriasis severity in clinical trials. A 75% reduction in PASI (PASI75) has been deemed clinically significant and new therapies for psoriasis have to demonstrate a significant higher percentage of patients achieving PASI75 compared to placebo in order to be approved for the treatment of psoriasis. However, the severity of the cutaneous involvement is only one aspect of psoriasis. Psoriasis may have a significant impact on patients' quality of life. In clinical trials and in practice, the PASI must be combined with a measure of the quality of life in order to assess the impact of the disease on each patient.

The Dermatology Quality of Life Index (DLQI) is the patient reported outcome measure that is used most frequently. The DLQI assesses the impact of psoriasis over the previous 7 days on a variety of activities and results in a score between 0 and 30. Values greater than 10 indicate a severe impact of the disease on a patient's quality of life [39].

There are now many more treatments available to treat people with moderate to severe psoriasis. These new treatments have had a tremendous impact on the severity of disease and quality of life for many patients. It would be very useful to have more topical options available for people with mild to moderate disease and for the persistent areas in people treated with systemic agents. Treatment for psoriasis is discussed in Chapters 26 to 31.

References

1. Parisi R, Symmons DP, Griffiths CE, et al. Global epidemiology of psoriasis: a systematic review of incidence and prevalence. J Invest Dermatol 2013;133(2):377–85.
2. Raychaudhuri SK, M.E., Raychaudhuri SP, Diagnosis and classification of psoriasis. Autoimmunity Review, 2014; 13:490–5.
3. Umezawa Y, Ozawa A, Kawasima T, et al., Therapeutic guidelines for the treatment of generalized pustular psoriasis (GPP) based on a proposed classification of disease severity. Arch Dermatol Res, 2003; 295 Suppl 1:S43–54.
4. Merola JF, Li T, Li W, Cho E, Qureshi AA. Prevalence of psoriasis phenotypes among men and women in the USA. Clin Exp Dermatol, 2016; 41(5):486–9.
5. Wilson FC, Icen M, Crowson CS, McEvoy MT, Gabriel SE, Kremers HM. Incidence and clinical predictors of psoriatic arthritis in patients with psoriasis: a population-based study. Arthritis Rheum, 2009;61(2):233–9.
6. Obeid G, DG, Latsahian S, Kirby L, Hughes C, LeLeach L. Interventions for chronic palmoplantar pustulosis. Cochrane Database Sytematic Reviews, 2015;25(CD001433).
7. Asumalahti K, Ameen M, Suomela S, et al., Genetic analysis of PSORS1 distinguishes guttate psoriasis and palmoplantar pustulosis. J Invest Dermatol, 2003;120(4):627–32.
8. O'Doherty CJ, MacIntyre, C. Palmoplantar pustulosis and smoking. Br Med J (Clin Res Ed), 1985; 291(6499):861–4.
9. Brunasso AM, Massone C. Can we really separate palmoplantar pustulosis from psoriasis? J Eur Acad Dermatol Venereol, 2010; 24(5):619–21; author reply 621.
10. Brunasso AM, Puntoni M, Aberer W, Delfino C, Fancelli L, Massone C. Clinical and epidemiological comparison of patients affected by palmoplantar plaque psoriasis and palmoplantar pustulosis: a case series study. Br J Dermatol, 2013; 168(6):1243–51.
11. Eder L, Haddad A, Rosen CF, et al., The incidence and risk factors for psoriatic arthritis in patients with psoriasis: a prospective cohort study. Arthritis Rheumatol, 2016; 68(4):915–23.
12. Langley RG, Dauden E. Treatment and management of psoriasis with nail involvement: a focus on biologic therapy. Dermatology, 2010; 221 Suppl 1:29–42.
13. de Vries AC, Bogaards NA, Hooft L, et al. Interventions for nail psoriasis. Cochrane Database Syst Rev, 2013(1):CD007633. DOI: 10.1002/14651858.CD007633.pub2.
14. Henseler T, Christophers, E. Psoriasis of early and late onset: characterization of two types of psoriasis vulgaris. J Am Acad Dermatol, 1985;13(3):450–6.
15. Springate DA., Parisi R, Kontopantelis E, Reeves D, Griffiths CE, Ashcroft DM. Incidence, prevalence and mortality of patients with psoriasis: a U.K. population-based cohort study. Br J Dermatol, 2016; 176(3):650–8.
16. White D, O'Shea SJ, Rogers S. Do men have more severe psoriasis than women? J Eur Acad Dermatol Venereol, 2012; 26(1):126–7.
17. Nestle FO, Kaplan DH, Barker J. Psoriasis. N Engl J Med, 2009; 361(5):496–509.
18. Arakawa A., Siewert K, Stöhr J, et al., Melanocyte antigen triggers autoimmunity in human psoriasis. J Exp Med, 2015; 212(13):2203–12.
19. Reich K, Papp KA, Matheson RT, et al. Evidence that a neutrophil-keratinocyte crosstalk is an early target of IL-17A inhibition in psoriasis. Exp Dermatol, 2015; 24(7):529–35.

20. Varricchi G, Granata F, Loffredo S, Genovese A, Marone G. Angiogenesis and lymphangiogenesis in inflammatory skin disorders. J Am Acad Dermatol, 2015; 73(1):144–53.

21. Saraceno R, Kleyn CE, Terenghi G, Griffiths CE. The role of neuropeptides in psoriasis. Br J Dermatol, 2006. 155(5):876–82.

22. Thorleifsdottir RH, Eysteinsdóttir JH, Olafsson JH, et al., Throat infections are associated with exacerbation in a substantial proportion of patients with chronic plaque psoriasis. Acta Derm Venereol, 2016; 96(6):788–91.

23. McFadden J, Valdimarsson H, Fry L. Cross-reactivity between streptococcal M surface antigen and human skin. Br J Dermatol, 1991; 125(5):443–7.

24. Sigurdardottir SL, Thorleifsdottir RH, Valdimarsson H, Johnston A. The association of sore throat and psoriasis might be explained by histologically distinctive tonsils and increased expression of skin-homing molecules by tonsil T cells. Clin Exp Immunol, 2013;174(1):139–51.

25. Chalmers RJ, O'Sullivan T, Owen CM, Griffiths CE. A systematic review of treatments for guttate psoriasis. Br J Dermatol, 2001; 145(6):891–4.

26. Rachakonda TD, Dhillon JS, Florek AG, Armstrong AW. Effect of tonsillectomy on psoriasis: a systematic review. J Am Acad Dermatol, 2015; 72(2):261–75.

27. Morar N, Willis-Owen SA, Maurer T, Bunker CB. HIV-associated psoriasis: pathogenesis, clinical features, and management. Lancet Infect Dis, 2010; 10(7):470–8.

28. Basavaraj KH, Ashok NM, Rashmi R, Praveen TK. The role of drugs in the induction and/or exacerbation of psoriasis. Int J Dermatol, 2010; 49(12):1351–61.

29. Sasaki JL,Koo JY. Skin therapies: dermatologic perspective on the rheumatology-dermatology interface. Clin Exp Rheumatol, 2015;33(5 Suppl 93):S78–81.

30. Guerra I, Pérez-Jeldres T, Iborra M, et al. Incidence, clinical characteristics, and management of psoriasis induced by anti-TNF therapy in patients with inflammatory bowel disease: a nationwide cohort study. Inflamm Bowel Dis, 2016; 22(4):894–901.

31. Ko JM, Gottlieb AM, Kerbleski JF. Induction and exacerbation of psoriasis with TNF-blockade therapy: a review and analysis of 127 cases. J Dermatolog Treat, 2009; 20(2):100–8.

32. Fortune DG, Richards HL, Griffiths CE. Psychologic factors in psoriasis: consequences, mechanisms, and interventions. Dermatol Clin, 2005; 23(4):681–94.

33. Rosen CF, Yilmaz Tasdelen O, Bodur H, et al. Patients with psoriatic arthritis have worse quality of life than those with psoriasis alone. Rheumatology (Oxford), 2012;51(3):571–6.

34. Rutter KJ, Watson RE, Cotterell LF, Brenn T, Griffiths CE, Rhodes LE. Severely photosensitive psoriasis: a phenotypically defined patient subset. J Invest Dermatol, 2009; 129(12):2861–7.

35. Camargo CM, Brotas AM, Ramos-e-Silva M, Carneiro S. Isomorphic phenomenon of Koebner: facts and controversies. Clin Dermatol, 2013; 31(6):741–9.

36. Eder L, Law T, Chandran V, et al., Association between environmental factors and onset of psoriatic arthritis in patients with psoriasis. Arthritis Care Res (Hoboken), 2011; 63(8):1091–7.

37. Armstrong AW, Harskamp CT, Dhillon JS, Armstrong EJ. Psoriasis and smoking: a systematic review and meta-analysis. Br J Dermatol, 2014; 170(2):304–14.

38. Qiu F, Liang CL, Liu H, et al. Impacts of cigarette smoking on immune responsiveness: Up and down or upside down? Oncotarget, 2017. 8(1):268–84.

39. Adamzik K, McAleer MA, Kirby B. Alcohol and psoriasis: sobering thoughts. Clin Exp Dermatol, 2013; 38(8):819–22.

40. Poikolainen K, Karvonen J, Pukkala E. Excess mortality related to alcohol and smoking among hospital-treated patients with psoriasis. Arch Dermatol, 1999; 135(12):1490–3.

41. McAleer MA, Mason DL, Cunningham S, et al. Alcohol misuse in patients with psoriasis: identification and relationship to disease severity and psychological distress. Br J Dermatol, 2011; 164(6):1256–61.

42. Kirby B, Richards HL, Mason DL, Fortune DG, Main CJ, Griffiths CE. Alcohol consumption and psychological distress in patients with psoriasis. Br J Dermatol, 2008; 158(1):138–40.

43. Ryan C, Kirby B. Psoriasis is a systemic disease with multiple cardiovascular and metabolic comorbidities. Dermatol Clin, 2015; 33(1):41–55.

44. Kumar S, Han J, Li T, Qureshi AA Obesity, waist circumference, weight change and the risk of psoriasis in US women. J Eur Acad Dermatol Venereol, 2013; 27(10):1293–8.

45. Tobin AM, Hackett CB, Rogers S, et al. Body mass index, waist circumference and HOMA-IR correlate with the Psoriasis Area and Severity Index in patients with psoriasis receiving phototherapy. Br J Dermatol, 2014; 171(2):436–8.

46. Upala S, Sanguankeo A. Effect of lifestyle weight loss intervention on disease severity in patients with psoriasis: a systematic review and meta-analysis. Int J Obes (Lond), 2015; 39(8):1197–202.

47. Mehta NN, Azfar RS, Shin DB, Neimann AL, Troxel AB, Gelfand JM. Patients with severe psoriasis are at increased risk of cardiovascular mortality: cohort study using the General Practice Research Database. Eur Heart J, 2010. 31(8):1000–6.

48. Lai YC, Yew YW, Psoriasis as an independent risk factor for cardiovascular disease: an epidemiologic analysis using a national database. J Cutan Med Surg, 2016; 20(4):327–33.

49. Roubille C, Richer V, Starnino T, et al. The effects of tumour necrosis factor inhibitors, methotrexate, non-steroidal anti-inflammatory drugs and corticosteroids on cardiovascular events in rheumatoid arthritis, psoriasis and psoriatic arthritis: a systematic review and meta-analysis. Ann Rheum Dis, 2015; 74(3):480–9.

50. Ahlehoff O, Skov L, Gislason G et al. Cardiovascular outcomes and systemic anti-inflammatory drugs in patients with severe psoriasis: 5-year follow-up of a Danish nationwide cohort. J Eur Acad Dermatol Venereol, 2015; 29(6):1128–34.

51. Ahlehoff O, Hansen PR, Gislason GH. Myocardial function and effects of biologic therapy in patients with severe psoriasis: a prospective echocardiographic study. J Eur Acad Dermatol Venereol, 2016; 30(5):819–23.

52. Hjuler KF, Bøttcher M, Vestergaard C, Bøtker HE, Iversen L, Kragballe K. Association between changes in coronary artery disease progression and treatment with biologic agents for severe psoriasis. JAMA Dermatol, 2016; 152(10):1114–21.

53. Fredriksson T, Pettersson U. Severe psoriasis–oral therapy with a new retinoid. Dermatologica, 1978; 157(4):238–44.

CHAPTER 10

Peripheral arthritis

Raffaele Scarpa, Francesco Caso, Luisa Costa,
Rosario Peluso, Nicola Matteo Dario Di Minno,
and Antonio Del Puente

Introduction

Clinical presentation of peripheral arthritis in patients with psoriatic arthritis (PsA), has been described by Moll and Wright who classified it into four subsets: symmetrical polyarthritis, asymmetrical oligoarthritis, distal interphalangeal (DIP) arthritis and arthritis mutilans [1].

The characteristics and the frequency of these subsets markedly vary in different populations, according to genetic, environmental, and geographic factors [2]. In addition, we have to consider that disease patterns naturally change over time [3] and that all subsets of peripheral arthritis (particularly DIP arthritis and polyarthritis) may overlap with axial disease [4]. Moreover, the frequency of patterns appears different in patients with an articular involvement of recent onset (early PsA) [5, 6] when compared to patients with a long-standing disease (established PsA) [7–9].

Finally, with the development of the CASPAR criteria [10], we should consider the case of patients with peripheral arthritis belonging to the subsets described above, but with the occurrence of psoriasis only in other members of the family. This is the subset classified as 'sine psoriasis' which has been recently characterized [11].

Symmetrical polyarthritis

In this subset, the distribution of articular involvement is similar that of rheumatoid arthritis (RA) and this clinical presentation has for many years justified the inappropriate use of term 'rheumatoid-like form', at present completely abandoned (Figure 10.1A ; 10.1B). Several clinical features differentiate psoriatic polyarthritis from RA. Apart from the usual absence of serum rheumatoid factor (RF), joint distribution of psoriatic polyarthritis includes DIP arthritis, anterior chest wall involvement, occurrence of enthesopathies, and the presence of few non-marginal syndesmophytes, randomly distributed along the spine, occurring in the absence of sacroiliac changes [4, 9]. All these clinical features would be non-characteristic findings of RA. In addition, in psoriatic polyarthritis, nodules, lymphadenopathy, vasculitis, and pulmonary and kidney involvement are generally not found [9].

Prevalence is not consistent in different populations. Data from an Italian cohort show polyarthritis as the second most frequent subset, accounting for 20% of the cases with an established form of arthritis, while in cases of early onset it is a very rare presentation

[5, 6]. However Kane et al. have identified polyarthritis as the most common pattern, occurring in more than 60% of the cases. Even in early arthritis, the authors found that polyarthritis was the most common pattern [12].

Symmetrical polyarthritis may be also recorded in overlap with spondylitis (accounting for 30% of all spondylitic cases) [4] with a marked involvement of cervical tract, nonmarginal and asymmetrical syndesmophytes, and unilateral sacroiliitis.

Asymmetrical oligoarthritis

Oligoarthritis is characterized by asymmetrical involvement of few joints (fewer than four), which include scattered DIP or proximal interphalangeal (PIP) joints (Figure 10.2) and/or metatarsophalangeal joints. Dactylitis (sausage digit) may be a typical feature of this pattern (see below) (Figure 10.3).In an Italian cohort the early subset was the usual presentation, accounting for over 75% of the cases studied. [5, 6]. However, Kane et al. show a reduced prevalence, accounting for 40% of subjects with oligoarthritis [12].

Oligoarthritis may be recorded as exclusive form in about 15% of all patients with established form of arthritis [7, 9].

In the time before the use of biological agents, the progression from asymmetric oligoarthritis to symmetric polyarthritis over time was the norm [3, 13]. Indeed, more than 60% of patients who were starting with mono-oligoarthritis ended up developing polyarthritis during follow-up. The number of involved joints was a function of disease duration, despite treatment with traditional DMARDs. Oligoarthritis may be also observed in overlap with spondylitic subset, in fewer than 10% of all cases [4, 14].

Distal interphalangeal arthritis

Among the articular patterns, DIP arthritis is the most classical presentation. It was first described by a French dermatologist, Charles Bourdillon, in 1888, in his doctoral thesis on 34 patients with psoriasis and a peculiar clinical pattern of arthritis [15]. In particular, Bourdillon reported the involvement of DIP joints of hands and feet and considered this localization a distinctive feature with respect to other rheumatic forms.

DIP arthritis may occur with symmetrical or asymmetrical features, and it is often in strict association with onycopathy (Figure 10.4A ; 10.4B) [7, 9, 16]. In fact, using magnetic resonance imaging (MRI) to study nail unit of patients with psoriatic nail involvement,

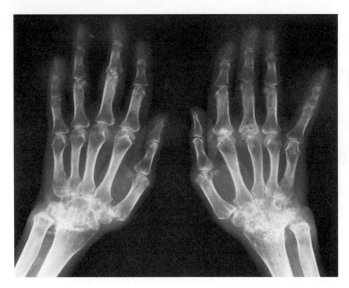

Figure 10.1A Psoriatic symmetrical polyarthritis resembling classical RA (rheumatoid-like form). The severe involvement of wrists, metacarpophalangeal and interphalangeal joints with the characteristic erosions is shown. (This image was obtained in the 'pre-biologic era').

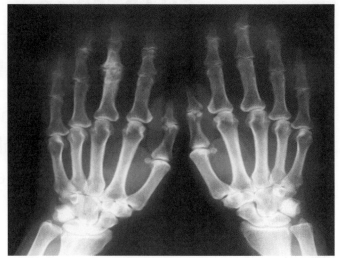

Figure 10.2 Typical aspect of oligoarthritis involving the third proximal interphalangeal joint of the left hand. Medical history of the patient reported that when symptoms began, that the finger was diffusely swollen (dactylitis). (This image has been realized in the 'pre-biologic era').

it was confirmed that initial lesions of nail induce the damage of distal phalanx and consequently of DIP joint [17, 18, 19].

Erosive changes initially affect the margins of DIP joint, but later on progress centrally (Figure 10.5) [9, 20].

As a unique pattern, DIP arthritis may occur in about 5% of all the arthritic cases of the established form, while in the case of early onset it is particularly rare [5–7].

In addition, DIP arthritis may occur with all the other peripheral subsets and the axial form [4, 9]. In particular, DIP arthritis may

overlap with spondylitis in over 15% of all axial cases. With time, an associated peripheral arthritis involving other joints develops. In these cases, while sacroiliitis may be absent, spinal involvement is striking and affects all vertebral tracts with the presence of non-marginal and asymmetrical syndesmophytes [5].

Arthritis mutilans

This pattern is characterized by the osteolysis of phalanx and metacarpals producing features defined by French authors as

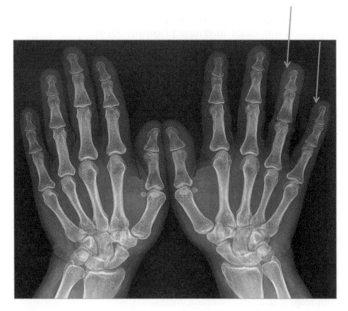

Figure 10.1B Psoriatic symmetrical polyarthritis. In this case, as compared to the subject in figure 10.1A, the involvement of all joints is moderate. This is a the more frequent and typical presentation of this subset. Note the involvement of distal interphalangeal joints which would be unusual in RA. (This image has been realized in the 'pre-biologic era').

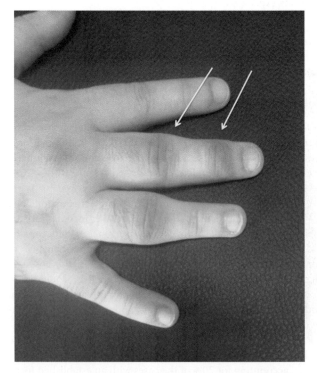

Figure 10.3 Typical appearance of dactylitis, involving the third finger of the right hand.

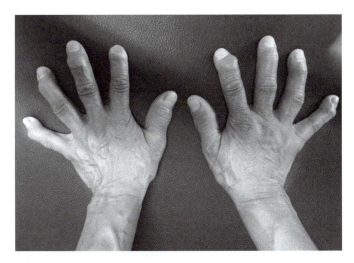

Figure 10.4A Marked distal interphalangeal joints involvement (DIP arthritis) symmetrically occurring at second, third and fourth fingers. The fifth finger shows bilaterally also the tendency to the subluxation.

'doigt en lorgnette' or by English authors as 'opera glass finger' [9] (Figure 10.6). It is very rare, occurring in less than 1% of patients with established form of arthritis [7, 9] It is also uncommon to observe the mutilans subset overlapping with other peripheral patterns of arthritis [9, 21–23].

Psoriatic arthritis 'sine psoriasis'

We know from epidemiological studies that in 15–20% of cases, the arthritis may precede the onset of the psoriatic skin rash [7, 8]. Consequently, PsA 'sine psoriasis' should not be considered a rare clinical finding. In this subset, although articular involvement is clinically expressed, cutaneous is apparently absent.

PsA 'sine psoriasis' is characterized by the co-occurrence of dactylitis, DIP arthritis, enthesitis, and tenosynovitis in the absence

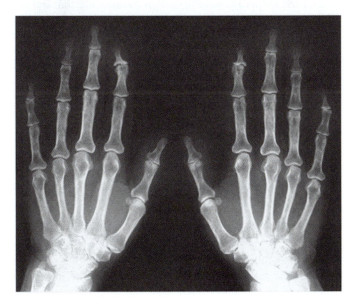

Figure 10.4B Symmetrical involvement of distal interphalangeal joints (DIP arthritis) affecting in particular the second fingers bilaterally. (This image has been realized in the 'pre-biologic era').

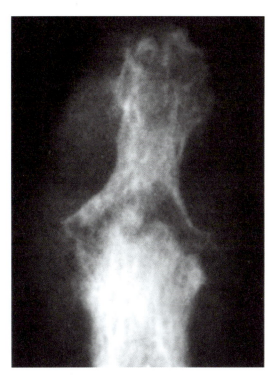

Figure 10.5 Erosive changes of the distal phalanx with osteitis. Clinical appearance of extensive changes in the distal interphalangeal joint in a patient with psoriatic arthritis and onychopathy. (This image has been realized in the 'pre-biologic era').

of overt psoriasis [11]. More rare is an axial involvement even in overlap with other peripheral patterns [11]. In their geographical area (Italy), a study of HLA haplotypes showed an increased frequency of HLA-Cw6 in 'sine psoriasis' subset [11].

As reported by Olivieri and coworkers, in the past these patients were diagnosed as having undifferentiated spondyloarthritis [24]. In 2003, on the basis of their clinical observations, in the absence of an overt skin and/or nail psoriasis, a familial history of psoriasis in first and/or second-grade relatives was considered a clinically equivalent element for a correct diagnosis [11]. In 2006 this conclusion has been confirmed by the CASPAR Criteria [10] which valued this clinical subset with the inclusion of familial psoriasis among classification criteria.

Laboratory tests and imaging for diagnosis

Although important for clinical differentiation, laboratory tests are of minor relevance to confirm the diagnosis of PsA. In fact, two of the most common tests used in clinical practice by rheumatologists, erythrocyte sedimentation rate (ESR) and C-reactive protein (CRP), are elevated in only half of the patients. This clinical observation has been confirmed in an Italian multicentre epidemiological study on a large cohort of patients [25]. Another characteristic finding is the usual absence of RF in the serum. This aspect plays a particularly relevant role in cases where the clinical presentation may mimic RA. Recently, in patients with the symmetrical polyarthritis subset the presence of anticyclic citrullinated peptide antibodies (anti-CCP), universally considered a characteristic and specific marker of RA [26, 27], has been reported [28, 29]. However, in the CASPAR study only 7% of the patients were anti-CCP positive [10].

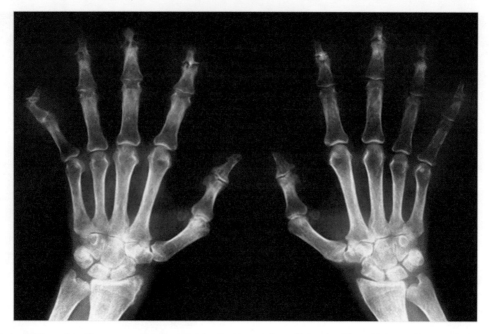

Figure 10.6 Symmetrical arthritis mutilans. The severe erosive disease of the distal interphalangeal joints is evident with intense bone resorption and subluxation. (This image has been realized in the 'pre-biologic era').

Anti-CCP antibodies seem to detect polyarticular cases with a more aggressive and erosive disease course. In a more extensive study, recently published by Espinoza and coworkers [30], the authors found anti-CCP positivity to be correlated with the polyarticular subset, female sex, more aggressive and erosive joint involvement, and higher use of TNF-blocking therapy. In this cohort, on the basis of the concurrent presence of dactylitis, enthesitis, axial and DIP joint involvement, and nail and cutaneous psoriasis, as well as typical radiological features including new bone formation, pencil-in-cup deformity, ankylosis, DIP involvement, and sacroileitis, Espinoza indicated a diagnosis of PsA anti-CCP positive, rather than an overlap syndrome (rheumatoid and psoriatic) or a co-occurrence of psoriasis with concomitant RA.

In the early PsA subset our recent observations outline seronegativity for RF and anti-CCP, with a moderate increase of ESR and CRP in only 25% of the cases (Table 10.1) [31].

Table 10.1 Laboratory findings of early arthritis patients with and without psoriasis

	Early arthritis patients with psoriasis (n; 24)	Early arthritis patients without psoriasis (n; 11)	p
Erythrocyte sedimentation rate >15 mm/1h (n; %)	6; 25%	11; 100%	ns
C-reactive protein > 0.5mg/dL (n; %)	6; 25%	11; 100%	ns
Rheumatoid factor positivity (n; %)	0	9; 81.8%	0.01
Anti-cyclic citrullinated peptide antibodies positivity (n; %)	0	4; 36.3%	ns

The analysis of synovial fluid may be helpful in supporting clinical diagnosis. Punzi and coworkers outlined the importance of the study of synovial fluid in PsA, describing as characteristic the abundance of effusion and the increased number of leukocytes, in the presence of normal levels of serum acute phase reactants [32, 33]. The overexpression of angiogenic factors (in particular transforming growth factor and vascular endothelial growth factor) has been also described [34].

In the diagnosis of peripheral arthritis, an essential role is surely played by radiology. Plain film radiography has markedly contributed to the affirmation of the concept of PsA as a disease entity different from RA. With regard to peripheral arthritis, characteristic aspects are the asymmetric joint involvement in hands and feet with the classic involvement of DIP joints of fingers and toes; the occurrence of marginal erosions with concomitant adjacent bone proliferation; the lack of prominent juxta-articular osteoporosis (although it does occur); the resorption of the tufts of terminal phalanx of hands and feet; the osteolysis of phalangeal, metacarpal, and metatarsal bone resulting in telescoping digits, in the case of arthritis mutilans; periarticular and shaft periostitis; and pencil-in-cup deformity.

An additional diagnostic support is offered by high-resolution ultrasonography, ultrasound combined with power Doppler, and MRI which have been validated as sensitive techniques to detect the involvement of synovial membrane but also of adjacent soft structures [35–40].

Differential diagnosis

Among the clinical features helpful in differentiating psoriatic polyarthritis from rheumatoid polyarthritis, is the important role played by articular presentation and laboratory tests [41–43]. In fact, RA usually tends to show a symmetric pattern involving, progressively and bilaterally small, medium, and large joints. Furthermore, in RA, the involvement of DIP as well of the spine is unusual, except for the cervical spine. Finally, laboratory findings can show an appreciable increase of inflammatory markers and in a large percentage of cases RF is present in the serum [41–43]. In addition, CCP (which occasionally may be found in PsA) antibodies, in high titre are characteristic and specific markers of RA [26–31].

In RA, one of the possible aspects of bone involvement is osteoporosis at a systemic level and bone erosion locally as expression of bone loss manifestations. The situation is not so clear-cut in PsA. In this disease, the involvement of bone is more complex because it affects not only mechanisms of bone loss but also of bone formation (ankylosis, periostitis, syndesmophytes) [44]. A recent study using X-ray evaluation of fragility fractures in subjects with PsA shows prevalence of vertebral fractures in a third of patients, correlating with duration of disease and with the presence of a peripheral subset of joint involvement [45].

Oligoarthritis, especially when occurring in the most frequent asymmetrical form, involving DIP, PIP, and/or MTP joints, could represent a diagnostic dilemma. Indeed, these findings which may coexist with inflammatory back pain, could be also present in other spondyloarthritides [46]. In these cases, a history of inflammatory bowel diseases and/or a recent gastrointestinal or urogenital infection for one to six weeks can be useful for addressing, respectively, a diagnosis of enteroarthritides or reactive arthritis [46]. Peripheral oligoarthritis occurring during the course of Crohn's disease and ulcerative colitis can often mimic PsA, in particular if concomitant with axial involvement and/or extra-intestinal manifestations, such as uveitis and episcleritis [46].

Actually, the presence of psoriasis in the context of a clinical picture characterized by arthritis/dactylitis/enthesitis prompts a definite change in the diagnostic approach. In these cases, the question is no longer the positioning of the clinical picture within the area of spondyloarthritis (peripheral and/or axial), but we are definitely in the PsA domain, with its profile of diagnostic criteria, prognosis, and specific treatment approaches. We believe this is of crucial importance not only because of the strength of the available clinical evidences but also in virtue of the pathogenetic characteristics of PsA, mainly related to the peculiarly pivotal role of TNF-α. These features are giving increasing confirmation of the need to shift for this disease, from a simple association of articular and cutaneous signs toward the concept of a systemic condition: psoriatic disease [47].

In mono-oligo arthritis, gout, or chondrocalcinosis have to be considered. Sometimes PsA patients may show increased serum levels of uric acid, particularly in cases with severe skin rash. This finding complicates the differential diagnosis. Only the detection of crystals of uric acid or pyrophosphate in synovial fluid with the improvement of articular symptoms using colchicine may support the suspicion of gout or chondrocalcinosis. Septic arthritis occurs most frequently as a monoarthritis often involving knee and hip. It generally presents with an acute onset of joint pain accompanied by fever. These signs, along with synovial fluid study, can be relevant to the diagnosis. A diagnosis of septic arthritis, in case of flare, needs to be ruled out even when PsA has already been diagnosed, especially in patients on immunosuppressive therapies [48].

Although PsA and osteoarthritis (OA) have clear distinguishing features, in some anatomical sites, such as DIP joints, clinical differentiation could be particularly difficult. Also erosive form of OA may be suspected in the presence of an associated scattered involvement of PIP joints [49–52]. Today, the support of MRI has permitted the demonstration in most cases of PsA of inflamed entheses with diffuse bone oedema while, in OA, entheses appear thickened and osteophytes, cartilage loss, and joint space narrowing are observed [53]. Notwithstanding, in some cases PsA and OA show similar clinical aspects and differential diagnosis is particularly complicated. In these cases we may imagine an overlap of the two diseases or the co-occurrence of two common arthropathies affecting the same anatomical site [53]. The presence of skin and/or nail psoriasis or, in their absence, a positive family history of psoriasis, in our opinion, may help in this differential diagnosis, which in particular conditions remains a demanding clinical exercise.

Prognosis

The outcome of peripheral pattern of PsA patients is unpredictable. This may be due, in part, to the heterogenous and very complex spectrum of peripheral phenotypes, ranging from mild oligo-entheso-arthritic forms to severe polyarthritis [54].

Genetic studies have not provided conclusive results on the clinical course of the disease and specific investigations on this topic are rare. In a study focusing on HLA alleles, a concomitant association of HLA-DR7 with HLA-B27 and B39 has been correlated with more severe disease progression [55]. It is not clear if HLA-DR4 positivity is also related to symmetrical polyarthritis and severe erosive course [56–60].

In a recent analysis by Eder et al., in which the authors studied data on clinical outcome of a large PsA cohort, they concluded that male sex and low burden of inflammation with small number of involved joints at first visit represent predictors of better outcome and, in several cases, of remission [61, 62].

On the other hand, delay in diagnosis, disability, and marked joint damage represent factors influencing worse long-term outcomes. In particular, the latter correlates with reduced physical function and work disability [63, 64].

Finally, recent studies have focused on correlation between PsA outcome and metabolic aspects including metabolic syndrome and overweight/obesity. An inverse association has been found between presence of metabolic syndrome and the likelihood of achieving minimal disease activity in PsA patients despite the use of TNF blockers [65]. In addition, obesity has been confirmed as a negative predictor of achieving and maintaining minimal disease activity in PsA patients, when results are compared with those obtained in subjects with normal weight [63, 66].

References

1. Moll JM, Wright V. Psoriatic arthritis. Semin Arthritis Rheum 1973;3: 55–78.
2. Bruce IN. Psoriatic Arthritis clinical features. In Hochberg, M., Silman, A., Smolen, J., Weinblatt M., and Weiseman, M (eds) Rheumatology. Mosby, St Louis 1165–75. 2008.
3. Jones SM, Armas JB, Cohen MG, Lovell CR, Evison G, McHugh NJ. Psoriatic arthritis: outcome of disease subsets and relationship of joint disease to nail and skin disease. Br J Rheumatol 1994;33:834–9.
4. Scarpa R, Oriente P, Pucino, A, et al. The clinical spectrum of psoriatic spondylitis. Br J Rheumatol 1988;27:133–7.
5. Scarpa R, Cuocolo A, Peluso R, et al. Early psoriatic arthritis: the clinical spectrum. J Rheumatol 2008;35:137–41.
6. Scarpa R, Atteno M, Costa L, et al. Early psoriatic arthritis. J Rheumatol 2009;Suppl 83, 26–7.

7. Scarpa R, Oriente P, Pucino A, et al. Psoriatic arthritis in psoriatic patients. Br J Rheumatol 1984;23:246–50.

8. Gladman DD, Shuckett R, Russell ML, Thorne JC, Schachter, RK. Psoriatic arthritis (PSA)—an analysis of 220 patients. Q J Med 1987;62: 127–41.

9. Oriente P, Biondi-Oriente C, Scarpa R. Psoriatic arthritis. Clinical manifestations. Baillieres Clin Rheumatol 1994;8:277–94.

10. Taylor W, Gladman D, Helliwell P, et al. Classification criteria for psoriatic arthritis: development of new criteria from a large international study. Arthritis 2006;Rheum 54: 2665–73.

11. Scarpa R, Cosentini E, Manguso F, et al. Clinical and genetic aspects of psoriatic arthritis 'sine psoriasis'. J Rheumatol 2003;30:2638–40.

12. Kane D, Stafford L, Bresnihan B, FitzGerald O. A classification study of clinical subsets in an inception cohort of early psoriatic peripheral arthritis—'DIP or not DIP revisited'. Rheumatology (Oxford) 2003;42:1469–76.

13. Khan M, Schentag C, Gladman DD. Clinical and radiological changes during psoriatic arthritis disease progression. J Rheumatol 2003;30:1022–6.

14. Helliwell PS, Hetthen J, Sokoll K, et al. Joint symmetry in early and late rheumatoid and psoriatic arthritis: comparison with a mathematical model. Arthritis Rheum 2000;43: 865–71.

15. Bourdillon C. Psoriasis et arthropaties. PhD thesis, University of Paris. 1888.

16. Wright V, Moll JMH. Seronegative Polyarthritis. Amsterdam. Elsevier North Holland. 1976.

17. Scarpa R, Ayala F, Caporaso N, Olivieri I. Psoriasis, psoriatic arthritis, or psoriatic disease? J Rheumatol 2006;33:210–2.

18. Soscia E, Scarpa R, Cimmino MA, et al. Magnetic resonance imaging of nail unit in psoriatic arthritis. J Rheumatol 2009;Suppl 83, 42–5.

19. Soscia E, Sirignano C, Catalano O, et al. New developments in magnetic resonance imaging of the nail unit. J Rheumatol 2012;Suppl 89, 49–53.

20. Scarpa R, Manguso F, Oriente A, Peluso R, Atteno M, Oriente P. Is the involvement of the distal interphalangeal joint in psoriatic patients related to nail psoriasis? Clin Rheumatol 2004;23, 27–30.

21. Haddad A, Johnson SR, Somaily M, et al. Psoriatic arthritis mutilans: clinical and radiographic criteria. a systematic review. J Rheumatol 2015;42:1432–8.

22. Jadon DR, Shaddick G, Tillett W, et al. Psoriatic arthritis mutilans: characteristics and natural radiographic history. J Rheumatol 2015;42:1169–76.

23. Gudbjornsson B, Ejstrup L, Gran JT, et al. Psoriatic arthritis mutilans (PAM) in the Nordic countries: demographics and disease status. The Nordic PAM study. Scand J Rheumatol 2013;42:373–8.

24. Olivieri I, Padula A, D'Angelo S, Cutro MS. Psoriatic arthritis sine psoriasis. J Rheumatol Suppl. 2009;83:28–9.

25. Cervini C, Leardini G, Mathieu A, Punzi L, Scarpa R. Psoriatic arthritis: epidemiological and clinical aspects in a cohort of 1,306 Italian patients. Reumatismo 2005;57: 283–90.

26. Schellekens GA, Visser H, de Jong BA, et al. The diagnostic properties of rheumatoid arthritis antibodies recognizing a cyclic citrullinated peptide. Arthritis Rheum 2000;43:155–63.

27. Nijenhuis S, Zendman AJ, Vossenaar ER, Pruijn GJ, vanVenrooij WJ. Autoantibodies to citrullinated proteins in rheumatoid arthritis: clinical performance and biochemical aspects of an RA-specific marker. Clin Chim Acta 2004;350:17–34.

28. Pasquetti P, Morozzi G, Galeazzi M. Very low prevalence of anti-CCP antibodies in rheumatoid factor-negative psoriatic polyarthritis. Rheumatology (Oxford) 2009;48:315–6.

29. Popescu C, Zofotă S, Bojincă V, Ionescu R. Anti-cyclic citrullinated peptide antibodies in psoriatic arthritis--cross-sectional study and literature review. J Med Life 2013;6:376–82.

30. Perez-Alamino R, Garcia-Valladares I, Cuchacovich R, Iglesias-Gamarra A, Espinoza LR Are anti-CCP antibodies in psoriatic arthritis patients a biomarker of erosive disease? Rheumatol Int 2014;34:1211–6.

31. Caso F, Costa L, Atteno M, et al. Simple clinical indicators for early psoriatic arthritis detection. Springerplus 2014;22,3:759.

32. Punzi L, Bertazzolo N, Pianon M, Michelotto M, Cesaro G, Gambari PF. The volume of synovial fluid effusion in psoriatic arthritis. Clin Exp Rheumatol 1995;13:535–6.

33. Punzi L, Podswiadek M, Oliviero F, et al. Laboratory findings in psoriatic arthritis. Reumatismo 2007;59:52–5.

34. Fearon U, Reece R, Smith J, Emery P, Veale DJ. Synovial cytokine and growth factor regulation of MMPs/TIMPs: implications for erosions and angiogenesis in early rheumatoid and psoriatic arthritis patients. Ann N Y Acad Sci 1999;30:619–21.

35. Olivieri I, Scarano E, Padula A, D'Angelo S. Imaging of psoriatic arthritis. Reumatismo 2007;59:73–6.

36. Filippucci E, De Angelis R, Salaffi F, Grassi W. Ultrasound, skin, and joints in psoriatic arthritis. J Rheumatol Suppl. 2009:83, 35–8.

37. Cimmino MA, Parodi M, Zampogna G, et al. Magnetic resonance imaging of the hand in psoriatic arthritis. J Rheumatol Suppl 2009;83:39–41.

38. Cimmino MA, Barbieri F, Boesen M, et al. Dynamic contrast-enhanced magnetic resonance imaging of articular and extraarticular synovial structures of the hands in patients with psoriatic arthritis. J Rheumatol Suppl 2012;89:44–8.

39. Grassi W, Gutierrez M. Psoriatic arthritis: need for ultrasound in everyday clinical practice. J Rheumatol Suppl 2012;89, 39–43.

40. Spadaro A, Lubrano E. Psoriatic arthritis: imaging techniques. Reumatismo 2012;64:99–106.

41. Jevtic V, Lingg G. Differential diagnosis of rheumatoid and psoriatic arthritis at an early stage in the small hand and foot joints using magnetic resonance imaging. Handchir Mikrochir Plast Chir 2012;44:163–70.

42. Balakrishnan C, Madnani N. Diagnosis and management of psoriatic arthritis. Indian J Dermatol Venereol Leprol 2013;79:18–24.

43. Olivieri I, D'Angelo S, Palazzi C, Padula A. Advances in the management of psoriatic arthritis. Nat Rev Rheumatol 2014;10:531–42.

44. Del Puente A, Esposito A, Parisi A, et al. Osteoporosis and psoriatic arthritis. J Rheumatol 2012;Suppl 89:36–8.

45. Del Puente A, Esposito A, Costa L, et al. Fragility fractures in patients with psoriatic arthritis. J Rheumatol Suppl 2015;93: 36–9.

46. van Tubergen A, Weber U. Diagnosis and classification in spondyloarthritis: identifying a chameleon. Nat Rev Rheumatol 2012;8: 253–61.

47. Scarpa R, Soscia E, Peluso R, et al. Nail and distal interphalangeal joint in psoriatic arthritis. J Rheumatol 2006;33:1315–9.

48. Colavite PM, Sartori A. Septic arthritis: immunopathogenesis, experimental models and therapy. J Venom Anim Toxins Incl Trop Dis 2014;6:20:19.

49. Crain DC. Interphalangeal osteoarthritis. JAMA 1961;175:1049–53.

50. Peter JB, Pearson CM, Marmor, L. Erosive osteoarthritis of the hands. Arthritis Rheum 1966;9:365–88.

51. Swezey RL, Alexander SJ. Erosive osteoarthritis and the main en lorgnette deformity (opera glass hand). Arch Intern Med 1971;128:269–72.

52. Smukler NM, Edeiken J, Giuliano VJ. Ankylosis in osteoarthritis of the finger joints. Radiology 1971;100:525–30.

53. McGonagle D, Hermann KG, Tan AL. Differentiation between osteoarthritis and psoriatic arthritis: implications for pathogenesis and treatment in the biologic therapy era. Rheumatology (Oxford) 2015;54: 29–38.

54. Boehncke WH, Qureshi A, Merola JF, et al. Diagnosing and treating psoriatic arthritis: an update. Br J Dermatol 2014;170:772–86.

55. Gladman DD, Farewell VT, Kopciuk KA, Cook RJ. HLA markers and progression in psoriatic arthritis. J Rheumatol 1998;25:730–3.

56. Gladmann DD, Anhorn KAB, Schachter RK, Mervant U. HLA antigens in psoriatic arthritis. J Rheumatol 1986;13:586–92.

57. Haroon M, Winchester R, Giles JT, Heffernan E, FitzGerald O. Certain class I HLA alleles and haplotypes implicated in susceptibility play a role in determining specific features of the psoriatic arthritis phenotype. Ann Rheum Dis. 2016;75;155–62.

58. Korendowych E, Dixey J, Cox B, Jones S, McHugh N. The influence of the HLA-DR B1 rheumatoid arthritis shared epitope on the clinical characteristics and radiological outcome of psoriatic arthritis. J Rheumatol 2003;30:96–101.

59. Queiro-Silva R, Torre-Alonso JC, Tinturé-Eguren T, Lopez-Lagunas I. The effect of HLA-DR antigens on the susceptibility to, and clinical expression of psoriatic arthritis. Scand J Rheumatol 2004;33:318–22.

60. Eder L, Chandran V, Pellet F, et al. Human leucocyte antigen risk alleles for psoriatic arthritis among patients with psoriasis. Ann Rheum Dis. 2012;71:50–5.

61. Eder L, Gladman DD. Predictors for clinical outcome in psoriatic arthritis—what have we learned from cohort studies? Expert Rev Clin Immunol. 2014;10:763–70.

62. Gladman DD, Hing EN, Schentag CT, Cook RJ. Remission in psoriatic arthritis. J Rheumatol. 2001;28:1045–8.

63. Eder L, Thavaneswaran A, Chandran V, Cook RJ, Gladman DD Obesity is associated with a lower probability of achieving sustained minimal disease activity state among patients with psoriatic arthritis. Ann Rheum Dis 2014;74:813–7.

64. Haroon M, Gallagher P, FitzGerald O. Diagnostic delay of more than 6 months contributes to poor radiographic and functional outcome in psoriatic arthritis. Ann Rheum Dis 2015;74:1045–50.

65. Costa L, Caso F, Ramonda R, et al. Metabolic syndrome and its relationship with the achievement of minimal disease activity state in psoriatic arthritis patients: an observational study. Immunol Res 2015;61:147–53.

66. di Minno MN, Peluso R, Iervolino S, et al. Obesity and the prediction of minimal disease activity: a prospective study in psoriatic arthritis. Arthritis Care Res (Hoboken) 2013;65:141–7.

CHAPTER 11

Enthesitis

Juan D. Cañete and Julio Ramírez

Dedication:
To Leonor Calvet Riatós for his permanent support full of love (*JDC*).

Definition, clinical evaluation and differential diagnosis

Definition, clinical relevance and prevalence

Enthesitis, that is inflammation of the attachment sites of tendons, ligaments, fascias, and joint capsule fibres into bone, is a hallmark of spondyloarthropathies (SpAs) and is a common feature in psoriatic arthritis (PsA). It combines inflammatory changes, such as thickening of the enthesis, oedema, and new vessel formation, and structural changes, such as cortical bone erosions and calcification of the fibrocartilage adjacent to bone. Chronic inflammation usually causes erosive changes in the bone where the tendons are inserted, followed by periosteal changes, the formation of spurs, new subperiosteal bone, and syndesmophytes [1].

Functional enthesitis is a concept that concerns areas of bone marrow oedema far away from the attachment of the enthesis to bone. This region has been called the 'functional enthesis unit', where the friction of the tendon/ligament against the bone appears to be related to inflammation [2] (Figure 11.1).

Enthesitis is one of the three inflammatory musculoskeletal manifestations required to fulfil the CASPAR (ClASsification criteria for Psoriatic ARthritis) criteria [3], equally important as synovitis or spondylitis. Enthesitis is also included in the OMERACT set of domains to be assessed in some but not all clinical trials in PsA [4].

Detecting enthesitis can be challenging especially when asymptomatic. It is often underestimated by clinical examination and requires imaging techniques [5]. On the other hand, many sites of enthesitis, particularly most of those in the spine and large joints, are clinically inaccessible. Enthesitis may be the initial inflammatory manifestation in PsA causing severe pain and high negative impact on function and quality of life [6]. In some patients with PsA enthesitis is the only clinical manifestation of the disease for months to years before affecting other sites, making it challenging to diagnose [7].

Clinically, enthesitis is reported in 25–78% of PsA patients [8–12] while Kane et al. found enthesitis in 38% of patients at initial presentation [13]. However, the true prevalence may be underestimated, and more abnormalities at entheseal sites may be detected using advanced imaging techniques such as musculoskeletal ultrasound [14]. However, the clinical implications of these findings remain to be studied further.

Enthesitis is more painful and frequent in the lower than the upper extremities, with the Achilles and plantar fascia insertions being the most affected sites. Other sites include the insertions of the quadriceps and patellar tendons, the rotator cuff, the epicondyles at the elbow, and ligament insertion sites around the pelvis and ribs [15]. Enthesitis often occurs in the spine at ligament insertion sites on the vertebrae. Patients complain of pain and tenderness at these sites and swelling can be present on examination. The clinical diagnosis in some of these sites requires a high level of suspicion. While polyenthesitis is a common feature in SpAs, several enthesitis sites are close to fibromyalgia (FM) tender points thus differential diagnosis can be difficult [16].

Clinical evaluation, including outcome measures

Enthesitis can be assessed by both clinical examination and imaging techniques. On clinical assessment, enthesitis may be defined as tenderness determined by applying sufficient pressure to blanch the tip of the examiner's thumb (approximately 4 kg/cm2) at entheseal sites. To improve discrimination between tenderness and hyperalgesia (increased sensitivity to painful stimuli), standard palpation of control sites [17] (thumb, nail, and volar side of forearm bilaterally) may be made at the beginning of each examination. Associated swelling, erythema, and diffuse tenderness may be present in superficial entheses, facilitating the diagnosis [18].

Patients may experience pain at entheseal sites, without a clear traumatic onset, but typically attributed to overuse. Morning pain and stiffness, acute onset, and persistent pain improving with activity and worsening with rest may suggest the inflammatory nature. Often the patients have difficulties in distinguishing between arthritis and enthesitis (e.g. patellar tendon pain vs knee joint pain). Diffuse chest pain may not be recognized as inflammation arising from the insertion of the ligament at the costochondral joints or ribs. The patient also may not recognize the presence of enthesitis until palpation elicits tenderness. Usually, there is a lack of response to physical therapy but it remains unclear whether entheseal pain typically improves with nonsteroidal anti-inflammatory drugs (NSAIDs) [15].

Enthesitis is recorded as either present or absent or graded in terms of severity. Effective clinical measurement of enthesitis is challenging due to the complex heterogeneity of tissue involvement, which includes both deep bone and superficial soft tissue inflammation [19]. On the other hand, a relatively low concordance

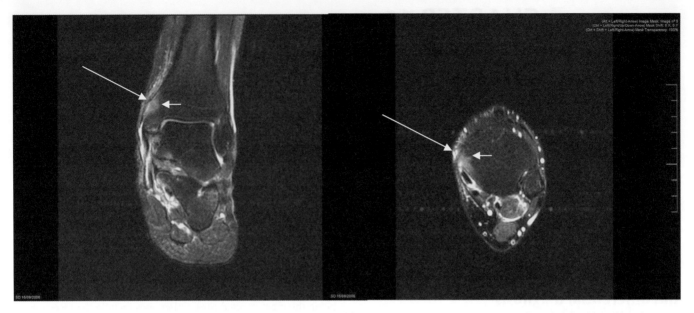

Figure 11.1 Fuctional enthesitis in a 38-year-old-male with severe pain and impaired function. Gadolinium-enhanced MRI image from the left ankle and foot showing increased signal in the posterior-tibialis tendon (long arrow) and the tibialis bone immediately under the tendon (short arrow) in sagittal (left) and axial (right) views.

between clinical and power Doppler ultrasound (PDUS) enthesitis was found in patients with PsA, suggesting that enthesitis may often be asymptomatic and that a more reliable definition of enthesitis would be welcomed [19].

The Leeds Enthesitis Index (LEI) is the only outcome measure that has been developed and validated specifically for PsA [18]. In addition to the LEI, three other indices, the Mander Enthesitis Index [20], its easier-to use modification MASES (Maastricht Ankylosing Spondylitis Enthesis Score) [21], and the SPARCC (Spondyloarthritis Research Consortium of Canada) [22] (Table 11.1), have been incorporated in the evaluation of enthesitis in some clinical trials. The INSPIRE study compared many of the enthesitis tools and demonstrated that the SPARCC and LEI are better for PsA while MASES is better for ankylosing spondylitis [23] Further work is needed to improve their value as diagnostic tools and outcome measures [24].

Differential diagnosis

Enthesitis involvement in the disease process is well recognized in SpAs and in rheumatoid arthritis (RA); however, various metabolic and endocrine conditions may manifest with enthesopathy features [25]. However, usually, the diagnostic considerations fall between inflammatory and degenerative/mechanical disease [15].

Enthesopathy defines all pathological abnormalities in the entheses due to metabolic, mechanical (including sports-related injury), and degenerative processes. Trauma, diabetes, gout, pseudogout, diffuse idiopathic skeletal hyperostosis (DISH), chronic retinoid toxicity, and hypercholesterolemia should be ruled out by medical history, physical examination, and appropriate complementary tests [25]. These conditions, which can elicit tenderness by palpation of the entheses should be differentiated from inflammatory enthesitis. Pain may sometimes be attributed to join pain and isolated enthesitis is often misdiagnosed as overuse-related enthesitis [25].

Erosive hand osteoarthritis (OA) may share clinical and imaging features with PsA, but there are more prominent inflammatory changes in ligament, tendon, enthesis and adjacent bone in the distal interphalangeal (DIP) joint in PsA patients with high-resolution magnetic resonance imaging (MRI) [26] Recently, a study using high-resolution peripheral quantitative computed tomography found that, although the overall number and size of bone spurs are similar in patients with PsA and those with hand OA, the anatomic sites of bone proliferation are different. Bone spurs dominated the radial side of the joints in PsA (entheseal regions), whereas the palmar and dorsal quadrants were the predilection sites in hand OA [27].

FM is a common cause of chronic widespread pain. Enthesitis may be very difficult to diagnose in PsA because its symptoms and signs are sometimes nonspecific and relatively indistinguishable from those of FM. Patients with primary FM and psoriasis or FM associated with PsA and those with psoriatic polyenthesitis may have almost identical clinical features and are at risk of misdiagnosis and management errors. Therefore, differentiating PsA enthesitis from FM can be challenging [16]. Marchesoni et al. studied 266 patients with PsA and 120 with FM and showed that FM patients had higher mean tender point and enthesitis scores, more somatic symptoms, and responded less to NSAIDs. Multivariate analysis showed that the presence of ≥6 FM-associated symptoms and ≥8 tender points were predictors of FM compared with PsA [16]. Evaluation of FM and PsA patients with PDUS revealed a high number of enthesopathic lesions in both disorders, which were more frequent and severe in PsA but not sufficient to distinguish the two disorders [28]. However, erosive changes, entheseal involvement at the plantar fascia insertion, and inflammation at the Achilles insertion were highly specific for PsA [28]. Furthermore, enthesitis may be the first symptom of PsA in patients with psoriasis [14].

Table 11.1 Enthesial sites assessed in outcome measures for enthesitis.

	MEI	MASES	LEI	SPARCC
Number sites (grades)	66 (0–3)	13 (0–1)	6 (0–1)	16 (0–1)
Nuchal crests (superior nuchal line along the insertion of the trapezius)	x			
C1–C7 (spinous process)	x			
T1–T12 (spinous process)	x			
L1–L4 (spinous process)	x			
L5 (spinous process)	x	x		
1st costochondral (R,L)	x	x		
2nd–6th costochondral (R,L)	x			
7th costochondral (R,L)	x	x		
Manubriosternal joint	x			
Greater tuberosity of humerus (R,L)	x			x
Lateral epicondyle humerus (R,L)	x		x	x
Medial epicondyle humerus (R,L)	x			x
Posterior superior iliac spine (R,L)	x	x		
Anterior posterior superior iliac spine (R,L)	x	x		
Iliac crest (R,L)	x	x		
Ischial tuberosity (R,L)	x			
Achilles insertion into calcaneus (R,L)	x	x	x	x
Greater trochanter (R,L)	x			x
Lateral condyle femur (R,L)	x			
Medial condyle femur (R,L)	x		x	
Insertion plantar fascia (R,L)	x			x
Quadriceps insertion patella (R,L)				x
Inferior pole patella (R,L)				x

MEI, Mander Enthesitis Index; MASES, Maastricht Ankylosing Spondylitis Enthesis Score; LEI, Leeds Enthesitis Index; SPARCC, Spondyloarthritis Research Consortium of Canada. R, right; L, left.

Pathogenesis

Based on an cross-sectional MRI study in ten RA and ten SpA patients with recent-onset knee effusion, which found more prominent entheseal abnormalities in SpA than in RA patients, McGonagle et al. hypothesized that the primary lesion of SpA is enthesitis, that enthesopathy may be the common link between all forms of SpA, and that enthesitis in synovial joints is frequent (Figure 11.2) [29].

Using anatomical and histopathological studies, McGonagle and Benjamin further delineated the heterogeneous structural and functional nature of entheses [30]. They proposed that entheses forms a functional unit with adjacent synovium termed the synovial–entheseal complex (SEC), which is composed of anatomically contiguous structures comprising the insertion of the tendon, adjacent tendon, bone, fat-pad and synovium, that continually respond to changing biomechanical loads [31].

The normal enthesis is avascular at the fibrocartilagionous point of attachment and lacks resident macrophages, but in the setting of high biomechanical stress or inflammation, danger signals released by shear forces or damaged entheses may trigger the production of cytokines by lining cells and infiltrating monocytes and lymphocytes in adjacent synovial tissue, initiating a local inflammatory response [32]. Therefore, the SEC represents a conceptual framework which may explain the tissue specificity and highlights the role of mechanical stress in the SpA, while at the same time providing a unifying pathophysiological concept for SpA based on the idea that specific tissues may be particularly sensitive to mechanical triggers [32, 33].

Challenging the hypothesis of enthesitis being the primary lesion in SpA leading to a secondary synovitis over time, an MRI and knee synovial biopsy study by Paramarta et al. [34] of 13 early SpA (4 with PsA) and 20 RA patients found that the MRI synovitis score was higher in SpA peripheral joints, and there was similar intensity of synovial immunopathology in SpA and RA, Furthermore, the number and distribution of enthesitis sites on MRI did not differ between the two diseases. The authors recognized certain limitations: enthesis was evaluated in the context of peripheral arthritis, but clinical enthesitis was not evaluated; only

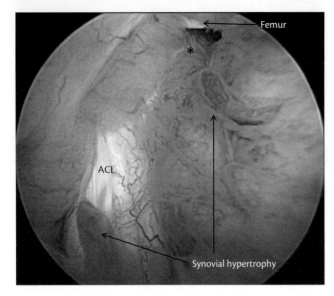

Figure 11.2 Arthroscopic view of left-knee intercondylar space in a patient with psoriatic arthritis showing anterior cruciate ligament (ACL) insertion (*). Synovial hypertrophy and red vessels around tendon insertion are shown.

large joints of the lower limbs were evaluated, and therefore the study did not exclude the possibility that the presence and/or the potential role of enthesitis may be different in small joints. The study also did not exclude the possibility that enthesitis may have a more prominent role in axial SpA than in peripheral SpA and did not question the idea that mechanical stress can lead to inflammation in SpA [34].

Overall, there is no definitive clinical evidence that enthesitis is the origin of inflammation in PsA, but definitive conclusions are difficult to reach due to the heterogeneity of disease manifestations, cross-sectional study designs, and the differences in the imaging techniques used [24].

Linking enthesitis and synovitis: the synovial-entheseal complex

The close anatomical relationship between the enthesis, prone to mechanical stress, and the vascularized synovium, in contact with a variety of immune mediators, may provide the pathogenic basis for joint inflammation in SpAs [32]. The concept of the SEC may be widely applicable at many sites in the body. Entheses are avascular structures composed of dense regular connective tissue with an avascular fibrocartilaginous attachment site. However, this site shows clear vascular invasion with aging, probably reflecting a tissue-repair response to accumulating microdamage [31]. In addition, it has been shown that, even in normally aged entheses and in SpA-related enthesitis, new bone formation and erosions occurred at different topographical locations, with new bone typically occurring at the distal part of the enthesis where the bone is under more tension, strongly suggesting a role for mechanical factors in physiological and pathological enthesis remodelling in humans [31].

Furthermore, soft tissue microdamage, which is widespread in the enthesis organ (Figure 11.3), is often accompanied by synovial changes and the presence of immune cells within the enthesis [31]. These findings would support the idea that biomechanical factors related to the enthesis and the wider SEC could play an important role in the genesis of synovial inflammation in both degenerative and inflammatory arthritis in humans [31].

Although the hypothesis of a mechanical-based origin of SpA may easily be appreciated from a conceptual point of view, formal proof is difficult to obtain from human research.

Immunogenetics of PsA enthesitis

Genes from MHC class I (HLA-Cw6, HLA-B27) have been long time known to be associated with PsA, as is discussed in Chapter 6. FitzgGerald and Winchester have reported that certain HLA-class I alleles are associated with different PsA clinical features [35]. Recently, this group reported an association between HLA class I alleles and clinical enthesitis [36] by examining HLA

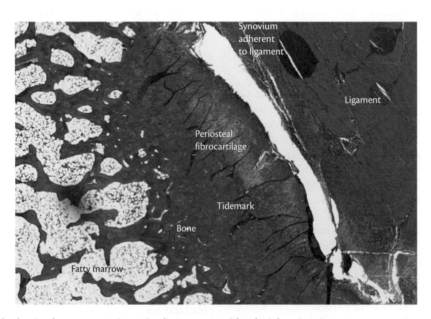

Figure 11.3 Microphotography showing damage at posterior cruciate ligamentat synovial-enthesis-bone junction
Courtesy of Prof. D McGonagle, University of Leeds, UK.

associations in a cohort of 282 clinically-phenotyped PsA patients. *HLA-B*27:05:02* was positively associated with enthesitis, dactylitis and symmetric sacroiliitis, whereas *HLA-B*08:01:01-C-07:01:01* and its component alleles were positively associated with joint fusion and deformities, asymmetrical sacroiliitis, and dactylitis. In contrast, *HLA-B*44* haplotypes were associated with the presence of milder disease and a decreased frequency of enthesitis, joint fusion, deformities, and dactylitis [36]. One small study found association between enthesitis and the *HLA-DR*17* in PsA [37]. These findings highlight the importance of stratifying PsA patients in more clinically homogeneous phenotypes in order to reveal the immunogenetic relationships contributing to the pathogenesis of enthesitis.

Immunopathology of human enthesitis

The difficulty in obtaining tissue from the entheses is a major obstacle to the study of its physiopathology. The few studies that have reported histopathological findings have found inflammatory cell infiltration within and adjacent to spinal enthesis in chronic ankylosing spondylitis [24]. Other studies focused on bone adjacent to the entheses of the sacroiliac [38, 39] and synovial joints [40], confirming the presence of inflammatory cell infiltrate containing macrophages and lymphocytes.

One study reported inflammatory infiltrates in the enthesis bone-marrow of all the eight SpA specimens included, in contrast with RA and OA specimens, using immunohistochemical techniques. The infiltrate was composed predominantly of CD8+ cells, which were five-fold more frequent than CD4+ cells. The most severely erosive lesions contained some CD68+ macrophages. These findings suggest that inflammation of the bone marrow beneath the enthesis may be a prominent feature of the disease process. All patients had long-standing disease, but information about whether or not the biopsied entheses were symptomatic was lacking [41].

In contrast, a study using ultrasound (US) guided biopsy of insertion points in four cases of symptomatic plantar fasciitis and one case of patellar tendon enthesis, all of <1 year of duration, reported increased vascularity in the fibrous part of the enthesis and predominantly CD68+ macrophages, mainly at sites of increased vascularity and cellularity. Unfortunately, insufficient tissue was collected to perform immunohistochemical analysis of the bone [42]. In conclusion, the few studies performed on human entheseal tissue samples confirm that inflammation of the bone marrow is a prominent feature of the disease process, thus complementing the information previously gained by MRI studies. However, these studies have yielded conflicting results as to what the major infiltrating cell type is. New studies are needed to delineate the cellular and molecular mechanisms of human enthesitis at early and established stages of the disease [43].

Animal models of enthesitis

The role of TNF and IL-23/IL-17 cytokine axis

Animal models have contributed greatly to the understanding of disease mechanisms relevant to rheumatic diseases, but they only mirror the activation of a single pathway of interest or some disease manifestations. Therefore, they should be considered as 'mechanisms of disease models' rather than 'disease-equivalent models'. This is especially relevant in the study of SpA, where the diversity of phenotypes and different grades of severity preclude the validity of a single model for the characterization of the disease [44].

Several models of SpA with pathological features of enthesitis have been developed and have been useful in building evidence on the key role of TNF and the interleukin (IL)-23/IL-17 cytokine axis in inflammatory and bone remodelling pathways [24].

Aging male DBA/1 mice share features with human SpAs including entheseal involvement, progressive ankylosis, but also dactylitis. In one study, male DBA/1 mice developed dermatitis, ankylosing enthesitis of the hind paws, and bone neoformation. The incidence of macroscopic arthritis was directly related to the degree of crowding of the animals, suggesting a pathogenic role for biomechanical stress; however, no clear enthesitis or inflammation in the paws could be detected by histomorphology [45].

A ground-breaking mechanistic study using minicircle technology provided evidence that IL-23 overexpression induces enthesitis (including involvement of the aortic root and valves, which are structurally similar to enthesitis) by activation of RORgt+CD3+CD4-CD8- entheseal-resident T-cells [46] (Figure 11.4). In a previous study, IL-23 overexpression in the same model induced a severely destructive polyarthritis [47]. These discrepancies demonstrate the difficulties in interpreting animal models and determining whether or not their findings reflect human disease.

The pivotal role of IL-23 in the pathogenesis of SpA was further supported by a study using the SKG mouse model. In response to systemic curdlan injections, intestinal IL-23 provoked local mucosa dysregulation and IL-17/IL-22 dependent-enthesitis [48]. Enthesitis was specifically dependent on IL-23, IL-17, and IL-22.

Two murine models provide additional support for common mechanistic pathways in the skin and joints in PsA [49, 50]. The F759 mice with the *K5.Stat3C* transgene manifested extensive psoriasis plaques and spontaneously developed arthritis, enthesitis and nail deformities as early as three weeks of age. Histopathology revealed enthesitis and bone erosions. Tissue analyses showed upregulation of IL-23/Th17 [49]. In the BI0Q inbred strain, a single intraperitoneal injection of mannan induced macrophage-associated acute inflammation with PsA-like features, including enthesitis. Neutralization of IL-17A inhibited these manifestations [50].

Generally, these models support the importance of the TNF and IL-23/IL-17 cytokine axis in enthesitis. They also suggest that cutaneous inflammation through the IL-23/IL-17 pathways promotes periarticular and articular joint inflammation with the potential to alter bone turnover. However, the relevance of these findings to enthesitis in PsA remains to be studied.

The role of mechanical stress

Mechanical stress and microdamage has been postulated to play a role in inflammatory enthesitis as a primary driver in SpA development, including PsA. The enthesitis-based model proposes that interactions between biomechanical factors and the innate immune response may lead to disease. In fact, several animal models have suggested that mechanical stress can induce experimental SpA [51].

In the aging DBA/1 mice stimulation of aggressive behaviour leads to spontaneous development of arthritis [45]. In the TNFΔARE mouse model, mechanical unloading of the hind limb for 14 days prevented the induction of clinical arthritis in the hind limbs and histology revealed only mild inflammatory infiltration.

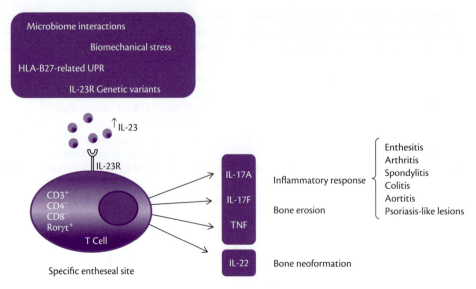

Figure 11.4 Schematic interpretation of the experimental model by Sherlock, et al., which supports a crucial role for IL-23 in inducing first enthesitis and after all manifestations of psoriatic arthritis. IL-23-R+ innate T lymphocytes, resident in entheseal sites, are activated, producing IL-17 and TNF, which induce inflammation and bone destruction, and IL-22, which produces bone neoformation. The source of IL-23 is hypothesized to derive from biomechanical stress, unfolded protein responses or microbiome- interactions. In addition, some IL-23R variants in humans could predispose to an increased response to IL-23.

The signalling pathway of mechanoreceptors was activated through ERK1/2 just a few minutes after reintroduction of mechanical strain in previously unloaded limbs. Inhibition of ERK1/2 was efficacious in treating enthesitis, thus showing that mechanical unloading ameliorated TNF-induced enthesitis and arthritis in this model. Moreover, tail suspension for 28 days reduced osteophyte size in collagen-antibody-induced arthritis in DBA/1 mice [51, 52], although the use of this model in studying the effect of mechanical stress and bone formation in SpA-like diseases has been questioned [53]. Direct evidence on the role of mechanical stress remains difficult to obtain in human SpA.

Imaging modalities

Imaging modalities for the assessment of psoriatic enthesitis include conventional radiographs, PDUS, MRI, bone scintigraphy, and 18 FDG PET CT scanning (see Chapters 16 to 19), with PDUS and MRI being the most used techniques in everyday clinical practice.

Conventional radiography can demonstrate chronic signs of enthesitis such as bony erosions, osteolysis, spurs, new bone formation, and periostitis, but provides no information about inflammatory activity, the early phase of the disease, or changes in soft tissues. The use of bone scintigraphy is limited by lack of anatomical detail and its ionizing radiation [54].

PDUS is preferred in daily practice due to its portability, good resolution, and the ability to detect increased blood flow/inflammation. Latest-generation machines with high frequency probes provide detailed assessment of superficial structures such as those most frequently involved in the entheses in PsA, including a sensitive assessment of the entheseal perfusion status. In the early stages of the disease, the enthesis and the adjacent structures may show several morphological and structural changes including entheseal thickening, hypoechogenicity, and fibrillar separation due to intra-tendinous oedema, with or without associated bursitis and different patterns of power Doppler signal distribution. In the

late stages, bony cortex changes may be related to the presence of enthesophytes and/or bone erosions [55] (see Figure 11.5).

MRI is also important in the assessment of enthesitis and is complementary to PDUS, as bone cannot be assessed by sonography. MRI visualizes both soft-tissue and bone marrow oedema using multiplanar views, but is mainly limited by the high cost [56].

High-resolution MRI studies have confirmed the intimate relationship between the nail bed, the distal phalanx, the DIP joint, and the insertion of the extensor tendon [57]. Whole body MRI is a promising new imaging modality for investigating axial and peripheral enthesis in patients with SpA and PsA, although its introduction as a clinical tool should be preceded by more research, including optimization of image acquisition [58].

A preliminary MRI scoring system for the evaluation of PsA (PsAMRIS) which focuses on inflammatory and destructive changes in PsA hands has been developed [59]. A few US scoring systems are available for quantifying severity of enthesitis. The most widely used are the Glasgow Ultrasound Enthesis Scoring

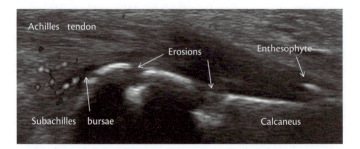

Figure 11.5 Longitudinal ultrasound image through the posterior heel of a patient with psoriatic arthritis. There is mild thickening and hypoechogenicity of the tendon. Erosions are evident in the proximal tendon and in the region of the superior tuberosity, with a small bone spur in the distal enthesis. Subachilles bursitis with power Doppler signal is also present.

System (GUESS) [60] and the MAdrid Sonographic Entheseal Index (MASEI) [61]. These scoring systems have moderate sensitivity and specificity in the identification of patients with SpA but have not been validated for PsA [62]. Composite-US scores sensitive for detection of inflammation and structural damage are under development [63].

Most studies have found that PDUS is more sensitive for the detection of enthesopathy than the clinical examination. PDUS has the potential to detect subclinical disease in patients with early PsA and in psoriasis with undiagnosed PsA [64].

Relatively large variations in the prevalence of subclinical enthesitis have been reported, with one recent study suggesting the clinical examination over-represented the degree of enthesitis [65]. A recent evaluation of symptomatic and asymptomatic entheses revealed increased vascularity on PDUS in PsA compared with psoriasis patients, even in sites without pain or tenderness, suggesting that development of a vascular phenotype may be an important step in the transition from psoriasis to PsA [66]. Also of importance are the findings of a recent study suggesting that subclinical enthesopathy in patients with psoriasis may predict future PsA [67]. Clinical enthesitis indices such as the LEI do not necessarily correlate well with US evaluation of enthesitis, partly because they do not measure all the sites included in the US assessment [68].

Innovative solutions to overcome these barriers might include the listed applications of both MRI and PDUS, and/or 3D US and US navigation to MRI studies. Furthermore, whole body MRI may be able to document the entire burden of enthesitis in a single scan [58].

Ultrasound findings in patients with psoriasis only: the preclinical phase of PsA?

Enthesitis can occur very early in the disease course, even before other manifestations of PsA. In patients with psoriasis, inflammatory lesions (synovitis, tenosynovitis, enthesitis, dactylitis, sacroiliitis, and spondylitis) can develop without clinical signs and symptoms [69]. Identification of patients having subclinical or 'occult' PsA represents a challenge to dermatologists and rheumatologists and may be of clinical importance.

US can detect enthesitis in patients with psoriasis without joint symptoms. In a large prospective study of patients with psoriasis without musculoskeletal manifestations, entheseal changes were detected in 62.5% and entheseal power Doppler signals in 7.4% of patients with psoriasis compared with 39.1% and 0% of age-matched controls with other skin diseases, respectively [5]. In another study, grey-scale thickness was detected in 32.9% and power Doppler signals in 0.9% of entheses in patients with psoriasis compared to 8.4% and 0% of entheses in sex-and age-matched healthy controls. Furthermore, grey-scale US enthesitis (increased thickness) at the distal patellar entheses was detected in 68.9% of patients with psoriasis compared to 6.7% of healthy controls [70]. The most frequent entheseal site with enthesitis was the Achilles tendon, followed by the proximal patellar entheses, the distal patellar entheses, and the plantar fascia entheses [70].

In line with previous studies, US enthesitis scores were higher in psoriasis patients with nail disease and no arthropathy compared to those without nail disease [71]. Nail disease involves the small entheses of the DIP joint, as the nail is anatomically attached to bone through several tendon and ligament fibres. Pathological US signs of enthesitis were significantly increased in patients with nail disease, not only with respect to nail related-entheses but also in other peripheral entheses [71]. These observations indicate a link between psoriatic onychopathy and musculo-skeletal disease [26, 71].

A recent study by McGonagle et al. suggests that soft-tissue involvement in psoriatic dactylitis is due to multiple enthesitis involving the finger ligaments and pulleys. Periarticular tissue oedema was also reported in asymptomatic fingers or toes from patients with psoriasis [72]. Another study using HR-pQCT at the ultradistal and periarticular radius showed that skin disease duration was associated with lower trabecular bone volume and the number of trabecules in patients with PsA [73], supporting the concept of subclinical musculoskeletal disease in psoriasis patients.

Overall, these studies suggest that asymptomatic patients with psoriasis often exhibit subclinical enthesitis. Further studies are required to elucidate if early detection of asymptomatic enthesitis in patients with psoriasis represents the preclinical phase of PsA.

A cohort of 30 psoriatic patients was assessed by clinical evaluation and using the GUESS score and followed-up for a mean duration of 3.5 years. At the end of follow-up, 23% of the patients had developed PsA. These patients had a significantly higher GUESS score at baseline, and the thickness of the quadriceps tendon was a predictor for subsequent development of PsA [67]. In addition, 10% of the patients with psoriasis developed PsA at 2-year's follow-up, and all three had a baseline GUESS score >9 [74]. These findings should be confirmed in larger, prospective studies.

A relevant and still unresolved question concerns the specificity of the PDUS findings in asymptomatic entheseal sites. Detection of vessels in entheses by power Doppler in at least one of 14 entheseal sites of patients with suspected SpA was highly predictive of SpA (sensitivity 75% and specificity 83.3%) [75]. Kocijan et al. studied the microstructural changes of the ultradistal and periarticular radius by HR-pQCT comparing psoriasis and PsA patients to healthy controls and found cortical alterations at the entheses even in the absence of PsA, providing evidence that structural joint alterations are present at the time of apparently exclusive skin involvement in psoriatic disease [73]. Enthesophytes were not related to erosions and erosions did not differ between psoriasis patients and healthy controls. This study found no relationship between enthesophytes and BMI, which is typically elevated in psoriasis patients [73]. It may emerge later during subclinical or clinical inflammation in psoriasis and PsA patients.

The exact prevalence of inflammatory findings in non-tender entheses requires further studies in order to determine its specificity and clinical significance as a predictor for future PsA development. Current evidence points to a high prevalence of subclinical findings in entheses of patients with psoriatic arthritis, but there is no clear evidence on its diagnostic utility [65]. Prospective studies are required to determine the exact relevance of these imaging findings in the long term, in particular their value in predicting future rheumatic disease in patients with psoriasis. New imaging indices like the MASEI should probably be used to find accurate cut-offs to identify patients at risk of developing PsA, as has already been demonstrated in SpA [76].

Treatment

Enthesitis has been traditionally a difficult-to-treat clinical manifestation of PsA. There remains a lack of strong evidence supporting the efficacy of NSAIDs and local glucocorticoid injection on enthesis, but they seem to work in some patients and reflected by international recommendations include both therapies as initial therapeutical approach. Since conventional synthetic (cs) disease modifying antirheumatic drugs (DMARDs), such as methotrexate, sulphasalazine, and leflunomide have not been proved efficacious in enthesis and have not been studied properly, they are not included in the recommendations for enthesis treatment [77, 78].

Advancements in TNF inhibitors (TNFi) have been heralded as a new era in the management of SpAs, led to successful treatment of the entire spectrum of clinical manifestations of PsA, including enthesis. Recently, the therapeutic armamentarium for PsA enthesis has been enriched with IL-23/IL-12 inhibitors, IL-17 inhibitors, and PDE4-inhibitors (see Chapters 26 to 32) [77, 78].

Although there is no direct evidence for the efficacy of glucocorticoid injections in PsA enthesis, this treatment can be an effective therapeutic approach. Given the potential risk of long-term harm to tendons exposed to glucocorticoid injections, it should be administered cautiously and ultrasound-guided when possible [79].

As enthesis may cause severe pain, dysfunction, and severely affects the quality of life, in patients with active enthesis and insufficient response to NSAIDs or local glucocorticoid injections, and in polyenthesis cases, therapy with a biological (b) DMARD should be initiated. Based on current data, bDMARDs may be administered even when no csDMARDs have been tried [77, 78]. Reports do not allow a definitive primary choice between a TNFi or bDMARDs targeting IL-12/IL-23 or IL-17 pathways, since there are no head-to-head comparisons and, based on the available data, all these agents appear to have similar efficacy on enthesis. Ustekinumab (anti-IL-23/IL-12) and sekunimumab (anti-IL-17A) have demonstrated high efficacy in phase III clinical trials of PsA, including enthesis [77, 78].

Once a bDMARD has failed, switching to another bDMARD is recommended. After the failure of one TNFi, switching to a secondary TNFi or to bDMARD with a distinct mode of action (antiIL-12/IL-23 or antiIL-17A) can be considered [77, 78].

The PDE4-inhibitor, apremilast, has also demonstrated efficacy in enthesis as well as other manifestation of PsA. Based on its efficacy and safety profile, apremilast could be used before or after a bDMARD, depending of the severity of enthesis (mild or severe) and the comorbidity/safety issues that could contraindicate bDMARDs [77, 78, 80].

Research agenda

Several points requiring further studies are highlighted here. These may have the potential to influence our understanding in detection and management of enthesis associated with PsA:

To develop a more-objective definition of enthesis, by integrating clinical examination and PDUS findings in large prospective cohorts of PsA patients and healthy controls.

To determine the specificity and clinical significance of the PDUS-changes seen in entheses from psoriatic patients without musculoskeletal manifestations. With appropriate design and biological sampling, such a prospective study with a long follow-up could be crucial in detecting biomarkers predicting the development of PsA.

To determine whether the role of double negative IL-23R+ RORgt+CD3+CD4-CD8- entheseal-resident T cells in mice is also applicable to human enthesis.

To better define patients with enthesis, genotypically, clinically and by imaging and to improve our understanding of these phenotypes in order to define specific therapeutic algorithms.

References

1. Francois RJ, Braun J, Khan MA. Entheses and enthesis: a histopathologic review and relevance to spondyloarthritides. Curr Opin Rheumatol 2001; 13:255–64.
2. Ritchlin CT. Psoriatic enthesis: an update from the GRAPPA 2013 Annual Meeting. J Rheumatol. 2014;41:1220–3.
3. Taylor W, Gladman D, Helliwell P, Marchesoni A, Mease P, Mielants H. CASPAR Study Group. Classification criteria for psoriatic arthritis: development of new criteria from a large international study. Arthritis Rheum. 2006; 54:2665–73.
4. Coates LC, Fitzgerald O, Mease PJ, et al. Development of a disease activity and responder index for psoriatic arthritis—report of the Psoriatic Arthritis Module at OMERACT 11. J Rheumatol 2014; 41:782–91.
5. Naredo E, Moller I, de Miguel E, et al. High prevalence of ultrasonographic synovitis and enthesopathy in patients with psoriasis without psoriatic arthritis: a prospective case–control study. Rheumatology (Oxford) 2011; 50:1838–48.
6. Turan Y, Duruöz MT, Cerrahoglu L. Relationship between enthesis, clinical parameters and quality of life in spondyloarthritis. Joint Bone Spine. 2009; 76:642–7.
7. Salvarani C, Cantini F, Olivieri I, et al. Isolated peripheral enthesis and/or dactylitis: a subset of psoriatic arthritis. J Rheumatol. 1997; 24: 1106–10.
8. Michet CJ, Mason TG, Mazlumzadeh M. Hip joint disease in psoriatic arthritis: risk factors and natural history. Ann Rheum Dis. 2005; 64: 1068–70.
9. Gladman DD, Chandran V. Observational cohort studies: lessons learnt from the University of Toronto Psoriatic Arthritis Program. Rheumatology (Oxford). 2011; 50: 25–31.
10. Kane D, Stafford L, Bresnihan B, FitzGerald O. A classification study of clinical subsets in an inception cohort of early psoriatic peripheral arthritis–'DIP or not DIP revisited'. Rheumatology (Oxford). 2003; 42:1469–76.
11. Helliwell PS, Porter G; CASPAR study group. Sensitivity and specificity of plain radiographic features of peripheral enthesopathy at major sites in psoriatic arthritis. Skeletal Radiol. 2007; 36: 1061–6.
12. Kavanaugh A, van der Heyde D, McInnes IB, et al. Golimumab in psoriatic arthritis: one-year clinical efficacy, radiographic, and safety results from a phase III, randomized, placebo-controlled trial. Arthritis Rheum 2012; 64:2504–17.
13. Kane D, Stafford L, Bresnihan B, FitzGerald O. A prospective, clinical and radiological study of early psoriatic arthritis: an early synovitis clinic experience. Rheumatology (Oxford). 2003; 42: 1460–8.
14. Gisondi P, Tinazzi I, El-Dalati G, et al. Lower limb enthesopathy in patients with psoriasis without clinical signs of arthropathy: a hospital-based case-control study. Ann Rheum Dis. 2008; 67: 26–30.
15. McGonagle D., Benjamin M. Enthesopathies. In Hochberg MC, Silman AJ, Smolen JS, Weinblatt ME, Weisman MH, Rheumatology, 5th edition, Elsevier, New York, 2011.
16. Marchesoni A, Atzeni F, Spadaro A, et al. Identification of the clinical features distinguishing psoriatic arthritis and fibromyalgia. J Rheumatol. 2012; 39: 849–55.
17. Wolfe F, Smythe HA, Yunus MB, Benne RM, Bombardier C, Goldenberg DL. The American College of Rheumatology 1990 criteria for the classification of fibromyalgia. Report of the multicenter criteria committee. Arthritis Rheum. 1990; 33:160–72.
18. Healy PJ, Helliwell PS. Measuring clinical enthesis in psoriatic arthritis: assessment of existing measures and development of an instrument specific to psoriatic arthritis. Arthritis Rheum. 2008; 59: 686–91.
19. Mandl P, Niedermayer DS, Balint PV. Ultrasound for enthesis: handle with care! Ann Rheum Dis. 2012; 71: 477–9.

20. Mander M, Simpson JM, McLellan A, Walker D, Goodacre JA, Dick WC. Studies with an enthesis index as a method of clinical assessment in ankylosing spondylitis. Ann Rheum Dis 1987; 46:197–202.

21. Heuft-Dorenbosch L, Spoorenberg A, van Tubergen A, et al. Assessment of enthesitis in ankylosing spondylitis. Ann Rheum Dis 2003; 62:127–32.

22. Maksymowych WP, Mallon C, Morrow S, et al. Development and validation of the Spondyloarthritis Research Consortium of Canada (SPARCC) Enthesitis Index. Ann Rheum Dis 2009; 68: 948–53.

23. Gladman DD, Inman RD, Cook RJ, et al. International spondyloarthritis interobserver reliability exercise--the INSPIRE study: II. Assessment of peripheral joints, enthesitis, and dactylitis. J Rheumatol 2007;34:1740–5.

24. Siegel EL, Orbai AM, Ritchlin CT. Targeting extra-articular manifestations in PsA: a closer look at enthesitis and dactylitis. Curr Opin Rheumatol. 2015; 27:111–7.

25. Slobodin G, Rozenbaum M, Boulman N, Rosner I. Varied presentations of enthesopathy. Semin Arthritis Rheum 2007; 37: 119–26.

26. Tan AL, Grainger AJ, Tanner SF, Emery P, McGonagle D. A high-resolution magnetic resonance imaging study of distal interphalangeal joint arthropathy in psoriatic arthritis and osteoarthritis: are they the same? Arthritis Rheum 2006; 54: 1328–33.

27. Finzel S, Sahinbegovic E, Kocijan R, Engelke K, Englbrecht M, Schett G. Inflammatory bone spur formation in psoriatic arthritis is different from bone spur formation in hand osteoarthritis. Arthritis Rheumatol. 2014; 66: 2968–75.

28. Marchesoni A, De Lucia O, Rotunno L, De Marco G, Manara M. Entheseal power Doppler ultrasonography: a comparison of psoriatic arthritis and fibromyalgia. J Rheumatol Suppl. 2012; 89:29–31.

29. McGonagle D, Gibbon W, O'Connor P, Green M, Pease C, Emery P. Characteristic magnetic resonance imaging entheseal changes of knee synovitis in spondylarthropathy. Arthritis Rheum. 1998; 41: 694–700.

30. Benjamin M, Moriggl B, Brenner E, Emery P, McGonagle D, Redman S. The 'enthesis organ' concept: why enthesopathies may not present as focal insertional disorders. Arthritis Rheum. 2004; 50: 3306–13.

31. Benjamin M, McGonagle D. Histopathologic changes at 'synovio-entheseal complexes' suggesting a novel mechanism for synovitis in osteoarthritis and spondylarthritis. Arthritis Rheum. 2007; 56: 3601–9.

32. McGonagle D, Lories RJ, Tan AL, Benjamin M. The concept of a 'synovio-entheseal complex' and its implications for understanding joint inflammation and damage in psoriatic arthritis and beyond. Arthritis Rheum. 2007; 56: 2482–91.

33. Lories RJ, de Vlam K. Is psoriatic arthritis a result of abnormalities in acquired or innate immunity? Curr Rheumatol Rep. 2012;14:375–82.

34. Paramarta JE, van der Leij C, Gofita I, et al. Peripheral joint inflammation in early onset spondyloarthritis is not specifically related to enthesitis. Ann Rheum Dis. 2014; 73: 735–40.

35. FitzGerald O, Haroon M, Giles JT, Winchester R. Concepts of pathogenesis in psoriatic arthritis: genotype determines clinical phenotype. Arthritis Res Ther. 2015;17:115.

36. Haroon M, Winchester R, Giles JT, Heffernan E, FitzGerald O. Certain class I HLA alleles and haplotypes implicated in susceptibility play a role in determining specific features of the psoriatic arthritis phenotype. Ann Rheum Dis 2016;75:155–62.

37. Queiro R, González S, Alperi M, et al. HLA-DR17 is associated with enthesitis in psoriatic arthritis. Joint Bone Spine. 2011; 78: 428–9.

38. Ball J. Enthesopathy of rheumatoid and ankylosing spondylitis. Ann Rheum Dis. 1971; 30: 213–23.

39. Braun J, Bollow M, Neure L, et al. Use of immunohistologic and in situ hybridization techniques in the examination of sacroiliac joint biopsy specimens from patients with ankylosing spondylitis. Arthritis Rheum. 1995; 38: 499–505.

40. Francois RJ, Gardner DL, Degrave EJ, Bywaters EG. Histopathologic evidence that sacroiliitis in ankylosing spondylitis is not merely enthesitis. Arthritis Rheum 2000;43:2011–24.

41. Laloux L, Voisin MC, Allain J, et al. Immunohistological study of entheses in spondyloarthropathies: comparison in rheumatoid arthritis and osteoarthritis. Ann Rheum Dis. 2001; 60: 316–21.

42. McGonagle D, Marzo-Ortega H, O'Connor P, et al. Histological assessment of the early enthesitis lesion in spondyloarthropathy. Ann Rheum Dis. 2002; 61: 534–7.

43. Paramarta JE, Baeten D. Spondyloarthritis: from unifying concepts to improved treatment. Rheumatology (Oxford). 2014;53:1547–59.

44. Vieira-Sousa E, van Duivenvoorde LM, Fonseca JE, Lories RJ, Baeten DL. Animal models as a tool to dissect pivotal pathways driving spondyloarthritis. Arthritis Rheumatol. 2015;67:2813–27.

45. Braem K, Carter S, Lories RJ. Spontaneous arthritis and ankylosis in male DBA/1 mice: further evidence for a role of behavioral factors in 'stress induced arthritis'. Biol Proced Online 2012; 14:10.

46. Sherlock JP, Joyce-Shaikh B, Turner SP, et al. IL-23 induces spondyloarthropathy by acting on ROR-γt+ CD3+CD4-CD8- entheseal resident T cells. Nat Med. 20121; 18: 1069–76.

47. Adamopoulos IE, Tessmer M, Chao CC, et al. IL-23 is critical for induction of arthritis, osteoclast formation, and maintenance of bone mass. J Immunol. 2011; 187:951–9.

48. Benham H, Rehaume LM, Hasnain SZ, et al. Interleukin-23 mediates the intestinal response to microbial β-1,3-glucan and the development of spondyloarthritis pathology in SKG mice. Arthritis Rheumatol. 2014; 66:1755–67.

49. Yamamoto M, Nakajima K, Takaishi M, et al. Psoriasis inflammation facilitates the onset of arthritis in a mouse model. J Invest Dermatol 2015;135:445–53.

50. Khmaladze I, Kelkka T, Guerard S, et al. Mannan induces ROS-regulated, IL-17A-dependent psoriasis arthritis-like disease in mice. Proc Natl Acad Sci (USA) 2014;111:E3669–78.

51. Jacques P, McGonagle D. The role of mechanical stress in the pathogenesis of spondyloarthritis and how to combat it. Best Pract Res Clin Rheumatol. 2014;28:703–10.

52. Jacques P, Lambrecht S, Verheugen E, et al. Proof of concept: enthesitis and new bone formation in spondyloarthritis are driven by mechanical strain and stromal cells. Ann Rheum Dis. 2014; 73: 437–45.

53. Van Duivenvoorde L, Baeten D. Comment on: 'Spondyloarthritis: may the forcé be with you', the Editorial by McGonagle et al. Ann Rheum Dis 2014;73:e38.

54. Tan AL, McGonagle D. Imaging of seronegative Spondyloarthritis. Best Pract Res Clin Rheumatol. 2008; 22: 1045–59.

55. Gutierrez M, Filippucci E, De Angelis R, Filosa G, Kane D, Grassi W. A sonographic spectrum of psoriatic arthritis: 'the five targets'. Clin Rheumatol. 2010; 29: 133–42.

56. Coates LC, Hodgson R, Conaghan PG, Freeston JE. MRI and ultrasonography for diagnosis and monitoring of psoriatic arthritis. Best Pract Res Clin Rheumatol. 2012; 26: 805–22.

57. Tan AL, Benjamin M, Toumi H, et al. The relationship between the extensor tendon enthesis and the nail in distal interphalangeal joint disease in psoriatic arthritis–a high-resolution MRI and histological study. Rheumatology (Oxford). 2007; 46:253–6.

58. Poggenborg RP, Eshed I, Østergaard M, et al. Enthesitis in patients with psoriatic arthritis, axial spondyloarthritis and healthy subjects assessed by 'head-to-toe' whole-body MRI and clinical examination. Ann Rheum Dis. 2015;74:823–9.

59. Ostergaard M, McQueen F, Wiell C, et al. The OMERACT psoriatic arthritis magnetic resonance imaging scoring system (PsAMRIS): definitions of key pathologies, suggested MRI sequences, and preliminary scoring system for PsA Hands. J Rheumatol 2009; 36:1816–1824.

60. Balint PV, Kane D, Wilson H, McInnes IB, Sturrock RD. Ultrasonography of entheseal insertions in the lower limb in spondyloarthropathy. Ann Rheum Dis 2002; 65:905–910.

61. de Miguel E, Cobo T, Muñoz-Fernandez S, Naredo E, et al. Validity of enthesis ultrasound assessment in spondyloarthropathy. Ann Rheum Dis 2009; 68:169–174.

62. Eder L, Jayakar J, Haddad A, Chandran V, et al. Is the Madrid Sonographic Enthesitis Index (MASEI) useful or differentiating psoriatic arthritis from psoriasis alone and healthy controls? J Rheumatology 2014; 41:466–472.

63. Ficjan A, Husic R, Gretler J, et al. Ultrasound composite scores for the assessment of inflammatory and structural pathologies in Psoriatic Arthritis (PsASon-Score). Arthritis Res Ther 2014; 16:476.

64. Bandinelli F, Prignano F, Bonciani D, et al. Ultrasound detects occult entheseal involvement in early psoriatic arthritis independently of clinical features and psoriasis severity. Clin Exp Rheumatol 2013; 31:219–224.

65. Frediani B, Falsetti P, Storri L, Allegri A, et al. Ultrasound and clinical evaluation of quadricipetal tendon enthesitis in patients with psoriatic arthritis and rheumatoid arthritis. Clin Rheumatol 2002; 21:203–206.

66. Aydin SZ, Ash ZR, Tinazzi I, et al. The link between enthesitis and arthritis in psoriatic arthritis: a switch to a vascular phenotype at insertions may play a role in arthritis development. Ann Rheum Dis 2013; 72:992–995.

67. Tinazzi I, McGonagle D, Biasi D, et al. Preliminary evidence that subclinical enthesopathy may predict psoriatic arthritis in patients with psoriasis. J Rheumatol. 2011;38:2691–2.

68. Husic R, Gretler J, Felber A, et al. Disparity between ultrasound and clinical findings in psoriatic arthritis. Ann Rheum Dis 2014; 73:1529–1536.

69. Palazzi C, Lubrano E, D'Angelo S, Olivieri I. Beyond early diagnosis: occult psoriatic arthritis. J Rheumatol 2010; 37:1556–8.

70. Gutierrez M, Filippucci E, De Angelis R, et al. Subclinical entheseal involvement in patients with psoriasis: an ultrasound study. Semin Arthritis Rheum 2011; 40: 407–12.

71. Ash ZR, Tinazzi I, Gallego CC, et al. Psoriasis patients with nail disease have a greater magnitude of underlying systemic subclinical enthesopathy than those with normal nails. Ann Rheum Dis 2012; 71: 553–6.

72. Tan AL, Fukuba E, Halliday NA, Tanner SF, Emery P, McGonagle D. High-resolution MRI assessment of dactylitis in psoriatic arthritis shows flexor tendon pulley and sheath-related enthesitis. Ann Rheum Dis. 2015;74:185–9.

73. Kocijan R, Englbrecht M, Haschka J, et al. Quantitative and qualitative changes of bone in psoriasis and psoriatic arthritis patients. J Bone Miner Res 2015; 30(10):1775–83.

74. Girolomoni G, Gisondi P. Psoriasis and systemic inflammation: underdiagnosed enthesopathy. J Eur Acad Dermatol Venereol 2009; 23(Suppl.1):3–8.

75. D´Agostino MA, Aegerter P, Bechara K, et al. How to diagnose spondyloarthritis early? Accuracy of peripheral enthesitis detection by power Doppler ultrasonography. Ann Rheum Dis 2011; 70:1433–40.

76. de Miguel E, Muñoz-Fernández S, Castillo C, Cobo-Ibáñez T, Martín-Mola E. Diagnostic accuracy of enthesis ultrasound in the diagnosis of early spondyloarthritis. Ann Rheum Dis. 2011;70:434–9.

77. Gossec L, Smolen JS, Ramiro S, et al. European League Against Rheumatism (EULAR) recommendations for the management of psoriatic arthritis with pharmacological therapies: 2015 update. Ann Rheum Dis 2016;75: 499–510.

78. Coates LC, Kavanaugh A, Mease PJ, et al. Group for research and assessment of psoriasis and psoriatic arthritis: Treatment recommendations for psoriatic arthritis 2015. Arthritis Rheumatol. 2016; 68(5):1060–71.

79. Dean BJ, Lostis E, Oakley T, et al. The risks and benefits of glucocorticoid treatment for tendinopathy: a systematic review of the effects of local glucocorticoid on tendon. Semin Arthritis Rheum 2014; 43:570–576.

80. Orbai AM, Weitz J, Siegel EL, et al. Systematic review of treatment effectiveness and outcome measures for enthesitis in psoriatic arthritis. J Rheumatol. 2014;41:2290–4.

CHAPTER 12

Dactylitis

Ignazio Olivieri[†], Enrico Scarano, Salvatore D'Angelo, Carlo Palazzi, and Angela Padula

Introduction

Dactylitis, also known as 'sausage-shaped' digit, is defined in medical dictionaries as inflammation of an entire digit (a finger or toe) [1]. This term is derived from the Greek word dactylos, which means a finger. Even though every inflammatory process involving the digits may be designated as dactylitis, the term is currently used only in some diseases including tuberculosis, syphilis, sickle cell anaemia, sarcoidosis, gout, spondyloarthritis (SpA), and infection of the fat pad of the distal phalanx [2].

These types of dactylitis differ in the precise tissues involved and in the type of involvement. Syphilitic dactylitis [3] and sickle cell dactylitis [4] involve only the bone; tuberculous dactylitis [5] and sarcoid dactylitis [6] extend from the bone to the adjacent soft tissues; gouty dactylitis [7, 8], SpA dactylitis [2], and blistering distal dactylitis [9] involve only the soft tissues of the digit. Regarding the aetiopathogenesis, the different forms may be classified as inflammatory infectious (syphilitic dactylitis, tuberculous dactylitis, and blistering distal dactylitis), inflammatory non-infectious (sarcoid dactylitis, gouty dactylitis, and SpA dactylitis) and non-inflammatory (sickle cell dactylitis) [2].

SpA dactylitis is known as sausage-shaped digit because there is diffuse swelling of the entire digit due to synovitis, tenosynovitis, and soft tissue inflammation, and it should be clearly differentiated from the other forms of 'false' dactylitis, described above. It is a specific manifestation of SpA, a group of interrelated diseases which includes, in addition to psoriatic arthritis (PsA), primary ankylosing spondylitis, reactive arthritis, arthritis associated with inflammatory bowel disease, and the undifferentiated forms [2, 10]. Sausage-like digit was included in the Amor criteria suggested for all forms of SpA in the early 1990s [11]. It was not included in the European Spondylarthropathy Study Group (ESSG) criteria suggested at that time due to the low sensitivity (17.9%) found in this study in spite of the high specificity (96.4%) [12]. However, dactylitis is present, due to its high specificity and satisfactory sensitivity, among the criteria suggested by the Assessment of SpondyloArthritis international Society (ASAS) for axial [13] and peripheral SpA [14] as well as in the ClASsification criteria for Psoriatic ARthritis (CASPAR) [15].

Clinical aspects

Dactylitis digit has been defined as 'uniform swelling such that the soft tissues between the metacarpophalangeal and proximal interphalangeal, proximal and distal interphalangeal joints, and/or distal interphalangeal joint and digital tuft are diffusely swollen to the extent that the actual joint swelling could no longer be independently recognized' [8] (Figures 12.1 and 12.2).

Dactylitis may be acute with painful inflammatory changes or chronic when the digit remains swollen despite the disappearance of acute inflammatory findings [16]. It has been proposed that chronic dactylitis occurs following an episode of acute dactylitis but this has not been proven. In acute dactylitis, physical examination of the involved finger or toe nearly always shows swelling and pain along the flexor tendons. In finger dactylitis, the swelling of the flexor tendon synovial sheaths is often so marked that the patient cannot flex his finger. Sometimes, there is also swelling and pain in one or more joints of the dactylitic digit. There is no need to obtain imaging evaluation for the clinical diagnosis of current dactylitis since physical examination has the same high specificity and sensitivity as magnetic resonance imaging (MRI) for the diagnosis of flexor tenosynovitis [17, 18]. Studies of the assessment of clinical evaluation of patients with PsA showed that there is agreement among rheumatologists on the assessment of dactylitis [19, 20]. One of these studies involving rheumatologists and dermatologists with expertise on psoriatic disease also demonstrated that there is poor reliability of the assessment of dactylitis by dermatologists [20]. Therefore, the training of dermatologists and other clinicians to recognize and to assess dactylitis is important to improve referral to the rheumatologist.

Diagnosis of SpA dactylitis by history taking is more difficult, especially when dactylitis occurred many years before the consultation. In this case, there are only two possibilities for diagnosing dactylitis: (a) to show a photograph of finger or toe dactylitis to the patient for confirmation; (b) to examine the routine radiograph obtained by the patient's physician at the time of the sausage-like swelling [21]. The typical diffuse soft tissue swelling should be present on X-rays if the patient truly had dactylitis (Figure 12.3).

Although dactylitis is more frequent in PsA, occurring in 16–48% of cases [16, 22–25], it may be observed in all forms of SpA [11–14]. In undifferentiated SpA, dactylitis usually occurs together with the other SpA features: peripheral arthritis, peripheral enthesitis, inflammatory spinal pain, buttock pain, chest wall pain, acute anterior uveitis, and aortic incompetence together with conduction abnormalities [26]. Like these, dactylitis may sometimes

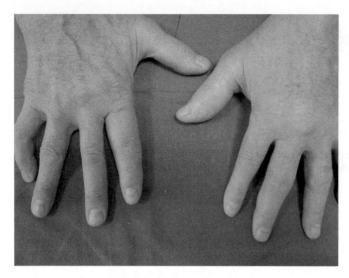

Figure 12.1 Dactylitis of the right index and of the left thumb.

occur for a long time in isolation as the only clinically apparent manifestation of the *HLA-B*27*-associated disease process [27–30]. This has been observed in children [27–28], in young and middle-aged adults [29], and in the elderly [30]. There are also patients with psoriatic changes or with a family history of psoriasis who exhibit dactylitis and/or enthesitis for months or years as the only musculoskeletal manifestations of psoriatic disease [31].

Usually dactylitis involves few fingers and/or toes asymmetrically [16–18, 32, 33]. Sometimes it may simultaneously involve most of the fingers [33]. Like other peripheral manifestations of SpA, i.e. enthesitis and arthritis, the onset of dactylitis may be triggered by a physical injury [34]. The involvement of the tenosynovial sheaths

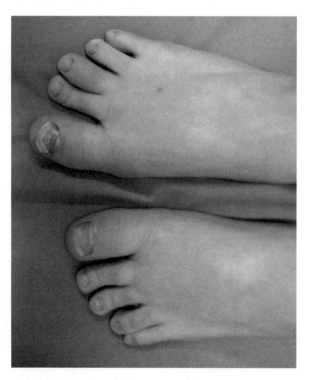

Figure 12.2 Dactylitis of the third digit of the right foot.

in finger dactylitis may extend beyond the digit [35–38]. The most frequent anatomic pattern of digital and palmocarpal synovial sheaths is as follows. The index, middle, and ring fingers have synovial sheaths separate from those of the radial and ulnar bursae, which communicate respectively with the synovial sheaths of the thumb and the little finger. However, variants showing communication of the sheaths of the index, middle, or ring fingers with the ulnar bursa occur frequently. When dactylitis involves a finger with synovial sheaths communicating with the ulnar bursa, the painful swelling also extends into the palm of the hand [35, 36]. In addition, in dactylitis of the first and fifth fingers, synovial inflammation may spread to the radial and ulnar bursa, respectively [37, 38].

According to Brockbank et al., dactylitis can be a marker of disease severity [16]. The authors followed prospectively 537 patients suffering from PsA with the aim of establishing if dactylitis is associated with a worse prognosis. They observed increased radiological progression of joint damage in digits showing dactylitis compared with those without dactylitis. In the authors' opinion, the presence of dactylitis should prompt the physician to start specific treatment.

Imaging

So far, the pathophysiology of SpA dactylitis has not been completely elucidated [39]. It is not clear which are the involved tissues and which is the primary lesion of the sausage-like digit [39, 40]. Since obtaining histologic samples of the digital structures is not feasible, ultrasound (US) and MRI have been used to examine the multiple tissue compartments (Figures 12.4 and 12.5). Before these studies, it was thought the 'sausage-like' appearance was due to concomitant involvement of the flexor tendon synovial sheaths and the metacarpophalangeal (or metatarsophalangeal) and interphalangeal joints. The first US and MRI studies established that dactylitis is due to flexor tenosynovitis and marked adjacent soft tissue swelling with a variable degree of joint synovitis [17, 18, 32, 41–43]. Flexor tenosynovitis was found to be nearly always present while joint synovitis occurred in 17–66% of the sausage-like digits [17, 18, 32, 41–43].

In the late 1990s and in the early years of the new century, McGonagle and his colleagues hypothesized that enthesitis is the primary lesion in SpA and that synovitis of the various structures (joint, tendon, and bursa) represents a secondary phenomenon due to the release of pro-inflammatory cytokines from the inflamed entheses [44–47]. In their opinion, the flexor tenosynovitis of dactylitis is due to enthesitis as a consequence of the diffusion of cytokines along the tenosynovial sheaths [47]. We demonstrated, by using fast spin echo-T2-weighted sequences with fat saturation, that in SpA dactylitis there is no evidence of enthesitis of the insertion of the flexor digitorum tendons or of the attachment of the capsule of the digit joints [32, 41]. However, Mc Gonagle and his colleagues further suggested that in dactylitis enthesitis could occur at the numerous 'functional entheses' that the digit flexor tendons form with retinacula or pulleys [47]. These functional entheses are frequently associated with the presence of fibrocartilage that reduces compression and shear. They advocated that this hypothesis could be tested by using high-resolution imaging.

In 2008, Healey and co-workers reported their MRI study on psoriatic dactylitis [48]. Scans were performed before and after treatment and pre- and post-gadolinium contrast. Joint synovitis

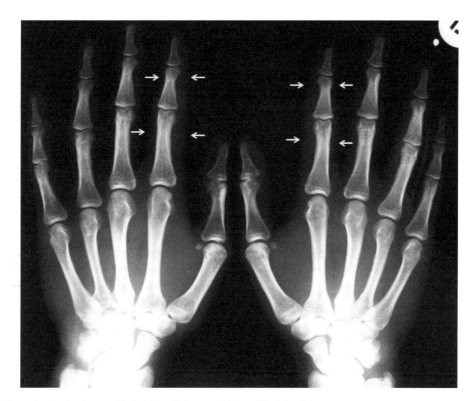

Figure 12.3 Plain film radiography showing 'sausage- like' swelling of the second finger of both hands.

and soft tissue oedema were the most frequent abnormalities. The oedema extended all around the circumference and was not associated with flexor tenosynovitis, which was, however, a common finding. Bone oedema ranged from small areas adjacent to the joint capsule insertions to oedema involving the whole phalanx. This last finding adds support to the hypothesis by McGonagle on a primary involvement of the entheses in dactylitis.

Recently, the Leeds group used high-resolution MRI to visualize the small entheses of the digit in dactylitis [49]. They found collateral ligament enthesitis, extensor tendon enthesitis, and functional enthesitis in most dactylitic fingers and in none of the normal digits of healthy volunteers.

In 75% of the dactylitic digits, there was flexor tenosynovitis together with flexor tendon pulley/flexor sheath microenthesitis

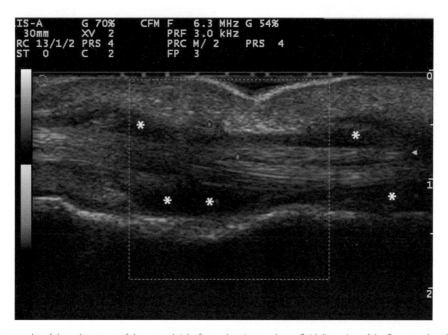

Figure 12.4 Longitudinal sonography of the volar aspect of the second right finger showing moderate fluid distension of the flexor tendon sheaths (white asterisks) without significant increased vascularity at power Doppler.

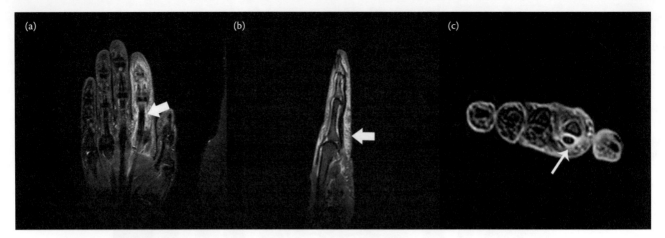

Figure 12.5 Coronal T2 STIR (A), sagittal DP SPAIR (B) and axial fat saturated contrast-enhanced T1 weighted images (C) showing moderate fluid distension of the flexor tendon synovial sheaths of the second right finger together with diffuse soft tissue oedema (big white arrows) and diffuse enhancement of the flexor tendon synovial sheaths (small white arrow).

suggesting a form of functional enthesitis. In the authors' opinion, the swelling along the digits observed in dactylitis is linked to polyenthesitis. The relationship between dactylitis and enthesitis was recently addressed by a paper on associations of clinical phenotypes with HLA genotype [50]. In this study enthesitis was associated with B27 while dactylitis was associated with both B27 and B08, the latter also associated with more synovial-based disease.

Further imaging US and MRI studies should develop a core set of elementary lesions that can discriminate dactylitic from normal digits and a composite valid and sensitive measure of activity to be used in clinical trials.

Clinimetric assessment

Dactylitis has been used in clinical trials of PsA performed in the past as a secondary outcome measure although no validated instruments were available [51]. Most studies used a simple count of dactylitic digits in which the presence of dactylitis was based on the clinician's opinion. Other studies utilized non-validated physician graded severity (0–3 or 1–4) which have been shown to have poor inter-observer reliability. In 2005, Helliwell and co-workers developed a clinically objective and validated instrument for dactylitis called the Leeds Dactylometer [52] (Figure 12.6). This instrument quantifies both the size and tenderness so that the score can differentiate between tender and non-tender dactylitis. Dactylitis was defined as an increase in circumference of the digit of more than 10% compared with the contralateral digit and, if both digits are involved, the circumference can be compared to the normative data provided. The tenderness score can range between 0 and 3 or can be dichotomous with 0 for non-tender and 1 for tender digit. An index was established, the Leeds Dactylitis Index (LDI), which was able to identify improvements in dactylitis in a randomized control trial where dactylitis was a secondary outcome measure [53].

Dactylitis is one of the domains of disease activity composite scores used for PsA such as the Composite Psoriatic Disease Activity Index (CPDAI) [54] and the Psoriatic Arthritis Disease Activity Score (PASDAS) [55].

Therapy

Treatment of dactylitis has been recently reviewed as part of the treatment update performed by the Group for Research and Assessment of Psoriasis and Psoriatic Arthritis (GRAPPA) [56].

Non-steroidal anti-inflammatory drugs (NSAIDs) and local corticosteroid injections, which are the most commonly used therapies, have not been formally assessed by randomized, double-blind placebo-controlled trials. Conventional synthetic disease-modifying anti-rheumatic drugs (DMARDs) such as methotrexate, cyclosporine, sulphasalazine, and leflunomide may be effective but trials have not been sufficiently powered. In an observational

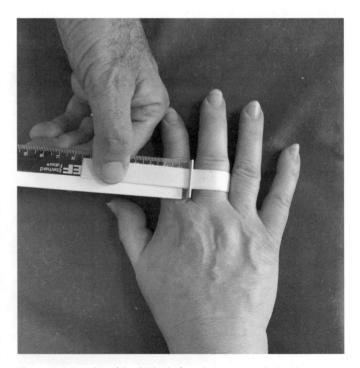

Figure 12.6 Dactylitis of the third right finger being measured using the dactylometer.

cohort, treatment with biologics was more effective than treatment with traditional DMARDs [25]. Among the biologic DMARDs infliximab, certolizumab pegol, and ustekinumab have appeared promising [53, 57, 58], with golimumab as another potential candidate [59]. Etanercept requires more dedicated studies to ascertain its efficacy on dactylitis [60], with adalimumab and apremilast showing some effect [61, 62]. The role of the new biologic agents is as yet uncertain. There are no head-to-head studies suggesting the superiority of one agent over another. So far, the longest experience exists for the tumor necrosis factor inhibitors, which are preferred by the updated European League Against Rheumatism (EULAR) recommendations for patients with predominant dactylitis [63]. Future randomized controlled trials using dactylitis as a primary outcome feature will establish the most appropriate treatment for this important and frequent manifestation of psoriatic disease.

References

1. Dorland's Illustrated Medical Dictionary, 30th Edition. Philadelphia: Saunders; 2000: 473.
2. Olivieri I, Scarano E, Padula A, Giasi V, Priolo F. Dactylitis, a term for different digit diseases. Scand J Rheumatol 2006;35:333–40.
3. Rasool MN, Govender S. The skeletal manifestations of congenital syphilis. A review of 197 cases. J Bone Joint Surg Br 1989;71:752–5.
4. Worrall VT, Butera V. Sickle-cell dactylitis. J Bone Joint Surg Am 1976;58:1161–3.
5. Andronikou S, Smith B. 'Spina ventosa'—tuberculous dactylitis. Arch Dis Child 2002;86:206.
6. Pitt P, Hamilton EBD, Innes EH, Morley KD, Monk BE, Hughes GR. Sarcoid dactylitis. Ann Rheum Dis 1983;42:634–9.
7. Andracco R, Zampogna G, Parodi M, Paparo F, Cimmino MA. Dactylitis in gout. Ann Rheum Dis 2010;69:316.
8. Rothschild BM, Pingitore C, Eaton M. Dactylitis: implications for clinical practice. Semin Arthritis Rheum 1998;28:41–7.
9. Hays GC, Mullard JE. Blistering dactylitis: a clinically recognizable streptococcal infection. Paediatrics 1975;56:129–31.
10. Olivieri I, Padula A, Scarano E, Scarpa R. Dactylitis or 'sausage-shaped' digit. J Rheumatol 2007;34:1217–22.
11. Amor B, Dougados M, Mijiyawa M. Criteria of the classification of spondylarthropathies. [French]. Rev Rhum Mal Osteoartic 1990;57:85–9.
12. Dougados M, van der Linden S, Juhlin R, et al. The European Spondylarthropathy Study Group preliminary criteria for the classification of spondylarthropathy. Arthritis Rheum 1991;34:1218–27.
13. Rudwaleit M, van der Heijde D, Landewé R, et al. The development of Assessment of SpondyloArthritis international Society classification criteria for axial spondyloarthritis (part II): validation and final selection. Ann Rheum Dis 2009;68:777–83.
14. Rudwaleit M, van der Heijde D, Landewé R, et al. The Assessment of SpondyloArthritis International Society classification criteria for peripheral spondyloarthritis and for spondyloarthritis in general. Ann Rheum Dis 2011;70:25–31.
15. Taylor W, Gladman D, Helliwell P, et al. Classification criteria for psoriatic arthritis: development of new criteria from a large international study. Arthritis Rheum 2006;54:2665–73.
16. Brockbank JE, Stein M, Schentag CT, Gladman DD. Dactylitis in psoriatic arthritis: a marker for disease severity? Ann Rheum Dis 2005;64:188–90.
17. Olivieri I, Barozzi L, Favaro L, , et al. Dactylitis in patients with seronegative spondylarthropathy: assessment by ultrasonography and magnetic resonance imaging. Arthritis Rheum 1996;39:1524–8.
18. Olivieri I, Barozzi L, Pierro A, De Matteis M, Padula A, Pavlica P. Toe dactylitis in patients with spondyloarthropathy: assessment by magnetic resonance imaging. J Rheumatol 1997;24:926–30.
19. Gladman DD, Cook RJ, Schentag C, et al. The clinical assessment of patients with psoriatic arthritis: results of a reliability study of the Spondyloarthrtitis Research Consortium of Canada. J Rheumatol 2004;31:1126–31.
20. Chandran V, Gottlieb A, Cook RJ, et al. International multicenter psoriasis and psoriatic arthritis reliability trial for the assessment of skin, joints, nails, and dactylitis. Arthritis Rheum 2009;61:1235–42.
21. Olivieri I, Montaruli M, Scarano E, Peruz G, Padula A. Usefulness of plain film radiography in the diagnosis of dactylitis by history taking. J Rheumatol 2005;32:1379.
22. Helliwell P, Marchesoni A, Peters M, Barker M, Wright V. A re-evaluation of the osteoarticular manifestations of psoriasis. Br J Rheumatol 1991;30:339–45.
23. Fournié B, Crognier L, Arnaud C, et al. Proposed classification criteria of psoriatic arthritis. A preliminary study in 260 patients. Rev Rhum Engl Ed 1999;66:446–56.
24. Carneiro JN, Paula AP, Martins GA. Psoriatic arthritis in patients with psoriasis: evaluation of clinical and epidemiological features in 133 patients followed at the University Hospital of Brasilia. An Bras Dermatol 2012;87:539–44.
25. Gladman DD, Ziouzina O, Thavaneswaran A, Chandran V. Dactylitis in psoriatic arthritis: Prevalence and response to therapy in the biologic era. J Rheumatol 2013;40:1357–9.
26. Olivieri I, Padula A, Pierro A, Favaro L, Oranges GS, Ferri S. Late onset undifferentiated seronegative spondyloarthropathy. J Rheumatol 1995;22:899–903.
27. Siegel DM, Baum J. HLA-B27 associated dactylitis in children. J Rheumatol 1988;15:976–7.
28. Padula A, Scarano E, Giasi V, Olivieri I. Juvenile onset isolated B27 associated dactylitis. Semin Arthritis Rheum 2003;32:341–2.
29. De Ceulaer K, van der Linden JM, Cats A. 'Sausage-like' toes (dactylitis) and HLA B27. J Rheumatol 1977;4 (Suppl 3):66–9.
30. Padula A, Giasi V, Olivieri I. Elderly onset isolated B27 associated dactylitis. Ann Rheum Dis 2002;61:759–60.
31. Salvarani C, Cantini F, Olivieri I, et al. Isolated peripheral enthesitis and/or dactylitis: a subset of psoriatic arthritis. J Rheumatol 1997;24:1106–10.
32. Olivieri I, Salvarani C, Cantini F, et al. Fast spin echo-T2-weighted sequences with fat saturation in dactylitis of spondylarthritis. No evidence of entheseal involvement of the flexor digitorum tendons. Arthritis Rheum 2002;46:2964–7.
33. Olivieri I, Scarano E, Padula A, Giasi V. Dactylitis involving most of the fingers. Clin Exp Rheumatol 2003;21:406.
34. Padula A, Belsito F, Barozzi L, et al. Isolated tenosynovitis associated with psoriasis triggered by physical injury. Clin Exp Rheumatol 1999;17:103–4.
35. Olivieri I, Favaro L, Pierro A, Frisoni M, Ferri S, Barozzi L. Dactylitis also involving the synovial sheaths in the palm of the hand. Ann Rheum Dis 1994;53:783–4.
36. Padula A, Salvarani C, Barozzi L, et al. Dactylitis also involving the synovial sheaths in the palm of the hand: two more cases studied by magnetic resonance imaging. Ann Rheum Dis 1998;57:61–2.
37. Olivieri I, Scarano E, Padula A, Giasi V. Dactylitis of the thumb extending to the radial bursa. J Rheumatol 2003;30:1626–7.
38. Olivieri I, Scarano E, Padula A, Giasi V. Dactylitis of the thumb and little finger extending to the carpal tunnel. J Rheumatol 2007;34:1155–6.
39. Bakewell CJ, Olivieri I, Aydin SZ, et al. Ultrasound and magnetic resonance imaging in the evaluation of psoriatic dactylitis: status and perspectives. J Rheumatol 2013;40:1951–7.
40. Olivieri I, D'Angelo S, Scarano E, Padula A. What is the primary lesion in SpA dactylitis? Rheumatology 2008;47:561–2.
41. Olivieri I, Scarano E, Padula A, et al. Fast spin echo-T2-weighted sequences with fat saturation in toe dactylitis of spondyloarthritis. Clin Rheumatol 2008;27:1141–5.
42. Kane D, Greaney T, Bresnihan B, Gibney R, FitzGerald O. Ultrasonography in the diagnosis and management of psoriatic dactylitis. J Rheumatol 1999;26:1746–51.

43. Wakefield RJ, Emery P, Veale D. Ultrasonography and psoriatic arthritis. J Rheumatol 2000;27:1564–5.

44. McGonagle D, Gibbon W, O'Connor P, Green M, Pease C, Emery P. Characteristic magnetic resonance imaging entheseal changes of knee synovitis in spondylarthropathy. Arthritis Rheum 1998;41:694–700.

45. McGonagle D, Gibbon W, Emery P. Classification of inflammatory arthritis by enthesitis. Lancet 1998;352:1137–40.

46. McGonagle D, Pease C, Marzo-Ortega H, O'Connor P, Emery P. The case for classification of polymyalgia rheumatica and remitting seronegative symmetrical synovitis with pitting edema as primarily capsular/entheseal based pathologies. J Rheumatol 2000;27:837–40.

47. McGonagle D, Marzo-Ortega H, Benjamin M, Emery P. Report on the second international enthesitis workshop. Arthritis Rheum 2003;48:896–905.

48. Healy PJ, Groves C, Chandramohan M, Helliwell PS. MRI changes in psoriatic dactylitis: extent of pathology, relationship to tenderness and correlation with clinical indices. Rheumatology 2008;47:92–5.

49. Tan AL, Fukuba E, Halliday NA, Tanner SF, Emery P, McGonagle D. High-resolution MRI assessment of dactylitis in psoriatic arthritis shows flexor pulley and sheath-related enthesitis. Ann Rheum Dis 2015;74:185–9.

50. Haroon M, Winchester R, Giles JT, Heffernan E, FitzGerald O. Certain class I HLA alleles and haplotypes implicated in susceptibility play a role in determining specific features of the psoriatic arthritis phenotype. Ann Rheum Dis 2016;75:155–62.

51. Ferguson EG, Coates LC. Optimisation of rheumatology indices: dactylitis and enthesitis in psoriatic arthritis. Clin Exp Rheumatol 2014;32(Suppl 85):S113–7.

52. Helliwell PS, Firth J, Ibrahim GH, et al. Development of an assessment tool for dactylitis in patients with psoriatic arthritis. J Rheumatol 2005;32:1745–50.

53. Mease PJ, Fleischmann R, Deodhar AA, et al. Effect of certolizumab pegol on signs and symptoms in patients with psoriatic arthritis: 24-week results of a phase 3 double-blind randomized placebo-controlled study (RAPID-PsA). Ann Rheum Dis 2014;73:48–55.

54. Mumtaz A, Gallagher P, Kirby B, et al. Development of a preliminary composite disease activity index in psoriatic arthritis. Ann Rheum Dis 2011;70:272–7.

55. Helliwell PS, FitzGerald O, Fransen J, et al. The development of candidate composite disease activity and responder indices for psoriatic arthritis (GRACE project). Ann Rheum Dis. 2013;72:986–91.

56. Rose S, Toloza S, Bautista-Molano W, Helliwell PS, GRAPPA Dactylitis Study Group. Comprehensive treatment of dactylitis in psoriatic arthritis. J Rheumatol 2014;41:2295–300.

57. Antoni CE, Kavanaugh A, van der Heijde D, et al. Two-year efficacy and safety of infliximab treatment in patients with active psoriatic arthritis: findings of the Infliximab Multinational Psoriatic Arthritis Controlled Trial (IMPACT). J Rheumatol 2008;35:869–76.

58. McInnes IB, Kavanaugh A, Gottlieb AB, , et al. Efficacy and safety of ustekinumab in patients with active psoriatic arthritis: 1 year results of the phase 3, multicentre, double-blind, placebo-controlled PSUMMIT 1 trial. Lancet 2013;382:780–9.

59. Kavanaugh A, van der Heijde D, McInnes IB, et al. Golimumab in psoriatic arthritis: one-year clinical efficacy, radiographic, and safety results from a phase III, randomized, placebo-controlled trial. Arthritis Rheum 2012,64:2504–17.

60. Sterry W, Ortonne JP, Kirkham B, et al. Comparison of two etanercept regimens for treatment of psoriasis and psoriatic arthritis: PRESTA randomized double blind multicentre trial. BMJ 2010;340:c147.

61. Mease PJ, Ory P, Sharp JT, et al. Adalimumab for long-term treatment of psoriatic arthritis: 2 year data from the Adalimumab Effectiveness in Psoriatic Arthritis Trial (ADEPT). Ann Rheum Dis 2009;68:702–9.

62. Gladman D, Kavanaugh A, Adebajo A, et al. Apremilast, an oral phosphodiesterase 4 inhibitor, is associated with long-term (104-week) improvements in enthesitis and dactylitis in patients with psoriatic arthritis: pooled results from the three phase 3, randomized controlled trials. Ann Rheum Dis 2015;74 (Suppl 2):133.

63. Gossec L, Smolen JS, Ramiro S, et al. European League Against Rheumatism (EULAR) recommendations for the management of psoriatic arthritis with pharmacological therapies: 2015 update. Ann Rheum Dis 2016;75:499–510.

CHAPTER 13

Axial disease

Ennio Lubrano

Introduction

Psoriatic arthritis (PsA) is a common disease with a broad spectrum of clinical and radiological features [1] and, sometimes, it can be indistinguishable from rheumatoid arthritis (RA) with a predominant peripheral arthritis or, less frequently, from ankylosing spondylitis (AS), with a true spinal involvement. Most of the time, an asymmetrical peripheral arthritis, with or without enthesitis, associated with some spinal manifestations is the commonest phenotypical subset of the disease. Thus, this overlap of peripheral and axial manifestations could be identified as a single entity belonging to the PsA disease or as a possible phenotypical expression of a quite wide group of diseases such as axial spondyloarthritis (SpA).

The concept of different diseases among the group of SpA, sharing some clinical, functional and radiological aspects is supported by the identity of conditions such as PsA. Similarly, the concept of just one broad disease, called SpA with predominant peripheral or axial involvement is supported by others, as recently suggested by ASAS (Assessment of SpondyloArthritis International Society) with the new classification criteria [2]. With regard to axial PsA, this debatable concept is important, since its main characteristics could be a predominant phenotypic expression of SpA in patients with coincidental psoriasis, or a subset of PsA [3]. Moreover, as the frequency of axial PsA patients is a function of the number, sensitivity of the diagnostic instruments, and of disease duration, it may vary between 25% (early disease and clinical assessment only) and 75% (late disease and sophisticated imaging) [4]. In fact, axial PsA could be defined according to either the Calin criteria for inflammatory back pain or those recently revised and proposed by ASAS; alternatively, the criteria used to define axial PsA in other studies were radiographic sacroiliitis grade 2 or greater and/or any other typical radiologic signs of spondylitis in psoriatic patients. The difficulties in defining axial PsA could also be related to the fact that PsA is not as painful as that in AS, which is the reason for identifying the radiographic criteria rather than inflammatory back pain criteria [5]. Thus, the uncertain definition of axial PsA [6] needs clinical, imaging, diagnostic, and therapeutic clarification. Indeed, there is about 15% of patients with PsA that develop axial disease late and this subset in not associated with *HLA-B*27* but is associated with more severe peripheral arthritis [7].

Clinical manifestations of axial PsA

The clinical picture of axial PsA can be indistinguishable from AS, when classical spinal involvement with functional impairment and without clear peripheral joint involvement is present. This clinical picture could be the coincidental presence of psoriasis in a patient with AS, mainly if *HLAB*27* positive. Alternatively, axial PsA is often characterized by an overlap of spinal manifestations, with or without sacroiliitis, and peripheral joint involvement. In fact, the clinical picture of axial PsA has been described in various ways, with the tendency of two different patterns of involvement: 1) 'pure' spondylitis with a male preponderance, higher prevalence of *HLA-B*27* positivity, and the radiological presence of sacroiliitis (at least grade 2 according to the New York criteria); 2) an overlap of asymmetrical arthritis associated with axial involvement, and with a tendency to be more frequent in female, lower prevalence of *HLA-B*27* and less radiological presence of sacroiliitis. All the studies, most of them with a small number of cases, described this tendency to characterize axial PsA phenotypically and, to a certain extent, to underline the clinical difference from AS. With regard to long-term follow-up studies, Hanly et al. in 1988 showed some results from a group of patients followed-up for at least 30 months. The authors identified PsA patients with inflammatory back pain or stiffness, inflammatory neck pain or stiffness, and clinical evidence of sacroiliitis, assessed by the Gaenslen Test, Patrick-FABER test, and/or direct compression of the sacroiliac joints. More recently, a study reported an update on a long-term prospective study and, interestingly, after ten follow-up patients with axial PsA had an improvement in neck and back pain, but lateral spinal flexion and cervical mobility deteriorated [8].

Axial PsA can affect patients in a more severe way depending on gender. The study by Gladman and colleagues, looking for variables discriminating between men and women with this condition, provided some evidence for more advanced axial PsA in men and independent of *HLA-B*27* [9]. Another study demonstrated that the extent of the spondylitic process was quite similar between men and women, even if women showed poorer functional performance and more aggressive peripheral disease. The same Spanish authors showed, a few years later, that asymptomatic spondylitis was observed in 20% of the group of patients examined [10]. The definition of axial involvement was based on radiographic grade 2 or greater and/or any other typical radiologic signs of spondylitis in psoriatic patients. These interesting results along with some others have led to the concept that occult PsA could be present especially in those with axial involvement [11].

An important aspect is the cervical involvement in axial PsA. To address this, in 1992, Salvarini and colleagues showed some data from a group of PsA patients in whom cervical involvement was present with two main radiological and clinical subset: a) 25 patients (44% of the total group) with a pattern similar to AS, and b) 15 patients who showed erosive and/or subluxing cervical rheumatoid-type lesions [12].

Another interesting topic is the relationship between musculo-skeletal involvement and severity of psoriasis. To address this point, a Spanish study showed that, among a group of PsA patients, the subgroup with axial involvement was significantly associated with moderate to severe psoriasis [13]. Finally, a study was conducted to describe differential characteristics of axial involvement in AS patients compared with that seen in PsA and inflammatory bowel disease-associated SpA. This study, which included 2044 consecutive patients with SpA, showed that primary AS had more severe axial involvement than those with spondylitis associated with psoriasis or inflammatory bowel disease, while functional capacity, disease activity, and quality of life were comparable among the groups studied [14]. Moreover, supporting the assumption that axial PsA and AS may not be similar, previous studies demonstrated that the Bath Ankylosing Spondylitis Disease Activity score (BASDAI) in PsA was significantly lower than in AS, correlated poorly with external indicators of disease activity [15], and may be influenced by the peripheral involvement. All these interesting data have confirmed, to some extent, that axial PsA is quite different from classical AS and is usually less severe [3].

In the last five years, a few studies have concentrated on other interesting aspects of axial PsA. In particular, the possible co-incidence of DISH (diffuse idiopathic skeletal hyperostosis) and axial PsA has been evaluated [16]. This study was undertaken to assess the prevalence of DISH, any association with clinical and/ or other factors (i.e. gender, BMI etc) and the possibility of co-occurrence of the two conditions. The results showed that DISH was recognized in 78 of 938 PsA patients (prevalence 8.3%). DISH was associated with older age and with higher BMI. Finally the authors concluded that DISH and axial PsA can co-exist in some PsA patients.

Another very interesting study showed that certain class I HLA alleles and haplotypes implicated in susceptibility can play a role in determining specific features of the PsA phenotype [17]. In particular, the allele HLA-B*27:05:02 and associated haplyotypes were associated with enthesitis, dactylitis and symmetrical sacroiliitis, while the haplotype HLA-B*08:01:01-C*07:01:01 was associated with asymmetrical sacroiliitis. Moreover, HLA-C*060201 was negatively associated with sacroiliitis. This interesting exploratory study strongly contributed to clarify some intriguing aspects of the possible links between immunogenetics and clinical manifestations of PsA (see Chapter 6).

Imaging of axial PsA

Radiographic features of axial PsA, such as asymmetrical sacroiliitis, non-marginal syndesmophytes, asymmetrical syndesmophytes, paravertebral ossification, and more frequent involvement of cervical spine seem to be characteristic and potentially helpful in diagnosing PsA and differentiating this condition from some cases of psoriasis with co-incidental AS [18, 19] (Table 13.1). In a retrospective study of 140 patients with PsA, 50 patients had both peripheral and axial changes, defined by bilateral stage 2 sacroiliitis or unilateral stage 3 or more sacroiliitis and/or syndesmophytes. This subgroup of patients with axial changes was characterized by more frequent and more severe peripheral lesions suggesting that both axial and peripheral changes contribute to the severity of the disease [20].

The radiological pattern of axial PsA, compared to that classically observed in AS patients, was first described by McEwen and

Table 13.1 Main radiological differences between axial PsA and ankylosing spondylitis (AS)

Radiological feature	Axial PsA	AS
Sacroiliitis	Unilateral or bilateral asymmetrical++	Severe and symmetrical
Vertebral squaring	Less frequent	More frequent
Osteoporosis	Less frequent	More frequent
Syndesmophytes	Less frequent, asymmetrical	More frequent, symmetrical
Progression of syndesmophytes	Random	From lumbar to cervical spine

colleagues [18] and later by Helliwell and colleagues [19], where the two studies showed a radiological picture with some peculiarities. For instance, the sacroiliac joint involvement was not so frequent and was mainly found to be asymmetrical in axial PsA compared to AS (Figure 13.1). A similar result was found in an our study in which an axial involvement at the cervical and lumbar spine without sacroiliac involvement was observed in 9.8% patients by using the Bath Ankylosing Spondylitis Radiology Index (BASRI) and in 4.28% by using the modified Stoke Ankylosing Spondylitis Spine Score (m-SASSS) [21]. This aspect, in turn, could suggest a different pathophysiology of PsA compared to AS, supporting the concept that among the SpA some identities should be considered separately but under the same umbrella.

Another radiological finding distinguishing axial PsA to AS is the type of syndesmophytes. In fact, since the studies by McEwen and Helliwell, non-marginal and asymmetrical syndesmophytes were found in patients with axial PsA, with a so-called 'chunky' shape, meaning a substantial structural difference to those 'coarse' marginal and symmetrical ones observed in classical AS. The radiological patterns of axial PsA, qualitatively might be completely different to that observed in AS patients. Even the distribution along the spine is not like AS, in which a progression of syndesmophytes from lumbar towards cervical is the rule, while a more random distribution is the most frequent finding in axial PsA. Indeed, sometimes

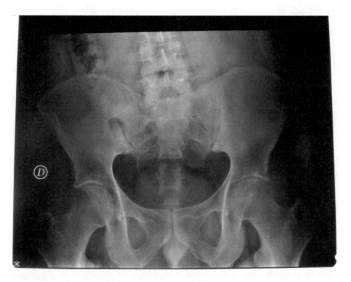

Figure 13.1 Asymmetrical sacroiliac joint involvement.

the type of syndesmophytes occurring in axial PsA patients could be so 'atypical' as to be quite difficult to distinguish from those occurring in AS, as well as from the osteophytes (spondylophytes) occurring in patients with degenerative spinal disease. A recent study proposed a way of differentiating the main two radiological findings, namely syndesmophytes and spondylophytes, by using a 45° angle cut-off on lateral views [22]. Syndesmophytes grow at an angle of < 45° to the vertebral edge, while spondylophytes grow at an angle of >45° to the vertebral edge. Using this methodology, it may therefore be possible to separate the inflammatory radiological findings from those that are truly degenerative.

Another feature which is commonly observed in clinical practice, is the frequent involvement of the zygo-apophyseal joints, with a tendency to be the only anatomical area of the vertebra to be involved in some patients (Figure 13.2). The radiological scoring systems developed and validated for AS do not take into account the posterior elements of the spine. In our study, we found that 28% of patients showed a fusion of the zygo-apophyseal joints at the cervical spine and this radiological finding is not considered by BASRI and m-SASSS [23]. The feature which is quite common and distinctive in axial PsA has led to development of a new radiological score tailored for axial PsA. This new index, called PASRI (Psoriatic Arthritis Spondylitis Radiology Index), was developed using a group patients with established PsA with axial involvement [23].

Following these studies, other groups reported some results on the radiological involvement of axial PsA. In particular, a study by Chandran and colleagues [24] assessed the reliability and the sensitivity to change of radiographic scoring instruments in axial PsA. The study was designed to test BASRI spine, m-SASSS, another score called Radiographic Ankylosing Spondylitis Spinal Score (RASSS) and PASRI, in a group of PsA patients with axial involvement, defined as grade 2 sacroiliitis or greater, inflammatory back pain, and/or restricted spinal mobility. The X-rays, two time points

(at least 2 years apart) were read by three rheumatologists, and the independent assessment by an independent assessor represented the true change (gold standard) [25]. The main results showed that the three scoring instruments had a moderate sensitivity to change but with high specificity to detect the true changes. All measures performed equally well in detecting change [24]. In contrast to X-ray studies, the assessment of axial involvement in PsA has been rarely evaluated by MRI dedicated studies. In fact, on MRI, sacroiliac joint abnormalities of PsA could be identical to those MRI abnormalities described in axial SpA. MRI features of sacroiliitis were found in 38% of 68 PsA patients and were not associated with HLA-B*27 [25]. However, the prevalence of bone oedema in symptomatic axial PsA, compared to that of a group of non-radiographic axial spondyloarthritis and AS, as well as any possible relationship with HLA-B*27 status, has been evaluated. The results showed that HLA-*B27 positivity defined a group of patients with more severe axial bone oedema that is likely related to the classic AS phenotype. On the other hand, HLA-*B27 negative PsA was more likely to be reported as 'negative' MRI result. These results are, to a certain extent, in keeping with different pathophysiology of PsA compared to AS [26]. Finally, the detection of inflammatory and structural lesions of PsA and SpA patients has been evaluated by whole-body MRI scan and compared to healthy subjects. This interesting study showed that whole-body MRI scan allowed simultaneous detection of the presence and the distribution of inflammatory /structural lesions in peripheral and axial joints. Moreover the authors proposed a global score and suggested a possible role for this new technique [27].

Diagnosis of axial PsA (including differential diagnosis)

The recognition of axial PsA has some uncertain aspects. The diagnosis may be very easy when radiological involvement of the spine (with or without sacroiliac joints) is clear. Therefore, the crucial point remains to assess whether a patient has AS with coincidental psoriasis or has true axial PsA. It remains to be seen whether the presence of HLA-*B27 can be helpful in answering this question. More complicated is the frequent situation of patients with PsA and some axial manifestations, either clinical or radiological, not totally in keeping with a real spinal involvement—in other words, some cases of possible osteoarthritis, DISH, or even a true mechanical back pain in PsA patients with peripheral joint involvement. These coincidences of degenerative and or mechanical disorders are crucial in the diagnostic process of axial PsA. In helping to clarify this complicated situation, the classification criteria for PsA could be useful. In terms of PsA classification criteria, different proposals have been made to define the axial PsA: Vasey and Espinoza defined axial PsA as any of: a) spinal pain and stiffness with the restriction of motion present for over 4 weeks; b) grade 2 symmetric sacroiliitis according to the New York criteria; c) grade 3 or 4 unilateral sacroiliitis. Bennett defined axial PsA as axial radiographs showing one or more of: sacroiliitis, syndesmophytes, paravertebral ossification.

The ClASsification of Psoriatic ARthritis (CASPAR) study aimed at finding diagnostic criteria which might distinguish PsA from RA and AS. The study found high specificity for inflammatory thoracic spinal pain, thoracic stiffness, clinical sacroiliitis, and particularly unilateral and marginal syndesmophytes for PsA. However,

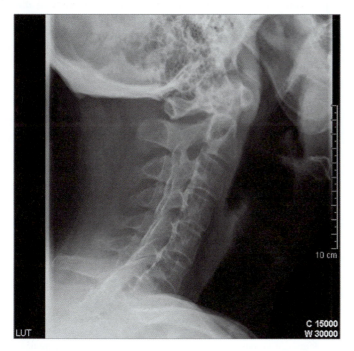

Figure 13.2 Cervical spine is often involved in axial PsA, with zygo-apophyseal joint involvement.

Table 13.2 Main characteristics and differences between axial PsA, ankylosing spondylitis (AS), and DISH

Features	Axial PsA	AS	DISH
Inflammatory back pain	++	+++	−
Symmetrical sacroiliitis	+	+++	−
Asymmetrical sacroiliitis	+++	+	−
Syndesmophytes classic ('Coarse')	+	+++	−
Syndesmophytes paramarginal ('Chunky')	+++	+	−
Thoracic hyperostostis	+/−	−	+++
Zygoaphophyseal cervical involvement	+++	+	−
HLA-B*27	+	+++	−

the mandatory criterion is the presence of inflammatory articular disease (joint, spine or entheseal) [28]. Therefore this latter aspect is the main clinical aspect to be taken into consideration to differentiate between inflammatory and degenerative or mechanical back pain.

PsA patients with axial involvement are often diagnosed late and they have less limited spinal mobility compared to that observed in AS patients. In fact, radiological sacroiliitis can be seen in the absence of spinal symptoms, suggesting that PsA may be an occult disease [11, 29].

Inflammatory back pain and the restricted spinal mobility are the main characteristics of AS. These two criteria, even if they are usually milder in PsA, have been adopted in the study on axial PsA and might still be considered the main criteria in detecting axial PsA in established disease.

Table 13.2 summarizes all main distinctive characteristics of axial PsA compared to AS and DISH.

Treatment of axial PsA

The treatment of axial PsA has been rarely investigated. In fact, no randomized controlled trials reported results separately for the axial subtype, whereas only two observational studies considered this pattern of involvement. The psoriatic arthritis cost evaluation (PACE) observational study evaluated spinal disease associated with PsA, although final results were pooled for patients with *or* without spinal involvement disease [30].

Another observational study focused on PsA patients with axial manifestations and suitable to begin tumor necrosis factor-α blocking (TNFα) treatment. This 12-month observational study was carried out to assess the effectiveness of biologic agents on axial manifestations in PsA patients with established disease. Effectiveness on axial involvement was defined according to the ASAS response criteria (BASDAI: 50% relative or absolute change of 20 mm and expert opinion in favour of continuation), and on the improvements of BASFI, BASMI, and anthropometric measures at 12 months. Efficacy was observed in all outcome measures, as well as on spinal mobility [31]. However, the paucity of data obtained from available literature can be explained by the assumption that treatment of axial PsA is the same as for AS patients. In fact, the GRAPPA (Group for Research and Assessment of Psoriasis and Psoriatic Arthritis) Group recommendations

proposed for axial involvement are based on a therapeutic approach using non-steroidal anti-inflammatory drugs (NSAIDs), physiotherapy and biologic agents derived from ASAS recommendations [32]. The lack of efficacy in AS of traditional oral disease modifying antirheumatic drugs (DMARDs), such as methotrexate, leflunomide, cyclosporine, and sulfasalazine, has been also extrapolated to the axial subset of PsA.

According to GRAPPA, treatment with NSAIDs, physiotherapy, education, analgesia, and injection of sacroiliac joints have been recommended in PsA patients with mild (mild pain and no loss of function) or moderate (loss of function or BASDAI >4) spinal involvement. The cut-off point (BASDAI score >4) for the definition of moderate to severe disease activity has been considered an appropriate criterion adopted from AS for axial disease in PsA, although the BASDAI in PsA may be influenced by the peripheral involvement.

For patients with severe disease who fail to respond to therapies recommended for mild to moderate disease, anti-TNFα treatment with infliximab, etanercept, adalimumab, golimumab, or certolizumab has been considered effective as observed in AS. A similar approach has been proposed by the European League Against Rheumatism (EULAR) recommendations for the management of PsA which state that TNFα inhibitors can be considered even if no synthetic DMARDs have been tried, suggesting that one should follow established recommendations for AS in PsA patients with predominant axial involvement. In fact anti-TNFα treatment can be started after the failure of two NSAIDs for 3 months. Recently ASAS recommendations for the use of anti-TNFα agents in patients with axial SpA have been updated and have defined treatment failure as inadequate response to a therapeutic trial of at least two NSAID over a 4-week period in total at the maximum recommended dose unless contraindicated. These recommendations suggest that the anti TNFα response, defined as 50% improvement in BASDAI or absolute change of 2 (0–10) and positive expert opinion in favour of continuation, should be evaluated after at least 12 weeks. In this context, controlled trials focusing on the treatment of PsA axial involvement should be performed. Finally new therapeutic targets have been recognized for the treatment of PsA, including axial PsA. In particular, targeting the IL-12/IL-23 axis and IL-17 with monoclonal antibodies and small molecules acting on intracellular pathways are potential new medication for axial PsA.

Conclusion

In conclusion, PsA is a heterogeneous disease with some aspects that must be focused on. In this context, axial PsA represents one of the domains which is considered important to be evaluated in order to resolve the intriguing dilemma of being a coincidental AS in patients with psoriasis or a defined subset of PsA. Probably, specific and validated clinical and instrumental tools should be developed for the correct management of axial PsA.

References

1. Moll JM, Wright V. Psoriatic arthritis. Semin Arthritis Rheum. 1973;3: 55–78.
2. Rudwaleit M, van der Heijde D, Landewe R, et al. The assessment of SpondyloArthritis international Society (ASAS) Classification Criteria

for peripheral spondyloarthritis and for sponyloarthritis in general. Ann Rheum Dis. 2011;70;1:25–31.

3. Lubrano E, Spadaro A. Axial psoriatic arthritis: an intriguing clinical entity or a subset of an intriguing disease? Clin Rheumatol. 2012;31:1027–32.

4. Hanly JG, Russell ML, Gladman DD. Psoriatic spondyloarthropathy: a long term prospective study. Ann Rheum Dis. 1988;47: 386–93.

5. Gladman DD, Brubacher B, Buskila D, et al. Psoriatic spondyloarthritis: a clinical, radiographic and HLA study. Clin Invest Med. 1993;15: 371–5.

6. Gladman DD. Axial disease in psoriatic arthritis. Curr Rheumatol Rep. 2007;9(6):455–60.

7. Chandran V, Tolusso DC, Schentag CT, Cook RJ, Gladman DD. Risk factors for axial inflammatory arthritis in patients with psoriatic arthritis. J Rheumatol. 2010;37:809–15.

8. Chandran V, Barrett J, Schentag CT, Farewell VT, Gladman DD. Axial psoriatic arthritis: update on a long-term prospective study. J Rheumatol. 2009;36:2744–50.

9. Gladman DD, Brubacher B, Buskila D, Langevitz P, Farewell VT. Differences in the expression of spondyloarthropathy: a comparison between ankylosing spondylitis and psoriatic arthritis. Clin Invest Med 1993;16: 1–7.

10. Queiro R, Belzunegui J, Gonzalez C, et al. Clinically asymptomatic axial disease in psoriatic spondyloarthropaty. Clin Rheumatol 2002;21:10–13.

11. Palazzi C, Lubrano E, D'Angelo S, Olivieri I. Beyond early diagnosis: occult psoriatic arthritis. J Rheumatol 2010;37 (8):1556–8.

12. Salvarani C, Macchioni P, Cremonesi T, et al. The cervical spine in patients with psoriatic arthritis: a clinical, radiological and immunogenetic study. Ann Rheum Dis. 1992;51: 73–7.

13. Busquets-Perez N, Rodriguez- Moreno J, Gomez-Vaquero C, Noalla-Solè JM. Relationship between psoriatic arthritis and moderate-severe psoriasis: analysis of a series of 166 psoriatic arthritis patients selected from a hospital population. Clin Rheumatol 2012;31:139–43.

14. Perez Alamino R, Maldonado Cocco JA, Citera G, et al. Differential features between primary ankylosing spondylitis and spondylitis associated with psoriasis and inflammatory bowel disease. J Rheumatol 2011;38:1656–60.

15. Taylor WJ, Harrison AA. Could the Bath Ankylosing Spondylitis Disease Activity Index (BASDAI) be a valid measure of disease activity in patients with Psoriatic Arthritis? Arthritis Rheum. 2004;51: 311–5.

16. Haddad A, Thavaneswaran A, Toloza S, Chandran V, Gladman DD. Diffuse idiopathic skeletal hyperostosis in psoriatic arthritis. J Rheumatol. 2013;40(8):1367–73.

17. Haroon M, Winchester R, Giles JT, Heffernan E, Fitzgerald O. Certain class I HLA alleles and haplotypes implicated in susceptibility play a role in determining specific features of the psoriatic arthritis phenotypes. Ann Rheum Dis. 2015;75(1):155–62.

18. McEwen C, Di Tata D, Lingg C, Porini A, Good A, Rankin T. A comparative study of ankylosing spondylitis and spondylitis accompanying ulcerative colitis, regional enteritis, psoriasis and Reiter's disease. Arthritis Rheum. 1971;14: 291–318.

19. Helliwell PS, Hickling P, Wright V. Do the radiological changes of classic ankylosing spondylitis differ from the changes found in the spondylitis associated with inflammatory bowel disease, psoriasis, and reactive arthritis? Ann Rheum Dis 1998;57:135–40.

20. Taccari E, Spadaro A, Riccieri V. Correlations between peripheral and axial radiological changes in patients with psoriatic polyarthritis. Rev Rhum Engl Ed. 1996;63:17–23.

21. Lubrano E, Marchesoni A, Olivieri I, et al. The radiological assessment of axial involvement in Psoriatic Arthritis: a validation study of the BASRI total and The Modified SASSS scoring system. Clin Exp Rheumatol 2009;27:977–80.

22. Baraliakos X, Listing J, Rudwaleit M, et al. Progression of radiographic damage in patients with ankylosing spondylitis: defining the central role of syndesmophytes. Ann Rheum Dis 2007;66: 910–5.

23. Lubrano E, Marchesoni A, Olivieri A, et al. Psoriatic arthritis spondylitis radiology index: a modified index for radiological assessment of axial involvement in psoriatic arthritis. J Rheumatol. 2009;36: 1006–11.

24. Biagioni BJ, Gladman DD, Cook RJ, et al. Reliability of radiographic scoring methods in axial psoriatic arthritis. Arthritis Care Res (Hoboken) 2014; 66(9):1417–22.

25. Williamson L, Dockerty JL, Dalbeth N, et al. Clinical assessment of sacroiliitis and HLA-B27 are poor predictors of sacroiliitis diagnosed by magnetic resonance imaging in psoriatic arthritis. Rheumatology (Oxford) 2004;43(1):85–8.

26. Castillo-Gallego C, Aydin SZ, Emery P, McGonagle DG, Marzo-Ortega H. Magnetic resonance imaging assessment of axial psoriatic arthritis: extent of disease relates to HLA-B27. Arthritis Rheum 2013;65:2274–8.

27. Poggenborg RP, Pedersen SJ, Eshed I, et al. Head-to-toe whole-body MRI in psoriatic arthritis, axial spondyloarthritis and healthy subjects: first steps towards global inflammation and damage scores of peripheral and axial joints. Rheumatology (Oxford) 2015;54(6):1039–49.

28. Taylor WJ, Gladman DD, Helliwell PS, et al. Classification criteria for Psoriatic Arthritis. Development of new criteria from a large international study. Arthritis Rheum 2006;54:2665–73.

29. Chandran V, O'Shea FD, Schentag CT, Inman RD, Gladman DD. Relationship between spinal mobility and radiographic damage in ankylosing spondylitis and psoriatic spondylitis: a comparative analysis. J Rheumatol 2007;34:2463–5.

30. Olivieri I, de Portu S, Salvarani C, et al. The psoriatic arthritis cost evaluation study: a cost-of-illness study on tumour necrosis factor inhibitors in psoriatic arthritis patients with inadequate response to conventional therapy. Rheumatology (Oxford) 2008;47(11):1664–70. doi: 10.1093/rheumatology/ken320.

31. Lubrano E, Spadaro A, Marchesoni A, et al. The effectiveness of a biologic agent on axial manifestations of psoriatic arthritis. A twelve months observational study in a group of patients treated with etanercept. Clin Exp Rheumatol 2011;29(1):80–4.

32. Ritchlin CT, Kavanaugh A, Gladman DD, et al. Treatment recommendations for psoriatic arthritis. Ann Rheum Dis. 2009;68: 1387–94.

CHAPTER 14

Extra-articular, extra-skin disease

Filip Van den Bosch

Introduction

Psoriatic arthritis (PsA) is a complex disorder in which psoriatic skin (and nail) involvement is accompanied by an inflammatory musculoskeletal condition, that can involve peripheral joints and entheses, as well as the axial skeleton. Besides the different rheumatological manifestations, which have been described in detail in previous chapters, patients with psoriatic disease might present with a variety of manifestations affecting other organ systems: these are summarized in Table 14.1. The problem is definitely not marginal: in a recent retrospective analysis of case records of 387 PsA patients, 190 showed at least one extra-articular manifestation, including bowel, ocular, cardiovascular, urogenital, skin (excl. psoriasis), pulmonary, or renal involvement [1]. These concomitant diseases could share a common pathogenetic pathway with psoriasis or PsA, be the consequence of a specific chronic inflammatory process, or simply be a random coincidence. Consequences of long-standing inflammation are often termed co-morbidities, and will be discussed in Chapter 15. The diseases that share a common pathogenetic pathway with PsA are usually called extra-articular (and extra-skin) manifestations. Some typical rheumatological manifestations, such as asymmetric, oligo-articular arthritis predominantly affecting the lower limbs, enthesitis, dactylitis, and inflammatory axial involvement, provide a rationale to consider psoriatic disease as part of the global spondyloarthritis (SpA) spectrum; the strikingly similar occurrence of SpA-concept-related extra-articular manifestations in psoriasis lends additional support to the inclusion. The interplay between the rheumatological manifestations and the different extra-articular manifestations (including psoriatic skin disease) is an important phenomenon that may play a prominent role in the recognition, diagnosis/classification and potentially also the therapeutic approach to these diseases, and supports the idea that—at least for the clinician in daily practice—it makes sense to consider grouping the different SpA-diseases under one umbrella.

In this chapter we will focus on ophthalmological (uveitis) and gastrointestinal (Crohn's disease, ulcerative colitis) manifestations.

Ophthalmological manifestations

Although we will mainly focus on uveitis as the hallmark ophthalmological manifestation in patients with SpA, a number of different ocular findings have been described in patients with psoriasis. The late Verna Wright, who recognized the clinical link between the different rheumatological entities now grouped in the SpA-concept [2], prior to the development of (genetic) laboratory tests that would later prove him correct, also published one of the first case series of 112 PsA patients in whom he investigated ocular inflammation [3]: ocular inflammation was detected in 35 patients, with conjunctivitis, iritis, keratoconjunctivitis sicca, and episcleritis being present in respectively 19.6%, 7.1%, 2.7%, and 1.8%; iritis was more prevalent in psoriatic patients with sacroiliitis (15%) and spondylitis (18%). Kilic et al. compared 100 patients with psoriasis to 100 healthy individuals and reported on the presence of all ophthalmological manifestations in both groups after performing a full eye exam, including Schirmer's test and tears break-up time (BUT) [4]. The majority of the psoriasis patients (93/100) were suffering from classic plaque psoriasis, precluding conclusions about other types of skin involvement. Eye abnormalities were detected in 58 patients with psoriasis compared to only 25 in the healthy control group. In decreasing frequency they observed blepharitis, conjunctivitis, corneal involvement, cataract, anterior uveitis, episcleritis, pigment dispersion, and cystoid macular oedema. The measured values for the Schirmer's test and BUT were also statistically significantly lower in the psoriasis patients, compatible with a tendency towards keratoconjunctivitis sicca. With logistic regression, the authors could not find any relationship with gender, age, extent of psoriasis, nail involvement, or associated PsA. There was also no link with the presence of psoriatic plaques on the eyelids, a feature observed in 13 eyelids. Of interest, no uveitis, episcleritis, or cystoid macular oedema was detected in the control group.

Uveitis: background, (differential) diagnosis and prevalence

Uveitis is the medical term that describes inflammation of the uveal tract. The uvea is located between the outer (cornea and sclera) and inner layer (retina) of the eye. The most anterior portion is the iris; therefore anterior uveitis and iritis are synonymes. Additional inflammation of the ciliary body is termed iridocyclitis. The posterior uvea is called choroid; when the retina is also involved in the inflammatory process, it is called retinochoroiditis. Panuveitis is used to describe inflammation involving the entire uveal tract. Inflammation in the eye is usually recognized by biomicroscopy or slit lamp examination, as there is an excellent correlation between cells in the anterior chamber and anterior uveitis, and leucocytes in the vitreous humour and intermediate uveitis. Immune-mediated arthritides can cause uveitis: an important proportion of this list of systemic diseases is made up by the diseases grouped in the SpA-concept. However, it should always be noted from a differential diagnostic point of view that intra-ocular inflammation defined by the presence of leucocytes in the eye could also result from infection or one of the so-called uveitis masquerade syndromes, such as lymphoma or leukaemia. Finally, a significant number of uveitis cases remain idiopathic.

Table 14.1 Extra-articular, extra-skin manifestations/co-corbidities

Organ system	Manifestation[s]
Extra-articular manifestations	
Skin [excl. Psoriasis]	Erythema nodosum, keratoderma blenorragicum, pyoderma gangrenosum
Eye	Uveitis, conjunctivitis
Gut	Crohn's disease, ulcerative colitis
Urogenital	Urethritis, prostatitis, balanitis, vaginitis, cervicitis
Co-morbidities	
Cardiovascular system	Metabolic syndrome and its components
	Atherosclerosis
	Aortic insufficiency, conduction disturbances
Bone	Osteoporosis
Lung	Apical pulmonary fibrosis, chronic obstructive lung disease [?]
Nervous system	Depression, anxiety
Miscellaneous	
Related to lifestyle	Smoking, alcoholism
Related to treatment	Hepatotoxicity, nephrotoxicity, hypertension, skin cancer

A systematic literature review of 126 articles including 29,877 SpA patients reports the prevalence of uveitis to be as high as 32.7% [5]. This varied with the type of SpA, with higher values for ankylosing spondylitis (AS) (33.2%) and the lowest percentage for undifferentiated SpA (13.2%). In PsA, a prevalence of 25.1% was found, based on ten articles including 1341 patients. Prevalence increased with disease duration: for a mean disease duration of <5 years the prevalence was 12.3%, whereas it was 43.0% for patients with >30 years of disease. A higher risk of uveitis was observed in HLA B27-positive patients (odds ratio [OR] 4.2).

Uveitis: clinical manifestations

The uveitis associated with AS is best studied and usually has a consistent pattern: there is a sudden onset of inflammation in the anterior uvea (acute anterior uveitis [AAU]), which is typically unilateral, but may be recurrent (then potentially also affecting the other eye) [6]. The above-mentioned literature review [5] reports that 737 of 1456 patients (50.6%) had more than one flare. Symptoms include acute redness, photophobia, ocular pain, and impairment of visual acuity, when inflammation leads to debris accumulating in the anterior chamber. Males are slightly more often affected than females. The iritis associated with AS can be intense with hypopyon (pus in the anterior chamber of the eye), or posterior synechiae (the pupil becoming attached to the lens). However, prognosis is generally excellent with full recovery of vision after the acute attack has subsided. The phenotype of uveitis in association with PsA and inflammatory bowel disease (IBD) is not as clearly characterized due to smaller numbers of patients compared to AS. Paiva et al. [7] reported that at least two patterns of eye disease seem to be present in patients with psoriatic disease:

1] approx. 50% of their patients developed a typical anterior uveitis with sudden onset, either unilateral or alternating which was indistinguishable from what is classically associated with AS; 2] some patients develop eye inflammation which was bilateral, insidious in onset, and sometimes involving the posterior uvea, with a much more persistent disease course that might be associated with cataract or glaucoma. In these patients vision loss is usually the only symptom. In this study, patients with peripheral PsA who developed uveitis were predominantly female, whereas PsA patients with axial involvement and uveitis were more likely to be male and HLA-B27 positive. Interestingly, a similar phenotype of more chronic bilateral uveitis is also observed in patients with IBD [8]. In a case–control study, Durrani et al. compared 36 patients with a diagnosis of uveitis and psoriasis to 30 randomly selected patients with either idiopathic anterior uveitis or with HLA-B27-associated anterior uveitis [9]. They found that—irrespective of the HLA-B27-status—the mean age at presentation of uveitis was significantly higher in patients with psoriasis, compared with the non-psoriatic groups: 48.0 years in patients with psoriasis compared to 35.9 and 35.7 years in respectively idiopathic uveitis and HLA-B27-positive uveitis. Thirteen of the 30 (43%) HLA-B27-associated uveitis patients were female, compared to 10 of 15 (67%) psoriatic patients that were also HLA-B27-positive. Regarding clinical characteristics of the uveitis, bilateral involvement occurred in 56% of psoriatic cases, compared to only 3% in the classic HLA-B27-positive AAU. Chronic uveitis, defined as an episode lasting for more than 3 months, was observed in 29% of psoriasis patients, compared to none in the control group; the mean duration of a uveitis attack was also significantly longer in psoriatic uveitis. Posterior involvement was a common occurrence in patients with psoriasis, with cystoid macular oedema in 22%, retinal vasculitis in 11%, and papillitis in 6% of cases. Consequently, supplemental therapy in addition to topical corticosteroids was also more common in these patients. These findings were confirmed in a small retrospective cohort study of 71 PsA patients in whom 13 patients (18%) had uveitis: while 9 patients had acute-onset uveitis, 4 had insidious onset, and 5 cases had bilateral-simultaneous involvement; in 3 cases there was posterior pole involvement [10]. In this small series, multivariate analysis identified bilateral sacroiliitis (OR 17), presence of syndesmophytes (OR 9.7), and HLA-DR13 (OR 24) as predictive factors for the appearance of uveitis. A similar pattern was also observed in a recent Japanese case series of 13 consecutive patients with psoriatic uveitis [11]: although all cases had acute, non-granulomatous anterior uveitis, 6 cases were bilateral, and the authors mention that macular oedema and hyperaemic disc, which are features of posterior pole involvement, were present in respectively 4 and 2 cases; there was also one case of panuveitis.

Even if it seems that a particular type of uveitis is present in most series of patients with psoriatic disease, the aforementioned studies are limited by a small sample size of selected patients. Therefore, further epidemiological studies are still needed to determine the strength of the association between psoriasis, PsA, and uveitis. In this regard, recently published results from a Danish nationwide cohort study provide strong evidence for a bidirectional association between both diseases [12]: from 1997 to 2011, a total study cohort of 5,508,878 patients revealed 74,129 cases with incident psoriasis and 13,114 with incident uveitis. The outcome of the study was the first occurrence of mild psoriasis, severe psoriasis, or psoriatic arthritis in patients with uveitis and the first occurrence of uveitis in patients with psoriasis or PsA. The results—adjusted for age, sex, socioeconomic status, and confounding comorbidities (such as IBD, herpes zoster, and sarcoidosis)—showed an overall increased risk for uveitis (reported as incidence rate ratios [IRR] with 95% confidence intervals [CI]) in mild psoriasis (IRR 1.38 [1.11–1.70]) and PsA (IRR 2.50 [1.53–4.08]); the model also showed a 40% increased risk for uveitis in patients with severe psoriasis (IRR 1.40), but this was not statistically significant probably due to the low number of events. In the subgroup of PsA patients with axial involvement (n=294), the IRR was 8.35 (2.09–33.38). Conversely, patients with uveitis also exhibited an increased risk of developing skin disease and associated arthritis, with IRRs for mild psoriasis, severe psoriasis, PsA, and psoriatic spondylitis, respectively being 1.59, 2.17, 3.77, and 8.03 (all statistically significant). This emphasizes the important role of the ophthalmologist in triggering a diagnostic work-up in case of typical uveitis. This was confirmed with the use of a recently developed and validated algorithm (DUET: Dublin Uveitis Evaluation Tool), which allowed the detection of about 40% of patients with previously undiagnosed SpA in a cohort of consecutive patients with idiopathic AAU [13].

Uveitis: treatment

Treatment of uveitis will of course be coordinated by the ophthalmologist, and in the case of a typical attack of AAU, will consist of topical corticosteroids and cycloplegic agents (mydriatics). Sometimes subconjunctival injections with corticosteroids are necessary to control inflammation in the anterior chamber. In most cases there is no residual visual impairment, and uveitis will subside over 6 to 12 weeks. In cases with severe posterior involvement, oral corticosteroids (up to 60 mg daily), and/or immunosuppressive drugs may become necessary. There seems to be consensus among ophthalmologists that in patients with three or more flares of AAU during a 1-year period or with recurrence of inflammation close to cessation of the topical therapy, further systemic treatment is indicated. This may consist of non-steroidal anti-inflammatory drugs (NSAIDs), conventional disease-modifying anti-rheumatic drugs (DMARDS) or biological DMARDs.

NSAIDs

NSAIDs are the cornerstone of pharmacologic treatment in patients with axial SpA. They were however also used (before the emergence of topical corticosteroids) in the treatment of uveitis [14–17]. In a study by Fiorelli et al., 59 patients with recurrent anterior uveitis were treated with continuous oral NSAID therapy (celecoxib: n=30; diflunisal: n=29) [18]. In both groups, the average number of relapses decreased from 2.84 attacks per person-year follow-up before start of systemic NSAID therapy to 0.53 attacks while on treatment (P<0.001). Patients remained in remission for an average of 18–22 months.

Sulfasalazine

There is some evidence that the use of sulfasalazine reduces the recurrence rate of AAU [19]: in an open, prospective study the number of uveitis flares decreased from 3.4 in the pre-treatment year to 0.9 (P=0.007). Benitez-del-Castillo et al. randomized 22 AS patients with recurrent attacks of AAU to receive either sulfasalazine (n=10) or no treatment (n=12) [20]. During a follow-up period of 36 months, a statistically significant difference in favour of sulfasalazine was observed regarding the number of recurrences; new episodes of uveitis in the sulfasalazine group were also less severe.

Methotrexate

In severe chronic, non-infectious uveitis, a number of immunomodulatory drugs are introduced by ophthalmologists in order to control inflammation and avoid undesirable side-effects of chronic high-dose, oral corticosteroid therapy. In a survey among uveitis specialists [21], inquiring about practice patterns regarding the prescription of corticoid-sparing therapy, methotrexate was the most commonly used initial treatment for anterior, intermediate, and posterior/panuveitis (85%, 57%, and 37%, respectively). This would seem to be a logical choice, given the fact that international treatment recommendations consider methotrexate also as an anchor drug for psoriatic skin and peripheral joint disease (the latter despite a lack of controlled studies on its efficacy).

Biological DMARDs

In the previous decade, the advent of TNF-blockers has dramatically changed the treatment algorithm of patients with active SpA, including psoriatic disease. At this moment, five different anti-TNF agents are indicated for the treatment of signs and symptoms of AS and PsA: etanercept (a soluble TNF-receptor fusion protein), infliximab, adalimumab, and golimumab (all anti-TNF monoclonal antibodies), and certolizumab (an anti-TNF Fab-fragment conjugated to PEG). Although a small case series of patients with HLA-B27-associated anterior uveitis showed that infliximab treatment resulted in fast and complete resolution of inflammation in the anterior chamber [22], treatment with anti-TNF agents is usually reserved to cases with severe, recurrent disease and/or additional sight-threatening involvement of the posterior uvea. Given the fact that the uveitis in PsA might be somewhat different with a more chronic presentation, bilateral involvement, and additional involvement of the posterior segment of the eye, the step towards biological treatment might be taken earlier. An analysis of four placebo-controlled and three open-label studies with TNF-blocking agents in AS showed a frequency of flares of anterior uveitis in the placebo-group of 15.6 per 100 patient-years, compared with 7.9 in the etanercept and only 3.4 in the infliximab-treated patients (both, however, significantly better than placebo) [23]. However, other studies and case reports have suggested that etanercept is less effective in the prevention of uveitis relapses [24], or might even trigger new attacks [25]. Reports on the efficacy of adalimumab for uveitis are based on a large, prospective study in 1,250 AS patients that received open-label treatment for up to 20 weeks [26]: 15 uveitis flares per 100 patient-years were noted before start of adalimumab treatment; the overall rate of flares was reduced with 51% in all patients with better results seen in those patients that had a prior history of uveitis. Preliminary data seem to indicate that golimumab and certolizumab would also decrease the number of recurrent flares of uveitis in patients with established AS.

Gastrointestinal manifestations

It is commonly recognized that patients with idiopathic inflammatory bowel diseases (IBD), both ulcerative colitis (UC) and Crohn's disease (CD), can present with locomotor manifestations, such as peripheral arthritis/enthesitis, as well as axial disease. As a consequence, the arthritis/spondylitis associated with IBD was from the start considered as an integral part of the SpA-concept [2]. Given the well-known association of rheumatological SpA-manifestations and psoriatic skin and nail disease, it would seem logical to search for a link between psoriasis and IBD as well. Surprisingly, there is only very limited literature data, which points, however—comparable to what is observed with uveitis—to a bi-directional relationship.

In 1982 Yates et al. observed an increased occurrence of psoriasis in patients with IBD [27]. They compared 204 patients (116 CD, 88 UC) with the same number of age- and sex-matched controls: an elevated prevalence of psoriasis was found in both CD and UC, with respectively 11.2% and 5.7% of patients, compared to only 1.5% in the control group. In another controlled study of 136 unselected patients with CD [28], psoriasis was present in 13 (9.6%) compared to 2.2% in the control population. In both studies, there were also significantly more IBD patients with a family history of psoriasis in first-degree relatives. A more recent study [29], confirmed that—compared to population controls—both UC and CD patients had a significantly greater likelihood of having other inflammatory disorders, such as arthritis, asthma, psoriasis, and pericarditis. Concerning the clustering of skin and gut disease, 9.19% of 3,873 UC cases and 9.39% of 4,187 CD cases had at least one patient contact for the indication of psoriasis. Conversely, patients with asthma, arthritis, or psoriasis had increased risks for having either CD or UC: for psoriasis, the age-adjusted prevalence ratios were respectively 1.52 (95% CI 1.22–1.89)] for CD and 1.56 (95% CI: 1.24–1.95) for UC. Of interest, 63% of chronic inflammatory diseases were already present before IBD was diagnosed. This elevated risk was also found in a cohort of 103 unselected patients with PsA from Oxford, UK [30]: in these patients a detailed history was taken for the presence of gastrointestinal (GI) disease, including a diagnosis of IBD, irritable bowel syndrome (IBS), and coeliac disease. While the prevalence of IBS was comparable to that of the general population and no patients were diagnosed with coeliac disease (all patients were negative for IgA antiendomysial antibodies), the investigators found that 4 of 103 (3.9%) patients had biopsy-proven IBD (compared to 0.4% in the general UK population). HLA-B27 results were available in three IBD patients: all were negative, pointing towards other potential susceptibility genes and/or environmental factors, underlying skin, joint, and gut disease. In a much larger study, Li et al. [31] investigated 174,476 women enrolled in the Nurses' Health Studies (NHS and NHS II): 2,755 reported psoriasis at baseline with an additional 1,634 women reporting psoriasis over the follow-up through 2005. In this pooled analysis, psoriasis was associated with a relative risk (RR) for developing CD of 3.86 (95% CI 2.23–6.67) (adjusted for age, body mass index, smoking, alcohol intake, physical activity, and NSAID-use); no such association was observed for UC (RR: 1.17, 95% CI 0.41–3.36). The risk of CD was especially pronounced among psoriatics with concomitant PsA (RR: 6.43, 95% CI 2.04–20.32). The importance of the association of skin and gut disease was highlighted in a publication from the same research group in 2012 [32]. Clearly patients with both psoriasis and IBD had higher rates of comorbidities compared to psoriasis-only patients: this was significant for autoimmune thyroiditis, hepatitis, and diabetes; there was also a higher objective inflammatory burden with raised erythrocyte sedimentation rate (33.5 vs 4.0 mm/h) and C-reactive protein (9.1 vs 2.3 mg/L). Most importantly—from a rheumatologist's point of view—60 of the 146 patients with psoriasis and IBD (41.1%) were also diagnosed with seronegative arthritis.

Besides overt IBD, Mielants et al. described—as early as the 1980s—that SpA patients without gastrointestinal symptoms could suffer from subclinical microscopic gut inflammation, detected in biopsies obtained through ileocolonoscopy (summarized in 33). More recently, similar percentages of microscopic gut lesions were confirmed in a prospective cohort of newly diagnosed SpA patients, classified according to the Assessment in SpondyloArthritis international Society (ASAS) criteria for axial and peripheral SpA [34]; in this cohort, presence of gut inflammation was linked to a higher degree of bone marrow oedema in the sacroiliac joints [visualized on magnetic resonance imaging], potentially indicating a more severe inflammatory phenotype [35]. The same research group also performed a prospective ileocolonoscopic study in 64 patients with PsA [36]: inflammatory gut lesions were observed in 10 patients (16%); interestingly, none of the 26 patients with polyarthritis showed these lesions, in contrast to 3/15 (20%) oligoarthritis PsA patients and 7/23 (30%) psoriatics with axial involvement. Scarpa et al. [37] confirmed these findings in a small study, comparing 15 patients with both active psoriasis and PsA (but without bowel symptoms) to 10 healthy subjects who had follow-up ileocolonoscopy after resection of benign polyps. All 15 psoriatic patients showed microscopic changes, with active neutrophilic inflammation evident in 9 patients; no abnormalities were observed in the control group. Taken together, these results support a pathogenetic link between skin, joints, and gut, probably a combination of genetic and environmental factors. In an animal model, Taurog et al. demonstrated that a germ-free environment prevented development of gut and joint inflammatory disease in HLA-B27 transgenic rats, with, however, the skin and genital lesions unaffected by the germ-free state [38]. There is now also preliminary evidence to suggest that the intestinal microbiome may play a role as a mediator of the inflammatory pathways in immune-mediated diseases belonging to the SpA-concept: in this regard a recent study comparing the gut microbiota in 16 patients with PsA, 15 patients with skin psoriasis-only, and 17 matched healthy controls, yielded interesting results as psoriasis and PsA patients had a lower relative abundance of multiple intestinal bacteria [39]. Samples from PsA patients were characterized by a significant reduction in reportedly beneficial bacterial species, resembling a gut microbiota profile previously described in patients with IBD [40]: however, it remains to be investigated whether this dysbiosis is a cause or consequence of systemic inflammation.

Inflammatory bowel disease: clinical manifestations

There is no data to suggest that the signs and symptoms of CD or UC secondary to SpA or PsA are different from what is observed in idiopathic IBD. Symptoms may vary depending on the severity of the inflammation as well as the specific part of the GI tract that is affected. The disease can come and go with episodes of acute, active illness ('flare-ups'), followed by long periods of more quiescent disease with few or even no symptoms at all ('remission'). The cardinal symptoms are diarrhoea, abdominal pain, and systemic features, such as (low-grade) fever, anaemia, fatigue, and weight loss. The diarrhoea in IBD presents as an increase of the frequency of the stools, which can be slimy (CD) or bloody (predominantly UC); it is accompanied by abdominal pain (which can be cramping in UC), and sometimes also nausea and vomiting. Ileocolonoscopy is performed to confirm the diagnosis: in UC the disease may affect different parts of the colon, such as the rectum, sigmoid colon, or descending colon, resulting in respectively proctitis, proctosigmoiditis, or left-sided colitis; pancolitis is the medical term for involvement of the entire colon. In CD, the entire GI tract may be involved from the mouth to the anus, but most commonly involvement of the ileum (terminal part of the small intestine) and colon is observed. In contrast to UC, the inflammation in CD can tunnel through the bowel wall, leading to fistulas. Narrowing of the intestine as a consequence of chronic inflammation may lead to strictures and the clinical picture of bowel obstruction. Given the aforementioned link between skin and [sub]clinical gut disease, it is important that the clinician who is taking care of patients with psoriatic disease, should have an increased awareness of the possibility of GI inflammation and should have a lower threshold to perform further investigations in case of suspicious signs and symptoms.

Inflammatory bowel disease: treatment

Concomitant active gut inflammation, both in CD and UC, may complicate the traditional treatment approach in patients with active axial and/or peripheral SpA or PsA.

NSAIDs

According to the recently updated EULAR recommendations [41], NSAIDs should be used as first-line agents for the symptomatic treatment of axial, but also peripheral joint involvement in patients with psoriatic disease. They should, however, be administered with caution because some data suggest that they may cause an exacerbation of intestinal symptoms, mainly in UC; these relapses of quiescent IBD in the large intestine may appear already after a few days of NSAID treatment in susceptible patients. The role of Cox-2 selective agents, such as celecoxib and etoricoxib, is not entirely clear. Whereas these agents seem to have a better safety profile regarding upper GI tract lesions, there are no systematic data on their safety regarding IBD. Nevertheless, two prospective, controlled studies concerning patients with IBD and rheumatic symptoms who were evaluated for IBD flares while under Cox-2 selective agents vs placebo, suggested no higher incidence of flares with the active drug compared to placebo [42, 43]. Based on these data, a short trial of a Cox-2 selective agent may be considered in patients with quiescent IBD that experience active rheumatological symptoms related to PsA.

Glucocorticoids

Intra-articular corticosteroid injections may be beneficial in mono- or oligoarticular flares of PsA. Oral corticosteroids have no effect on axial symptoms, but may reduce peripheral synovitis. Their systematic use could be justified if they are also required for control of the bowel disease. Controlled ileal release (CIR) budesonide, a corticosteroid that has high affinity for the glucocorticoid receptor but low systemic activity due to extensive first-pass hepatic metabolism, may be used as an alternative to prednisone when treating bowel symptoms; no trials in SpA have yet been performed, and the effect of CIR budesonide on peripheral arthritis or spondylitis was not examined in the CD trials. However, a placebo-controlled trial comparing prednisolone 7.5 mg vs CIR budesonide 3 or 9 mg daily in patients with rheumatoid arthritis yielded similar efficacy results for the prednisolone and the budesonide 9 mg group [44]; this might suggest that if CIR budesonide is prescribed for active gut disease, there might also be beneficial effects on peripheral arthritis.

Disease-modifying anti-rheumatic drugs

DMARDs have been used by clinicians for the treatment of peripheral arthritis associated with IBD, but comparable to the situation in PsA, well designed, controlled studies are lacking. Azathioprine and its principal metabolite 6-mercaptopurine have been successfully used for the treatment of patients with CD; the drug has not been systematically studied in relation to PsA, although a small case series of 18 PsA patients concluded that it may be safely used as an alternative therapy (albeit not superior to other treatments used at the time of the study) [45]. Sulfasalazine, which showed efficacy (albeit with a modest effect size) in the treatment of peripheral joint manifestations of PsA in a number of randomized controlled trials, has been successfully used in the past to treat colonic inflammation in IBD, but is nowadays not recommended as first-line DMARD treatment for active CD or UC. Three systematic Cochrane reviews looked at the efficacy of methotrexate in inducing and maintaining remission in CD and UC [46–48]: in CD, there is some evidence that weekly administration of 25 mg intramuscular methotrexate would provide a benefit for induction of remission and withdrawal from steroids, with a lower dose of 15 mg being superior to placebo regarding maintenance of remission. In contrast, no such benefit was observed in patients suffering from UC; this was recently confirmed in a large placebo-controlled trial (METEOR) [49]. Finally, two small studies explored the effect of leflunomide on CD disease activity [50, 51]: these preliminary data suggest a beneficial effect, but would need to be confirmed in larger controlled trials.

Biological DMARDs

In the 1990s, it was shown that treatment with a single infusion of infliximab is highly effective in the short-term treatment of intestinal involvement in treatment-resistant CD, even resulting in the closure of enterocutaneous fistulae. Later on, multiple placebo-controlled, phase III studies were performed to study the efficacy and safety of anti-TNF monoclonal antibodies in active IBD, investigating both induction schedules and maintenance regimens. Currently, infliximab and adalimumab are approved for the treatment of CD and UC worldwide, whereas golimumab has received approval for the treatment of UC alone. Despite the fact that phase III studies with certolizumab in CD showed efficacy, the drug was only approved for use in the USA, but not the European Union.

The first observations that anti-TNF monoclonal antibodies might also be useful for the treatment of resistant joint or spine manifestations in patients with CD, came from an open pilot study [52]: patients with treatment-resistant or fistulizing CD, but at the same time also active axial and/or peripheral SpA, exhibited a significant improvement of their rheumatological symptoms upon treatment with 5 mg/kg infliximab. Although no formal, placebo-controlled studies with TNF-blocking agents have been performed in PsA associated with IBD, there is little doubt that monoclonal antibodies targeting TNF, are also highly efficacious in this indication. A curious observation is the fact that more TNF-blocking agents are effective in psoriasis and PsA than in the field of IBD. Etanercept is an example of a biological with such differential efficacy: while it is comparable in effectiveness on skin and joint disease to monoclonal antibodies targeting TNF, a proof-of-concept trial in active CD yielded negative results [53]. Given the potential flare of GI disease when patients are treated with NSAIDs, and the limited efficacy of conventional DMARDs mentioned above, it seems logical that in cases where there is active arthritis and/or spondylitis in a patient with psoriatic disease, in whom there is also active IBD, the threshold for starting a biological DMARD would be definitely lower compared to uncomplicated PsA.

Regarding non-TNF biological treatments, one can look at the currently available treatments in gastroenterology and dermatology. For CD, anti-alpha4-integrins have been approved for clinical use in adult patients [54]: currently, there is no data with regard to the efficacy of these drugs on skin disease and/or arthritis in SpA. On the contrary, a recently published small case series even suggested flare of arthritis/spondylitis in CD patients treated with vedolizumab [55]. In skin psoriasis, antibodies targeting the interleukin (IL)-17 axis have been extensively studied, resulting in the approval of ustekinumab (which targets the common p40-subunit of IL-12 and IL-23) and secukinumab (targeting IL-17A). For ustekinumab, a recent Cochrane review suggested that the drug may be effective for induction of clinical improvement in CD [56]; phase III trials in patients with active CD reached its endpoints resulting in the recent FDA-approval of ustekinumab for treatment of CD [57]. However, like etanercept, secukinumab is an example of a biological drug with differential efficacy on skin and joint symptoms on one hand and inflammatory GI symptoms on the other. Whereas the drug has now been approved for treatment of psoriasis, PsA, and AS, a small pilot study exhibited unexpected results when CD patients were treated with this IL-17A blocker: not only was the drug ineffective, but higher rates of adverse events were noted compared with placebo, an effect that seemed to be driven by patients with elevated inflammatory markers [58].

Finally, there is now a new class of targeted synthetic DMARDs, of which apremilast, an oral phosphodiesterase-4 inhibitor, is the first to be approved for treatment of psoriasis and PsA. Clinical trials for the treatment of IBD have not been initiated, but preliminary evidence suggested reduced TNF and MMP-3 production by gut lamina propria mononuclear cells when exposed to apremilast, providing a mechanistic rationale for the evaluation of this drug as a novel oral therapy in the treatment of CD and UC [59].

Conclusion

Psoriasis is a common dermatological disorder that is often accompanied by an inflammatory arthritis that might affect peripheral joints, entheses as well as the spine and sacroiliac joints. As with other diseases belonging to the SpA-concept, there is an important role for the so-called concept-related extra-articular manifestations: in this chapter we discussed the important role of inflammatory ophthalmological and gastroenterological manifestations and their role in recognition and diagnosis, as well as the impact that these diseases might have on therapeutic decisions.

References

1. Peluso R, Iervolino S, Vitiello M, Bruner V, Lupoli G, Di Minno MND. Extra-articular manifestations in psoriatic arthritis patients. Clin Rheumatol 2015;34:745–53.
2. Wright V. Seronegative polyarthritis. A unified concept. Arthritis Rheum 1978;21:619–33.
3. Lambert JR, Wright V. Eye inflammation in psoriatic arthritis. Ann Rheum Dis 1976;35:354–6.
4. Kilic B, Dogan U, Parlak AH, et al. Ocular findings in patients with psoriasis. Int J Dermatol 2013;52:554–9.
5. Zeboulon N, Dougados M, Gossec L. Prevalence and characteristics of uveitis in the spondyloarthropathies: a systematic literature review. Ann Rheum Dis 2008;67(7):955–9.
6. Rosenbaum JT. Uveitis in spondyloarthritis including psoriatic arthritis, ankylosing spondylitis, and inflammatory bowel disease. Clin Rheumatol 2015;34:999–1002.
7. Paiva ES, Macaluso DC, Edwards A, Rosenbaum JT. Characterisation of uveitis in patients with psoriatic arthritis. Ann Rheum Dis 2000;59(1):67–70.
8. Lyons JL, Rosenbaum JT. Uveitis associated with inflammatory bowel disease compared with uveitis associated with spondyloarthropathy. Arch Ophthalmol 1997;115:61–4.
9. Durrani K, Foster CS. Psoriatic uveitis: a distinct clinical entity? Am J Ophthalmol 2005;139:106–11.
10. Queiro R, Torre JC, Belzunegui J, et al. Clinical features and predictive factors in psoriatic arthritis-related uveitis. Semin Arthritis Rheum 2002;31:264–70.
11. Tanaka R, Takamoto M, Komae K, Ohtomo K, Fujino Y, Kaburaki T. Clinical features of psoriatic uveitis in Japanese patients. Graefes Arch Clin Exp Ophthalmol 2015;253:1175–80.
12. Egeberg A, Khalid U, Gislason GH, Mallbris L, Skov L, Hansen PR. Association of psoriatic disease with uveitis: a Danish nationwide cohort study. JAMA Dermatol 2015;151:1200–5.
13. Haroon M, O'Rourke M, Ramasamy P, Murphy CC, FitzGerald O. A novel evidence-based detection of undiagnosed spondyloarthritis in patients presenting with acute anterior uveitis: the DUET (Dublin Uveitis Evaluation Tool). Ann Rheum Dis 2015;74:1990–5.
14. Perkins ES, MacFaul PA. Indomethacin in the treatment of uveitis: a double blind trial. Trans Ophthalmol Soc UK 1965;85:53–8.
15. March W, Coniglione TC. Ibuprofen in the treatment of uveitis. Ann Ophthalmol 1985;17:103–4.
16. Hunter PJ, Fowler PD, Wilkinson P. Treatment of anterior uveitis: comparison of oral oxyphenbutazone and topical steroids. Br J Ophthalmol 1973;57:892–6.
17. Olson NY, Lindsley CB, Godfrey WA. Non-steroidal anti-inflammatory drug therapy in chronic childhood iridocyclitis. Am J Dis Child 1988;142:1289–92.
18. Fiorelli VM, Bhat P, Foster CS. Nonsteroidal anti-inflammatory therapy and recurrent acute anterior uveitis. Ocul Immunol Inflamm 2010;18(2):116–20.
19. Munoz-Fernandez S, Hidalgo V, et al. Sulfasalazine reduces the number of flares of acute anterior uveitis over a one-year period. J Rheumatol. 2003;30:1277–9.
20. Benitez-del-Castillo JM, Garcia-Sanchez J, Iradier R, et al. Sulfasalazine in the prevention of anterior uveitis associated with ankylosing spondylitis. Eye 2000; 14:340–3.
21. Esterberg E, Acharya NR. Corticosteroid-sparing therapy: practice patterns among uveitis specialists. J Ophthalmic Inflamm Infect 2012;2:21–8.
22. El-Shabrawi Y, Hermann J. Anti-tumor necrosis factor-alpha therapy with infliximab as an alternative to corticosteroids in the treatment of human leukocyte antigen B27-associated acute anterior uveitis. Ophthalmology 2002;109:2342–6.
23. Braun J, Baraliakos X, Listing J, Sieper J. Decreased incidence of anterior uveitis in patients with ankylosing spondylitis treated with the anti-tumor necrosis factor agents infliximab and etanercept. Arthritis Rheum 2005;52:2447–51.
24. Guignard S, Gossec L, Salliot C, et al. Efficacy of tumour necrosis factor blockers in reducing uveitis flares in patients with spondylarthropathy: a retrospective study. Ann Rheum Dis 2006;65:1631–4.
25. Rosenbaum JT. Effect of etanercept on iritis in patients with ankylosing spondylitis. Arthritis Rheum 2004;50:3736–7.
26. Rudwaleit M, Rødevand E, Holck P, Vanhoof J, Kron M, Kary S, Kupper H. Adalimumab effectively reduces the rate of anterior uveitis flares in patients with active ankylosing spondylitis: results of a prospective open-label study. Ann Rheum Dis 2009;68:696–701.
27. Yates VM, Watkinson G, Kelman A. Further evidence for an association between psoriasis, Crohn's disease and ulcerative colitis. Br J Dermatol 1982;106:323–30.
28. Lee, FI, Bellary SV, Francis C. Increased occurrence of psoriasis in patients with Crohn's disease and their relatives. Am J Gastroenterol 1990;85:962–3.

29. Bernstein CN, Wajda A, Blanchard JF. The clustering of other chronic inflammatory diseases in inflammatory bowel disease: a population-based study. Gastroenterology 2005;129:827–36.

30. Williamson L, Dockerty JL, Dalbeth N, Wordsworth P. Gastrointestinal disease and psoriatic arthritis. J Rheumatol 2004;31(7):1469–70.

31. Li W, Han J, Chan AT, Qureshi AA. Psoriasis, psoriatic arthritis and increased risk of incident Crohn's disease in US women. Ann Rheum Dis 2013;72:1200–5.

32. Binus AM, Han J, Qamar AA, Mody EA, Holt EW, Qureshi AA. Associated comorbidities in psoriasis and inflammatory bowel disease. J Eur Acad Dermatol Venereol 2012;26:644–50.

33. Mielants H, Veys EM, Cuvelier C, et al. The evolution of spondyloarthropathies in relation to gut histology. II. Histological aspects. J Rheumatol 1995;22:2273–8.

34. Van Praet L, Van den Bosch F, Jacques P, et al. Microscopic gut inflammation in axial spondyloarthritis: a multiparametric predictive model. Ann Rheum Dis 2013;72:414–7.

35. Van Praet L, Jans L, Carron P, et al. Degree of bone marrow oedema in sacroiliac joints of patients with axial spondyloarthritis is linked to gut inflammation an male sex: results from the GIANT cohort. Ann Rheum Dis 2014;73:1186–9.

36. Schatteman L, Mielants H, Veys EM, et al. Gut inflammation in psoriatic arthritis: a prospective ileocolonoscopic study. J Rheumatol 1995;22:680–3.

37. Scarpa R, Manguso F, D'Arienzo A, et al. Microscopic inflammatory changes in colon of patients with both active psoriasis and psoriatic arthritis without bowel symptoms. J Rheumatol 2000;27:1241–6.

38. Taurog JD, Richardson JA, Croft JT, et al. The germfree state prevents development of gut and joint inflammatory disease in HLA-B27 transgenic rats. J Exp Med 1994;180:2359–64.

39. Scher JU, Ubeda C, Artacho A, et al. Decreased bacterial diversity characterizes the altered gut microbiota in patients with psoriatic arthritis, resembling dysbiosis in inflammatory bowel disease. Arthritis Rheum 2015;67:128–39.

40. Manichanh C, Rigottier-Gois L, Bonnaud E, et al. Reduced diversity of faeca microbiota in Crohn's disease revealed by a metagenomic approach. Gut 2006;55:205–11.

41. Gossec L, Smolen JS, Ramiro S, et al. European League Against Rheumatism (EULAR) recommendations for the management of psoriatic arthritis with pharmacological therapies: 2015 update. Ann Rheum Dis 2016;75:499–510.

42. Sandborn WJ, Stenson WF, Brynskov J, et al. Safety of celecoxib in patients with ulcerative colitis in remission: a randomized, placebo-controlled, pilot study. Clin Gastroenterol Hepatol 2006;4:203–11.

43. El Miedany Y, Youssef S, Ahmed I, El Gaafary M. The gastrointestinal safety and effect on disease activity of etoricoxib, a selective cox-2 inhibitor in inflammatory bowel diseases. Am J Gastroenterol 2006;101:311–7.

44. Kirwan JR, Hällgren R, Mielants H, et al. A randomised placebo controlled 12 week trial of budesonide and prednisolone in rheumatoid arthritis. Ann Rheum Dis 2004;63:688–95.

45. Lee JCT, Gladman DD, Schentag CT, Cook RJ. The long-term use of azathioprine in patients with psoriatic arthritis. J Clin Rheumatol 2001;7:160–5.

46. McDonald JW, Wang Y, Tsoulis DJ, et al. Methotrexate for induction of remission in refractory Crohn's disease. Cochrane Database Syst Rev 2014 Aug 6;8:CD003459.

47. Patel V, Wang Y, MacDonald JK, McDonald JW, Chande N. Methotrexate for maintenance of remission in Crohn's disease. Cochrane Database Syst Rev 2014 Aug 26;8:CD006884.

48. Chande N, Wang Y, MacDonald JK, McDonald JW. Methotrexate for induction of remission in ulcerative colitis. Cochrane Database Syst Rev 2014 Aug 27;8:CD006618.

49. Carbonnel F, Colombel JF, Filippi J, et al. Methotrexate is not superior to placebo for inducing steroid-free remission, but induces steroid-free clinical remission in a larger proportion of patients with ulcerative colitis. Gastroenterology 2016;150:380–8.

50. Prajapati DN, Knox JF, Emmons J, Saeian K, Csuka ME, Binion DG. Leflunomide treatment of Crohn's disease patients intolerant to standard immunomodulator therapy. J Clin Gastroenterol 2003;37:125–8.

51. Holtmann MH, Gerts A, Weinman A, Galle PR, Neurath MF. Treatment of Crohn's disease with leflunomide as second-line immunosuppression. Dig Dis Sci 2008;53:1025 32.

52. Van den Bosch F, Kruithof E, De Vos M, De Keyser F, Mielants H. Crohn's disease associated with spondyloarthropathy: effect of TNF-alpha blockade with infliximab on articular symptoms. Lancet 2000;356:1821–2.

53. Sandborn WJ, Hanauer SB, Katz S, et al. Etanercept for active Crohn's disease: a randomized, double-blind, placebo-controlled trial. Gastroenterology 2001;122:1088–94.

54. Chandar AK, Singh S, Murad MH, Peyrin-Biroulet L, Loftus EV. Efficacy and safety of natalizumab and vedolizumab for the management of Crohn's disease: a systematic review and meta-analysis. Inflamm Bowel Dis 2015;21:1695–708.

55. Varkas G, Thevissen K, De Brabanter G, et al. An induction or flare of arthritis and/or sacroiliitis by vedolizumab in inflammatory bowel disease: a case series. Ann Rheum Dis 2017;76:878–81.

56. Khanna R, Preiss JC, MacDonald JK, Timmer A. Anti-IL-12/23p40 antibodies for induction of remission in Crohn's disease. Cochrane Database Syst Rev 2015;5: CD007572. DOI: 10.1002/14651858. CD007572.pub2.

57. Feagan BG, Sandborn WJ, Gasink C, et al. Ustekinumab as induction and maintenance therapy for Crohn's disease. N Engl J Med 2016;375:1946–60.

58. Hueber W, Sands BE, Lewitzky S, et al. Secukinumab, a human anti-IL-17A monoclonal antibody, for moderate to severe Crohn's disease: unexpected results of a randomised, double-blind placebo-controlled trial. Gut 2012;61:1693–700.

59. Gordon JN, Prothero JD, Thornton CA, et al. CC-10004 but not thalidomide or lenalidomide inhibits lamina propria mononuclear cell TNF-alpha and MMP-3 production in patients with inflammatory bowel disease. J Crohn's Colitis 2009;3:175–82.

CHAPTER 15

Co-morbidities

Muhammad Haroon

Introduction

Psoriatic arthritis (PsA) is a chronic immune-mediated inflammatory disease which affects peripheral joints, entheses, and axial sites in addition to both skin and nails. There is considerable evidence to support the assertion that PsA is actually a multisystem disease. In addition to the characteristic extra-articular features, such as uveitis and inflammatory bowel disease, patients with PsA may also suffer from conditions which do not belong to the concept of PsA or spondyloarthritis (SpA) but are related to the consequences of the disease or its treatment. Such co-existing diseases are referred to as comorbidities. Examples of comorbidities in PsA are hypertension, hypercholesterolaemia, diabetes mellitus, obesity, depression, and malignancy. The presence of both extra-articular manifestations and comorbidities may have consequences for the treatment, prognosis, and outcome of the disease, which frequently go unrecognized or undertreated, causing a significant clinical burden for patients and an economic burden for the healthcare system.

Cardiovascular diseases

There has been a growing interest in the identification of cardiovascular disease risks in psoriasis and PsA, with much of the initial data and pathogenic hypotheses extrapolated from the rheumatoid arthritis (RA) literature. There is considerable evidence from large observational cohorts, both retrospective and prospective, and also studies using different imaging techniques, which demonstrate that both psoriasis and PsA are associated with heightened cardiovascular risk [1–7].

Conventional cardiovascular diseases

Similar to patients with psoriasis, PsA patients have an increased prevalence of conventional cardiovascular risk factors compared to the normal population. Interestingly, PsA patients may also have increased risk from non-conventional risk factors such as raised levels of homocysteine, increased burden of inflammation, and excessive alcohol consumption [8].

Hypertension

The prevalence of hypertension has been reported to be higher in patients with PsA compared to that in the general population [3, 9–13] and also in comparison to those patients with psoriasis only [14]. In a recent study, Haroon et al. have shown in a cross-sectional assessment of 283 PsA patients that 74% of them had elevated blood pressure [15]. In another recent study, it was shown that 55% of 158 PsA patients had arterial hypertension, and this was significantly associated with the presence of cardiovascular disease (defined on the basis of the occurrence of coronary artery disease or cerebrovascular ischaemic disease events) with an odds ratio of 21.0 [16]. Not surprisingly, the presence of hypertension was also found to be independently associated with subclinical left ventricular dysfunction in patients with PsA [17].

Hypercholesterolaemia

Hypercholesterolemia is an established important risk factor for cardiovascular disease. Interestingly, hypercholesterolaemia, through the involvement of the immune system, can induce inflammation in each segment of microvasculature, and it also promotes a pro-inflammatory phenotype in large vessels [18]. One of the early immune cell types activated by hypercholesterolaemia [19] is the T-lymphocyte, which has been proposed as having an important role in PsA pathogenesis [20].

There have been some controversies regarding the prevalence of lipid profile abnormalities among PsA patients. For example, the prevalence of hyperlipidaemia was found to be higher in patients with PsA in comparison to the general population [7] and to healthy controls [3]. Another study showed however that the prevalence of hypertriglyceridaemia or hypercholesterolaemia was not increased in PsA [13]. Similarly, significantly reduced high-density lipoprotein (HDL) levels have been reported among PsA patients, and notably significantly lower total cholesterol and high-density lipoprotein cholesterol among patients with active synovitis [21, 22]; however, higher HDL cholesterol levels have also been reported in patients with PsA [13].

A recent important study has evaluated whether a history of hypercholesterolaemia is associated with the risk of developing psoriasis and PsA in a cohort of 95,540 US women. The fully adjusted hazard ratios (HRs) of incident psoriasis and PsA associated with hypercholesterolaemia were 1.25 (95% CI 1.04–1.50) and 1.58 (95% CI 1.13–2.23), respectively. Participants with hypercholesterolaemia duration time ≥ 7 years were at a higher risk of developing psoriasis (fully adjusted HR=1.29, 95% CI1.03–1.61) (Ptrend=0.0002) and PsA (fully adjusted HR=1.68, 95% CI 1.12–2.52) (Ptrend=0.002). Importantly, this association was noted to be independent of cholesterol-lowering medication use. The authors conclude that hypercholesterolaemia, as a well-known risk factor of cardiovascular disease, may also increase the risk of incident psoriasis/PsA [23].

Diabetes

The reported association of psoriatic disease with diabetes mellitus dates back to 1966, when it was noted that psoriasis patients are at increased risk of developing this condition [24]. A recent meta-analysis which included 557,697 patients with psoriasis and

5,186,485 controls has shown that the pooled odds ratio (OR) for the association between psoriasis and the risk of type-2 diabetes mellitus was 1.76, 95% CI 1.59–1.96. It was also noted that there was a dose effect of psoriasis on diabetes risk among patients with severe psoriasis compared to pooled OR (OR 2·10, 95% CI 1·73–2·55, vs 1·76, 95% CI 1·59–1·96) (pooled OR is the combined data on OR from multiple studies). Importantly, it was observed that the risk of diabetes mellitus was highest among PsA patients compared to pooled OR (OR 2·18, 95% CI 1·36–3·50 vs. OR 1·76, 95% CI 1·59–1·96) [25]. Similarly, another population-based cross-sectional study used logistic multivariate models and found a possible association between PsA and diabetes in women. This led to the authors to conclude that women with PsA might be candidates for regular diabetes screening [26].

One plausible explanation is that patients with psoriasis have high visceral fat and non-alcoholic fatty liver both of which are associated with insulin resistance. Moreover, psoriasis and PsA are inflammatory diseases and there is increasing acceptance of inflammation-induced insulin resistance [27]. It has been postulated that insulin resistance (IR) possibly explains the increased cardiovascular co-morbidity associated with systemic inflammatory conditions, such as psoriasis and other immune-mediated inflammatory diseases [28]. IR in turn causes endothelial cell dysfunction, subsequently leading to atherosclerosis and finally to end-organ damage with stroke or myocardial infarction.

There is paucity of data regarding the effect of drugs or adequate disease control on the risk of developing diabetes among patients with PsA. It has been postulated that the drugs used to treat immune-mediated diseases, such as psoriasis or RA, by suppressing the immune system may also reduce the risk of developing diabetes. Interestingly, a retrospective cohort study of 121,280 patients with a diagnosis of either RA or psoriasis has found that the use of a TNF inhibitor or hydroxychloroquine, but not methotrexate, is associated with a reduced risk of diabetes mellitus compared with other non-biologic disease-modifying antirheumatic drugs (DMARDs) [29]. This study shows only an association and does not establish any cause and effect relationship. Further studies are needed to confirm these findings.

Metabolic syndrome

Metabolic syndrome (MetS) is a cluster of five classic cardiovascular risk factors. Under current guidelines, revised in 2005 by the National Heart, Lung, and Blood Institute (NHLBI) and the American Heart Association (AHA), MetS is diagnosed when a patient has at least three of the following five conditions: fasting glucose ≥100 mg/dL, or receiving drug therapy for hyperglycemia; blood pressure ≥130/85 mm Hg, or receiving drug therapy for hypertension; triglycerides ≥150 mg/dL, or receiving drug therapy for hypertriglyceridaemia; HDL-C < 40 mg/dL in men or < 50 mg/dL in women, or receiving drug therapy for reduced HDL-C; and for Caucasians the waist circumference ≥40 inches (≥102 centimetres) in men or ≥ 35 inches (≥88 centimetres) in women [30]. Recent studies have estimated that the prevalence of MetS in the Western population is 15–24% [31, 32]. MetS is a well-recognized risk factor for coronary artery disease, and as a group, may confer a cardiovascular risk higher than the individual components. It has been shown that men with MetS are almost three times more likely to die of coronary artery disease after adjustment for conventional cardiovascular risk factors [32]. Interestingly, it has been shown

that MetS is associated with a state of chronic, low-grade inflammation [33, 34].

There are established links between psoriasis and MetS [35], and it has been even suggested that patients with severe psoriasis in particular, should be screened for metabolic disorders and cardiovascular risk factors. Haroon et al. have recently examined in detail the prevalence and its clinical correlations of MetS and IR among patients with PsA. They found that 44% (111 out of 283) and 16% (41 out of 263) of consecutive PsA patients attending rheumatology clinics had MetS and IR, respectively [15]. These results are in agreement with the published literature of relatively small studies reporting a prevalence of MetS in PsA of 27–58% [36–39]. Haroon et al. have since recruited an age, gender, and race/ethnicity matched control group attending rheumatology clinics with non-inflammatory rheumatologic conditions. Their objective was to compare the prevalence of MetS in this control group (100 patients) with their earlier published cohort of patients with PsA (283 patients) to further test the inflammation–cardiovascular disease hypothesis. This is unpublished data as of yet. They found that the prevalence of MetS is much higher in patients with PsA compared to a well matched control group (44% vs 29%, P=0.009). Among the components of MetS, increased waist circumference and hypertension were statistically more common among patients with PsA (submitted for publication). Moreover, in a recent small study of 91 patients (40 patients with PsA and 51 patients with RA), significantly higher prevalence of the MetS in patients with PsA was noted compared to patients with RA (67.5% vs. 37.2%). The psoriatic patients had a higher prevalence of impaired fasting glucose (52.5% vs 27.4%, P=0.018), and elevated triglyceride values as compared to those presenting with RA (25% vs 11% P=0.0004) [40].

Cardiovascular morbidity

There are limited data regarding cardiovascular morbidity in patients with PsA [9–12, 14], but recent important studies have examined this aspect in greater detail, especially by comparing with different population groups.

Compared to general population

A cross-sectional cohort study has examined the prevalence of cardiovascular disease (CVD) in 3,066 patients with PsA compared to 12,264 healthy controls [11]. Significantly higher age and sex adjusted prevalence of chronic heart failure, ischaemic heart disease, peripheral vascular disease, CVD, type II diabetes, hyperlipidaemia, and hypertension was found when compared to healthy controls. A recent meta-analysis has also concluded that despite heterogeneity among studies, PsA appears significantly associated with markers of subclinical atherosclerosis and CV risk [41].

Compared to patients with psoriasis

The prevalence of cardiovascular morbidities has been compared between 611 patients with PsA and 449 patients with psoriasis only, in a cross-sectional study [14]. Significantly increased prevalence of the following CVDs has been noted among patients with PsA compared to those with psoriasis: hypertension (37.1% vs 19.6%), obesity (30% vs 26.5%), hyperlipidaemia (20.7% vs 14.5%), type 2 diabetes mellitus (12% vs 6.7%), and at least one cardiovascular event (8.2% vs 3.3%, including angina, myocardial infarction, cardiomyopathy, congestive heart failure, and cerebrovascular accident).

Compared to patients with RA and ankylosing spondylitis

In a cross-sectional study of 489 patients with PsA and 353 patients with RA, it has been shown that the age- and sex-adjusted OR of CVD (including myocardial infarction, stroke, and/or transient ischaemic attack) in PsA (10%) was noted to resemble that in RA (12%) [44]. In a recently published 10-year prospective study [CARdiovascular in rheumatology (CARMA) project], it was noted that PsA patients had more commonly classic CV risk factors and MetS features than did the patients with RA and AS [43].

Cardiovascular risk profile and disease duration

Generally it is considered that cardiovascular risks are linked with longer disease duration. However, a recent population-based study has investigated the cardiovascular risk profile at the onset of PsA. It was noted that the majority of newly diagnosed PsA patients have a >10% risk of CVD within 10 years of PsA onset, which is higher than expected and was found to be underestimated by the Framingham Risk Score [44]. Another study has also shown that among patients with early PsA (disease duration of <2 years), the prevalence of comorbidities (hypercholesterolaemia, obesity, hypertension, diabetes mellitus, anxiety/depression, and coronary heart disease was 61.6, 59.7, 32.7, 13.8, 13.8, and 8.7%, respectively) was not only high, but was also comparable to those with established PsA [10].

Cardiovascular outcomes and the effect of treatments

There has been no study to date which has specifically assessed the cardiovascular risk related to nonsteroidal anti-inflammatory drugs (NSAIDs) in patients with PsA. However, there is a large body of evidence showing that NSAIDs (both 'traditional', such as diclofenac or ibuprofen, and selective cyclooxygenase inhibitors, COX-2) are associated with a significant increased risk of cardiovascular events, both fatal and nonfatal. Clearly, the choice of using NSAIDs and its class, traditional or coxibs, should be based on individual patient risk factors.

There is evidence that the use of DMARDs, including methotrexate, sulphasalazine, and leflunomide, was not associated with abnormal carotid intimal medial thickness [45]. Although, there is some data on the cardioprotective effect of methotrexate in rheumatoid arthritis [46, 47], the effect of methotrexate on psoriasis and PsA patients with regards to cardiovascular outcomes is inconclusive at present [48].

It has been found that the use of a TNF inhibitor (TNFi) or hydroxychloroquine but not methotrexate is associated with a reduced risk of diabetes mellitus compared with other non-biologic DMARDs [29]. The CaRRDs study group has interestingly shown in a cross-sectional assessment that among PsA individuals, the C-IMT (carotid intimal medial thickness) was higher in subjects on DMARDs than in those on TNFi. This effect of TNFi was related to treatment duration, which inversely (β=-0.317, P<0.0001) predicted C-IMT in PsA subjects on TNFi but not in those on DMARDs (P=0.313) [41]. In a 2-year prospective study, Tam et al. have shown that TNFi are associated with significant reduction in carotid IMT and further regression of the maximum IMT was possible only in patients who were continued on long-term TNFi therapy [49]. These results are consistent with the concept that reduction of systemic inflammation may hamper the cascade that leads to enhanced vascular risk in immune-mediated disease. For example, in ankylosing spondylitis, a recent study has shown that among frequent COX II users, the risks for all types of CVDs were ten times lower than non-users at 24 months (OR, 0.08; 95% CI 0.01–0.92). The authors conclude that long-term frequent use of NSAIDs might protect AS patients from CVDs; however, NSAIDs still carried higher short-term risk in the non-frequent users [50]. Endothelial dysfunction, which is considered an early feature in atherogenesis, has been consistently associated with cardiovascular risk [51] and TNFi has been shown to modify the endothelial function [52].

A recent systematic review has investigated the effects of biologic agents and other DMARDs on cardiovascular outcomes in PsA. Preliminary evidence suggest that the use of TNFi may be associated with reduced risk of adverse cardiovascular events; however, epidemiological data is insufficient to reach definitive conclusions with regards to the effects of biologics and other DMARDs on cardiovascular outcomes in patients with PsA [53]. Another recent systematic review and meta-analysis has shown that among patients with psoriasis/PsA, biologics and other DMARDs may be associated with a decreased risk of cardiovascular events, but also acknowledged that evidence is less conclusive than in RA and that further studies are needed [53].

Since CVDs are the top leading cause of mortality in PsA patients, regular screening and vigorous control of these metabolic and cardiovascular risk factors cannot be over-emphasized.

Obesity

Obesity affects 35% of adults in United States [54, 55]. There are various ways to measure different aspects of obesity including body mass index (BMI), skin fold thickness, waist circumference, and waist to hip ratio. BMI provides an easy way to measure obesity and is calculated as weight in kilograms divided by height in meters squared. BMI between 25 and 29.99 indicates patients are overweight, BMI≥30 indicates obesity, and BMI ≥ 40 shows severe obesity. A recent study provides US national estimates of childhood obesity and analyses trends in childhood obesity between 2003 and 2012, along with the detailed obesity trend analyses among adults. It was noted that the adult obesity rates remained high overall, but childhood obesity has more than doubled in children and quadrupled in adolescents in the past 30 years [55, 56].

Adipose tissue is now increasingly considered a pro-inflammatory state since adipose tissue has been found to secrete more than 50 cytokines and other molecules that play an important role in the inflammatory cascade and are known as adipokines. These adipokines include adiponectin, leptin, plasminogen activator inhibitor-1 (PAI-1), IL-6, and TNF-a [57]. Adipokines engage, through endocrine, paracrine, autocrine, or juxtacrine mechanisms of action, in a wide variety of physiological or pathological processes, including immunity and inflammation [58].

Leptin is mainly produced by adipocytes, and circulating leptin levels directly correlate with adipose tissue mass [59]. Apart from its known effects of causing reduction of food intake and increased energy consumption through a number of complicating pathways, it is remarkable to note the pro-inflammatory effects of leptin on immune system. It has been shown that a number of common inflammatory signals, for example, IL-1, IL-6, and lipopolysaccharide, increase circulating leptin levels [60]. Interestingly, in an animal model, mouse deficient in leptin were less likely to develop autoimmune diseases [58] and less severe arthritis [61].

Adiponectin is another important molecule, which has anti-inflammatory properties and has been shown to have protective role against obesity-related metabolic disease and CVDs. In obese patients, its levels inversely correlates with the inflammatory marker C-reactive protein. Moreover, typical inflammatory cytokines, IL-6 and TNF-α, may reduce adiponectin production, which in turn can contribute to insulin resistance. Similarly, IL-6 and TNF, which have well proven pro-inflammatory properties, are also produced by adipose tissue [62].

Obesity in patients with PsA increases the burden of inflammation, but it is also an established significant risk factor for the development of skin psoriasis. A number of case-controlled studies have shown that patients with skin psoriasis have higher prevalence of overweight and obesity than the general population, and the ORs for this association have been reported to range from 1.6–2.05 [63–66]. Not only is psoriasis prevalence is higher among obese patients, but also such patients are more likely to have more severe skin disease [67–68]. This makes the potential link between obesity and PsA even complex given a high prevalence of PsA among psoriasis patients, and there are inherent difficulties to examine whether obesity is simply a comorbid condition of psoriasis/PsA or a real factor for the development of PsA. A case series of 943 psoriasis patients has revealed that people who are obese by the age of 18 or earlier are more likely to develop PsA as compared to those with a normal weight, and is independent of other risk factors. Each unit increase in BMI at 18 years of age was associated with a 5.3% increase in the risk of PsA [69]. Although, there were important limitations to this study, two other large prospective studies published in 2012 concluded with the similar findings of the dose-dependent link of obesity with the diagnosis of PsA even in different population settings [70, 71].

Interventional studies are required to confirm whether preventing or treating obesity may serve as a preventive and/or concomitant therapeutic measure for PsA. Interestingly, a study of Di Minno et al. has shown that losing 5–10% of total body weight is associated with a higher achievement of minimal disease activity in people taking TNFi in patients with PsA (OR=3.75, 95% CI 1.36–10.36, P=0.011). Furthermore, those who lost more weight (>10%) had even better achievement of minimal disease activity (OR=6.67, 95% CI 2.41–18.41, P<0.001) [72].

Given obesity is a modifiable risk factor, it provides a unique opportunity to reduce the occurrence of this potentially destructive PsA by simply reducing the body weight.

Depression

Depression is quite common in patients with chronic pain. A number of studies have shown a higher prevalence of behavioural disorders among patients with psoriasis [73, 74], and, not surprisingly, the same has been the case in patients with PsA. Furthermore, a recent study has shown that patients with PsA are twice as likely to be depressed as those with psoriasis alone. This study included 306 patients with PsA and 135 people with psoriasis. The depression and anxiety was studied using the Hospital Anxiety and Depression Scale (HADS). More than a third of PsA patients (36.6%) reported anxiety, compared to just a quarter (24.4%) of patients with psoriasis alone. However, the presence of depression in PsA patients was more than twice as high compared to patients without joint involvement (22.2% vs 9.6%). In this study, neither the use of DMARDs nor NSAIDs had any significant effect on the mood disorders; however, depression and anxiety were related to unemployment, and were more common among those with greater disability, pain, and fatigue [75]. Another recent study has shown that the prevalence of moderate to severe levels of depressive symptoms as measured by Patient Health Questionnaire 9 (PHQ-9 score >10) was 21.7% in PsA patients, 25.1% in RA patients, and 36.7% in those PsA patients with polyarthritis. Interestingly, it was noted that after adjustment for severity of disease and pain, the factors that correlated independently with physical health related quality of life (HRQoL) in PsA were anxiety (ß=-0.28) and concern about bodily symptoms attributed to the illness (ß=-0.33) [76]. A large epidemiological, cross-sectional, multi-centre Spanish study (including 495 patients with PsA) has shown that when defining anxiety or depression as the presence of the disorder according to a score ≥11 points on the HADS or as receiving prescription drug treatment for such disorders, the prevalence of anxiety was estimated to be 29.7% (95% CI 25.7% to 33.7%) and the prevalence of depression was 17.6% (95% CI 14.2% to 21.0%). It is interesting to note that among the individuals receiving biological treatment, in monotherapy or in combination with DMARDs, a lower prevalence of anxious symptomatology is seen vs patients being treated with other drugs or combinations (P<0.05) [77]. The prevalence of behavioural disorders is comparable to that found in other rheumatic diseases. For example, there is 25% prevalence of depression among patients with RA [76], 19% prevalence of depression in systemic sclerosis [78], and 17–22% in lupus [79, 80].

It seems that cross talk between the immune system and the central nervous system occurs with resultant neuropsychiatric symptoms, such as depression and anxiety in patients with chronic inflammatory diseases, such as PsA. Interestingly, a recent study has investigated the molecular mechanisms by which inflammation originating in the periphery can induce transcriptional modulation in the brain leading to neuropsychiatric symptoms, such as depression and anxiety. This study showed the increased transcription of a range of interferon-stimulated genes in the brain as a consequence of peripheral toll-like-receptor-induced inflammation. Since type I interferons are linked to psychiatric disorders, this interferon production in the brain could represent an important mechanism linking peripheral inflammation with behavioural changes [81].

Autoimmune ophthalmic disease

Autoimmune ophthalmic disease has been shown to have a significant prevalence of up to 25% in PsA patients. Such occular manifestations include uveitis, keratitis, blepharitis, conjunctivitis, episcleritis, and scleritis, but uveitis appears to have the strongest association [82]. Uveitis affects approximately 7% of patients with PsA [83, 84]. There is some data to suggest that the presence of PsA in patients with psoriasis increases their risk of having uveitis [85, 86] Uveitis associated with PsA is usually atypical in that it follows a more insidious course, more likely to be continuous, bilateral, and to be situated behind the crystalline lens compared to cases of uveitis among ankylosing spondylitis patients [87]. It has also been shown that axial disease affects about one fifth of patients with PsA but has been found to account for 50% of the patients with PsA and uveitis [88].

A need for a close collaboration between rheumatologists and ophthalmologists is certainly recommended. A novel evidence-based algorithm called DUET (Dublin Uveitis Evaluation Tool) has been recently proposed to guide ophthalmologists to refer appropriate anterior uveitis patients to rheumatology [89] that will aid the early detection of undiagnosed SpA (including PsA) in patients presenting with anterior uveitis. In this large 2 phase study, approximately 40% of patients presenting with idiopathic anterior uveitis were noted to have undiagnosed SpA, and DUET algorithm was noted to have excellent sensitivity (96%) and specificity (97%). It has a positive likelihood ratio (LR) 41.5 and negative LR 0.03 [89].

Malignancy

Psoriasis is well known to predispose patients to malignancy and studies have so far found increased rates of skin cancers, especially non-melanoma, lung cancer [90], and haematologic malignancy [91]. Rates of malignancy among patients with RA are higher than the general population, and it is not yet clear whether this malignancy risk seen in RA and psoriasis is applicable to PsA. In PsA, it has been reported that 10% of patients developed malignancy during a prospective follow up from 1978 to 2004, and this incidence of malignancy in the large PsA cohort did not differ from that in the general population [92]. Similarly, another recent study has shown that in PsA, the overall cancer risk was not significantly increased in comparison to the general population, whereas the risk of haematologic malignancies appeared significantly higher in RA patients (SIR 4.94, 95% CI 1.35–12.64), particularly in females [93]. However, when the data from Consortium of Rheumatology Researchers of North America (CORRONA) registry was studied to compare the incidence rates of malignancy in PsA and RA, it was found that the overall malignancy incidence per 100 patient-years was similar, which indirectly suggests higher risk of malignancy among patients with PsA compared to the general population [94]. Importantly, this study also showed no association between TNFi exposure and cancer in this cohort of patients with inflammatory arthropathies. Clearly, more data is needed to understand this association better, with to date a paucity of studies evaluating the malignancy risk among patients with PsA.

Inflammatory bowel disease

A possible overlap in pathogenic mechanisms has been suggested since common genetic associations between psoriasis, Crohn's disease (CD), and ulcerative colitis (UC) [95] have been found. It is common that patients with inflammatory bowel disease (IBD) have extra intestinal manifestations, such as psoriasis, but the risk of subsequent development of psoriasis among patients with IBD remains less clear and the nature of such association is debatable. Lee et al. in 1990 reported an incidence of psoriasis in patients with CD of 9.6%, while in the control group it was only 2.2% (P<0.02). The incidence of psoriasis in the relatives of patients with CD was 10%, compared to 2.9% in the control group (P<0.02) [96]. The question as to whether individuals with established psoriasis and PsA have an increased risk of subsequently developing CD or UC was addressed in a prospective study of 174,476 women in the United States. It was found that women with psoriasis, particularly with concomitant PsA, had a significantly increased risk of developing CD, but there was no significant increased risk of UC development associated with psoriasis [97].

Burden of inflammation and co-morbidities

In PsA, skin and musculoskeletal inflammation coexist. It has been hypothesized therefore, that there might be a greater burden of co morbidities in PsA compared to psoriasis only, such as MetS and IR, and consequently of CVD due to a greater inflammatory load [15]. Haroon et al. have shown that severity of PsA is significantly linked to the presence of MetS not only on univariate analysis but also after adjusting for IR, severity of skin psoriasis, and the usual confounders. Severe PsA was defined as having both of the following features present: a) the presence of one or more of the PsA-related radiographic damage features (peripheral joint erosions, osteolysis, sacroiliitis); and b) PsA requiring TNFi therapy [15].

Similarly, another study has shown that the increased burden of inflammation over time is associated with the extent of atherosclerotic plaques in patients with PsA. The cumulative effect of inflammation was measured by a time-adjusted arithmetic mean of all measurements from the first visit to the clinic, which included: Psoriasis Activity and Severity Index (PASI), erythrocyte sedimentation rate (ESR), white blood cell, tender and swollen joint counts, C-reactive protein, PsA Disease Activity Score (PASDAS), and Disease Activity for PsA (DAPSA). However, these associations were not significant after adjustment for traditional cardiovascular risk factors, which suggests that this association may be mediated by the traditional risk factors [98]. In another study, the cumulative inflammatory burden, as reflected by cumulative averages of repeated measures of ESR (ca-ESR), was associated with increased arterial stiffness in PsA patients even after adjustment for cardiovascular risk factors, emphasizing the important role of chronic inflammation in accelerating the development of cardiovascular risks in PsA patients [99] Moreover, Lin at al. have shown that incremental increases in inflammatory pathways in PsA may contribute to a higher cardiovascular risk as compared to patients with psoriasis only. PsA patients with MetS had the greatest carotid intimal medial thickness measurements compared to PsA patients without MetS and psoriasis patients with or without MetS [100].

Screening and treating co-morbidities

The comorbidities associated with PsA have been under-appreciated and under-reported. The Group for Research and Assessment of Psoriasis and Psoriatic Arthritis (GRAPPA) has recently published guidelines to raise the awareness about the need to screen patients with PsA for conditions that often accompany this disease [101]. It was found that the CVD is top of the list of comorbidities, and the guidelines recommend that all PsA patients should be screened for it. Since a likely link has been established with PsA/psoriasis, the guidelines also recommend screening for IBD, obesity, diabetes, and ophthalmic conditions, such as uveitis. Although they do not recommend any particular treatment, the treatment guidelines do include information on what medications to use for various comorbidities. The patient's and treating physician's awareness of these comorbidities remains critical not only for its early detection but also to improve the overall outlook of the patients with PsA.

The impact of comorbidities

The impact of comorbidity on different aspects of patient's life and disease course has been discussed above. Comorbidities tend to increase with age and in psoriasis patients, it has been shown that nearly half of patients aged over 65 years have at least three comorbidities and worryingly, two thirds of patients have two or more comorbidities [102]. In PsA, the prevalence of comorbidity is even higher with 42% of patients having three or more comorbid conditions in a study involving 631 patients [103]. As the number of comorbidities increases, so does the healthcare utilization and healthcare costs. In PsA, the incremental effects of comorbidity on quality of life have been studied. It was found that the added effect of comorbidity on patient-reported physical and mental health in PsA was more related to type of comorbidity than number of comorbidities [104].

Conclusions

PsA is a multisystem chronic inflammatory condition, and the patients are at a higher risk for a number of major systemic comorbidities contributing further to significant adverse outcomes. It is important to conduct periodic comprehensive assessments to identify and monitor the comorbidities of PsA. The importance of close, multispecialty cooperation, and multidisciplinary assessments cannot be overstated.

References

1. Ahlehoff O, Gislason GH, Charlot M, et al. Psoriasis is associated with clinically significant cardiovascular risk: a Danish nationwide cohort study. J Intern Med 2011;270:147–57.
2. Ludwig RJ, Herzog C, Rostock A, et al. Psoriasis: a possible risk factor for development of coronary artery calcification. Br J Dermatol 2007;156:271–6.
3. Kimhi O, Caspi D, Bornstein NM, et al. Prevalence and risk factors of atherosclerosis in patients with psoriatic arthritis. Semin Arthritis Rheum 2007;36:203–9.
4. Soltani-Arabshahi R, Wong B, Feng BJ, Goldgar DE, Duffin KC, Krueger GG. Obesity in early adulthood as a risk factor for psoriatic arthritis. Arch Dermatol 2010;146:721–6.
5. Setty AR, Curhan G, Choi HK. Obesity, waist circumference, weight change, and the risk of psoriasis in women: Nurses' Health Study II. Arch Intern Med 2007;167:1670–5.
6. Prey S, Paul C, Bronsard V, Puzenat E, Gourraud PA, Aractingi S. Cardiovascular risk factors in patients with plaque psoriasis: a systematic review of epidemiological studies. J Eur Acad Dermatol Venereol 2010;24 Suppl 2:23–30.
7. Han C, Robinson DW Jr, Hackett MV, Paramore LC, Fraeman KH, Bala MV. Cardiovascular disease and risk factors in patients with rheumatoid arthritis, psoriatic arthritis, and ankylosing spondylitis. J Rheumatol 2006;33:2167–72.
8. Zhu TY, Li EK, Tam LS. Cardiovascular risk in patients with psoriatic arthritis. Int J Rheumatol. 2012;2012:714321.
9. Kondratiouk S, Udaltsova N, Klatsky AL. Associations of psoriatic arthritis and cardiovascular conditions in a large population. Perm J. 2008;12(4):4–8.
10. Khraishi M, MacDonald D, Rampakakis E, Vaillancourt J, Sampalis JS. Prevalence of patient-reported comorbidities in early and established psoriatic arthritis cohorts. Clin Rheumatol. 2011;30(7):877–85.
11. Han C, Robinson DW Jr, Hackett MV, Paramore LC, Fraeman KH, Bala MV. Cardiovascular disease and risk factors in patients with rheumatoid arthritis, psoriatic arthritis, and ankylosing spondylitis. J Rheumatol. 2006;33(11):2167–72.
12. Gladman DD, Ang M, Su L, Tom BD, Schentag CT, Farewell VT. Cardiovascular morbidity in psoriatic arthritis. Ann Rheum Dis. 2009;68(7):1131–5.
13. Tam LS, Tomlinson B, Chu TT, et al. Cardiovascular risk profile of patients with psoriatic arthritis compared to controls —the role of inflammation. Rheumatology 2008;47:718–23.
14. Husted JA, Thavaneswaran A, Chandran V, et al. Cardiovascular and other comorbidities in patients with psoriatic arthritis: a comparison with patients with psoriasis. Arthritis Care Res (Hoboken). 2011;63(12):1729–35.
15. Haroon M, Gallagher P, Heffernan E, FitzGerald O. High prevalence of metabolic syndrome and of insulin resistance in psoriatic arthritis is associated with the severity of underlying disease. J Rheumatol 2014;41:1357–65.
16. Favarato MH, Mease P, Gonçalves CR, et al. Hypertension and diabetes significantly enhance the risk of cardiovascular disease in patients with psoriatic arthritis. Clin Exp Rheumatol. 2014;32(2):182–7.
17. Shang Q, Tam LS, Yip GW, et al. High prevalence of subclinical left ventricular dysfunction in patients with psoriatic arthritis. J Rheumatol. 2011;38(7):1363–70.
18. Stokes KY, Calahan L, Hamric CM, Russell JM, Granger DN. CD40/CD40L contributes to hypercholesterolemia-induced microvascular inflammation. Am J Physiol Heart Circ Physiol. 2009;296(3):H689–97.
19. Stokes KY. Microvascular responses to hypercholesterolemia: the interactions between innate and adaptive immune responses. Antioxid Redox Signal. 2006; 8:1141–1151.
20. Haroon M, Fitzgerald O. Pathogenetic overview of psoriatic disease. J Rheumatol Suppl. 2012;89:7–10.
21. Jones SM, Harris CP, Lloyd J, Stirling CA, Reckless JP, McHugh NJ. Lipoproteins and their subfractions in psoriatic arthritis: identification of an atherogenic profile with active joint disease. Ann Rheum Dis. 2000;59(11):904–9.
22. Skoczyñska AH, Turczyn B, Barancewicz-Losek M, Martynowicz H. High-density lipoprotein cholesterol in patients with psoriatic arthritis. J Eur Acad Dermatol Venereol. 2003 May;17(3):362–3.
23. Wu S, Li WQ, Han J, Sun Q, Qureshi AA. Hypercholesterolemia and risk of incident psoriasis and psoriatic arthritis in US women. Arthritis Rheumatol. 2014;66(2):304–10.
24. Brownstein MH. Psoriasis and diabetes mellitus. Arch Dermatol 1966; 93:654–5.
25. Shoelson SE, Lee J, Goldfine AB. Inflammation and insulin resistance. J Clin Invest. 2006;116(7):1793–801.
26. Boehncke WH, Boehncke S, Tobin AM, Kirby B. The 'psoriatic march': a concept of how severe psoriasis may drive cardiovascular comorbidity. Exp Dermatol. 2011;20(4):303–7.
27. Coto-Segura P, Eiris-Salvado N, González-Lara L, et al. Psoriasis, psoriatic arthritis and type 2 diabetes mellitus: a systematic review and meta-analysis. Br J Dermatol. 2013;169(4):783–93.
28. Dreiher J, Freud T, Cohen AD. Psoriatic arthritis and diabetes: a population-based cross-sectional study. Dermatol Res Pract. 2013;2013:580404.
29. Solomon DH, Massarotti E, Garg R, Liu J, Canning C, Schneeweiss S. Association between disease-modifying antirheumatic drugs and diabetes risk in patients with rheumatoid arthritis and psoriasis. JAMA. 2011;22:305(24):2525–31.
30. Grundy SM, Cleeman JI, Daniels SR, et al. Diagnosis and management of the metabolic syndrome: an American Heart Association/National Heart, Lung, and Blood Institute Scientific Statement. Circulation. 2005;112(17):2735–52.
31. Ford ES, Giles WH, Dietz WH. Prevalence of the metabolic syndrome among US adults: findings from the Third National Health and Nutrition Examination Survey. JAMA. 2002;287(3):356–9.
32. Hu G, Qiao Q, Tuomilehto J, Balkau B, Borch-Johnsen K, Pyorala K; DECODE Study Group. Prevalence of the metabolic syndrome and its relation to all-cause and cardiovascular mortality in nondiabetic European men and women. Arch InternMed. 2004;164(10):1066–76.
33. Lakka HM, Laaksonen DE, Lakka TA, et al. The metabolic syndrome and total and cardiovascular disease mortality in middle-aged men. JAMA 2002; 288:2709–16.
34. Hotamisligil GS. Inflammation and metabolic disorders. Nature. 2006 14;444(7121):860–7.

35. Armstrong AW, Harskamp CT, Armstrong EJ. Psoriasis and metabolic syndrome: a systematic review and meta-analysis of observational studies. J Am Acad Dermatol. 2013;68(4):654–62.

36. Mok CC, Ko GT, Ho LY, Yu KL, Chan PT, To CH. Prevalence of atherosclerotic risk factors and the metabolic syndrome in patients with chronic inflammatory arthritis. Arthritis Care Res (Hoboken). 2011;63(2):195–202.

37. Raychaudhri SK, Chatteriee S, Nguyen C, Kaur M, Jialal I, Raychaudhri SP. Increased prevalence of the metabolic syndrome in patients with psoriatic arthritis. Metab Syndr Relat Disord. 2010;8(4):331–4.

38. Bahce-Altuntas A, Schwartzman-Morris JS, et al. Higher frequency of metabolic syndrome in psoriatic arthritis compared with rheumatoid arthritis may be explained by high triglycerides and increased rates of obesity and diabetes [abstract]. Arthritis Rheum 2011;63 Suppl 10:2634.

39. Eder L, Jayakar J, Pollock R, Pellett F, Thavaneswaran A, Chandran V. Serum adipokines in patients with psoriatic arthritis and psoriasis alone and their correlation with disease activity. Ann Rheum Dis. 2013;72(12):1956–61.

40. Crăciun L, Crăciun P, Buicu F. Prevalence of metabolic syndrome in psoriatic arthritis and rheumatoid arthritis. Acta Medica Marisiensis 2014;60(5):196–9.

41. Di Minno MN, Ambrosino P, Lupoli R, et al. Cardiovascular risk markers in patients with psoriatic arthritis: A meta-analysis of literature studies. Ann Med. 2015;47(4):346–53.

42. Jamnitski A, Visman IM, Peters MJ, Boers M, Dijkmans BA, Nurmohamed MT. Prevalence of cardiovascular diseases in psoriatic arthritis resembles that of rheumatoid arthritis. Ann Rheum Dis. 2011;70(5):875–6.

43. Castañeda S, Martín-Martínez MA, González-Juanatey C, et al. Cardiovascular morbidity and associated risk factors in Spanish patients with chronic inflammatory rheumatic diseases attending rheumatology clinics: Baseline data of the CARMA Project. Semin Arthritis Rheum. 2015;44(6):618–26.

44. Ernste FC, Sánchez-Menéndez M, Wilton KM, Crowson CS, Matteson EL, Maradit Kremers H. Cardiovascular Risk Profile at the Onset of Psoriatic Arthritis: A Population-Based Cohort Study. Arthritis Care Res (Hoboken). 2015;67(7):1015–21.

45. Mazlan SA, bin Mohamed Said MS, Hussein H, binti Shamsuddin K, Shah SA, Basri H. A study of intima media thickness and their cardiovascular risk factors in patients with psoriatic arthritis. Acta Medica (Hradec Kralove). 2009;52(3):107–16.

46. Westlake SL, Colebatch AN, Baird J, et al. The effect of methotrexate on cardiovascular disease in patients with rheumatoid arthritis: a systematic literature review. Rheumatology (Oxford) 2010;49:295–307.

47. Micha R, Imamura F, Wyler von Ballmoos M, et al. Systematic review and meta-analysis of methotrexate use and risk of cardiovascular disease. Am J Cardiol 2011;108:1362–70.

48. Armstrong AW, Brezinski EA, Follansbee MR, Armstrong EJ. Effects of biologic agents and other disease-modifying antirheumatic drugs on cardiovascular outcomes in psoriasis and psoriatic arthritis: a systematic review. Curr Pharm 2014;20(4):500–12.

49. Tam LS, Li EK, Shang Q, et al. Tumour necrosis factor alpha blockade is associated with sustained regression of carotid intima-media thickness for patients with active psoriatic arthritis: a 2-year pilot study. Ann Rheum Dis. 2011;70(4):705–6.

50. Tsai WC, Ou TT, Yen JH, Wu CC, Tung YC. Long-term frequent use of non-steroidal anti-inflammatory drugs might protect patients with ankylosing spondylitis from cardiovascular diseases: a nationwide case-control study. PLoS One. 2015;10(5):e0126347.

51. Brunner H, Cockcroft JR, Deanfield J, et al. Endothelial function and dysfunction. Part II: Association with cardiovascular risk factors and diseases. A statement by the Working Group on Endothelins and Endothelial Factors of the European Society of Hypertension. J Hypertens. 2005;23(2):233–46.

52. Mazzoccoli G, Notarsanto I, de Pinto GD, et al. Anti-tumor necrosis factor-α therapy and changes of flow-mediated vasodilatation in psoriatic and rheumatoid arthritis patients. Intern Emerg Med. 2010;5(6):495–500.

53. Roubille C, Richer V, Starnino T, McCourt C, et al. The effects of tumour necrosis factor inhibitors, methotrexate, non-steroidal anti-inflammatory drugs and corticosteroids on cardiovascular events in rheumatoid arthritis, psoriasis and psoriatic arthritis: a systematic review and meta-analysis. Ann Rheum Dis. 2015;74(3):480–9.

54. World Health Organization. Obesity: preventing and managing the global epidemic. Report of a WHO Consultation. World Health Organ Tech Rep Ser 2000;894:ixii, 1253.

55. Ogden CL, Carroll MD, Kit BK, Flegal KM. Prevalence of childhood and adult obesity in the United States, 2011-2012. JAMA 2014;311(8):806–14.

56. National Center for Health Statistics. Health, United States, 2011: With Special Features on Socioeconomic Status and Health. Hyattsville, MD; U.S. Department of Health and Human Services; 2012.

57. Rondinone CM. Adipocyte-derived hormones, cytokines, and mediators. Endocrine. 2006;29(1):81–90.

58. Otero M, Lago R, Lago F, et al. Leptin, from fat to inflammation: old questions and new insights. FEBS Lett. 2005;579(2):295–301.

59. Lago F, Dieguez C, Gómez-Reino J, Gualillo O. Adipokines as emerging mediators of immune response and inflammation. Nat Clin Pract Rheumatol. 2007 ;3(12):716–24.

60. Faggioni R, Feingold KR, Grunfeld C. Leptin regulation of the immune response and the immunodeficiency of malnutrition. FASEB J. 2001;15(14):2565–71.

61. Bernotiene E, Palmer G, Gabay C. The role of leptin in innate and adaptive immune responses. Arthritis Res Ther. 2006;8(5):217.

62. Aprahamian TR, Sam F. Adiponectin in cardiovascular inflammation and obesity. Int J Inflam 2011;2011:376909.

63. Henseler T, Christophers E. Disease concomitance in psoriasis. J AmAcad Dermatol. 1995;32(6):982–6.

64. Naldi L, Chatenoud L, Linder D, et al. Cigarette smoking, body mass index, and stressful life events as risk factors for psoriasis: results from an Italian case control study. J Invest Dermatol. 2005;125(1):61–7.

65. Cohen AD, Gilutz H, Henkin Y, et al. Psoriasis and the metabolic syndrome. Acta Derm Venereol. 2007;87(6):506–9.

66. Cohen AD, Sherf M, Vidavsky L, Vardy D, Shapiro J, Meyerovitch J. Association between psoriasis and the metabolic syndrome: a cross-sectional study. Dermatology. 2008;216(2):152–5.

67. Marino MG, Carboni I, De Felice C, Maurici M, Maccari F, Franco E. Risk factors for psoriasis: a retrospective study on 501 outpatients clinical records. Ann Ig. 2004;16(6):753–8.

68. Murray ML, Bergstresser P, Adams-Huet B, Cohen J. Relationship of psoriasis severity to obesity using same-gender siblings as controls for obesity. Clin Exp Dermatol. 2009;34(2):140–4.

69. Soltani-Arabshahi R, Wong B, Feng BJ, Goldgar DE, Duffin KC, Krueger GG. Obesity in early adulthood as a risk factor for psoriatic arthritis. Arch Dermatol. 2010;146(7):721–6.

70. Love TJ, Zhu Y, Zhang Y, Wall-Burns L, et al. Obesity and the risk of psoriatic arthritis: a population-based study. Ann Rheum Dis. 2012;71(8):1273–7.

71. Li W, Han J, Qureshi AA. Obesity and risk of incident psoriatic arthritis in US women. Ann Rheum Dis. 2012;71(8):1267–72.

72. Di Minno MN, Peluso R, Iervolino S, et al. Weight loss and achievement of minimal disease activity in patients with psoriatic arthritis starting treatment with tumour necrosis factor α blockers. Ann Rheum Dis. 2014;73(6):1157–62.

73. Korkoliakou P, Christodoulou C, Kouris A, et al. Alexithymia, anxiety and depression in patients with psoriasis: a case-control study. Ann Gen Psychiatry. 2014;13(1):38.

74. Dowlatshahi EA, Wakkee M, Arends LR, Nijsten T. The prevalence and odds of depressive symptoms and clinical depression in psoriasis patients: a systematic review and meta-analysis. J Invest Dermatol. 2014 ;134(6):1542–51.

75. McDonough E, Ayearst R, Eder L, et al. Depression and anxiety in psoriatic disease: prevalence and associated factors. J Rheumatol. 2014;41(5):887–96.

76. Kotsis K, Voulgari PV, Tsifetaki N, et al. Anxiety and depressive symptoms and illness perceptions in psoriatic arthritis and associations with physical health-related quality of life. Arthritis Care Res (Hoboken). 2012;64(10):1593–601.

77. Freire M, Rodríguez J, Möller I, Valcárcel A, et al. Prevalence of symptoms of anxiety and depression in patients with psoriatic arthritis attending rheumatology clinics. Reumatol Clin. 2011;7(1):20–6.

78. Julian LJ, Gregorich SE, Tonner C, et al. Using the Center for Epidemiologic Studies Depression Scale to screen for depression in systemic lupus erythematosus. Arthritis Care Res (Hoboken) 2011;63:884–90.

79. Nery FG, Borba EF, Hatch JP, Soares JC, Bonfa E, Neto FL. Major depressive disorder and disease activity in systemic lupus erythematosus. Compr Psychiatry 2007;48:14–9.

80. Bachen EA, Chesney MA, Criswell LA. Prevalence of mood and anxiety disorders in women with systemic lupus erythematosus. Arthritis Rheum 2009;61:822–9.

81. Thomson CA, McColl A, Cavanagh J, Graham GJ. Peripheral inflammation is associated with remote global gene expression changes in the brain. J Neuroinflammation. 2014;11:73.

82. Au SC, Yaniv S, Gottlieb AB. Psoriasis Forum. 2011;17(3):169–79.

83. Niccoli L, Nannini C, Cassara E et al. Frequency of iridocyclitis in patients with early psoriatic arthritis: a prospective, follow up study. Int J Rheum Dis 2012;15:414–418.

84. Lambert JR, Wright V. Eye inflammation in psoriatic arthritis. Ann Rheum Dis 1976;35:354–356.

85. Casarou-Catsari A, Katsambas A, Theodoropoulos P, Stratigos J Ophthalmological manifestations in patients with psoriasis. Acta Derm Venereol 1984;64:557–559.

86. Ijima S, Iwata M, Otsuka F. Psoriatic arthritis and hypopion-iridocyclitis. Dermatology 1996;193:295–299.

87. Paiva ES, Macaluso DC, Edwards A, Rosenbaum JT. Characterisation of uveitis in patients with psoriatic arthritis. Ann Rheum Dis. 2000;59(1):67–70.

88. Fraga NA, Oliveira Mde F, Follador I, Rocha Bde O, Rêgo VR. Psoriasis and uveitis: a literature review. An Bras Dermatol. 2012;87(6):877–83.

89. Haroon M, O'Rourke M, Ramasamy P, Murphy CC, FitzGerald O. A novel evidence-based detection of undiagnosed spondyloarthritis in patients presenting with acute anterior uveitis: the DUET (Dublin Uveitis Evaluation Tool). Ann Rheum Dis. 2015; 74(11): 1990–5.

90. Frentz G, Olsen JH. Malignant tumours and psoriasis: a follow-up study. Br J Dermatol 1999;140:237–42.

91. Gelfand JM, Berlin J, Van Voorhees A, Margolis DJ. Lymphoma rates are low but increased in patients with psoriasis: results from a population-based cohort study in the United Kingdom. Arch Dermatol 2003;139:1425–9.

92. Rohekar S, Tom BD, Hassa A, Schentag CT, Farewell VT, Gladman DD. Prevalence of malignancy in psoriatic arthritis. Arthritis Rheum. 2008;58(1):82–7.

93. Fantò M, Peragallo MS, Pietrosanti M, et al. Risk of malignancy in patients with rheumatoid arthritis, psoriatic arthritis and ankylosing spondylitis under immunosuppressive therapy: a single-center experience. Intern Emerg Med. 201511(1):31–40.

94. Gross RL, Schwartzman-Morris JS, Krathen M, et al. A comparison of the malignancy incidence among patients with psoriatic arthritis and patients with rheumatoid arthritis in a large US cohort. Arthritis Rheumatol. 2014;66(6):1472–81.

95. Wolf N, Quaranta M, Prescott NJ, et al. Psoriasis is associated with pleiotropic susceptibility loci identified in type II diabetes and Crohn disease. J Med Genet. 2008;45:114–16.

96. Lee FI, Bellary SV, Francis C. Increased occurrence of psoriasis in patients with Crohn's disease and their relatives. Amer J Gastroenterol, 1990; 85:962–963.

97. Li WQ, Han JL, Chan AT Qureshi AA Psoriasis, psoriatic arthritis and increased risk of incident Crohn's disease in US women. Ann Rheum Dis. 2013;72(7):1200–5.

98. Eder L, Thavaneswaran A, Chandran V, Cook R, Gladman DD. Increased burden of inflammation over time is associated with the extent of atherosclerotic plaques in patients with psoriatic arthritis. Ann Rheum Dis. 2015; 74(10):1830–5.

99. Shen J, Shang Q, Li EK, et al. Cumulative inflammatory burden is independently associated with increased arterial stiffness in patients with psoriatic arthritis: a prospective study. Arthritis Res Ther. 2015;;17:75.

100. Lin YC, Dalal D, Churton S, et al. Relationship between metabolic syndrome and carotid intima-media thickness: cross-sectional comparison between psoriasis and psoriatic arthritis. Arthritis Care Res (Hoboken). 2014;66(1):97–103.

101. Ogdie A, Schwartzman S, Eder L, et al. Comprehensive treatment of psoriatic arthritis: managing comorbidities and extraarticular manifestations. J Rheumatol. 2014;41(11):2315–22.

102. Gulliver WP. Importance of screening for comorbidities in psoriasis patients. Expert Rev Dermatol. 2008;3(2):133–5.

103. Husted JA, Thavaneswaran A, Chandran V, Gladman DD. Incremental effects of comorbidity on quality of life in patients with psoriatic arthritis. J Rheumatol. 2013;40(8):1349–56.

Imaging

CHAPTER 16

Plain radiography

William Tillett and Neil McHugh

Introduction

The purpose of this chapter is to discuss the role of plain radiography in psoriatic arthritis (PsA). In an era of modern imaging techniques such as computed tomography, magnetic resonance imaging, and musculoskeletal ultrasound plain radiography may seem obsolete. Plain radiography is, however, simple, accessible, and inexpensive, and, as such, remains the standard measure for the determination of disease progression and prognosis. We will briefly discuss the role plain radiography has had in establishing PsA as a distinct clinical entity, describe the radiographic features of peripheral and axial disease, the measurement techniques available, and finally prognostic value and natural history.

Historical perspective and the role of plain radiography in defining psoriatic arthritis

The association between psoriasis and arthritis was first made by Alibert in 1822 but PsA was only formally recognised by the American Rheumatology Association (ARA) as a distinct disease entity in 1964. The varying definitions of PsA and a suspicion it was simply concurrent rheumatoid arthritis (RA) and psoriasis delayed progress in our understanding of the disease. Two factors in particular influenced the acceptance of PsA as a distinct disease, the development of the Rose–Waller agglutination test [1], to which most patients with PsA were found to be negative [2], and the development of modern radiology. With the routine use of plain radiographs in clinical practice, it became apparent that there were clear distinguishing features between RA and PsA.

Case series of distinguishing radiographic features in PsA were reported in the 1950s [3, 4] but the first large prospective, study came from Wright in 1961 comparing the radiographic features of 103 cases with PsA with cases of RA and gout [5]. Wright reported that radiographic damage amongst those with PsA was characterized by more frequent involvement of the distal interphalangeal and sacroiliac joints, terminal tuft resorption, and was generally less severe than RA. With the advent of more robust classification criteria, terminology and modern epidemiology, our understanding of radiographic damage in PsA has been refined [6]. Subsequent sections of this chapter will address the characteristics of radiographic damage in peripheral and axial PsA, modern measurement techniques, and the natural history of radiographic damage.

Radiographic features of peripheral psoriatic arthritis

Soft tissue swelling is the first radiographic feature in early disease, either per-articular or affecting the whole digit in the presence of dactylitis. Periarticular osteopenia is recognized in PsA but felt to be less frequent than RA [7]. Subsequent features include erosions (articular or entheseal), joint space narrowing, osteolysis (bone resorption), osteoproliferation, and ankylosis. The order in which these features occur has not been established. The pattern of joints affected radiographically follows the recognized clinical phenotypes of asymmetrical oligoarthritis (in early disease), distal interphalangeal joint involvement, polyarthritis (in established disease), and less frequently monoarthritis and arthritis mutilans (phenotypes are discussed in more detail in Chapter 10) [8]. Joints typically affect a digital 'ray' rather than 'rows' of joints (as is typical in RA) and the distal interphalangeal joints are commonly affected, illustrated in Figure 16.1 [9].

Articular erosion

PsA is an erosive arthritis [6, 8, 10, 11]. One early study estimated the level of destruction to be equivalent to RA [12]. A large study from the Consortium of Rheumatology Researchers of North America (CORRONA) database of 2481 patients with PsA and 17,107 patients with RA showed a higher prevalence of erosions (47.4% vs 37.6%, $P=0.020$) and deformity (25.2% vs 21.6%, $P=0.021$) amongst patients with RA vs PsA [13]. The burden of erosive disease is, however, substantial: approximately half (47%) patients with early PsA have erosive disease within two years of diagnosis and up to two thirds have radiographic damage at their first visit to a PsA specialist [10, 14]. A longitudinal study of 139 patients with established PsA demonstrated progressive damage in established disease. Fifty-eight percent of patients had radiographic damage at baseline (median 5 years disease duration) progressing to 78% at follow up (median 12 years disease duration) [15].

Differentiating erosions from PsA and RA or erosive osteoarthritis (particularly at the distal interphalangeal joints) can be particularly challenging as the morphology is similar. Erosions typically occur slightly away from the joint margin at the site of the joint capsule/enthesis rather than at the joint margin as seen in RA (Figure 16.2a).

The presence of osteoproliferation adjacent to the erosion is more likely to be related to PsA. Erosions at the distal interphalangeal

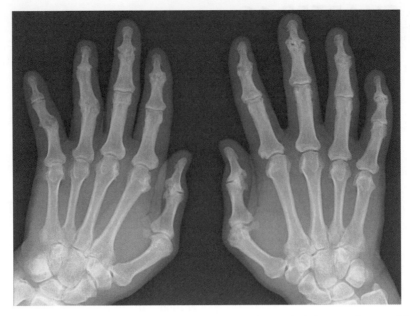

Figure 16.1 Hand Radiographs of a patient with psoriatic arthritis demonstrating asymmetric, erosive and ankylosing involvement of digital 'rays' rather than 'rows' of joints.

joints can be difficult to distinguish from erosive osteoarthritis, especially as the two diseases often co-exist. Central erosions, the absence of proliferation, and presence of joint space narrowing can be useful indicators of osteoarthritis. Taylor and colleagues defined the radiographic features of PsA in a study of 164 radiographs from 62patients [6]. PsA erosions can be defined as 'clearly defined marginal erosions with juxtaarticular periostitis or the absence of osteophytes, joint space narrowing or central erosions' (Figure 16.2b) [6].

Extra-articular erosions

Entheseal erosions may affect tendon insertions at the calcaneus, patellar, iliac crests, humeral tuberosity, or greater trochanters [16, 17]. Entheseal ossification may occur at the same entheses in the form of irregular bony proliferation detectible on plain radiographs.

Osteolysis and psoriatic arthritis mutilans

Osteolysis (bone resorption) can occur at the joint or tuft and is the radiographic characteristic of the most destructive phenotype of PsA—psoriatic arthritis mutilans [16, 18–20]. Psoriatic arthritis mutilans was originally described in 1913 by Marie et al., who clinically described the telescoping of affected digits [21]. Psoriatic arthritis mutilans is currently defined radiographically by the presence of

osteolysis affecting >50% of the articular surface on both sides of the joint, illustrated in Figure 16.3 [22–24]. Moll and Wright estimated an approximately 5% prevalence [25] which has been confirmed in subsequent studies [26–28]. The natural history of psoriatic arthritis mutilans has only recently been reported in a study of 39 patients over a median duration of ten years. Psoriatic arthritis mutilans typically presents as a monoarticular phenomenon initially with progressive destruction within the affected joint and progression to polyarticular involvement during follow-up [29]. Patients with arthritis mutilans had earlier disease onset, worse physical function, and greater nail and axial involvement than patients without mutilans.

Osteolysis can also affect the phalange tufts resulting in a 'whittled' appearance. The combination of osteolysis on one side of a joint leading to 'cup' formation and 'whittling' to a 'pencil' form on the other side creates the 'pencil-in-cup' appearance recognized in PsA Figure 16.3.

Osteoproliferation (juxtaarticular/periosteal) and ankylosis

Osteoproliferation is a characteristic feature in PsA and, although seen in other diseases such as peripheral spondyloarthritis, was found to be sufficiently specific to PsA to be included in the

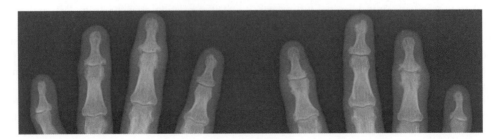

Figure 16.2a Marginal erosions of the distal interphalangeal joints with juxtaarticular periostitis.

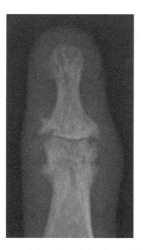

Figure 16.2b Close up view of the right 3rd distal interphalangeal joints demonstrating erosion and juxtaarticular periostitis.

CLASsification of Psoriatic Arthritis (CASPAR) criteria [30]. As such the use of plain radiography remains an important component in the diagnosis of PsA. Osteoproliferation can occur both at the metaphysis and the diaphysis and is considered likely to be related to enthesitis. Irregular, speculated osteoproliferation is seen at entheseal sites (Figure 16.4). Erosions can occur at the same site as osteoproliferation and this phenomenon has contributed to the leading hypothesis of disease aetiology in PsA of the synovio-entheseal complex [31]. Generalized thickening of the bony cortex can give rise to the 'ivory phalanx' which is a rare phenomenon, most commonly see in the feet.

Bony ankyloses is defined as trabeculae crossing the joint space [6] and was recognized as a feature in many of the early radiographic reports in PsA Figure 16.5 [19, 20, 32]. Ankylosis is most frequently seen at the interphalangeal joints [6] and has been seen to occur in the same way as osteolysis in arthritis mutilans [29].

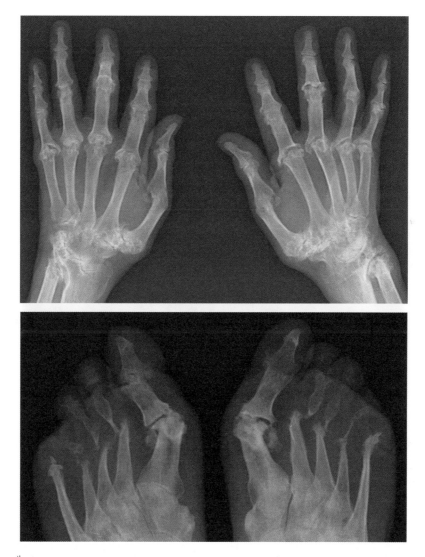

Figure 16.3 Psoriatic arthritis mutilans.
An example of osteolysis and subsequent digital shortening in the hands and feet of the same patient. There is osteolysis and 'whittling' of the MTPjoints resulting in the 'pencil in cup' pattern.

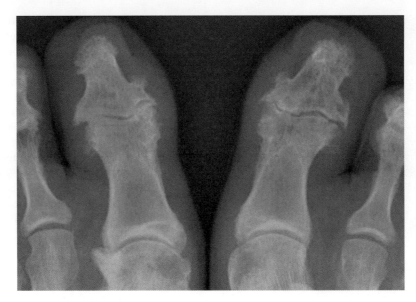

Figure 16.4 Irregular, 'spiculated' osteoproliferation at the hallux interphalangeal joints.

Radiographic features of psoriatic spondyloarthritis

History of psoriatic spondyloarthritis

Axial disease in PsA was first described by Zellner in 1928 but it was not until 1955 when the phrase 'psoriasis spondylytica' (PsSpA)was first used [33]. Wright reported sacroiliitis occurring more commonly in PsA than RA [5], and Dixon found a higher prevalence than in healthy controls [34]. Kaplan reported a higher prevalence of facet joint sclerosis and anterior ligamental calcification of the cervical spine amongst patients with psoriasis, noting that the sacroiliac joints and the lumbar spine were not always affected [35]. Jajic reported a case series in 1968 commenting that amongst 23 cases of PsA the majority had radiographic evidence of spondyloarthritis yet the mobility of the spine was maintained [36].

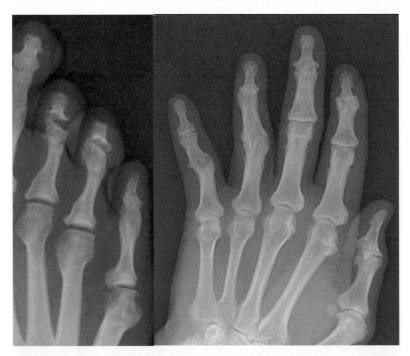

Figure 16.5 Ankylosis.

Hands: Ankylosis of the left hand little and ring finger proximal interphalangeal joints and index, ring and middle distal interphalangeal joints.

Feet: Ankylosis of the right 3rd, 4th and 5th proximal interphalangeal joints with erosion and osteolysis in the same ray at the 3rd and 4th distal interphalangeal joints (also seen in the feet radiograph of Figure 16.3).

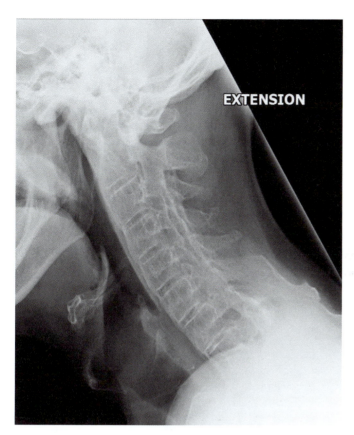

Figure 16.6 Psoriatic spondyloarthritis; Cervical spine involvement with flowing syndesmophytes similar to ankylosing spondylitis.

Prevalence and associations of psoriatic spondyloarthritis

Estimates of the prevalence of radiographic psoriatic spondyloarthritis (PsSpA) amongst patients with PsA range between 25% and 70%, depending upon cohorts and classification used. The burden of subclinical disease has yet to be fully determined. Studies in early PsA have shown ~20% of patients with PsA have radiographic evidence of SpA, in the absence of clinical symptoms [37]. Lambert and Moll first reported the association between *HLAB27* and PsSpA in 1976 and the association of several

HLA-B27 variants with PsSpA is now well established [38, 39]. Different HLA susceptibility genes may be associated with different radiographic phenotypes. A recent study of 282 patients with PsA by Haroon et al. showed *HLAB27* to be associated with symmetrical sacroileitis and *HLAB08* with asymmetrical sacroileitis [40]. Other risk factors for radiographic axial disease in PsA are male sex, nail dystrophy, worse peripheral joint damage, and elevated erythrocyte sedimentation rate (ESR) [39, 41].

Distribution and distinguishing features of psoriatic spondyloarthritis and ankylosing spondylitis

In comparison with ankylosing spondylitis, psoriatic spondyloarthritis has more frequent involvement of the cervical spine (Figure 16.6) [44, 45], asymmetrical and less severe sacroiliitis (Figure 16.7) [41], asymmetrical/ chunky and para-marginal syndesmophytes and paravertebral ossification (Figure 16.8) [42, 43]. Overall radiographic features are less severe in comparison to ankylosing spondylitis, where sacroiliitis tends to be higher grade and accompanied by bilateral, marginal syndesmophytes [46]. Table 16.1 summarizes the distinguishing features between AS and PsSpA.

Measurement of radiographic outcome in psoriatic arthritis

Measures of peripheral radiographic damage

There are several scoring methods that have been validated for use in PsA including the modified Sharp score [47, 48], the Sharp–van der Heijde modified method [48, 49], the modified Steinbrocker [50], and the PsA Ratingen score [51]. With the exception of the Ratingen method, these scoring systems were designed and validated for use in RA and subsequently modified for use in PsA.

The modified Steinbrocker is a global method that assesses 42 joints of the hands and feet (considering the wrist as a single joint) for soft tissue swelling or osteopenia, erosion, erosion and joint space narrowing, and total destruction (osteolysis or ankyloses) in a single global score for each joint [50]. The modified Steinbrocker is straightforward to learn, reliable, and the quickest of the existing methods to perform but is less sensitive to change than the modified Sharp, Sharp–van der Heijde, or Ratingen [52]. The Sharp–van der Heijde is a composite score that assesses 52 joints (including

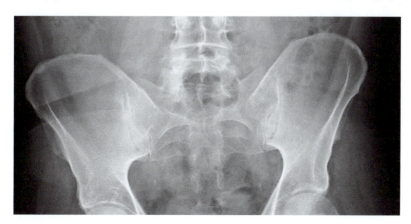

Figure 16.7 Psoriatic spondyloarthritis; mild asymmetrical sacroiliitis of the right sacroiliac joint.

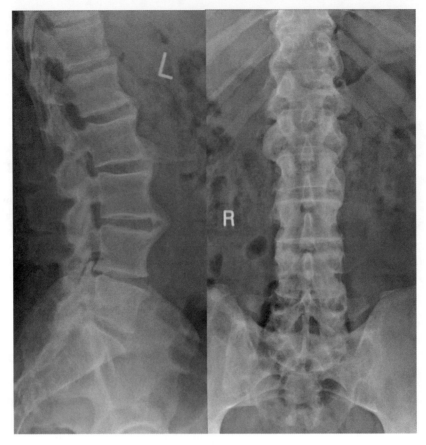

Figure 16.8 Psoriatic spondyloarthritis; 'chunky' syndesmophytes and asymmetric sacroiliac involvement.

the small joints of the wrists) for erosion and joint space narrowing separately [49]. The Sharp–van der Heijde is reliable, readily learned, and is the most sensitive to change of all the methods discussed but the most time consuming to perform [52]. The PsA Ratingen method assesses for erosion or osteoproliferation characteristic for PsA at 40 joints in the hands and feet [51]. The method is reliable and sensitive to change and through the inclusion of osteoproliferation (the radiographic feature found to be sufficiently specific to PsA to warrant inclusion in the CASPAR classification criteria) arguably is the most specific to PsA.

A recent study has compared the sensitivity to change of each method including the smallest detectable differences [52]. These data confirmed the high sensitivity of the Sharp–van der Heijde

method which has become the standard in randomized controlled trials. Radiographic change occurs slowly and most studies report small changes in each of these scores (Table 16.2). The minimally clinically important differences have not been established. Until such a study is undertaken the smallest detectable difference is regarded as relevant.

Outcome measurement in psoriatic spondyloarthritis

As with peripheral arthritis, a number of scoring methods have been developed to measure axial damage in psoriatic spondylitis [53]. Three scores, the Bath Ankylosing Spondylitis Radiology Index (BASRI), the modified Stoke Ankylosing Spondylitis Spinal Score (mSASSS), and the Radiographic Ankylosing Spondylitis Spinal Score (RASSS) were originally developed for use in ankylosing spondylitis. A fourth method, the Psoriatic Arthritis Spondylitis Radiology Index (PASRI) was developed specifically to measure psoriatic spondylitis. These four methods have recently been compared in PsSpA and were all found to perform well [53].

Natural history/prognosis

Cohort studies have shown than PsA is destructive and progressive [10, 11] even in established disease [15]. One study used the modified Steinbrocker to assess the severity of a cohort of patients with PsA and RA and found the overall level of severity of peripheral arthritis to be comparable at a mean of seven years disease duration [12]. Approximately half patients will have erosive disease by two years disease duration [14]. Radiographic damage has

Table 16.1 Comparison of radiographic axial features of ankylosing spondylitis and psoriatic spondyloarthritis

Feature	Ankylosing spondylitis	Psoriatic spondylitis
Sacroiliitis	More severe	Less severe
	Bilateral	Asymmetrical
Syndesmophytes	Progress from lumbar to cervical spine	Cervical spine more frequently involved
	Symmetrical	Asymmetrical
	Marginal	Para-marginal
Ossification	Ligamental	Para-vertebral

Table 16.2 Sensitivity to change of the modified Steinbroker, modified Sharp, Sharp–van der Heijde, or Ratingen methods in PsA

Method	Mean change	SD of change	SEM	SRM	SDD	SDC	SDD as % of total score	SDC as % of total score
Steinbrocker	2.3	4.91	3.49	0.46	8.11	4.83	4.82	2.87
Psoriatic Rating	3.3	7.61	5.46	0.44	12.71	7.57	3.53	2.10
Destruction	1.6	3.46	2.51	0.45	5.83	3.48		
Proliferation	1.8	4.28	3.15	0.43	7.34	4.37		
Modified Sharp	5.5	7.15	5.06	0.77	11.77	7.01	2.42	1.44
Erosion	2.4	4.15	2.97	0.57	6.90	4.11		
JSN	3.3	5.10	3.64	0.64	8.47	5.05		
Sharp van der Heijde	5.2	6.53	4.66	0.79	10.83	6.45	2.05	1.22
Erosion	2.3	4.41	3.14	0.52	7.31	4.36		
JSN	3.0	4.36	3.14	0.68	7.29	4.35		

Modified Steinbroker method (STB), Sharp–van der Heijde modified method (VDH), Modified Sharp method (MSS), psoriatic arthritis Ratingen score (PARS), joint space narrowing (JSN), standard deviation (SD), standard error of means (SEM), standardized response mean (SRM), smallest detectable difference (SDD), smallest detectable change (SDC).

Reproduced from Tillet et al. Feasibility, Reliability, and Sensitivity to Change of Four Radiographic Scoring Methods in Patients With Psoriatic Arthritis (2014) Arthritis Care and Research 66(2) 311–317 with permission from Wiley.

been proven to be progressive in the majority even in established disease [15, 29, 54]. Polyarticular involvement, high ESR, *HLA-B*27* positivity and high drug use predict radiographic progression [11, 54–57].

Radiographic damage has historically been considered irreversible although a recent report of dramatic improvement seen in a patient treated with anti-tumour necrosis factor inhibitor for four years challenges this viewpoint [58]. Radiographic damage was assessed with three methods: Steinbrocker, Ratingen and van der Heijde and all showed dramatic improvement, notably erosion scores (van der Heijde method) improved from 36 to 16 over four years. Improvements of this nature have been seen in RA but are considered rare [59]. Nevertheless it is likely that the natural history of radiographic damage in PsA will alter with increasing awareness of the disease, earlier diagnosis, tighter control of inflammatory disease, and the increasing availability of novel biological agents proven to reduce radiographic damage.

References

1. Greenbury CL. Elution of the rheumatoid-arthritis factor from red-cell agglutinates. Lancet 1956; 271(6944): 644–6.
2. Ball J. Sheep cell agglutination test for rheumatoid arthritis; a clinico-pathological study. Ann Rheum Dis 1952; 11(2): 97–111.
3. Fawcitt J. Bone and joint changes associated with psoriasis. Br J Radiol 1950; 23(271): 440–53.
4. Carrier JW. Psoriatic arthritis. Am J Roentgenol Radium Ther Nucl Med. 1958; 79(4): 612–7.
5. Wright V. Psoriatic arthritis. A comparative radiographic study of rheumatoid arthritis and arthritis associated with psoriasis. Ann Rheum Dis 1961; 20: 123–32.
6. Taylor WJ, Porter GG, Helliwell PS. Operational definitions and observer reliability of the plain radiographic features of psoriatic arthritis. J Rheumatol 2003; 30(12): 2645–58.
7. Harrison BJ, Hutchinson CE, Adams J, Bruce IN, Herrick AL. Assessing periarticular bone mineral density in patients with early psoriatic arthritis or rheumatoid arthritis. Ann Rheum Dis 2002; 61(11): 1007–11.
8. Siannis F, Farewell VT, Cook RJ, Schentag CT, Gladman DD. Clinical and radiological damage in psoriatic arthritis. Ann Rheum Dis 2006; 65(4): 478–81.
9. Green FA. Distal interphalangeal joint disease and nail abnormalities. Ann Rheum Dis 1968; 27(1): 55–9.
10. Gladman DD, Shuckett R, Russell ML, Thorne JC, Schachter RK. Psoriatic arthritis (PSA)–an analysis of 220 patients. QJM 1987; 62(238): 127–41.
11. Gladman DD, Stafford-Brady F, Chang CH, Lewandowski K, Russell ML. Longitudinal study of clinical and radiological progression in psoriatic arthritis. J Rheumatol 1990; 17(6): 809–12.
12. Rahman. Comparison of radiological severity in psoriatic arthritis and rheumatoid arthritis. J Rheumatol 2001; 28(5): 1041–4.
13. Reddy SM, Anandarajah AP, Fisher MC, et al. Comparative analysis of disease activity measures, use of biologic agents, body mass index, radiographic features, and bone density in psoriatic arthritis and rheumatoid arthritis patients followed in a large U.S. disease registry. J Rheumatol 2010; 37(12): 2566–72.
14. Kane D, Stafford L, Bresnihan B, FitzGerald O. A prospective, clinical and radiological study of early psoriatic arthritis: an early synovitis clinic experience. Rheumatology (Oxford) 2003; 42(12): 1460–8.
15. Ravindran J, Cavill C, Balakrishnan C, Jones SM, Korendowych E, McHugh NJ. A modified Sharp score demonstrates disease progression in established psoriatic arthritis. Arthritis Care Res (Hoboken) 2010; 62(1): 86–91.
16. Peterson CC, Jr., Silbiger ML. Reiter's syndrome and psoriatic arthritis. Their roentgen spectra and some interesting similarities. Am J Roentgenol Radium Ther Nucl Med.1967; 101(4): 860–71.
17. Resnick D, Niwayama G. Entheses and enthesopathy. Anatomical, pathological, and radiological correlation. Radiology 1983; 146(1): 1–9.
18. Wright V. Psoriasis and arthritis; a study of the radiographic appearances. Br J Radiol 1957; 30(351): 113–9.
19. Avila R, Pugh DG, Slocumb CH, Winkelmann RK. Psoriatic arthritis: a roentgenologic study. Radiology 1960; 75: 691–702.
20. Fournie B, Crognier L, Arnaud C, et al. Proposed classification criteria of psoriatic arthritis. A preliminary study in 260 patients. Rev Rhum Engl Ed 1999; 66(10): 446–56.
21. Marie P, Leri A. Une variete rare de rhumatisme chronique: La main en lorgnette. Bull Soc Med Hosp Paris 1913; 36: 104–7.
22. Tan YM, Ostergaard M, Doyle A, et al. MRI bone oedema scores are higher in the arthritis mutilans form of psoriatic arthritis and correlate

with high radiographic scores for joint damage. Arthritis Res Ther 2009; 11(1): R2.

23. Marsal S, Armadans-Gil L. Clinical, radiographic and HLA associations as markers for different patterns of psoriatic arthritis. Rheumatology (Oxford) 1999; (38): 332–7.

24. Haddad A, Chandran V. Arthritis mutilans. Curr Rheumatol Rep 2013; 15(4): 321.

25. Moll J, Wright V. Psoriatic arthritis. Semin Arthritis Rheum 1973; 3(1): 55–78.

26. Gladman DD. Psoriatic arthritis: epidemiology, clinical features, course, and outcome. Ann Rheum Dis 2005; 64(suppl_2): ii14–ii7.

27. Reich K, Kruger K, Mossner R, Augustin M. Epidemiology and clinical pattern of psoriatic arthritis in Germany: a prospective interdisciplinary epidemiological study of 1511 patients with plaque-type psoriasis. Br J Dermatol 2009; 160(5): 1040–7.

28. Nossent JC, Gran JT. Epidemiological and clinical characteristics of psoriatic arthritis in northern Norway. Scand J Rheumatol 2009; 38(4): 251–5.

29. Jadon DR, Shaddick G, Tillett W, et al. Psoriatic arthritis mutilans: characteristics and natural radiographic history. J Rheumatol 2015; 42(7):1169–76.

30. Taylor W, Gladman D, Helliwell P, Marchesoni A, Mease P, Mielants H. Classification criteria for psoriatic arthritis: development of new criteria from a large international study. Arthritis Rheum 2006; 54(8): 2665–73.

31. Mcgonagle D, Aydin SZ, Tan AL. The synovio-entheseal complex and its role in tendon and capsular associated inflammation. J Rheumatol 2012; 89: 11–4.

32. Baker H, Golding DN, Thompson M. Psoriasis and arthritis. AnnIntern Med 1963; 58: 909–25.

33. Fletcher E, Rose FC. Psoriasis spondylitica. Lancet 1955; 268(6866): 695–6.

34. Dixon AS, Lience E. Sacro-iliac joint in adult rheumatoid arthritis and psoriatic arthropathy. Ann Rheum Dis 1961; 20: 247–57.

35. Kaplan D, Plotz CM, Nathanson L, Frank L. Cervical spine in psoriasis and in psoriatic arthritis. Ann Rheum Dis 1964; 23: 50–6.

36. Jajic I. Radiological changes in the sacro-iliac joints and spine of patients with psoriatic arthritis and psoriasis. Ann Rheum Dis 1968; 27(1): 1–6.

37. Khan M, Schentag C, Gladman DD. Clinical and radiological changes during psoriatic arthritis disease progression. J Rheumatol 2003; 30(5): 1022–6.

38. Lambert JR, Wright V, Rajah SM, Moll JM. Histocompatibility antigens in psoriatic arthritis. Ann Rheum Dis 1976; 35(6): 526–30.

39. Chandran V, Tolusso DC, Cook RJ, Gladman DD. Risk factors for axial inflammatory arthritis in patients with psoriatic arthritis. J Rheumatol 2010; 37(4): 809–15.

40. Haroon M, Winchester R, Giles JT, Heffernan E, FitzGerald O. Certain class I HLA alleles and haplotypes implicated in susceptibility play a role in determining specific features of the psoriatic arthritis phenotype. Ann Rheum Dis 2015; 75(1):155–62.

41. Gladman DD, Brubacher B, Buskila D, Langevitz P, Farewell VT. Differences in the expression of spondyloarthropathy: a comparison between ankylosing spondylitis and psoriatic arthritis. Clin Invest Med 1993; 16(1): 1–7.

42. Helliwell PS, Hickling P, Wright V. Do the radiological changes of classic ankylosing spondylitis differ from the changes found in the spondylitis associated with inflammatory bowel disease, psoriasis, and reactive arthritis? Ann Rheum Dis 1998; 57(3): 135–40.

43. McEwen C, DiTata D, Lingg C, Porini A, Good A, Rankin T. Ankylosing spondylitis and spondylitis accompanying ulcerative colitis, regional enteritis, psoriasis and Reiter's disease. A comparative study. Arthritis Rheum 1971; 14(3): 291–318.

44. Jenkinson T, Armas J, Evison G, Cohen M, Lovell C, McHugh NJ. The cervical spine in psoriatic arthritis: a clinical and radiological study. Br JRheumatol 1994; 33(3): 255–9.

45. Salvarani C, Macchioni P, Cremonesi T, et al. The cervical spine in patients with psoriatic arthritis: a clinical, radiological and immunogenetic study. Ann Rheum Dis 1992; 51(1): 73–7.

46. Perez Alamino R, Maldonado Cocco JA, Citera G, et al. Differential features between primary ankylosing spondylitis and spondylitis associated with psoriasis and inflammatory bowel disease. J Rheumatol 2011; 38(8): 1656–60.

47. Sharp JT, Bluhm GB, Brook A, et al. Reproducibility of multiple-observer scoring of radiologic abnormalities in the hands and wrists of patients with rheumatoid arthritis. Arthritis Rheum 1985; 28(1): 16–24.

48. van der Heijde D, Sharp J, Wassenberg S, Gladman DD. Psoriatic arthritis imaging: a review of scoring methods. Ann Rheum Dis 2005; 64 Suppl 2: ii61–4.

49. van der Heijde D. How to read radiographs according to the Sharp/van der Heijde method. J Rheumatol 2000; 27(1): 261–3.

50. Rahman P, Gladman DD, Cook RJ, Zhou Y, Young G, Salonen D. Radiological assessment in psoriatic arthritis. Br J Rheumatol 1998; 37(7): 760–5.

51. Wassenberg S, Fischer-Kahle V, Herborn G, Rau R. A method to score radiographic change in psoriatic arthritis. Z Rheumatol 2001; 60(3): 156–66.

52. Tillett W, Jadon D, Shaddick G, et al. Feasibility, reliability, and sensitivity to change of four radiographic scoring methods in patients with psoriatic arthritis. Arthritis Care Res (Hoboken) 2014; 66(2): 311–7.

53. Biagioni BJ, Gladman DD, Cook RJ, et al. Reliability of radiographic scoring methods in axial psoriatic arthritis. Arthritis Care Res (Hoboken) 2014; 66(9): 1417–22.

54. McHugh NJ, Balachrishnan C, Jones SM. Progression of peripheral joint disease in psoriatic arthritis: a 5-yr prospective study. Rheumatology (Oxford) 2003; 42(6): 778–83.

55. Gladman DD. Natural history of psoriatic arthritis. Baillieres Clin Rheumatol 1994; 8(2): 379–94.

56. Gladman DD, Farewell VT. Progression in psoriatic arthritis: role of time varying clinical indicators. J Rheumatol 1999; 26(11): 2409–13.

57. Queiro-Silva R, Torre-Alonso JC, Tinture-Eguren T, Lopez-Lagunas I. A polyarticular onset predicts erosive and deforming disease in psoriatic arthritis. Ann Rheum Dis 2003; 62(1): 68–70.

58. Eder L, Chandran V, Gladman DD. Repair of radiographic joint damage following treatment with etanercept in psoriatic arthritis is demonstrable by 3 radiographic methods. J Rheumatol 2011; 38(6): 1066–70.

59. van der Heijde D, Landewe RB. Dramatic repair of joint damage in psoriatic arthritis. J Rheumatol 2011; 38(6): 969–70.

CHAPTER 17

Use of ultrasound in psoriatic arthritis

Gurjit S. Kaeley

Introduction

Clinically psoriatic arthritis (PsA) has been categorized into distinct clinical entities, first described by Moll and Wright [1]. Since these manifestations can overlap and change in time, further classification systems such as the Classification of Psoriatic Arthritis (CASPAR) have been developed. However, this system does not take into account subclinical enthesitis and synovitis detected by advanced imaging such as magnetic resonance imaging (MRI) and ultrasound [2]. Furthermore, these modalities have demonstrated that non-axial disease has many overlapping features of enthesitis and soft tissue involvement. In this chapter, the ultrasound (US) imaging characteristics of enthesitis, synovitis, nail disease, and dactylitis in PsA will be reviewed.

Enthesitis

Enthesitis is a cardinal manifestation of PsA, and its importance is denoted by inclusion in the stem of the ClASsification of Psoriatic ARthritis (CASPAR) criteria [3] as well as its presence associated with significant negative impact on the quality of life [4]. Traditionally, enthesitis has been regarded as merely the inflammation of the junction of the tendon/ligament to osseous junction. However, this does not explain the site specificity of the entheses involved with spondyloarthritis including PsA. Histological examination of commonly involved entheses revealed that the majority of these are fibrocartilaginous entheses [5]. Tendon fibres can be attached directly to bone by Sharpey's fibres (fibrous entheses) or transition into a zone of fibrocartilage which is attached to bone (fibrocartilaginous entheses). The fibrocartilaginous junction assists in stress dissipation. In addition, many entheses have adjacent fat pads and bursae which also help in dissipating mechanical force. The realization that the enthesis is not only an anchor but also serves to dissipate mechanical stresses has led to recognition of the importance of adjacent tissues in the pathology of enthesitis. The alterations in the surrounding tissues are readily demonstrated by advanced imaging techniques such as MRI or ultrasound. Benjamin and McGonagle have proposed the concept of an enthesis organ or synovio-entheseal complex encompassing these tissues. This view also recognizes the juxtaposition of synovial tissue in many entheses leading to the idea that inflammation of the enthesis may lead to underlying synovitis.

US imaging can provide high resolution imaging of the enthesis, leading tendon or ligament, as well as adjacent tissues. In addition,

it can provide information about vascularity of the tissues utilizing Doppler methods and not requiring use of intravenous contrast material. The Outcome Measures in Rheumatology (OMERACT) group have recently suggested an update of the elementary lesions observed by sonography at a protypical enthesis such as the Achilles tendon [6]. Although these alterations are not specific to PsA, they nevertheless serve as a useful reference and are likely to be revised as further investigations proceed. A summary of the elementary lesions is given in Table 17.1 and Figure 17.1. Although, there was consensus to define active and chronic enthesitis based on structural abnormalities, agreement was not reached on which lesions could categorize these two states. One other important limitation is that it may be difficult to distinguish mechanical enthesopathy from inflammatory enthesitis based just on findings at one enthesis. However, the presence of these findings at multiple entheses would suggest the presence of peripheral enthesitis. Instead of defining findings as acute inflammatory or chronic damage, it may make more sense to classify them by type and site of pathology since the disease and cytokine pathways may be different and there may be confounding with mechanical factors at some of these sites and hence differences in responsiveness.

- ◆ Tendon/enthesis—ultrastructural changes
  - Hypoechogenecity, loss fibrillar echo texture, thickening
- ◆ Tendon/enthesis—calcification
  - Intratendinous, enthesophyte formation
- ◆ Entheseal vascularity (defined as within 2 mm from bone)—tendon hypervascularity may occur in mechanical tendinosis and may not signify enthesitis
- ◆ Fibrocartilagenous entheseal involvement, e.g. paratenonitis, medial malleolar erosions, adjacent tenosynovitis
- ◆ Bursitis—synovial lining proliferation, fluid in the bursa, increased vascularity
- ◆ Bone
  - Destructive—erosions
  - Osteoproliferative—periostitis, bone irregularities

Sonographic indices

The choice of which entheses to examine has been variable in the clinical indices and sonographic indices utilized by various

Table 17.1 Entheseal Structural Abnormalities Observed by Sonography and OMERACT US subgroup consensus level (A consensus of greater than 80% is required for adoption of the definition.)

Structural abnormality	Description	Consensus Level
Tendon thickening or hypoechogenecity	Loss of homogeneous fibrillary pattern, increased thickness distally compared to body of tendon	>80%
Tendon hypervascularity	Increased Doppler signal within tendon body	<80%
Entheseal hypoehogenecity	Hypoechogenicity and loss of homogeneous fibrillar echo texture of the tendon or ligament or capsule at the enthesis attachment.	>80%
Entheseal hypervascularity	Doppler signal present at the enthesis (within 2mm of the bone attachment)	>80%
Entheseal calcifications	Intra-tendinous calcification at the level of the enthesis and or enthesophyte formation.	>80%
Entheseal irregularities	Cortical irregularities at enthesis junction to bone	<80%
Erosions	Cortical break seen in orthogonal planes at enthesis insertion	>80%
Adjacent bursitis	Distension of adjacent bursa with fluid or hypoechogenic material with or without vascularity	<80%
Bone pulley enthesitis	Tenosynovitis with or without adjacent bony irregularity eg posterior tibial tendon at medial malleolus	Not tested
Tenonitis or paratenonitis	Hypoechogenicity and increased vascularity around tendons without synovial sheaths eg extensor tendon at the metacarpophalangeal joint, or thickening and increased vascularity of the paratenon at larger tendons such as Achilles Tendon.	Not tested

Reproduced from Terslev L, et al. Outcome Measures in Rheumatology Ultrasound Task F. Defining enthesis in spondyloarthritis by ultrasound: results of a Delphi process and of a reliability reading exercise. Arthritis care & research. 2014;66(5):741–8. doi: 10.1002/acr.22191. PubMed PMID: 24151222 with permission from Wiley.

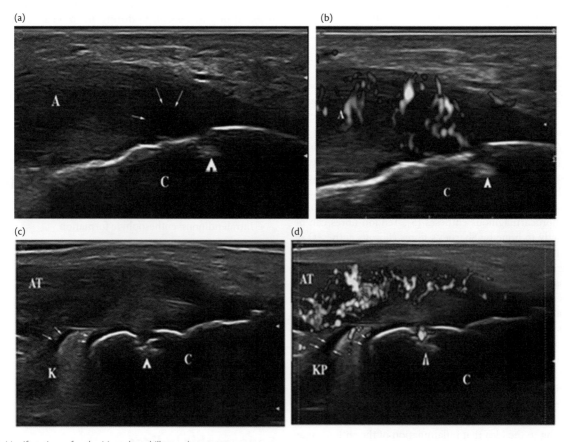

Figure 17.1 Manifestations of enthesitis at the achilles tendon.

1A and B: A—Swollen Achilles enthesis (A) with loss of fibrillary echo pattern (arrows), active power Doppler adjacent to the enthesis, as well as a calcaneal (C) erosion (arrow head). 1C and D: Swollen Achilles tendon (AT) with significant intra-tendinous vascularity. Erosion (arrow head) in superior pole of calcaneus (C) with abutting retrocalcaneal bursitis (arrows) which is present in a complex manner within Kagers fat pad (K).

investigators (See Table 17.2). Of note, the majority of these entheseal schemes have included lower extremity enthesis and all of them in particular have included the Achilles tendon. Some of the earlier schemes had a smaller number of entheses and their ultrastructural components included. Later schemes expanded on the ultrastructural components that were included as well as adding Doppler examination of these tissues. These indices were not tailored to PsA in particular and may not include commonly affected typical and atypical entheseal areas. For example, the posterior tibial tendon is not included in any of these schemes, but Galuzzo et al. have demonstrated that it may be involved in up to one third of PsA patients [7]. Similarly, periextensor tendinitis or tenonitis has been reported by several investigators in PsA as well as psoriasis patients but are not included in standardized indices [8–10].

One important purpose of developing sonographic entheseal indices is to be able to identify patients with psoriasis who may have occult PsA. De Fillipis et al. studied 24 patients with psoriasis and examined bilateral Achilles tendon insertions as well as flexor and extensor tendons at the level of the metacarpophalangeal joints [8]. Although all the patients were asymptomatic, a third of the patients had occult findings on sonography, the majority of which were in the hands. Inflammation was seen both at the extensor and flexor tendons. Subsequent investigators chose to use entheseal indices which did not include the hand and favoured the lower extremity. Gisondi et al. utilized the GUESS (Glasgow Ultrasound Enthesitis Scoring system) scoring system (without power Doppler) to examine asymptomatic psoriasis patients compared to controls [18]. They found that the mean GUESS score was higher in psoriasis patients compared with controls. Of note, the GUESS score correlated with age, body mass index (BMI), waist circumference, but not duration or severity of psoriasis.

Since the GUESS system examines only lower extremity entheses, there is likely a mechanical, weight-bearing interaction in combination with psoriasis. (Psoriasis and control groups were not different in BMI or waist circumference.) Guiterrez et al. reported on a similar study utilizing GUESS with power Doppler and found higher GUESS scores and power Doppler incidence in asymptomatic psoriasis patients [9]. In contrast to the Gisondi et al. study, they did not find any correlation with BMI, or severity or duration of psoriasis. Aydin et al. used the GUESS scoring system in conjunction with power Doppler to examine 100 patients with psoriasis and PsA in comparison to healthy controls [19]. Entheseal hypoechogenicity, thickening, and bursal enlargement grey scale changes were categorized as related to inflammation and added for a grey scale inflammation score whilst all Doppler scores were added to create a Doppler inflammation score. Grey scale changes of calcifications, erosions, and enthesophytes were added to create a chronicity score. Compared to healthy controls, patients with psoriasis or PsA had higher grey scale inflammation scores. PsA patients had higher grey scale inflammatory and chronic scores compared to psoriasis patients. The overall incidence of Doppler signal was low and found only at the retrocalcaneal bursa. PsA patients had a higher prevalence of power Doppler at the bursa compared to psoriasis patients. Although the authors report that PsA patients are more likely to have a vascular phenotype, this would only be supported at the bursa level. There was no analysis by BMI. Eder et al. utilized MASEI (Madrid Sonographic Enthesitis Index) to examine patients with psoriasis, PsA, and healthy controls [20]. Elements of the scoring system were categorized into grey scale inflammatory and chronic scores, in addition to power Doppler. Of note, the PsA patients were heavier and older than the psoriasis and healthy cohorts. Patients with PsA had the highest grey scale inflammatory and damage scores, followed by psoriasis patients when compared to healthy controls. However, in the subgroup of

Table 17.2 Sonographic indices utilized by various investigators

Entheses	GUESS	MASEI	SEI	Spanish School	'Sono' MASES	D'Agostino
Knee (quadriceps and patellar)	+	+	+	+		+
Achilles tendon	+	+	+	+	+	+
Plantar fascia	+	+	+	+		+
Triceps		+				
Elbow—medial and lateral epicondyle				+		+
1st and 7th costosternal joints					+	
Ant & post iliac spines, iliac crests					+	
5th lumbar spinous process					+	
Greater trochanter, pubis, tibialis anterior						+
DOPPLER		+		+	+	+

GUESS—Glasgow Ultrasound Enthesitis Scoring system—Balint et al. [11]

MASEI—Madrid Sonographic Enthesitis Index - de Miguel et al. [12]

SEI—Sonographic Enthesitis Index—Alcade et al. [13]

Spanish School—Naredo et al. [14]

'Sono' MASES—Maastricht Ankylosing Spondylitis Entheses Score (Klauser et al.; Kiris et al. [15, 16])

D'Agostino et al. [17]

patients with a BMI of greater than 30, no differences were seen between the PsA, psoriasis, and healthy control groups. Power Doppler signal was higher in the PsA group compared to the psoriasis group. There were no differences in the prevalence of power Doppler between the psoriasis and healthy control group. Overall the MASEI system had 30% sensitivity and 89% specificity in distinguishing PsA from psoriasis. In a recent study, response to lower extremity entheseal abnormalities to systemic therapies was reported by Acquacalda et al. [21]. Patients with psoriasis and PsA were recruited. In this small prospective study, no Doppler signal was reported in the entheses. In addition, active grey scale lesions were defined as tendon hypoechogenicity and thickening which were reported dichotomously. Tendon hypoechogenicity may be subjective and in the absence of direct tendon measurements and absence of Doppler signal, possibility of reporting bias by time, the validity of the findings are unclear.

Utilizing instruments that address anatomical areas that specifically affected by PsA may help improve the sensitivity as well as predictive value of US. Miedany et al. examined 126 patients with psoriasis clinically and with US at baseline, 6, and 12 months [22]. These variables were used to predict X-ray progression from baseline to 6 months (Modified Sharp score including distal interphalangeal [DIP] joints). Factors that were associated with progression of joint damage included baseline grey scale and Doppler synovitis of greater than grade 2, presence of baseline enthesitis as well as increased vascularity at entheses, baseline sonographic onychopathy as well as persistent synovitis, and enthesitis at 6 months. Several studies have been published following response to therapy in heterogeneous populations which included PsA patients. These studies demonstrated responsiveness to enthesitis after treatment with anti-TNF agents [23]. Litinsky et al. reported on responses in 43 consecutive PsA patients treated with either methotrexate (MTX) or adalimumab [24]. US areas examined included bilateral 2nd and 3rd finger extensor and flexor tendon thickness, plantar fascia, and Achilles tendon entheses. Decrease in tendon thickness was seen in the 24 patients treated with adalimumab, but not in the patients in the MTX arm. Overall several US parameters responded better to adalimumab than MTX.

In summary, US can depict granular manifestations of peripheral enthesitis and has a high level of sensitivity. The majority of published studies have utilized entheseal scores which were not developed a priori for PsA. Furthermore, since these systems are heavily weighted to lower extremity entheses, obesity is a significant confounding factor. Future studies should include entheseal sites such as the metacarpophalangeal periextensor region, as well as the posterior tibial tendon at the medial malleolus which may increase specificity and sensitivity. Sonography has a role in identifying early PsA patients as well as an outcome measure to follow response to therapeutic agents.

Nail disease

Nail disease in psoriasis and PsA can present as nail plate disorders such as pitting as well as onycholysis which is associated with nail bed pathology. The presence of nail disease is correlated with an increased incidence of joint disease as well as enthesitis [25]. In order to understand the basis of this, it is worth reviewing the anatomy of the nail complex. Although the nail is thought to be an epidermal appendage, it is closely related to the enthesis of the distal digits.

At the proximal portion of the nail, the nail matrix forms keratinocytes which later give rise to the hardened keratin of the nail [26]. Originally, it was thought that the nail matrix attaches to the periosteum of the bone. However, detailed gross and microanatomic studies have shown that the matrix terminates superficially and is enveloped by fibres of the extensor slip/tendon. Furthermore deep extensor tendon fibres insert distally in a fan-like fashion underneath the nail bed at the fingers and large toe [27, 28]. The extended insertion likely has a better mechanical advantage than if the fibres inserted just distal to the distal interphalangeal joint. The vascular and fibrous nail bed is attached to the periosteum and presumably the distal superficial fibres of the extensor fibres. Superficially, it is connected to the nail plate vial a corrugated interface. Finally, the collateral ligament which stabilizes the DIP joint, gives fibres that blend with the edges of the nail plate. The close proximity of extensor fibres as well as collateral ligament fibres to the nail may imply mechanical and proprioception for the nail. Reports of the right thumb being the commonest and worst afflicted nail adds evidence for a Koebner phenomenon also contributing to the pathogenesis of nail disease [29].

High resolution US can readily demonstrate the ultrastructural features of the nail. The nail plate is depicted as an apparent bi-layer with ventral and dorsal hyperechoic lines and an anechoic centre. (Figure 17.2) It can be followed proximally where it is seen to end as a sharp angulated edge cupped by fibres of the extensor tendon. The extensor fibres can be further followed proximally to the attachment on the proximal dorsal aspect of the distal phalange. In some cases, fibres can also be followed distally, diving deep to attach in the periosteum of the bone underneath the nail bed. Care needs to be taken in interpreting Doppler signal at the level of the distal phalanx and extensor tendon insertion. The dorsal aspect of this region is richly supplied with venous and capillary blood vessels. Short axis views may depict these distinctly. The nail bed appears as a homogeneous hypo-echoic area. Vascularity in the nail bed itself is demonstrated in a variable fashion.

Nail plate abnormalities demonstrated on US can range from pitting to complete obliteration of the apparent bi-layer as well as thickening of the nail plate. Thickening of the nail bed can also be observed. However, since vascularity is very variable in normal individuals, its assessment in abnormal nail beds is difficult to interpret. Increased thickness can also be seen in the extensor slip/tendon insertion at the base of the phalanx and in some cases abutting the nail matrix and deep to the nail bed. (Figure 17.3) Tan et al. studied the nail apparatus of the long and ring fingers in patients with PsA, osteoarthritis, and healthy controls [28]. They demonstrated enhancement in the pericapsular area as well distal to the DIP joint on water sensitive and contrast sequences in patients with PsA. Similar but less prominent changes were detected less frequently in patients with osteoarthritis. Thickened contrast enhancing tissue was also shown under the nail bed in PsA patients. In a sonographic study of patients with psoriasis and PsA, compared to controls, Aydin et al. demonstrated increased extensor slip/tendon at the level of the base of the phalange in psoriasis patients with nail disease [30]. Thickness of the nail plate and nail matrix, as well as skin, was higher in psoriatic patients compared to healthy controls. Extensor slip/tendon thickening was associated with increased skin thickness and oedema. These findings also occurred in a higher frequency in patients with clinical DIP disease. The importance of nail involvement was further emphasized by Ash

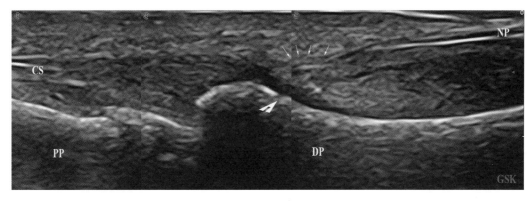

Figure 17.2 Sonographic appearances of the normal nail apparatus.

2: High resolution composite figure of the nail apparatus. Nail plate (NP) appears as an apparent bilayer. Distally, the nail bed is inferior to the nail plate. Proximally, the origin of the nail is at the nail matrix (arrows), which does not insert into bone and does receive fibres from the central slip/extensor (CS) complex. Of note the extensor apparatus fibers do not just insert on the base of the distal phalange (DP), but also continue further under the nail. (arrow head). PP—proximal phalange.

et al. in a study comparing psoriasis patients with and without nail disease to healthy controls [31]. Peripheral lower extremity as well elbow common extensor origin entheses were examined with sonography. Higher scores of both inflammatory and chronic entheseal changes were found in psoriasis patients with nail disease. Using modified NAPSI, the severity of the nail disease moderately correlated with both inflammation and chronicity scores, as did the duration of psoriasis. However, no correlation was found between skin PASI scores and US enthesitis scores.

Synovitis

In contrast to rheumatoid arthritis (RA), PsA can present with different clinical patterns of involvement as originally described by Moll and Wright. The differences between PsA and RA go beyond the detection of the pattern of synovitis. There are important differences in how the surrounding tissues are involved, morphology of

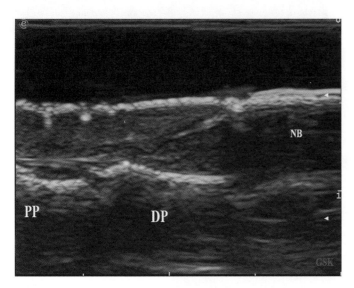

Figure 17.3 Sonographic manifestations of psoriatic nail disease.

Sonographic appearance of a severely affected nail. Note the complete obliteration and thickening of the nail plate causing posterior acoustic shadowing. The nail bed (NB) is markedly thickened. In this example, the extensor fibres travelling to the base of the nail at the nail matrix seem more obvious.

bone erosions, and, in contrast, the presence of osteoproliferation. Early investigations compared populations of patients with RA, PsA, and healthy subjects with multiple imaging modalities. Of note, earlier MRI equipment not only had less resolution but also used thicker cuts whilst earlier US machines operated a lower frequency with minimal post image processing resulting in relatively low resolution images compared to modern equipment. In a study comparing 25 fingers of RA patients, compared to 25 patients with PsA, Fournier et al. did not report extra-articular changes in RA patients. In contrast, patients with PsA had capsular enthesophytes, juxta-articular periosteal reaction, and enthesopathy at the profundus tendon attachment [32]. Weill et al. compared five patients each with RA, PsA, and healthy controls by using contrast-enhanced MRI, US and X-rays of the hands and feet. Bone proliferation as well as DIP involvement was reported to be more common than tenosynovitis in PsA patients. No other major differences were reported between the two groups. MRI and US were also more sensitive than plain X-rays in detecting inflammatory and destructive changes [33]. In a subsequent study of 13 patients with PsA examined with US, MRI, plain X-rays, and scintigraphy, Weiner et a. found plain radiography to be the least sensitive in detecting overall joint pathology. However, US and radiography detected more erosions and osteoproliferation than MRI did [34]. Marzo-Ortega et al. were not able to distinguish patients with PsA from those with RA based on contrast-enhanced MRI. One third of the PsA patients, however, had diffuse extracapsular involvement [35]. In a more contemporary investigation, Lin et al. reported higher prevalence of tenosynovitis, periosteal reaction, fluid around tendon insertions, and diffuse soft tissue swelling in PsA patients comparted to RA patients [36]. In an attempt to delineate PsA from RA, several authors have proposed that inflammation around the extensor tendons may be unique to PsA [37–39]. This is manifested by thickening of the extensor tendon often with an anechoic region around it associated with increased power Doppler signal. The extensor tendon at the level of the metacarpophalangeal does not have a synovial sheath, and hence enthesitis is invoked as a possible cause of this finding. Unfortunately, this finding is not unique to PsA, and it has been reported by several authors as also occurring in RA [40–43].

Sonography may be useful in the diagnosis and classification of articular manifestations of early PsA. In a study of 49 early PsA patients, Freeston et al. found that subclinical synovitis occurred often and most frequently at the wrists, knees, metatarsophalangeal joints, and metacarpophalangeal joints when examined by sonography. Furthermore, a significant proportion of individuals were reclassified from an oligoarticular presentation to polyarthritis [44].

Although much progress has been made in characterizing the unique findings of articular and periarticular manifestations in

PsA, (Figure 17.4) an US outcome tool has not yet been validated for therapeutic studies.

Dactylitis

Dactylitis, defined as a uniformly swollen digit, is a cardinal manifestation of PsA. It can present as an acutely swollen and tender

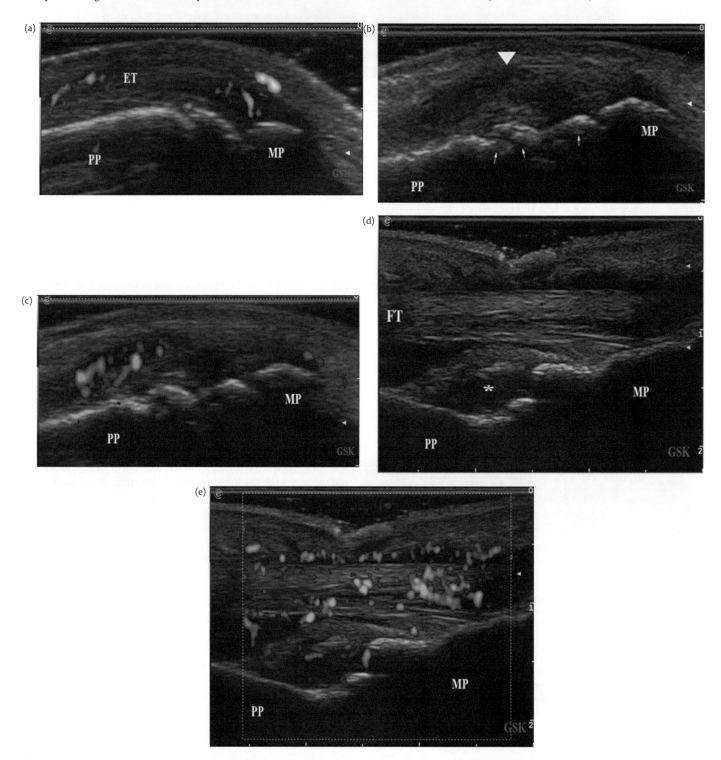

Figure 17.4 Articular and periarticular manifestations of PsA.
Sonographic examination of the third PIP in a patient with PsA. (a)—Dorsal views demonstrate edema and vascularity of the extensor tendon (ET) with mild underlying synovitis. Lateral views (b, c) reveal lateral collateral ligament thickening (arrow head), vascularity with underlying osteoproliferation. (Arrows). (d, e) Volar aspect of the same third PIP 3 joint reveals marked distension of the volar recess (asterix) as well as marked tenosynovitis of the flexor tendons (FT). PP proximal phalange, MP middle phalange.

Table 17.3 Elementary components of dactylitis and their demonstration by MRI or US

Elementary components	MRI	US
Soft tissue thickening, oedema	+	+
Flexor tendon tenosynovitis	+	+
Extensor tendon inflammation, thickening	+	+
Collateral ligament inflammation	+	-
Volar and plantar plate inflammation	+	-
Synovitis	+	+
Osteoproliferation—intra and extra-articular	-	+
Sesamoid abnormalities	-	+
Erosions	+	+
Nail—plate, matrix or bed abnormalities	-	-

digit or as an asymptomatic swollen digit. Its prevalence in PsA ranges from 16% to 48%. Its presence is associated with an increased disease severity as well as increased prevalence of erosive disease [45, 46]. Views of the pathophysiology of dactylitis have shifted from being caused solely by tenosynovitis [47–49] to involving multiple tissues in the digit [50–52]. The involvement of the digit is considered to be a form of enthesitis due to multiple tendon/ ligament connections to bone. A review of imaging studies in dactylitis categorized the various tissues involved (Table 17.3) as well as its documentation by imaging modality. Of note, abnormalities of smaller structures were documented by MRI imaging and not US possibly due to lack of insight into the involvement of these structures. In a recent high resolution MRI of dactylitic digits in 12 PsA patients compared to healthy controls, the prevalence of collateral ligament enthesitis was 75%, extensor tendon enthesitis 50%, volar plate enhancement 40%, and plantar plate enhancement 20%; 75% of the PsA cases demonstrated flexor tenosynovitis [53]. It is striking that the nail apparatus has largely not been studied in context with dactylitis.

The US subgroup of OMERACT (outcome measures in clinical Rheumatology clinical trials) has been working on developing an US outcome tool for dactylitis. Results of the first round Delphi were presented at OMERACT 12. It was proposed that the following areas should be prioritized in developing an instrument: soft tissue thickening, oedema, tenosynovitis, extensor tendon alterations, synovitis, nail plate abnormalities, and intracapsular calcification. Although there is agreement regarding inclusion of soft tissue thickening, there was little consensus as to how to measure or document it [54]. In summary, dactylitis epitomizes the many tissue compartments involved in the musculoskeletal manifestations of PsA. US has the ability to examine most of these compartments.

Conclusion

PsA is a fascinating inflammatory arthropathy with heterogeneous musculoskeletal manifestations. Sonography is able to depict the majority of non-spinal pathologies in the joints, tendons, tendon sheath, entheses, and the integumentary system. In some manifestations such as dactylitis, several tissue compartments are involved contemporaneously. Since many PsA patients have higher BMIs,

findings at lower extremity entheses should be interpreted with care. The future research agenda includes fine tuning the selection of entheses with the least confounding with age and BMI, as well as further developing and validating composite indices that may include different tissue compartments.

References

1. Moll JM, Wright V. Psoriatic arthritis. Semin Arthritis Rheum. 1973;3(1):55–78. PubMed PMID: 4581554.
2. Eder L, Gladman DD. Psoriatic arthritis: phenotypic variance and nosology. Current rheumatology reports. 2013;15(3):316. doi: 10.1007/s11926-013-0316-4. PubMed PMID: 23371481.
3. Taylor W, Gladman D, Helliwell P, et al. Classification criteria for psoriatic arthritis: development of new criteria from a large international study. Arthritis Rheum. 2006;54(8):2665–73. doi: 10.1002/art.21972. PubMed PMID: 16871531.
4. Turan Y, Duruoz MT, Cerrahoglu L. Relationship between enthesitis, clinical parameters and quality of life in spondyloarthritis. Joint, Bone, Spine. 2009;76(6):642–7. doi: 10.1016/j.jbspin.2009.03.005. PubMed PMID: 19464222.
5. Benjamin M, McGonagle D. The anatomical basis for disease localisation in seronegative spondyloarthropathy at entheses and related sites. JAnat. 2001;199(Pt 5):503–26. PubMed PMID: 11760883; PMCID: PMC1468363.
6. Terslev L, Naredo E, Iagnocco A, et al. Defining enthesitis in spondyloarthritis by ultrasound: results of a Delphi process and of a reliability reading exercise. Arthritis Care Res. 2014;66(5):741–8. doi: 10.1002/acr.22191. PubMed PMID: 24151222.
7. Galluzzo E, Lischi DM, Taglione E, et al. Sonographic analysis of the ankle in patients with psoriatic arthritis. ScandJ Rheumatol. 2000;29(1):52–5. PubMed PMID: 10722258.
8. De Filippis LG, Caliri A, Lo Gullo R, et al. Ultrasonography in the early diagnosis of psoriasis-associated enthesopathy. Int J Tissue React. 2005;27(4):159–62. PubMed PMID: 16440579.
9. Gutierrez M, Filippucci E, De Angelis R, et al. Subclinical entheseal involvement in patients with psoriasis: an ultrasound study. Semin Arthritis Rheum. 2011;40(5):407–12. doi: 10.1016/j.semarthrit.2010.05.009. PubMed PMID: 20688358.
10. Husic R, Gretler J, Felber A, et al. Disparity between ultrasound and clinical findings in psoriatic arthritis. Ann Rheum Dis. 2014;73(8):1529–36. doi: 10.1136/annrheumdis-2012-203073. PubMed PMID: 23740228.
11. Balint PV, Kane D, Wilson H, McInnes IB, Sturrock RD. Ultrasonography of entheseal insertions in the lower limb in spondyloarthropathy. Ann Rheum Dis. 2002;61(10):905–10. PubMed PMID: 12228161.
12. de Miguel E, Cobo T, Munoz-Fernandez S, et al. Validity of enthesis ultrasound assessment in spondylarthropathy. Ann Rheum Dis. 2009; 68(2):169–74. PubMed PMID: 18390909.
13. Alcalde M, Acebes JC, Cruz M, Gonzalez-Hombrado L, Herrero-Beaumont G, Sanchez-Pernaute O. A Sonographic Enthesitic Index of lower limbs is a valuable tool in the assessment of ankylosing spondylitis. Ann Rheum Dis. 2007;66(8):1015–9. doi: 10.1136/ard.2006.062174.
14. Naredo E, Batlle-Gualda E, García-Vivar ML, et al. Power Doppler Ultrasonography assessment of entheses in spondyloarthropathies: response to therapy of entheseal abnormalities. JRheumatol. 2010;37(10):2110–7. doi: 10.3899/jrheum.100136.
15. Kiris A, Kaya A, Ozgocmen S, Kocakoc E. Assessment of enthesitis in ankylosing spondylitis by power Doppler ultrasonography. Skeletal Radiol. 2006;35(7):522–8. doi: 10.1007/s00256-005-0071-3.
16. Klauser AS, Wipfler E, Dejaco C, Moriggl B, Duftner C, Schirmer M. Diagnostic values of history and clinical examination to predict ultrasound signs of chronic and acute enthesitis. Clin ExperRheumatol. 2008;26(4):548–53. doi: 2387 [pii]. PubMed PMID: 18799083.

17. D'Agostino MA, Said-Nahal R, Hacquard-Bouder C, Brasseur JL, Dougados M, Breban M. Assessment of peripheral enthesitis in the spondylarthropathies by ultrasonography combined with power Doppler: a cross-sectional study. Arthritis and rheumatism. 2003;48(2):523–33. doi: 10.1002/art.10812. PubMed PMID: 12571863.

18. Gisondi P, Tinazzi I, El-Dalati G, et al. Lower limb enthesopathy in patients with psoriasis without clinical signs of arthropathy: a hospital-based case-control study. Ann Rheum Dis. 2008;67(1):26–30. doi: 10.1136/ard.2007.075101. PubMed PMID: 17720726.

19. Aydin SZ, Ash ZR, Tinazzi I, et al. The link between enthesitis and arthritis in psoriatic arthritis: a switch to a vascular phenotype at insertions may play a role in arthritis development. Ann Rheum Dis. 2013;72(6):992–5. doi: 10.1136/annrheumdis-2012-201617. PubMed PMID: 22863575.

20. Eder L, Jayakar J, Thavaneswaran A, et al. Is the MAdrid Sonographic Enthesitis Index useful for differentiating psoriatic arthritis from psoriasis alone and healthy controls? J Rheumatol. 2014;41(3):466–72. doi: 10.3899/jrheum.130949. PubMed PMID: 24488414.

21. Acquacalda E, Albert C, Montaudie H, et al. Ultrasound study of entheses in psoriasis patients with or without musculoskeletal symptoms: A prospective study. Joint Bone Spine. 2015;82(4):267–71. doi: 10.1016/j.jbspin.2015.01.016. PubMed PMID: 25881759.

22. El Miedany Y, El Gaafary M, Youssef S, Ahmed I, Nasr A. Tailored approach to early psoriatic arthritis patients: clinical and ultrasonographic predictors for structural joint damage. Clin Rheumatol. 2015;34(2):307–13. doi: 10.1007/s10067-014-2630-2. PubMed PMID: 24794490.

23. Kaeley GS. Review of the use of ultrasound for the diagnosis and monitoring of enthesitis in psoriatic arthritis. Current Rheumatol Reports. 2011;13(4):338–45. Epub 2011/05/11. doi: 10.1007/s11926-011-0184-8. PubMed PMID: 21556844.

24. Litinsky I, Balbir-Gurman A, Wollman J, et al. Ultrasound assessment of enthesis thickening in psoriatic arthritis patients treated with adalimumab compared to methotrexate. Clin Rheumatol. 2016 5(2):363–70. doi: 10.1007/s10067-014-2753-5. PubMed PMID: 25073614.

25. Wilson FC, Icen M, Crowson CS, McEvoy MT, Gabriel SE, Kremers HM. Incidence and clinical predictors of psoriatic arthritis in patients with psoriasis: a population-based study. Arthritis Rheum. 2009;61(2):233–9. doi: 10.1002/art.24172. PubMed PMID: 19177544; PMCID: PMC3061343.

26. McGonagle D, Tan AL, Benjamin M. The nail as a musculoskeletal appendage--implications for an improved understanding of the link between psoriasis and arthritis. Dermatology. 2009;218(2):97–102. doi: 10.1159/000182250. PubMed PMID: 19060455.

27. Palomo Lopez P, Becerro de Bengoa Vallejo R, Lopez Lopez D, Prados Frutos JC, Alfonso Murillo Gonzalez J, Losa Iglesias ME. Anatomic relationship of the proximal nail matrix to the extensor hallucis longus tendon insertion. J Eur Acad Dermatol Venereol. 2015; 29(10):1967–71. doi: 10.1111/jdv.13108. PubMed PMID: 25807869.

28. Tan AL, Benjamin M, Toumi H, et al. The relationship between the extensor tendon enthesis and the nail in distal interphalangeal joint disease in psoriatic arthritis--a high-resolution MRI and histological study. Rheumatology (Oxford). 2007;46(2):253–6. doi: 10.1093/rheumatology/kel214. PubMed PMID: 16837473.

29. Rich P, Griffiths CE, Reich K, et al. Baseline nail disease in patients with moderate to severe psoriasis and response to treatment with infliximab during 1 year. J Am Acad Dermatol. 2008;58(2):224–31. doi: 10.1016/j.jaad.2007.07.042. PubMed PMID: 18083272.

30. Aydin SZ, Castillo-Gallego C, Ash ZR, et al. Ultrasonographic assessment of nail in psoriatic disease shows a link between onychopathy and distal interphalangeal joint extensor tendon enthesopathy. Dermatology. 2012;225(3):231–5. doi: 10.1159/000343607. PubMed PMID: 23128597.

31. Ash ZR, Tinazzi I, Gallego CC, et al. Psoriasis patients with nail disease have a greater magnitude of underlying systemic subclinical enthesopathy than those with normal nails. Ann Rheum Dis. 2012;71(4):553–6. doi: 10.1136/annrheumdis-2011-200478. PubMed PMID: 22156725.

32. Fournie B, Margarit-Coll N, Champetier de Ribes TL, et al. Extrasynovial ultrasound abnormalities in the psoriatic finger. Prospective comparative power-doppler study versus rheumatoid arthritis. Joint, Bone, Spine 2006;73(5):527–31. PubMed PMID: 16942893.

33. Wiell C, Szkudlarek M, Hasselquist M, Moller JM, et al. Ultrasonography, magnetic resonance imaging, radiography, and clinical assessment of inflammatory and destructive changes in fingers and toes of patients with psoriatic arthritis. Arthritis Res Ther. 2007;9:R119. PubMed PMID: doi:10.1186/ar2327.

34. Weiner SM, Jurenz S, Uhl M, et al. Ultrasonography in the assessment of peripheral joint involvement in psoriatic arthritis: a comparison with radiography, MRI and scintigraphy. Clin Rheumatol. 2008;27(8):983–9. doi: 10.1007/s10067-008-0835-y. PubMed PMID: 18259687.

35. Marzo-Ortega H, Tanner SF, Rhodes LA, et al. Magnetic resonance imaging in the assessment of metacarpophalangeal joint disease in early psoriatic and rheumatoid arthritis. Scand J Rheumatol. 2009;38(2):79–83. doi: 10.1080/03009740802448833. PubMed PMID: 19177263.

36. Lin Z, Wang Y, Mei Y, Zhao Y, Zhang Z. High-frequency ultrasound in the evaluation of psoriatic arthritis: a clinical study. Am J Med Sci. 2015;350(1):42–6. doi: 10.1097/MAJ.0000000000000504. PubMed PMID: 26110744.

37. Gutierrez M, Filippucci E, Salaffi F, Di Geso L, Grassi W. Differential diagnosis between rheumatoid arthritis and psoriatic arthritis: the value of ultrasound findings at metacarpophalangeal joints level. Ann Rheum Dis. 2011;70(6):1111–4. doi: 10.1136/ard.2010.147272. PubMed PMID: 21406459.

38. Filippou G, Di Sabatino V, Adinolfi A, et al. No enthesis should be overlooked when psoriatic arthritis is suspected: enthesitis of the extensor digitorum tendons. J Rheumatol. 2013;40(3):335. Epub 2013/03/05. doi: 10.3899/jrheum.121123. PubMed PMID: 23457399.

39. Husic R, Gretler J, Felber A, et al. Disparity between ultrasound and clinical findings in psoriatic arthritis. Ann Rheum Dis. 2013. doi: 10.1136/annrheumdis-2012-203073. PubMed PMID: 23740228.

40. Nieuwenhuis WP, Krabben A, Stomp W, et al. Evaluation of magnetic resonance imaging-detected tenosynovitis in the hand and wrist in early arthritis. Arthritis Rheumatol. 2015;67(4):869–76. doi: 10.1002/art.39000. PubMed PMID: 25510520.

41. Ramrattan LA, Kaeley GS. Ultrasound characteristics of extensor tendon abnormalities and peritendinous fluid in rheumatoid arthritis. Arthritis Rheum. 2013;65(SUPPL. 10):(S2686).

42. Backhaus M, Ohrndorf S, Kellner H, et al. Evaluation of a novel 7-joint ultrasound score in daily rheumatologic practice: a pilot project. Arthritis Rheum. 2009;61(9):1194–201. doi: 10.1002/art.24646. PubMed PMID: 19714611.

43. Wakefield RJ, O'Connor P J, Conaghan PG, et al. Finger tendon disease in untreated early rheumatoid arthritis: A comparison of ultrasound and magnetic resonance imaging. Arthritis Rheum 2007;57(7):1158–64. PubMed PMID: 17907233.

44. Freeston JE, Coates LC, Nam JL, et al. Is there subclinical synovitis in early psoriatic arthritis? A clinical comparison with gray-scale and power Doppler ultrasound. Arthritis Care Res 2014;66(3):432–9. doi: 10.1002/acr.22158. PubMed PMID: 24022986; PMCID: 4282111.

45. Helliwell PS. Established psoriatic arthritis: clinical aspects. J Rheumatol Supplement. 2009;83:21–3. doi: 10.3899/jrheum.090215. PubMed PMID: 19661532.

46. Brockbank JE, Stein M, Schentag CT, Gladman DD. Dactylitis in psoriatic arthritis: a marker for disease severity? Ann Rheum Dis. 2005;64(2):188–90. doi: 10.1136/ard.2003.018184. PubMed PMID: 15271771; PMCID: PMC1755375.

47. Olivieri I, Padula A, Scarano E, Scarpa R. Dactylitis or 'sausage-shaped' digit. J Rheumatol. 2007;34(6):1217–22. PubMed PMID: 17552053.

48. Wakefield RJ, Emery P, Veale D. Ultrasonography and psoriatic arthritis. J Rheumatol. 2000;27(6):1564–5. PubMed PMID: 10852294.

49. Kane D, Greaney T, Bresnihan B, Gibney R, FitzGerald O. Ultrasonography in the diagnosis and management of psoriatic dactylitis. J Rheumatol. 1999;26(8):1746–51. PubMed PMID: 10451072.

50. Bakewell CJ, Olivieri I, Aydin SZ, et al. Ultrasound and magnetic resonance imaging in the evaluation of psoriatic dactylitis: status and perspectives. J Rheumatol 2013;40(12):1951–7. doi: 10.3899/jrheum.130643. PubMed PMID: 24187105.

51. Olivieri I, Scarano E, Padula A, et al. Fast spin echo-T2-weighted sequences with fat saturation in toe dactylitis of spondyloarthritis. Clin Rheumatol. 2008;27(9):1141–5. doi: 10.1007/s10067-008-0882-4. PubMed PMID: 18528727.

52. Healy PJ, Groves C, Chandramohan M, Helliwell PS. MRI changes in psoriatic dactylitis—extent of pathology, relationship to tenderness and correlation with clinical indices. Rheumatology (Oxford). 2008;47(1):92–5. doi: 47/1/92 [pii] 10.1093/rheumatology/kem315. PubMed PMID: 18077498.

53. Tan AL, Fukuba E, Halliday NA, Tanner SF, Emery P, McGonagle D. High-resolution MRI assessment of dactylitis in psoriatic arthritis shows flexor tendon pulley and sheath-related enthesitis. Ann Rheum Dis. 2015;74(1):185–9. doi: 10.1136/annrheumdis-2014-205839. PubMed PMID: 25261575; PMCID: 4283670.

54. Bruyn GA, Naredo E, Iagnocco A, et al. The OMERACT Ultrasound Working Group 10 Years On: Update at OMERACT 12. J Rheumatol. 2015. doi: 10.3899/jrheum.141462. PubMed PMID: 25774059.

CHAPTER 18

MRI

Dennis McGonagle and Iris Eshed

Introduction

Radiographic imaging studies contributed to the formal recognition of psoriatic arthritis (PsA) as a unique entity, distinct from rheumatoid arthritis (RA). Given that the clinical phenotype of PsA may be so distinctive, radiographic imaging in clinical diagnosis is not always necessary. Nevertheless, there is a longstanding precedent for the use of conventional radiographic imaging in PsA assessment [1]. In the past two decades, there has been increasing use of both magnetic resonance imaging (MRI) and ultrasound in the evaluation of PsA with the focus of this chapter being MRI.

Unlike RA, which has a consistent phenotype of periarticular bone erosion and joint destruction and associated local and systemic osteoporosis, the imaging phenotypes of PsA are highly diverse [2]. These include periarticular joint destruction but also new bone formation including periostitis and where changes can sometimes be present in the same digit. (Figure 18.1) Although RA is generally viewed as a more destructive disease than PsA, the PsA-related arthritis mutilans phenotype is arguably the most destructive inflammatory arthritis of all. Also PsA is associated with many radiographic changes which are relatively unique to that condition including periostitis and a wealth of abnormalities including pencil-in-cup deformities. The aforementioned radiographic changes were seen during a time when patients presented with chronic end stage disease and where no effective therapies were available. This chapter on MRI will explain how the heterogeneity of radiographic findings might have a unified basis.

In the modern era, there is a need for prompt early diagnosis with effective treatment to prevent damage and also a need for prognostication [3]. The need for prognostic factors is particularly relevant given the lack of serological biomarkers comparable to early RA-associated autoantibodies. Also the extreme clinical heterogeneity in PsA ranging for monoarthritis to polyarticular arthritis, from axial involvement to peripheral involvement, and also including isolated polyenthesitis and isolated severe dactylitis underlines the need for good imaging biomarkers for early disease. Thus far, the best imaging biomarker for PsA has been radiographic erosions which predict progressive joint damage and even mortality [4, 5].

The anatomical inaccessibility of psoriatic inflammation in the axial skeleton and diffuse osteitis in the peripheral skeleton renders ultrasound of limited value in some settings. It is set against this background that this chapter covers MRI in its current role in the diagnosis and monitoring of PsA and its ongoing role in the assessment of prognosis.

History of MRI and psoriatic arthritis

The first MRI study to clearly highlight anatomical differences between PsA and RA was at the proximal interphalangeal (PIP) joints of the hands where capsular inflammation was more common in PsA [6]. Given the aforementioned differences between RA and PsA, it was surprising to note that initial MRI studies of knee involvement in PsA and RA did not reveal any significant difference between the diseases [7]. This occurred because the original MRI T1-weighted sequences, before the advent of fat suppression techniques, were not sensitive enough to show differences. It was the advent of such fat saturation or fat suppression methods that first allowed the typical diffuse bone marrow oedema pathology or osteitis to be appreciated. Indeed, fat suppressed MRI, with its ability to delineate sites of osteitis, has transformed the role of MRI in the assessment of PsA and the spondyloarthropathies (Figure 18.2).

From the original MRI protocols scanning single joints, there has been progress in several directions, including a move to whole body MRI to assess the extent of the disease and also high resolution MRI to delineate small joint structures that are not readily visualized on conventional techniques. Furthermore, specialist ultra-short echo time (UTE) MRI techniques have been developed to image both fibrocartilage and the entheses [8].

MRI interpretation considerations

The interpretation of MRI is dependent on three factors: firstly, knowledge of tissue anatomy; second, an understanding of the imaging technique; and third an understanding of disease pathological processes. As well reviewed in the literature, MRI, in particular fat suppression techniques, are useful for delineating sites of inflammation and it was the advent of fat suppression MRI that resulted in present day protocols for the rheumatic disorders [9]. Whilst an anatomical knowledge of disease is a pre-requisite for the proper radiological interpretation of imaging, the actual anatomical basis for PsA has emerged from MRI studies, which is briefly discussed here at the outset.

Psoriatic arthritis is increasingly recognized to localize at sites of high mechanical stress and tissue microdamage. These sites in the skeleton include the entheses and immediately adjacent bones to which the enthesis are functionally anchored. As reviewed elsewhere, there are several other structures including fibrocartilaginous synovial joints such as the sternoclavicular and sacroiliac joints which PsA not uncommonly involves. Because these entheseal structures are relatively avascular, inflammation of knee structures, as depicted on conventional MRI, may

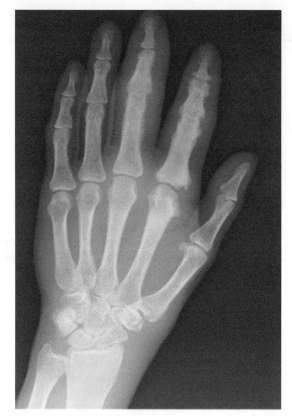

Figure 18.1 This is a right hand radiograph of a 54-year-old female with PsA. There is soft tissue swelling of the 2nd and 3rd digits compatible with 'sausage digits' or dactylitis. In addition, marginal erosions can be detected in the DIP and PIP of these fingers and the MCP joint of the 2nd finger. Another typical finding is periostitis along the proximal phalanges of these fingers. Prior to the advent of MRI, a unifying concept for these disparate radiographic features had not been defined. The adoption of MRI contributed to the realization that the PsA disease spectrum localised to the enthesis organ, including the synovio-entheseal complex and adjacent bone and other sites of high levels of biomechanical stressing in the skeleton.

show as high signal in the soft tissues including the joint cavity or synovium, periarticular soft tissues, or the bone marrow itself. The relatively avascular enthesis with a paucity of immune cells is functionally integrated with adjacent synovium forming a synovio-entheseal complex and as a result of this anatomical configuration entheseal-associated pathology may manifest as synovitis on MRI [10]. Therefore, juxta-articular entheseal inflammatory change may be impossible to appreciate and may thus manifest as synovitis and joint effusion [10]. Several animal models have convincingly shown the primacy of enthesitis and the secondary nature of synovitis in psoriatic-like disease but it is obviously not possible to do this in humans. Nevertheless, the entheseal concept which emerged from MRI studies in humans, serves as a key pathological consideration when interpreting MRI in PsA.

Evaluation of different joints in psoriatic arthritis

Knee joint and other large joints

The knee joint is especially important in PsA because it may be involved as part of monoarticular, oligoarticular, or polyarticular disease. Since knee joint swelling has such a wide differential diagnosis and may co-exist with osteoarthritis (OA) and since some psoriatic cases may not have psoriasis at disease onset, or occasionally never, an ability to define the PsA phenotype at onset would be of considerable value. The original MRI studies, using T1-weighted imaging, showed no differences between RA and PsA [7]. Fat suppression MRI showed a high prevalence of clinically non detectable enthesitis and osteitis in PsA and other forms of spondyloarthritis but not in RA [7]. Given the multiplicity of entheses within and around the knee and given the large extent of synovial tissue around the knee, MRI has not proven a reliable tool in the differentiation between PsA and other arthropathies around the knee (Figure 18.3). Nevertheless, the enthesitis/osteitis lesion may be very useful for recognizing PsA in large joints such as the knee (Figure 18.4). In

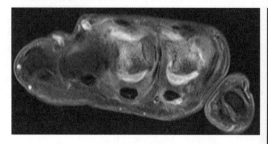

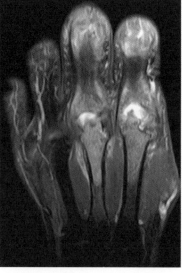

Figure 18.2 Coronal and axial T1-w with fat saturation images after gadolinium injection in a 54-year-old woman with PsA. Diffuse osteitis of the involved fingers as well as erosions of the 2nd MCP joint and synovitis of the 2nd and 3rd MCP joints. Tenosynovitis of the flexor tendon of the 2nd finger is also observed.

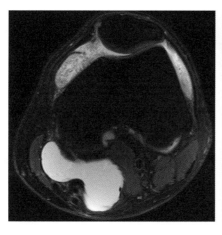
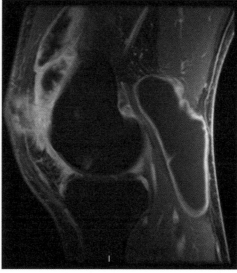

Figure 18.3 Axial T2W with fat suppression and sagittal T1W with fat saturation post gadolinium injection images of the left knee of a 43-year-old male with PsA demonstrating pronounced synovitis in the suprapatellar bursa and a large amount of fluid in a baker cyst. MRI studies of the knee which has numerous entheses and synovio-entheseal complexes often makes it difficult to recognize sites of enthestitis in large joints.

the spine, osteitis lesions are associated with progressive sacroiliac joint destruction so it was hypothesized that MRI-determined osteitis in knee joint disease equated with a poor prognosis. A study looked at the value of osteitis in the knee joint and prognosis of knee arthritis. The presence of psoriasis but not MRI-determined osteitis at that site at baseline was the best predictor of knee joint disease chronicity [11].

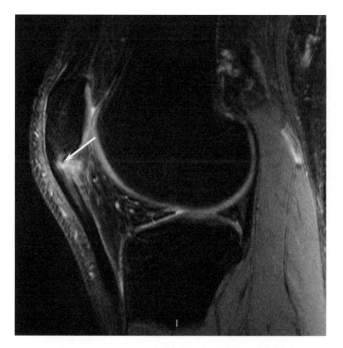

Figure 18.4 Sagittal T2w with fat suppression image of a 21-year-old male with psoriasis demonstrating patellar tendon enthesitis including patellar tendon thickening and high signal intensity as well as peri-entheseal soft tissue inflammation and insertional osteitis at the lower patellar pole.

Imaging studies of osteitis pre and post anti-TNF have shown that the lesions improve significantly following biological therapy [12]. This rapid improvement in osteitis, which is a forerunner of radiographic erosion, is likely relevant for explaining why biological therapy is so effective for stopping X-ray progression in PsA.

Entheseal changes have also been described in other large joints including the shoulder joint in spondyloarthritis and PsA. A typical location for such lesions to occur is at the supraspinatus insertion but lesions are also described at other entheseal sites including the deltoid muscle origin (Figure 18.5).

Imaging of hand metacarpophalangeal and proximal interphalangeal joints disease

The original study of hand disease in PsA showed a high prevalence of extra capsular and entheseal abnormalities compared to RA [6]. This raised the hope that seronegative RA could be distinguished from polyarticular PsA on the basis of entheseal abnormalities. Several other studies have shown a higher prevalence of extra capsular and bone oedema reactions in the hand joints in PsA [13]. These are statistical associations, and although not proven to be useful at an individual patient level, they can be used to robustly support a diagnosis of PsA [14]. A particular problem encountered was that some groups of generalized hand OA had a pattern of pathology centred on the enthesis making differentiation between PsA and OA difficult [14, 15]. Likewise, a large number of juxtaposed joints in the wrists with multiple areas of synovium and enthesis has limited the utility of MRI in the differentiation between these diseases in the wrist.

The PIP joint is unusual in that the three major categories of arthritis, namely RA, OA, and PsA, have a tendency to afflict this joint. In the modern era early differentiation is increasingly important between these conditions. Analogous to DIP joint arthropathy, MRI studies showed that PIP OA and PIP PsA may be impossible to tell apart due to a common entheseal and capsular basis and because the early stages of hand OA may have a marked inflammatory

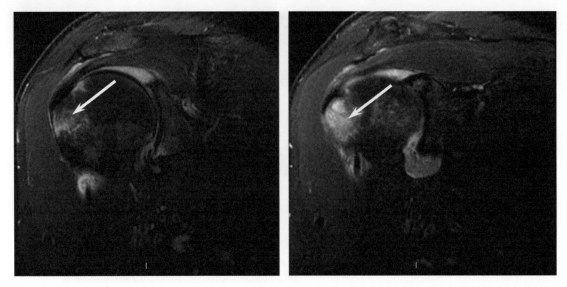

Figure 18.5 Coronal T2w with fat suppression images of a 63-year-old male with PsA. There is enthesitis of the supraspinatus tendinous insertion at the greater tuberosity. With pronounced bone marrow oedema (osteitis) at the insertional site (white arrow). Synovitis can also be detected in the axillary pouch.

component. On the other hand, most cases of RA could be delineated based on the synovial centric pattern of disease [14].

Imaging of hand distal interphalangeal joint disease

It has been known for 60 years that PsA is strongly associated with nail disease and that DIP joint disease showed an especially strong association. An explanation for this came from MRI studies showing that DIP joint inflammation was associated with extension of the inflammatory process to the nail matrix region. A consistent feature of DIP disease on MRI is extracapsular oedema, diffuse osteitis, and entheseal changes which was first demonstrated on high resolution MRI [16] (Figure 18.6).

Given that DIP joint disease can be associated with the most progressive and destructive form of PsA, namely arthritis mutilans, it could have been envisaged a few decades ago that MRI would have transformed the recognition of this group. However, arthritis mutilans is now comparatively rare, but MRI has nevertheless contributed to our understanding of the disease [17]. Disease of the DIP joint is associated with florid osteitis as inferred from MRI but proof that this is a forerunner of mutilans has not been furnished. MRI-determined DIP joint osteitis was associated with the

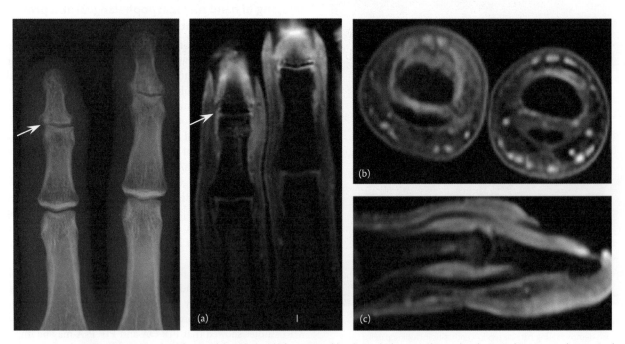

Figure 18.6 An AP radiograph of the 2nd and 3rd fingers of the right hand of a 37-year-old male in which a typical PsA related marginal erosion can be seen in the 2nd DIP joint (arrow). The MRI shows, coronal (A) , axial (B) and sagittal (C) T1W with fat suppression after gadolinium injection images of these fingers. The same joint erosion can be detected as well as marrow oedema at the proximal phalynx is also evident.

development of subsequent nail changes which underscores the close functional inter-relationship between the nail and the bone at that site [18]. In animal models, osteitis at other sites in the skeleton is associated with progressive joint destruction, so it is conceivable that MRI osteitis may be a forerunner of a more destructive arthritis. However, in an era of effective biological therapy, the issue of mutilans arthritis is less of a clinical problem.

DIP joint disease in psoriatic arthritis and osteoarthritis

Of note, the other major category of DIP arthropathy is OA. Given that psoriasis affects approximately 2% of the population and given that OA is very common, accurate diagnosis between these arthropathies in early disease is important. This may be more difficult than one might think since the early phases of OA often has an inflammatory nature and lacks the characteristic late disease features of Heberden's nodes. When MRI was applied to the study of early DIP disease in PsA and OA, the findings were somewhat unexpected. It was hypothesized that the entheseal centric nature of PsA DIP disease would be readily differentiated from the cartilage centric pathology of DIP OA. Whilst inflammatory changes were more common in PsA and cartilage damage was more common in OA, it was impossible to consistently differentiate between the disease groups [16]. Unexpectedly the OA cases also showed prominent entheseal abnormalities and adjacent bone marrow oedema changes which pointed to a classification of an OA subgroup as being enthesis associated [15].

These MRI observations indicate that enthesopathy may also be crucial for some types of OA and contribute to an anatomical classification of OA where the diffuse generalized hand variety is entheseal related. Given that entheses are sites of high mechanical stress and are the largest structures in the small joints of the hand, it is hardly surprising that OA, a disease of 'wear and tear' affects these entheses.

The nail

In the original description of PsA, it was noted that up to 90% of cases had nail disease which was significantly higher than the prevalence of nail disease in psoriasis [19]. Furthermore, a link between DIP arthropathy and involvement of the immediately adjacent nail is well recognized [20]. In the last decade, nail disease and scalp and genital disease have been recognized as predictors for the future development of PsA among patients with psoriasis [21]. The application of MRI to DIP joint disease showed that nail matrix and joint disease were virtually indistinguishable [16].

Subsequently, ultrasound imaging studies showed that nail disease was associated with enthesopathy in the adjacent extensor tendon in subjects with psoriasis. Moreover, nail psoriasis in subjects without PsA is associated with remote systemic enthesopathy [22, 23]. These observations relating to nail disease could be of great relevance for the early identification of PsA and stem from MRI research studies.

Studies using high resolution MRI in subjects with early PsA show that DIP/IP arthropathy was extremely diffuse with extensive entheseal involvement, diffuse osteitis, and diffuse extracapsular changes that extended to the nail matrix region (Figure 18.7). This prompted histological studies of cadaveric tissues in the same sagittal orientations and showed that the extensor tendon enthesis split with fibres anchoring directly to the nail. This elaborate enthesis organ helps explain the link between the nail, enthesis and bone disease [17].

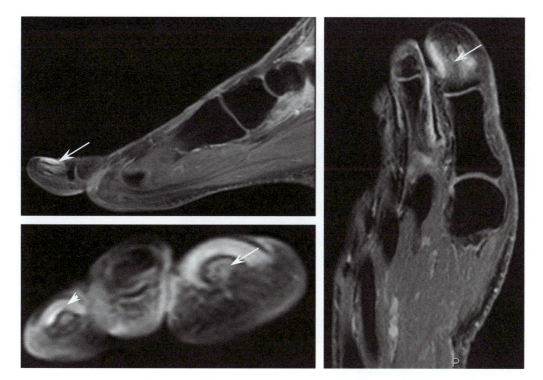

Figure 18.7 Post contrast T1w with fat suppression images of the left foot of a 59-year-old female with PsA. Osteitis of the distal phalange of the 1st toe is present (arrows) as well as enthesitis of the nail bed of the same toe and of the 3rd toe (arrowhead). Given that diffuse underlying osteitis is such a common finding at sites of nail disease, it is suspected but not proven, that such osteitis may be a forerunner of radiographic arthritis mutilans.

Dactylitis

Dactylitis or sausage digits are a characteristic feature of PsA. Whilst this lesion in the context of psoriasis is clinically diagnostic, there is probably little use for routine clinical MRI. However, imaging is important in cases where there may be no psoriasis and other differential diagnoses such as osteomyelitis, abscess formation, gout, pseudogout, or tissue infiltration by tumour or sarcoid need excluding. The lack of focal collections or tissue destruction point towards inflammatory dactylitis rather than an alternative diagnosis. Diffuse post contrast agent enhancement without tissue destruction in early diseases also supports such a diagnosis.

Of note, MRI has played an especially important role in elucidating the microanatomical basis for dactylitis. The first MRI study of dactylitis showed that flexor tenosynovitis rather than enthesitis was the most striking lesion [24]. Until recently, it was hard to reconcile dactylitis with associated enthesitis especially in the context of the dominant flexor tendon lesion which ostensibly appeared to point towards a synovial centric disease [25] (Figure 18.8). High resolution MRI studies showed diffuse inflammation adjacent to entheses around the finger joints pointing directly towards entheseal involvement [26]. Other studies also reported diffuse bone osteitis—a lesion that typically occurs in bones at sites of high mechanical stress and typically associated with enthesitis in PsA [27].

Recent high resolution MRI studies have helped improve the understanding of PsA-related dactylitis. The flexor tendons have a network of pulleys including the A1, A2, and A3 pulleys in addition to several others. These are ring like mini entheses that anchor the flexor tendons to the bone. In PsA, but not normal pulley anchorage points, these exhibited high signal on fat suppression MRI that is indicative of pulley enthesitis [16]. It is likely that this MRI abnormality may be linked to the abnormality evident on ultrasound termed 'pseudotenosynovitis'. This depicts inflammation outside of the tendon sheath and is not seen in RA and mechanistically it could be consequent to inflammation outside the actual tenosynovial sheath related to the pulleys. It is possible that digital tenosynovitis without clinical dactylitis in early PsA may have the same micro-anatomical basis. Further imaging studies are needed to evaluate whether US or MRI could be used to differentiate between these conditions.

The SAPHO syndrome

The term SAPHO syndrome denotes synovitis, acne, pustulosis, hyperostosis, osteitis. Patients with psoriasis and pustular lesions on the hands and feet in particular may present with sternoclavical joint involvement with impressive swelling of this region and associated loss of motion. In the modern era, patients tend to present early in the course of disease and at a stage when X-ray assessment is usually normal. The major differential diagnoses include osteomyelitis and sternoclavicular joint septic arthritis. These lesions may be relatively asymptomatic in PsA and SAPHO type lesions may occur in subjects with psoriasis and without arthritis [28]. Historically many of these cases have been sent for open biopsy procedures which reported neutrophilic-related osseous inflammation, frequently interpreted as supporting the concept of infection at that site. The advent of fat suppression MRI has transformed the recognition of SAPHO with the characteristic feature of diffuse bone oedema of the clavicular head near the sternum and adjacent manubrium (Figure 18.9). Quite often there is diffuse adjacent soft tissue inflammation and diffuse inflammation within the sternoclavicular joint synovial compartment. With more chronic or advanced disease MRI evidence of erosion may be evident.

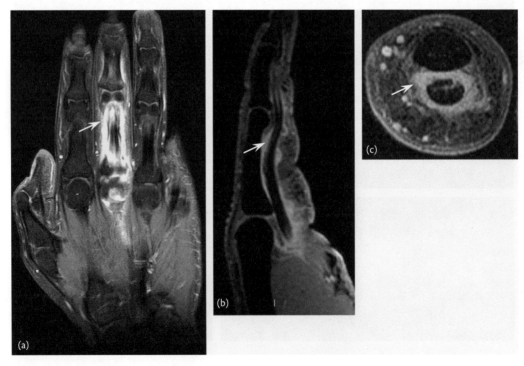

Figure 18.8 Post contrast coronal (A), sagittal (B) and axial (C) T1w with fat suppression images of the left hand of a 34-year-old male with PsA demonstrating flexor tenosynovitis of the 3rd finger (white arrows). Very high resolution MRI has shown a link between such tenosynovitis and the A1–3 minienthesis pulleys.

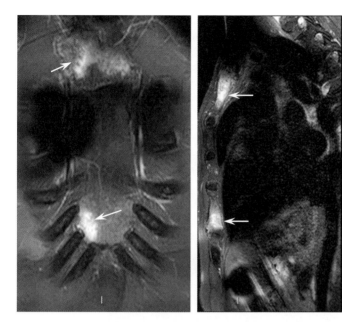

Figure 18.9 Coronal and sagittal T2 fat suppression images of the sternum of a 43-year-old male with PsA. Enthesitis of the costo-sternal junction of the 1st and 11th ribs on the right as evidenced by bone marrow oedema (arrows).

The SAPHO syndrome is another example of how MRI pointed towards a unifying concept in PsA. Just like the entheses and other fibrocartilaginous joints including the sacroiliac joints, it exhibits the peri-fibrocartilageous diffuse osteitis [29]. In the present era,

the early use of steroids and other strategies for SAPHO have likely changed the natural history of this condition and the later phases of disease with osteolysis are now infrequently seen in our practice. This is reminiscent of osteolysis in peripheral joints such as the terminal phalanges of the hands and feet where osteolysis is less often seen. With respect to the SAPHO syndrome, it needs to be borne in mind that this can occur at other fibrocartilaginous joints including the temporomandibular and acromioclavicular jointsand in the spine [30]. In a patient presenting with arthropathy of these sites a careful clinical history for psoriasis should be sought in order to support the diagnosis.

Spine and sacroiliac joints

Axial PsA showed two basic patterns of disease—a diffuse 'bamboo spine' appearance reminiscent of AS and a more PsA-specific pattern including an asymmetrical pattern of sacroiliitis, a propensity for neck involvement, and 'chunky syndesmophytes' [31]. Compared to other areas of the body, there has been a relative dearth of imaging reported in the spine in PsA and a lot of imaging data is extrapolated from AS and axial spondyloarthropathies. The neck is a common site of involvement in PsA axial disease, but there is little MRI data reported on this region in the literature (Figure 18.10). The MRI changes in PsA may be similar to those seen in axial SpA and AS. These include the acute changes of enthesitis/osteitis and also chronic post-inflammatory fatty corner lesions (Figure 18.11). Spinal MRI may also show the large chunky syndesmophytes that were first described using

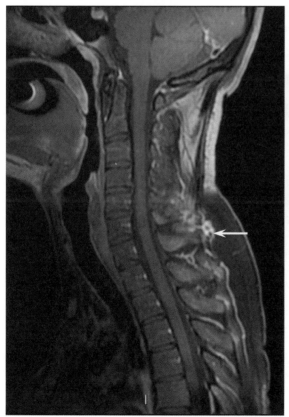

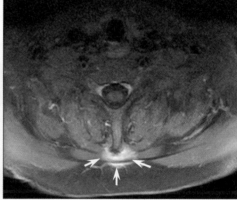

Figure 18.10 Sagittal and axial post contrast T1w with fat suppression images of a 28-year-old male with PsA. This demonstrates focal enthesitis of the supraspinous ligament of C7 vertebra (arrows).

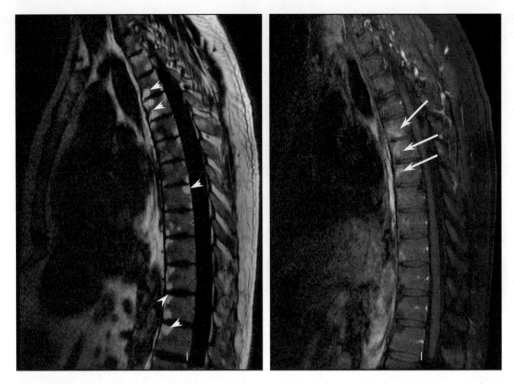

Figure 18.11 Sagittal T1w and STIR images of the thoracic spine of a 48-year-old male with longstanding PsA. This shows numerous corner fatty lesions (white arrows on left panel depicts a small proportion of these). Multiple fatty lesions are linked to spondylarthritis but not degenerative arthritis. In this case there is also acute inflammatory enthesitis/osteitis lesions compatible with spondyloarthropathy (arrows on the right panel).

radiographic techniques. These probably are a post-inflammatory tissue repair response and may be present at the same time as on-going active areas of osteitis at the same location or at different sites (Figure 18.12).

Clinical and imaging studies are increasingly supporting the concept that HLA-B27 axial PsA with psoriasis is simply anky-losing spondylitis (AS) in a patient with psoriasis. Firstly, when subjects with psoriasis are *HLA-B27* positive they tend to develop

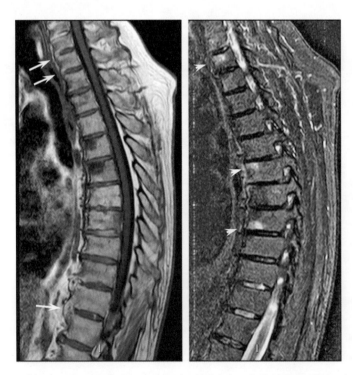

Figure 18.12 Sagittal T1w and STIR images of the thoracic spine of a 67-year-old male with PsA. Anterior bridging syndesmophytes are present in the upper and lower thoracic vertebrae (arrows on left panel). Corner inflammatory bone marrow edema compatible with peri-entheseal osteitis is noted in several vertebras (arrowheads).

PsA around the same time as psoriasis which is usually at a younger age. Secondly, MRI studies have looked at known AS, *HLA-B27* positive and *HLA-B27* negative axial PsA. It was already reported that carriage of the *HLA-B27* gene was associated with more diffuse enthesitis in the heel, shoulder, and spine in AS [32]. Studies in axial PsA showed that the *HLA-B27* positive axial group had a pattern of disease indistinguishable from AS [33]. However, the *HLA-B27* negative axial PsA group had a much lower frequency of peri-entheseal osteitis [33].

These observations are also of clinical relevance. About 30% of patients with AS with symptomatic spinal disease have a normal MRI. This does not exclude disease as it may be soft tissue inflammation without osteitis that is the driving forces for pain in these situations but this remains to be proven. However, in *HLA-B27* negative axial PsA with symptoms, the majority of cases may have normal MRI imaging [33]. Also normal MRI of the spine may be prognostically relevant based on extrapolations from AS. In AS, diffuse osteitis or post inflammatory fatty changes in the vertebral bodies may be prognostically relevant for future spinal fusion. Such changes in a *HLA-B27* positive axial PsA cases probably have the same relevance and might point towards a low probability of spinal fusion at a later date but this remains largely conjectural due to the absence of data from axial PsA.

The sacroiliac joint

Most of the information pertaining to the diagnostic and prognostic imaging of the sacroiliac joint (SIJ) comes from AS and early axial SpA [34]. Although the diagnostic and prognostic implications of early SIJ PsA disease have not been carefully evaluated in PsA, it is probably safe to extrapolate from axial SpA data especially in relationship to PsA SIJ disease, especially in *HLA-B27* positive cases. For SIJ osteitis, it has been shown that this is a forerunner of later radiographic sacroiliitis [34]. Similar patterns of MRI determined bone marrow oedema are well recognized in PsA (see Figure 18.13). Likewise, the chronic erosive changes noted in AS and SpA are also evident in some cases of PsA SIJ disease (Figure 18.14).

Given the increasing evidence that PsA is a biomechanical-stress-associated disease and given that PsA cases often have high BMIs, it is important to understand that all MRI-determined bone oedema in the SIJ may not be due to active disease. Normal subjects do occasionally have focal areas of bone oedema in the SIJ and in the spine. On their own, such lesions cannot be taken as proof of a positive MRI scan and detailed clinical consideration imperative for diagnosis.

The foot

The foot and ankle is commonly involved in PsA. Some abnormalities including plantar fasciitis and Achilles enthesitis are readily recognizable from the clinical perspective. However, MRI is commonly used for confirmation of the diagnosis at such sites of disease and typically shows soft tissue inflammatory changes and bone oedema (Figure 18.15).

Other disease features such as diffuse foot swelling may cause diagnostic confusion. Like the MRI changes at other sites in the body, diffuse bone marrow oedema may occur at entheses, the bones of the foot, and regions where tendons wrap around bones that have been dubbed as 'functional entheses' [29] (Figure 18.16).

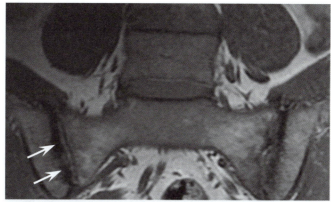
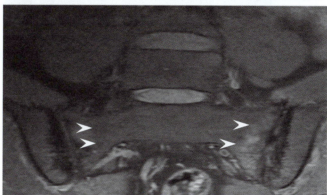

Figure 18.13 Semicoronal T1w and STIR images of the sacroiliac joints of a 44-year-old male with PsA. Structural and acute inflammatory lesions of the sacroiliac joints are evident. These include erosions and subchondral bone on the upper panel (arrows) and periarticular bone marrow edema on the lower panel (arrowheads).

Other manifestations

PsA is associated with several other patterns of disease that are rare and given that psoriasis itself may be overlooked then a reporting radiologist may not suggest PsA as part of the differential diagnosis. One such arthropathy is the psoriatic onychopachydermoperiostitis (POPP) syndrome. This may be completely missed and put down to fungal nail disease and osteomyelitis. The MRI in this condition shows diffuse digital osteitis and CT scanning may show wisps of new bone around the digit or a more diffuse periosteal reaction. (Figure 18.17). A prompt diagnosis will prevent needless open biopsies and prolonged antibiotic therapy or possibly surgical debridement or even amputation. For resistant cases, anti TNF may be effective and the diffuse MRI bone oedema resolves thereafter [35]. Periostitis is another well-recognized feature of PsA on radiographic assessment. MRI in PsA showing diffuse high signal along the periosteum and adjacent soft tissues and associated diffuse bone marrow oedema is the likely imaging forerunner of this radiographic abnormality.

Measuring MRI changes

In RA, synovitis is the primary lesion and erosion is secondary so the measurement of synovitis as determined by MRI is relatively easy because a line can be drawn around the joint capsule pre and

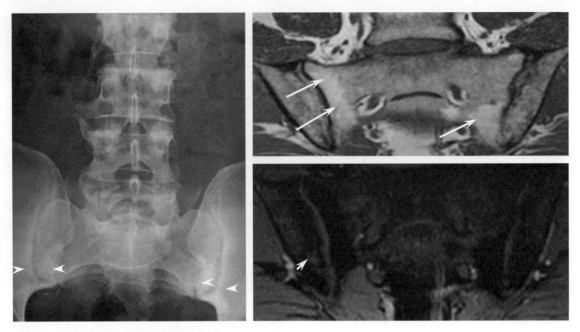

Figure 18.14 Frontal radiograph of the lumbar spine of a 56-year-old male with low back pain in which bilateral sacroiliitis (arrowheads) is evident. Semicoronal T1w and post contrast T1w with fat suppression images of the sacroiliac joints demonstrating changes of predominant chronic sacroiliac joint disease with fatty replacement and bone bridging (long arrows). There is minimal osteitis (short arrow).

post therapy. However, given the diffuse pathological process in PsA, including extensive subcutaneous oedema and diffuse osteitis related to disease localization to sites of high mechanical stress, it can be extremely difficult to measure such lesions. MRI certainly has a role for determining which patients who are in clinical remission actually have imaging remission with a complete absence of synovitis, osteitis, and enthesitis, and this is an area of ongoing research [36].

Other MRI techniques

Whole body MRI can detect the full extent and burden of disease and may have a role in the diagnostic evaluation of PsA and SpA. However, it is more time consuming to perform and also to evaluate and score. Its role in diagnosis and monitoring awaits further exploration and will undoubtedly be complicated by the fact that subclinical MRI entheseal changes are not uncommon in normals [37]. UTE imaging is another technique that has been applied in the last decade and is useful for the imaging of enthesis fibrocartilage that otherwise returns a signal void on conventional MRI. At this time UTE techniques are a research tool and its current use is geared towards understanding early fibrocartilage changes rather than having proven clinical application [38].

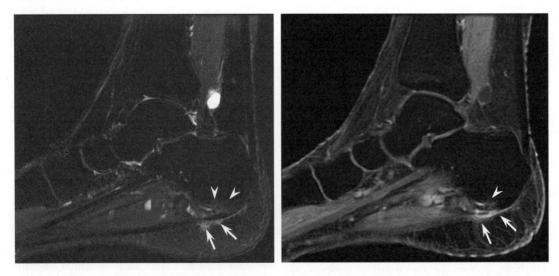

Figure 18.15 Sagittal T2 with fat suppression and post contrast T1w with fat suppression images of the ankle of a 55-year-old female with PsA demonstrating enthesitis of the plantar fascia including insertional bone marrow oedema (arrowheads), entheseal and perientheseal soft tissue inflammation (arrows).

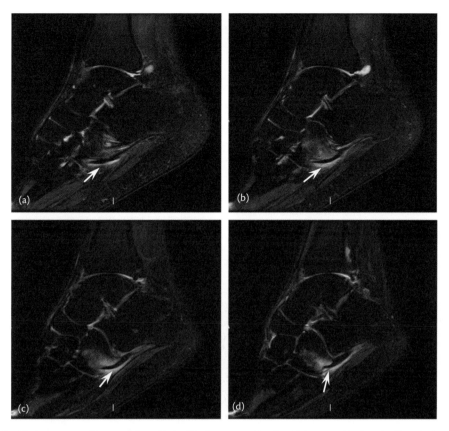

Figure 18.16 Sequential sagittal T2 fat suppressed images of the ankle (A-D) of a 53-year-old male with long-standing lateral ankle pain demonstrating tenosynovitis of the peroneus longus. There is tendon and bone marrow edema of the cuboid bone, findings compatible with 'functional enthesitis'—the site where tendons change direction and exert complex biomechanical forces on the bone analogous to those exerted at the enthesis.

Summary

The use of MRI has transformed the micro-anatomical understanding of PsA. The insights gained from such studies in humans have been used to show the primacy of enthesitis in animal models. MRI has been pivotal to showing the link between nail psoriasis and arthritis and also the basis for dactylitis. The ability of MRI to determine prognosis in PsA has not yet added significantly to the literature where, thus far, persistent swelling, elevation of C-reactive protein and radiographic damage are the best

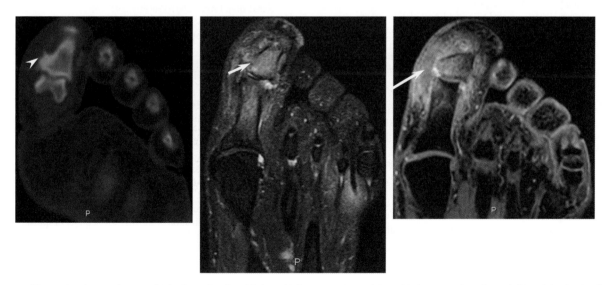

Figure 18.17 CT scan showing new bone at IP joint (arrowhead). Axial T2w with fat suppression and T1w with fat suppression after gadolinium injection in which diffuse osteitis of the proximal and distal phalanges of the 1st toe can be seen (arrow). Pronounced peri-articular inflammation is also seen around the IP joint (long arrow).

predictors for further joint destruction. The use of MRI as a tool to monitor therapy should increase in the coming years, especially with the wealth of new treatment in the clinic or on the horizon.

References

1. Moll JM, Wright V. Psoriatic arthritis. Semin Arthritis Rheuma. 1973;3(1):55–78.
2. Tan AL, McGonagle D. Psoriatic arthritis: correlation between imaging and pathology. Joint, Bone, Spine 2010;77(3):206–11.
3. Tan AL, Mc GD. The need for biological outcomes for biological drugs in psoriatic arthritis. J Rheumatol. 2016;43(1):3–6.
4. Gladman DD, Farewell VT, Husted J, Wong K. Mortality studies in psoriatic arthritis. Results from a single centre. II. Prognostic indicators for mortality. Arthritis Rheum 1998;41:1103–10.
5. Bond SJ, Farewell VT, Schentag CT, Gladman DD. Predictors for radiological damage in psoriatic arthritis. Results from a single centre. Ann Rheum Dis 2007;66:370–6.
6. Jevtic V, Watt I, Rozman B, Kos-Golja M, Demsar F, Jarh O. Distinctive radiological features of small hand joints in rheumatoid arthritis and seronegative spondyloarthritis demonstrated by contrast-enhanced (Gd-DTPA) magnetic resonance imaging. Skeletal Radiol. 1995;24(5):351–5.
7. McGonagle D, Gibbon W, O'Connor P, Green M, Pease C, Emery P. Characteristic magnetic resonance imaging entheseal changes of knee synovitis in spondylarthropathy. Arthritis Rheum. 1998;41(4):694–700.
8. Benjamin M, Bydder GM. Magnetic resonance imaging of entheses using ultrashort TE (UTE) pulse sequences. J Magn Reson Imaging. 2007;25(2):381–9.
9. Mirowitz SA, Apicella P, Reinus WR, Hammerman AM. MR imaging of bone marrow lesions: relative conspicuousness on T1-weighted, fat-suppressed T2-weighted, and STIR images. Am J Roentgenol. 1994 Jan;162(1):215–21.
10. McGonagle D, Lories RJ, Tan AL, Benjamin M. The concept of a 'synovio-entheseal complex' and its implications for understanding joint inflammation and damage in psoriatic arthritis and beyond. Arthritis Rheum. 2007;56(8):2482–91.
11. Bennett AN, Marzo-Ortega H, Tan AL, et al. Ten-year follow-up of SpA-related oligoarthritis involving the knee: the presence of psoriasis but not HLA-B27 or baseline MRI bone oedema predicts outcome. Rheumatology (Oxford). 2012;51(6):1099–106.
12. Marzo-Ortega H, McGonagle D, Rhodes LA, et al. Efficacy of infliximab on MRI-determined bone oedema in psoriatic arthritis. Ann Rheum Dis. 2007;66(6):778–81.
13. Marzo-Ortega H, Tanner SF, Rhodes LA, et al. Magnetic resonance imaging in the assessment of metacarpophalangeal joint disease in early psoriatic and rheumatoid arthritis. Scand J Rheumatol. 2009;38(2):79–83.
14. Braum LS, McGonagle D, Bruns A, et al. Characterisation of hand small joints arthropathy using high-resolution MRI–limited discrimination between osteoarthritis and psoriatic arthritis. Eur Radiol. 2013;23(6):1686–93.
15. McGonagle D, Tan AL, Carey J, Benjamin M. The anatomical basis for a novel classification of osteoarthritis and allied disorders. J Anat. 2010;216(3):279–91.
16. Tan AL, Grainger AJ, Tanner SF, Emery P, McGonagle D. A high-resolution magnetic resonance imaging study of distal interphalangeal joint arthropathy in psoriatic arthritis and osteoarthritis: are they the same? Arthritis Rheum. 2006;54(4):1328–33.
17. McGonagle D, Tan AL, Benjamin M. The nail as a musculoskeletal appendage–implications for an improved understanding of the link between psoriasis and arthritis. Dermatology. 2009;218(2):97–102.
18. Dalbeth N, Pui K, Lobo M, et al. Nail disease in psoriatic arthritis: distal phalangeal bone edema detected by magnetic resonance imaging predicts development of onycholysis and hyperkeratosis. J Rheumatol. 2012;39(4):841–3.
19. Gladman DD, Anhorn KB, Schachter RK, Mervart H. HLA antigens in psoriatic arthritis. J Rheumatol 1986;13:586–92.
20. Jones SM, Armas JB, Cohen MG, Lovell CR, Evison G, McHugh NJ. Psoriatic arthritis: outcome of disease subsets and relationship of joint disease to nail and skin disease. Br J Rheumatol. 1994 Sep;33(9):834–9.
21. Wilson FC, Icen M, Crowson CS, McEvoy MT, Gabriel SE, Kremers HM. Incidence and clinical predictors of psoriatic arthritis in patients with psoriasis: a population-based study. Arthritis Rheum. 2009;61(2):233–9.
22. Aydin SZ, Castillo-Gallego C, Ash Z, et al. Ultrasonographic assessment of nail in psoriatic disease shows a link between onychopathy and distal interphalangeal joint extensor tendon enthesopathy. Dermatology. 2012;225(3):231–5.
23. Ash ZR, Tinazzi I, Gallego CC, et al. Psoriasis patients with nail disease have a greater magnitude of underlying systemic subclinical enthesopathy than those with normal nails. Ann Rheum Dis. 2012;71(4):553–6. doi: 10.1136/annrheumdis-2011-200478.
24. Olivieri I, Salvarani C, Cantini F, et al. Fast spin echo-T2-weighted sequences with fat saturation in dactylitis of spondylarthritis. No evidence of entheseal involvement of the flexor digitorum tendons. Arthritis Rheum. 2002;46(11):2964–7.
25. Olivieri I, D'Angelo S, Scarano E, Padula A. What is the primary lesion in SpA dactylitis? Rheumatology (Oxford). 2008;47(5):561–2.
26. Eshed I1, Bollow M, McGonagle DG, et al. MRI of enthesitis of the appendicular skeleton in spondyloarthritis. Ann Rheum Dis. 2007 Dec;66(12):1553–9.
27. Healy PJ, Groves C, Chandramohan M, Helliwell PS. MRI changes in psoriatic dactylitis–extent of pathology, relationship to tenderness and correlation with clinical indices. Rheumatology (Oxford). 2008;47(1):92–5.
28. Helliwell P, Marchesoni A, Peters M, Barker M, Wright V. A re-evaluation of the osteoarticular manifestations of psoriasis. Br J Rheumatol. 1991;30(5):339–45.
29. Benjamin M, McGonagle D. The anatomical basis for disease localisation in seronegative spondyloarthropathy at entheses and related sites. J Anat. 2001;199(Pt 5):503–26.
30. Magrey M, Khan MA. New insights into synovitis, acne, pustulosis, hyperostosis, and osteitis (SAPHO) syndrome. Curr Rheumatol Rep. 2009;11(5):329–33.
31. Lubrano E, Parsons WJ, Marchesoni A, et al. The definition and measurement of axial psoriatic arthritis. J Rheumatol Suppl. 2015;93:40–2.
32. McGonagle D, Marzo-Ortega H, O'Connor P, et al. The role of biomechanical factors and HLA-B27 in magnetic resonance imaging-determined bone changes in plantar fascia enthesopathy. Arthritis Rheum. 2002;46(2):489–93.
33. Castillo-Gallego C, Aydin SZ, Emery P, McGonagle DG, Marzo-Ortega H. Magnetic resonance imaging assessment of axial psoriatic arthritis: extent of disease relates to HLA-B27. Arthritis Rheum. 2013;65(9):2274–8.
34. Bennett AN, Rehman A, Hensor EM, Marzo-Ortega H, Emery P, McGonagle D. Evaluation of the diagnostic utility of spinal magnetic resonance imaging in axial spondylarthritis. Arthritis Rheum. 2009;60(5):1331–41.

35. Bongartz T, Härle P, Friedrich S, et al. Successful treatment of psoriatic onycho-pachydermo periostitis (POPP) with adalimumab. Arthritis Rheum. 2005;52(1):280–2.

36. Glinatsi D, Bird P, Gandjbakhch F, et al. Validation of the OMERACT Psoriatic Arthritis Magnetic Resonance Imaging Score (PsAMRIS) for the hand and foot in a randomized placebo-controlled trial. J Rheumatol. 2015;42(12):2473–9.

37. Poggenborg RP, Eshed I, Østergaard M, et al. Enthesitis in patients with psoriatic arthritis, axial spondyloarthritis and healthy subjects assessed by 'head-to-toe' whole-body MRI and clinical examination. Ann Rheum Dis. 2015;74(5):823–9.

38. Hodgson RJ, Menon N, Grainger AJ, et al. Quantitative MRI measurements of the Achilles tendon in spondyloarthritis using ultrashort echo times. Br J Radiol. 2012;85(1015):e293–9.

CHAPTER 19

Assessment of joint and bone structure in PsA patients: Using high-resolution computed tomography

Camille Figueiredo and Georg Schett

Introduction

Psoriatic arthritis (PsA) is characterized by chronic inflammation of the synovial membrane and the insertion sites of tendons (entheses). Inflammation of these anatomical structures is associated with sustained joint pain and swelling, which are the key clinical features of patients affected by PsA. In addition to symptoms related to inflammation, PsA also triggers progressive structural changes in the adjacent bone as well as distant to the inflamed synovium and the entheses [1]. While local bone damage is associated with deterioration of the normal physiological architecture of the joints, systemic bone changes are associated with the development of premature osteoporosis and increased fracture risk. Assessing the impact of PsA on bone structure is therefore considered important. Imaging of structural bone changes in PsA has considerably improved over the recent years due to introduction of high-resolution computed tomography (CT). In this chapter the main findings related to investigations of PsA patients using high-resolution CT assessment are summarized.

Local bone erosions in PsA

Radiographic studies in patients with PsA have supported the concept that chronic inflammation of the joints precipitates structural bone damage [2]. This concept is well established in rheumatoid arthritis (RA), where the duration and intensity of inflammation determines progression of bone erosion. PsA seems to be similar in this respect with more severe erosions in patients with longer disease duration or in those with inadequate control of inflammation [1]. Arthritic bone erosions form in the context of osteoclast-mediated bone resorption. Seminal studies by Ritchlin and colleagues [3] have shown that large numbers of osteoclasts are found in the joints of PsA patients and contribute to bone erosion. In this respect, RA and PsA are highly similar and share the process of osteoclast-mediated bone erosion. Clinical studies with cytokine blockers have highlighted the importance of inflammation in driving the progression of bone erosions in PsA. Hence, inhibition

of tumour necrosis factor alpha, interleukin-23, and interleukin-17 retard the progression of bone erosion in PsA [4–6].

High-resolution (CT) has allowed the characterization of bone erosions in PsA patients in much more detail (see Fig 19.1). Comparative analysis of bone erosions in PsA and RA revealed a similar erosion burden in both inflammatory arthritides [7]. Nonetheless, clear qualitative differences in bone erosions between PsA and RA could be identified. Hence, erosions in PsA are usually characterized by small cortical breaks with a larger erosion of trabecular bone underneath the cortical bottleneck. This Ω-shaped appearance with a cortical bottleneck and a larger subcortical bone resorption is typical of PsA erosions and usually not found in patients with RA. The appearance is most likely based on enhanced periosteal responsiveness of bone in PsA patients, which translates to more pronounced periosteal sclerosis next to the cortical break as an attempt to repair the erosion. This process is highly specific to PsA and not found in other forms of arthritis. Small bone erosions can be also identified in patients with cutaneous psoriasis, which suggests that subclinical inflammation may precede the onset of joint disease [8].

Enthesiophyte formation in PsA

Although bone erosions are the best-investigated structural lesion, the most pronounced bone pathology in PsA is new bone formation. Clinical observations as well as radiographic data have clearly shown that structural damage in PsA is different from in RA. While erosions occur in both diseases, only PsA is characterized by pronounced bony proliferations at enthesial sites. These enthesophytes impact joint function, but were inadequately characterized until recently.

High-resolution CT studies have shown a high burden of enthesophytes in PsA patients (see Fig 19.2) [7]. These lesions emerge from proliferation of bone adjacent to the enthesial insertion sites. If severe, the entire periarticular bone can be covered by a new bony corona. Importantly, bone proliferations are distinct from those found on hand osteoarthritis, which primarily emerge from the cartilage–bone interphase [8]. Hence, enthesophytes in

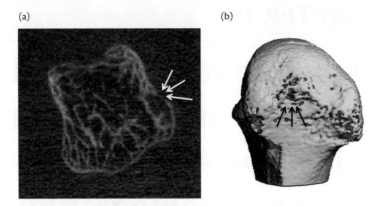

Figure 19.1 Bone erosion in psoriatic arthritis.
(A) High resolution quantitative CT section through the metacarpal head of a patient with PsA. White arrows indicate the cortical break with a larger erosion of trabecular bone underneath the break; (B) 3D-reconstruction of the metacarpal head showing the cortical break (black arrows).

PsA are associated with a very characteristic picture in high-resolution CT scans, which is not found in other rheumatic disease. Furthermore, longitudinal investigations have shown that progression of enthesophytes formation over one year is not significantly changed by methotrexate treatment or by tumour necrosis factor alpha inhibitors [9]. Hence, it will be interesting to study, whether newer drugs used in PsA can affect enthesophyte formation and retard the development of bony ankylosis.

Studies in patients with psoriatic skin disease but no PsA have shown that enthesophytes are the first structural bone pathology in PsA [10]. Hence, more than 30% of psoriasis patients show evidence for enthesophytes, indicating the existence of a so-called 'deep Koebner' phenomenon in the joints of psoriasis patients. It can be speculated that mechanical stress precipitates exaggerated inflammatory responses in the skin and the entheseal tissue, which is followed by the formation of a psoriatic plaque or an enthesiophyte, respectively.

Systemic bone loss in PsA

Chronic inflammation is linked to the development of premature osteoporosis and enhanced fracture risk. Although PsA may follow this concept, standard parameters of inflammation are usually not highly elevated in PsA patients. Furthermore, until

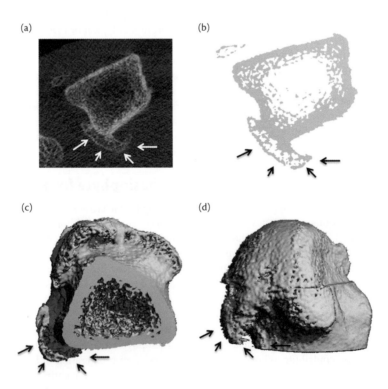

Figure 19.2 Enthesiophyte in psoriatic arthritis.
(A,B) High resolution quantitative computed tomography section through the metacarpal head of a patient with psoriatic arthritis. White and black arrows indicate the enthesiophyte as a bony spur; (C,D) 3D-reconstruction of the metacarpal head showing the enthesiophyte (black arrows).

recently data on systemic bone loss in PsA were confined to DXA (dual energy X-ray absorptiometry) studies, which yielded conflicting results. In contrast, high-resolution CT allows the separate analysis of cortical and trabecular bone and also allows the assessment of bone microarchitecture [11, 12]. These analyses showed that PsA is associated with a significantly reduction of trabecular bone based on a reduction of trabecular number [12]. The factor most strongly associated with trabecular bone loss in PsA was the duration of skin disease suggesting that long-term inflammation of the skin affects bone. Still, psoriasis patients without joint involvement do not develop significant bone loss, it seems that joint involvement is still the key step towards systemic bone loss in psoriasis patients.

Summary

High-resolution CT has improved the understanding of structural bone changes in PsA. It allows the detection and monitoring of bone erosions as well as enthesiophytes in PsA. In the future a better understanding of the dynamics of enthesiophyte formation in PsA patient is needed, not only because it represents the dominant joint pathology in PsA but also because we need to learn how different anti-rheumatic drugs affect joint remodelling. High-resolution CT also allows the early detection of systemic bone loss in patients with PsA and therefore represents a valuable tool to define patients at risk for fragility fractures. It thereby complements imaging techniques such as ultrasound, bone densitometry, or magnetic resonance imaging, which are highly valuable for the detection of inflammatory changes in patients with PsA.

References

1. Gladman DD, Stafford-Brady F, Chang CH, et al. Longitudinal study of clinical and radiological progression in psoriatic arthritis. J Rheumatol. 1990; 17:809–12.

2. Poggenborg RP, Bird P, Boonen A, et al. Pattern of bone erosion and bone proliferation in psoriatic arthritis hands: a high-resolution computed tomography and radiography follow-up study during adalimumab therapy. Scand J Rheumatol. 2014;43:202–8.

3. Ritchlin CT, Haas-Smith SA, Li P, Hicks DG, Schwarz EM. Mechanisms of TNF-alpha- and RANKL- mediated osteoclastogenesis and bone resorption in psoriatic arthritis.J Clin Invest. 2003;111:821–31.

4. Kavanaugh A, Antoni CE, Gladman D, et al. The Infliximab Multinational Psoriatic Arthritis Controlled Trial (IMPACT): results of radiographic analyses after 1 year. Ann Rheum Dis. 2006;65(8):1038–43.

5. Kavanaugh A, Ritchlin C, Rahman P, et al. Ustekinumab, an IL-12/23 monoclonal antibody, inhibits radiographic progression in patients with active psoriatic arthritis: results of an integrated analysis of radiographic data from the phase 3, multicentre, randomised, double-blind, placebo-controlled PSUMMIT-1 and PSUMMIT-2 trials. Ann Rheum Dis. 2014;73(6):1000–6.

6. Mease, P McInnes, IB, Kirkham, B, et al. Secukinumab inhibition of interleukin-17A in patients with psoriatic arthritis. N Engl J Med 2015; 373:1329–39.

7. Finzel S, Englbrecht M, Engelke K, et al. A comparative study of periarticular bone lesions in rheumatoid arthritis and psoriatic arthritis. Ann Rheum Dis. 2011; 70:122–7.

8. Finzel S, Sahinbegovic E, Kocijan R, et al. Inflammatory bone spur formation in psoriatic arthritis is different from bone spur formation in hand osteoarthritis. Arthritis Rheumatol. 2014;66:2968–75.

9. Finzel S, Kraus S, Schmidt S, et al. Bone anabolic changes progress in psoriatic arthritis patients despite treatment with methotrexate or tumour necrosis factor inhibitors. Ann Rheum Dis. 2013;72:1176–81.

10. Simon D, Faustini F, Kleyer A, et al. Analysis of periarticular bone changes in patients with cutaneous psoriasis without associated psoriatic arthritis. Ann Rheum Dis. 2016;75(4):660–6.

11. Zhu TY, Griffith JF, Qin L, et al. Density, structure, and strength of the distal radius in patients with psoriatic arthritis: the role of inflammation and cardiovascular risk factors. Osteoporos Int. 2015;26:261–72.

12. Kocijan R, Englbrecht M, Haschka J, et al. Quantitative and qualitative changes of bone in psoriasis and psoriatic arthritis patients. J Bone Miner Res. 2015;30:1775–83.

Diagnosis and classification

CHAPTER 20

Diagnosis and classification criteria

Laura C. Coates and William J. Taylor

The difference between diagnosis and classification

It is important to distinguish between diagnosis and classification. [1, 2] Diagnosis is what clinicians do in the clinic when they want to be able to name the pathological process that is affecting the patient in order to come to an effective treatment plan and provide accurate advice to the patient about what is wrong and what is likely to happen in the future. The diagnostic process brings to bear all available pieces of evidence in order to assign or not assign a particular diagnostic label. Such labels can vary in the level of detail or precision, but the process is the same and useful information may include aspects of the pathology itself but also the propensity of the patient to incur this pathology (e.g. age, gender, background prevalence, or other risk factors). Since physicians differ in the informational database available to them or how the same pieces of data are weighed (e.g. in different contexts, the report of mouth ulcers may have different meaning) and yet are still able to make the same diagnoses, standardization in diagnosis is not feasible unless the diagnosis/disease is of a very precise nature.

Although the diagnostic process usually results in a dichotomous output: the disease is present or not present, underneath this output is a probability exercise. The physician comes to an implicit judgement about the probability of the disease being present and almost at the same time whether this level of probability justifies the application of the diagnostic label. For some diseases with relatively trivial implications, a low probability of disease may be acceptable (e.g. 'muscle strain') whereas other diseases with implications of severe morbidity and potential toxic therapy may require a higher probability (e.g. cancer). The correct analytic framework for considering diagnosis is the joint distribution of all variables that might influence the probability of disease being present [3].

In rheumatology, the 'gold standard' of diagnosis is usually expert opinion. For clinical research, expert opinion may not always be obtainable. Furthermore, expert opinion is not only fallible, it is un-measurably fallible. That is, diagnostic errors are probably made from time to time but the extent of the error is unknown. For clinical research purposes, such a process is not adequate.

In contrast, classification is the process of defining case-ness for the purpose of studying the condition, that is, for research. In such a setting, standardization is very important since it is necessary for the same condition to be studied to make sense of all the research that considers this condition. The process of standardization inevitably means that only a limited part of the informational database is used to define whether the patient has the disease or not, but the critical issue is that the same segment of information is used in the same way in every research study to ensure homogeneity of the population under study. In addition, it is inevitable that the criteria will not agree with the 'gold standard' of diagnosis, but in this case it is possible to quantify the degree of disagreement: the false positive rate and the false negative rate.

Classification therefore resolves to a problem of finding the smallest informational database that leads to the smallest false positive rate and false negative rate. The correct analytic framework for classification criteria is the receiver operating characteristic (ROC) curve whereby different combinations of variables can be assessed against a 'gold standard' determination of the presence/absence of disease.

Clues to the diagnosis of psoriatic arthritis in a clinical setting

The diagnosis of psoriatic arthritis (PsA), particularly in the early stages of disease, is difficult. The majority of patients develop psoriasis prior to the onset of arthritis, although this may not have been previously diagnosed by a physician. However, up to 20% of patients develop arthritis first and are often labelled as undifferentiated SpA until the psoriasis becomes apparent [4].

In patients with psoriasis, the key issue is to identify whether the patient has inflammatory arthritis, enthesitis, or spondylitis. The majority of patients with inflammatory arthritis and psoriasis are likely to have a diagnosis of PsA, particularly if they show other typical features such as rheumatoid factor (RF) negativity and dactylitis. Whilst the identification of an inflammatory arthritis is also key in rheumatology clinics, once this is established, the aim is to make a diagnosis of PsA within the class of other inflammatory arthritides.

Symptoms and signs

There is little research into the reported symptoms and signs in initial presentations of PsA. A systematic review of symptoms of PsA identified 27 papers published that contained information on clinical phenotypes and symptoms in PsA. These symptoms were grouped together if they related to similar clinical forms of PsA and a Delphi exercise amongst psoriasis experts identified four key features: peripheral inflammatory pain, axial inflammatory pain, dactylitis, and buttock/sciatic pain [5]. However, they did

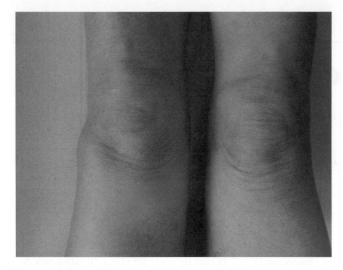

Figure 20.1 Knee swelling observed in a patient with PsA.

not include any patients in the discussion on common presenting symptoms; this is all described from the doctors' viewpoint.

In terms of the peripheral arthritis, the signs and symptoms related to individual joints are similar to any inflammatory arthritis, although the pattern of articular involvement may vary. In many modern series, patients presenting to rheumatology clinics more commonly have a polyarticular involvement (60–70%) rather than oligoarthritis (30–40%) [6–9]. Although in some series this trend is reversed with higher proportions of oligoarthritis, this seems to be more common in cohorts reporting patients with a very short disease duration before diagnosis [10–16].

Other patterns of peripheral arthritis are also reported in PsA cohorts. The prevalence of distal interphalangeal (DIP) joint disease in PsA varies from 5.4 to 41% in different cohorts but most people agree that it is a more typical finding in PsA than in rheumatoid arthritis (RA) [6–9, 11, 13, 16]. The most commonly involved joints at presentation of PsA are the knees (Figure 20.1), metacarpophalangeal and proximal interphalangeal joints (Figure 20.2) [9, 13].

Early morning stiffness (EMS) is a feature often used by rheumatologists to differentiate inflammatory arthritis although there is little data on this included in the early PsA cohorts. In an Italian study with only 33 new PsA patients (<1 year symptoms), 28 reported EMS over 45 minutes [6]. In Dublin, 50% of patients reported EMS >30 minutes but 23% denied any significant EMS (<10 minutes) [8].

At the GRAPPA 2013 meeting, a nominal group exercise was performed to identify descriptive elements of inflammatory joint disease. A group consisting of predominantly healthcare professionals interested in rheumatology, but also patient research partners identified possible signs and symptoms of inflammation in the peripheral joints. Symptoms included EMS >30 minutes, joint tenderness, pain aggravated by rest and relieved by exercise, symptoms improved by nonsteroidal anti-inflammatory drugs (NSAIDs) or steroid use, joint erythema or warmth, and related fatigue. Possible clinical signs included joint swelling (Figure 20.1), limited joint motion, and joint deformity [17].

The presence of enthesitis is considered a characteristic feature of PsA. Presence of clinical enthesitis at presentation is reported to vary from 8.6% to 67% [6–8, 11, 12]. Symptoms and signs suggested include pain near the joint possibly with associated swelling, functional limitations, and tenderness at typical entheseal insertion

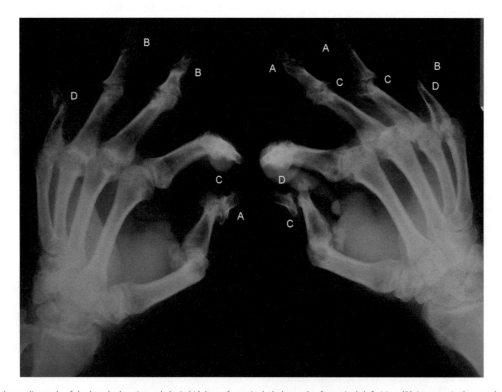

Figure 20.2 Ball catcher radiograph of the hands showing ankylosis (A), loss of terminal phalangeal tuft cortical definition (B), juxta-articular new bone formation (C),and joint osteolysis (D); the 5th fingers and thumbs demonstrate mutilans type changes.

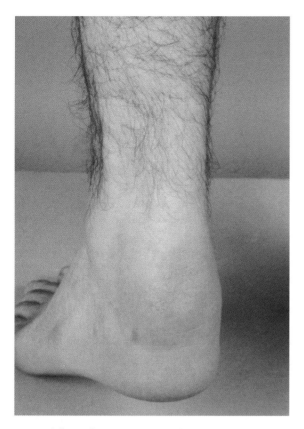

Figure 20.3 Achilles tendonitis in a patients with PsA.

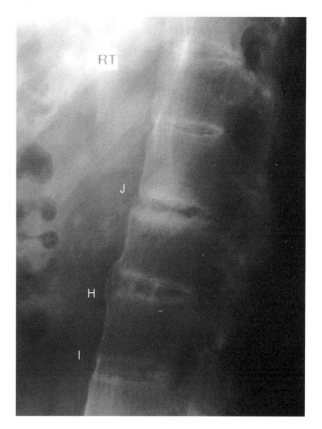

Figure 20.5 Lateral radiograph of the lumber spine showing chunky syndesmophyte (H), Andersson lesion of the disk (J) and classical syndesmophyte (I).

sites (Achilles, plantar fascia, quadriceps tendon, patellar ligament, iliac crest) (Figure 20.3) [17]. Dactylitis (Figure 20.4) is an almost pathognomic feature of PsA although it is usually reported as less common than enthesitis. At presentation, cohorts report that 12–29% have dactylitis [6–9, 11, 12]. Signs and symptoms seen in dactylitis are digital swelling, tenderness, warmth, and erythema. The swelling can be focal or diffuse and often results in decreased mobility. The digit should have a 'sausage'-like appearance typical in dactylitis with fusiform swelling [17].

Axial involvement in PsA is also recognized as part of the spondyloarthritis phenotype although there is difficulty in classifying this. Involvement of the spine confirmed by modified New York (mNY) criteria changes can take many years to develop. Cohorts have reported a prevalence of 5–28% of patients with some spinal involvement (Figure 20.5) alongside peripheral arthritis [7, 11–13, 16, 18]. Prevalence for pure axial disease is less commonly reported but seems to be 7–17% [12, 18].

Typical clinical features of axial involvement or inflammatory back pain (IBP) have been well researched in ankylosing spondylitis (AS), but less so in psoriatic patients. IBP is considered in patients who describe chronic back pain for over 3 months. Typically this is an insidious onset at a younger age. Typical features of the pain, suggested by patients and experts in PsA, include hip/buttock pain, pain that improves with activity and worsens with rest, night pain, NSAID-responsive pain, and axial morning stiffness ≥ 30 min. Patients may also have limited motion and sacroiliac joint tenderness on examination [17]. Presence of IBP in new PsA cohorts is also not commonly reported but may be around 15% [6]. Even in a cohort of patients with psoriatic SpA (meeting mNY criteria), IBP was only reported in 19% [14].

Predictors of PsA within psoriasis patients

Epidemiological studies of cohorts with psoriasis have attempted to identify which patients are more likely to develop PsA. A retrospective review of medical records identified a cohort of 1,633 patients with psoriasis. In this study approximately 10% of patients were diagnosed with PsA over a 30-year period. However, given the retrospective nature of the study and the lack of specific evaluation

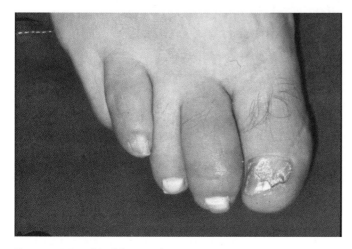

Figure 20.4 Dactylitis of the second toe.

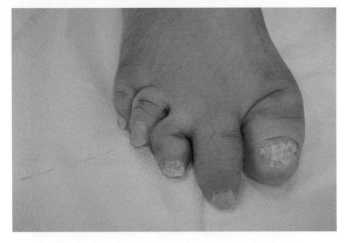

Figure 20.6 Nail dystrophy of each toenail with dactylitis of the second toe.

for PsA, this incidence is likely to be an underestimate. Nonetheless this study did identify a higher chance of PsA development in those with psoriatic nail changes (Figures 20.6 and 20.7), scalp psoriasis, and intergluteal/perianal psoriasis [19]. A prospective study in Canada is ongoing with 579 patients who were recruited up to December 2013 and has found an annual incidence of 3.1% (95% CI 2.2–4.0). They confirmed that nail lesions seemed to be associated with a higher incidence of PsA, but also found that flexural psoriasis, lower educational level, and obesity predicted the development of PsA [20].

Investigations—blood tests and imaging

In cohorts of early PsA patients, levels of acute phase markers such as erythrocyte sedimentation rate and C-reactive protein are typically raised [8]. However, many patients with PsA will never have raised inflammatory markers in their blood despite active disease. At presentation, 36–69% of patients have a raised erythrocyte sedimentation rate and 33–89% have raised C-reactive protein [6, 11, 15, 18]. While raised inflammatory markers may be helpful, normal inflammatory markers do not exclude a diagnosis of PsA.

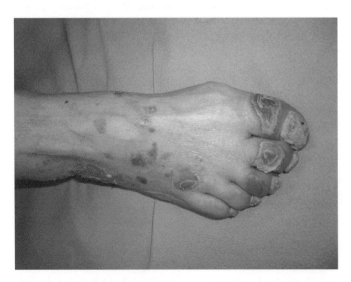

Figure 20.7 Psoriasis and severe nail dystrophy.

Typically, PsA is thought of a seronegative disease and the majority of patients do not have the rheumatoid factor (RF) or anti-citrullinated peptide antibodies (ACPA). However, a minority of patients are positive for one or both of these and a diagnosis of PsA should not be excluded. Series have shown prevalence of RF to be 5–8% compared to 76% in an RA control group [18, 21]. Interestingly, patients with polyarticular PsA were no more likely to be RF positive than those with oligoarthritis [21]. In most series, the titres of RF are not reported, but one of these series does say that only low titres were seen [18].

The estimates for prevalence of ACPA in PsA vary from 6 to 16% in different cross-sectional studies [23–26]. There is a trend towards a higher prevalence of ACPA in patients with PsA when compared to healthy controls or patients with psoriasis, however the prevalence is significantly lower than that seen in RA [23, 25, 26]. The significance of ACPA in PsA is uncertain. Nearly all of the smaller studies have shown a significant association with a polyarthritic phenotype [23, 25, 26], but interestingly an analysis of the larger CASPAR cohort (n=588) showed ACPA positivity in 7% of polyarticular PsA and 10% of oligoarticular PsA or psoriatic spondylitis [21]. Some have identified an association with erosive disease [25, 26] but not all studies demonstrate this [23].

Radiographic changes in PsA are seen more commonly in advancing disease, so at initial presentation radiographs are often normal. At presentation, around 27% have evidence of erosions on X-ray and this increases to 47% at 2 years despite conventional treatment with disease modifying anti-rheumatic drugs (DMARDs) [8]. However, the level of erosive disease seen is low with erosions typically seen in only one joint in these cases.

In addition to radiographs of the hands and feet, imaging the sacroiliac (SI) joint and spine is also common in patients presenting with possible PsA. Wright et al. recognized the frequent SI joint changes (erosions, sclerosis, and ankylosis) in patients with PsA compared to rheumatoid controls [27]. Spondylitis is seen in approximately 25% of PsA patients although as with peripheral radiographs, in early disease identifying significant changes is less likely. Even higher rates of SI disease are observed if specifically looked for and it may be that SI disease is often not symptomatic in PsA [28]. SI joint involvement in PsA looks similar to AS but with more frequent unilateral or asymmetrical involvement and subtle differences in the morphology of syndesmophytes (Figure 20.5) [29].

Historical development of classification criteria for psoriatic arthritis

Moll and Wright

The careful clinical observations of Moll and Wright led to the recognition of PsA as a distinct disease and also the seminal identification of the spondyloarthritis concept, as a disease group quite different from RA [30, 31]. This helped to establish that PsA was not simply co-incidental RA and psoriasis, an idea that was promoted as late as the 1980s [32].

The original criteria of Moll and Wright are the simplest and the most frequently used in studies prior to 2006. The criteria were expressed as: an inflammatory arthritis (peripheral arthritis and/or sacroiliitis or spondylitis) in the presence of psoriasis with the (usual) absence of serological tests for RF. These criteria were probably designed to be sensitive without being too specific but it is possible that Moll and Wright were using other (non-explicit) features of the disease to make their diagnosis in the clinic and subsequent clinical research. As a consequence of omitting from the criteria what would now be regarded as characteristic features of PsA (such as enthesitis, spondylitis, dactylitis, nail disease), it is possible that many of the patients included in later studies (by just applying the criteria alone) had seronegative RA with co-incidental psoriasis, since the ratio of patients with polyarthritis to oligoarthritis became reversed in cohorts subsequent to Moll and Wright.

Later modifications

The issue with using RF as an exclusion criterion was highlighted by Gladman, who found that 12% of her cohort with PsA had a positive RF. The criteria that she used to define PsA in the Toronto cohort was therefore less rigid concerning RF positivity, but still excluded patients with rheumatoid nodules or other kinds of inflammatory arthritis [33].

Other proposed classification criteria have not been widely adopted. They are of interest mainly in terms of the selection of features included, which highlight salient features of PsA. Bennett's criteria combined the clinical features unique to PsA together with characteristic radiologic features [34]. In addition, two pathological criteria, one based on synovial fluid analysis and the other based on synovial histology, were included. Vasey and Espinoza simplified the Bennett criteria recognizing that there are two principle manifestations of PsA; only two criteria are required—psoriasis and one manifestation of either peripheral joint disease or spinal disease [35]. Although the European Spondyloarthropathy Study Group (ESSG) developed criteria for the classification of the spondyloarthropathy (SpA) group as a whole, particular types of SpA can be identified from the published classification criteria, including PsA [36]. These criteria meant for the first time that it was possible for PsA to be classified in the absence of psoriasis, if a family history of psoriasis was present. McGonagle et al. proposed a definition of PsA based on enthesopathy [37].

As the first proper attempt to define and validate criteria from actual patient data, the study by Fournié represented an important step [38]. In this study, the criteria items and weighting were selected using discriminant function and logistic regression analysis. The data were derived from a population of patients diagnosed by rheumatologists from a single clinic as having PsA, AS, or RA. A score of 11 points is required for the diagnosis of PsA (sensitivity 95%, specificity 98%, LR + 47.5) and, although the criteria include HLA data, it is possible to attain this threshold on clinical data alone.

Some studies have sought to identify the best performing classification criteria. A retrospective study using data from clinical records and existing radiographs in 343 patients with PsA and 156 with RA found that the criteria of Vasey and Espinoza had the best combination of specificity, sensitivity, and feasibility, although there was no statistically significant difference between Vasey, Gladman, and McGonagle [39]. The CASPAR study also found that the criteria of Vasey and Espinoza performed the best of all the pre-CASPAR classification criteria [40]. Another small study of patients with PsA found that the CASPAR criteria had the best sensitivity compared to Bennett's criteria, Moll and Wright, ESSG, Vasey and Espinoza, and Fournié with the proportion of PsA patients who did not fulfil each criteria being 90%, 10%, 31%, 44%, 46%, and 79% respectively [41]. In Han Chinese patients with inflammatory arthritis, the performance (sensitivity/specificity) of Moll and Wright,

ESSG, Vasey and Espinoza and CASPAR criteria were 85/100, 81/99, 98/100, 98/100 respectively [42]. In another study, the performance (sensitivity/ specificity) of CASPAR, Moll and Wright and ESSG criteria was 92/99, 86/100, 63/94 respectively [43, 44].

The development of the CASPAR criteria

The **Cla**ssification of **P**soriatic **Ar**thritis (CASPAR) criteria, published in 2006, arose from an international collaboration of interested rheumatologists, motivated by the multiplicity of classification criteria for PsA and the clear need to have internationally agreed criteria that were data-driven and validated [40]. The project was initially discussed at a meeting in Brussels during 2000 but later expanded to include non-European investigators at the International League Against Rheumatism (ILAR) meeting in Edmonton, 2001. The development study was conducted across 13 countries and involved over 1000 patients consecutively recruited from rheumatology clinics.

A large number of potential items were examined. These were identified from literature review and from existing classification criteria. Plain radiographic features of PsA were also evaluated. The technique of latent class analysis was employed to construct an alternative 'gold-standard' to physician diagnosis. This was possible by examining the joint distribution of the multiple existing classification criteria sets.

Patients with other inflammatory arthritis were controls—these included RA (70% of controls), AS, undifferentiated arthritis, and a smaller number of other diseases. Using items derived from two different statistical techniques (classification and regression tree, logistic regression), new criteria were derived (Table 20.1).

Accuracy of the CASPAR criteria in established and early disease

Accuracy in development

In the development study, the accuracy of the new proposed CASPAR criteria was impressive with a sensitivity of 0.914 and specificity of 0.987 [40]. This compared favourably to the other previous classification criteria investigated in the study with only the Vasey and Espinoza criteria showing a higher sensitivity. Given their use as classification criteria, it was felt that a higher specificity was crucial to ensure that homogenous populations are recruited for clinical trials. However, testing the criteria in the cohort in which they were developed is always going to provide high estimates of their accuracy. To really test the abilities of the CASPAR criteria, they needed validation in other independent cohorts.

Testing in prospective studies of established disease

A prospective single centre study in the UK applied five of the existing PsA criteria (Moll and Wright [30], Vasey and Espinoza [35], Bennett [34], Fournie [38], ESSG [36]) with the CASPAR criteria. They found that only 21 of 60 patients with PsA fulfilled all of the criteria and then analysed the criteria sets further to investigate that discordance. The CASPAR criteria were positive in the highest number of these patients (35/39). Whilst the majority of patients fulfilling the CASPAR criteria did so with a 'typical' picture of current psoriasis and a negative RF, the additional sensitivity of these criteria was attributable to the fact that PsA could be classified

Table 20.1 The CASPAR criteria

Inflammatory articular disease (joint, spine, or entheseal)			
With 3 or more points from the following:			
1. Evidence of psoriasis (one of a, b, c)	(a) Current psoriasis*	Psoriatic skin or scalp disease present today as judged by a rheumatologist or dermatologist	
	(b) Personal history of psoriasis	A history of psoriasis that may be obtained from patient, family doctor, dermatologist, rheumatologist or other qualified health-care provider	
	(c) Family history of psoriasis	A history of psoriasis in a first or second degree relative according to patient report	
2. Psoriatic nail dystrophy		Typical psoriatic nail dystrophy including onycholysis, pitting and hyperkeratosis observed on current physical examination	
3. A negative test for rheumatoid factor		By any method except latex but preferably by ELISA or nephelometry, according to the local laboratory reference range	
4. Dactylitis (one of a, b)	(a) Current	Swelling of an entire digit	
	(b) History	A history of dactylitis recorded by a rheumatologist	
5. Radiological evidence of juxta-articular new bone formation		Ill-defined ossification near joint margins (but excluding osteophyte formation) on plain xrays of hand or foot	

Specificity 0.987, sensitivity 0.914
* Current psoriasis scores 2 whereas all other items score 1
Data sourced from Taylor et al. Classification criteria for psoriatic arthritis: development of new criteria from a large international study (2006) Arthritis and Rheumatism 54(8) 2655–2673.

without a personal history of psoriasis and in those with a positive RF [41].

Despite the CASPAR criteria being developed within an international cohort from 13 countries, the majority of patients were Caucasian and further validation has been performed in other ethnic groups. A study in Hong Kong assessed the utility of the criteria in the Han Chinese population recruiting 108 cases and 195 controls. Using clinical diagnosis as a gold standard, the best performing criteria were the CASPAR and the Vasey and Espinoza criteria with sensitivities of 98.2% and specificities of 98.5% [42]. Again they found that the majority of patients fulfilled the current psoriasis and negative RF items.

A single centre study in Istanbul recruited 86 patients with PsA to compare multiple classification criteria. They found that the CASPAR criteria had a sensitivity of 86% [45]. This was slightly lower than the criteria of Moll and Wright and Vasey and Espinoza. A multicentre study in Turkey also assessed the CASPAR criteria in comparison with multiple existing PsA criteria and the ASAS criteria for peripheral SpA. The sensitivity of the CASPAR criteria was 96.1% and was higher than all of the other criteria. Of the 128 patients, 30 had a disease duration of less than 12 months

and the CASPAR criteria still performed well (sensitivity 96.7%) in this early subgroup [46]. A Serbian study examined PsA criteria in 120 cases and two separate control groups: one group diagnosed with RA (n=123), and one with non-inflammatory musculoskeletal complaints (n=113). The CASPAR criteria had a sensitivity of 91.7% and a specificity of 99.2% and 99.1% in the RA and non-inflammatory control groups respectively. They found that the CASPAR criteria performed the best, with a slightly lower sensitivity in the Moll and Wright criteria (although 100% specific) and a much lower sensitivity/specificity in the ESSG criteria [44].

In addition to many studies assessing the CASPAR criteria in rheumatology populations, one study has tested their use in a family medicine clinic, where 175 consecutive attendees were assessed by a rheumatologist to apply the CASPAR criteria and establish whether any patients had PsA. As expected the prevalence of inflammatory arthritis was low (21%) with only two patients diagnosed with PsA. Both of these patients did fulfil the CASPAR criteria, and only two others fulfilled these criteria (one with AS and psoriasis, one with IBP and psoriasis). This gave a high sensitivity (100%) and high specificity (98.8%) [47]. This shows that the criteria can be applied in other clinic settings, but it must be noted that the patients were still assessed by a rheumatologist in this study.

Retrospective application in registries

A number of registries have retrospectively applied the CASPAR criteria to their data. Using 456 patients from the Bath PsA cohort and 115 controls with inflammatory arthritis recruited from clinics, they showed a high sensitivity and specificity in established disease (over 99%) and also showed that the criteria were relatively easy to apply retrospectively to existing cohorts [48]. The majority of patients achieved the CASPAR criteria as they had skin psoriasis and a negative RF which allowed a very quick assessment of the medical records. There were eight PsA patients who did not meet the criteria but in the majority (7/8) they had missing radiographs and/or RF status which prevented a full assessment of the criteria. There was very high agreement between two assessors showing that the objective nature of the criteria made classification straightforward with minimal training.

The Toronto PsA cohort also investigated the CASPAR criteria in a subset of their patients. The CASPAR criteria were applied to the patient's entry visit into the cohort (n=288) and they were subdivided into an early subgroup with <2.5 years duration (n=107) or established disease (n= 81). The sensitivity was high in both cohorts (early disease 99.1%, established disease 97.2%) [49]. This study showed a very high sensitivity even in the early disease subgroup, but it should be noted that these patients are recruited from those referred to a tertiary referral PsA service so they may not represent a standard early arthritis population.

Use in early disease study

A single centre study in Italy attempted to investigate the validity of the CASPAR criteria in classifying early disease. They recruited consecutive new referrals and reported that 34/44 PsA patients fulfilled the CASPAR criteria giving a sensitivity of 77.3%. The sensitivity of the CASPAR criteria was slightly lower in patients with a predominant tenosynovitis/enthesitis/dactylitis pattern (13/19, 68.4%) compared to those with peripheral arthritis (21/25, 84%). Only two patients showed typical radiographic changes for the CASPAR criteria. They concluded that the reduction in sensitivity in early disease could be principally related to this lower prevalence of radiographic change [50].

A further multicentre study was also ongoing in Italy led by the same authors. No full publication has become available, only an abstract reporting interim results in 2007. The study had recruited 78 patients with early PsA and 68 controls. In this study, the sensitivity and specificity appeared much higher with 71 PsA patients fulfilling the CASPAR criteria (91.0%) and only 2 control patients meeting the criteria (specificity 97.1%). However no further information are published concerning the pattern of disease in this cohort and which aspects of the criteria were fulfilled [51]. A similar study in the UK recruited 111 cases and 111 controls to compare the accuracy of the CASPAR criteria and the Moll and Wright criteria. They found identical specificities of 99.1% for both Moll and Wright and CASPAR criteria. However, the sensitivity of the CASPAR criteria was higher as classification was also possible in the case of no current psoriasis or a positive RF. As in the Italian studies, only two patients showed typical radiographic features. A group in Spain applied the CASPAR classification criteria alongside ASAS criteria for axial and peripheral SpA to consecutive patients attending a psoriasis dermatology clinic. Of 100 patients assessed, 17 were found to have peripheral arthritis and the median duration of arthritis was 6 years. The authors do not state if their arthritis had previously been diagnosed. All 17 patients with arthritis fulfilled the CASPAR criteria and the ASAS peripheral SpA criteria. In addition five of them also fulfilled the ASAS axial SpA criteria although it was noted that nine additional patients had sacroiliitis on plain radiography of grade 2 or higher [52]. The largest study to examine the CASPAR criteria in early disease was an analysis of the Leiden Early Arthritis Cohort. This cohort recruits patients referred to Leiden rheumatology with inflammatory arthritis of less than 2 years' duration. Of 2011 patients included in this study, they analysed 226 patients with SpA of whom 150 had PsA. They also used a matched control group who had diagnoses of RA, undifferentiated arthritis, OA, reactive arthritis, gout, sarcoid and other arthritides. The CASPAR criteria had a relatively high sensitivity of 88.7% in PsA and clearly outperformed the ESSG, Amor, and ASAS peripheral SpA criteria in identifying PsA patients. The specificity of all of these criteria was good with a specificity of 95.6% for the CASPAR criteria compared to the control group. Interestingly, they also had good specificity compared to the SpA group with only four SpA patients being positive for the CASPAR criteria [53]. The authors do identify one specific limitation which is that all of these patients were referred based on the presence of inflammatory arthritis and do not represent the full spectrum of PsA and SpA patients who may present with enthesitis, dactylitis, or inflammatory axial disease.

Proposed modifications to the CASPAR criteria

One of the issues identified with the CASPAR criteria has been the heavier weighting given to those with current psoriasis. Whilst multiple studies have shown that the majority of people do fulfil this item, there are a significant proportion of patients with PsA who have had psoriasis in the past but with effective therapy, this has gone into remission. This was identified as a problem within a cross-sectional study where patients had definite documented psoriasis in the past, but this resulted in a lower CASPAR score than those with current psoriasis [54]. To investigate the impact this has, the authors of the Serbian study discussed a previously applied

modification of the CASPAR criteria where similar weighting was given to a previous history of skin psoriasis or typical nail changes if this had been documented by a rheumatologist or dermatologist. With this modification the sensitivity increased from 91.7% to 95% with only one more control patient from the RA group being incorrectly classified as PsA [44].

Psoriatic arthritis and axial/peripheral spondyloarthritis

Psoriatic arthritis within the umbrella of spondyloarthritides

Although it is not clear whether SpA is a single disease with different phenotypic expressions, or whether it is a collection of different diseases with shared features, it is clear that PsA fits within the SpA concept. Moll and Wright formulated this by means of careful clinical observations, including family studies. They introduced the terms 'seronegative polyarthritis' and 'seronegative spondarthritis' to emphasize the profound differences between these conditions and RA [31]. Later, genetic and pathophysiological similarities were shown to exist amongst patients with different types of SpA. Shared clinical features include sacroiliitis and spondylitis, enthesitis, anterior uveitis, and bowel inflammation. The *HLA-B27* gene is found in 20% of UK patients with PsA [55] studies and although this is less frequent than is observed in AS, it is more frequent than in the general population.

Moll and Wright described axial disease as a subtype of PsA but there are difficulties with rigid sub-categories since spinal involvement is not uncommon in patients with peripheral disease involvement, who might otherwise be categorized as one of the peripheral patterns of disease. This is especially true given the high rate of subclinical spinal disease observed both by magnetic resonance imaging (MRI) and radiography. There is not much known about the natural history of non-symptomatic spinal involvement in PsA and so it is unclear whether precise identification of axial PsA contributes much to clinical management decisions.

For people with psoriasis and symptomatic spinal or sacroiliac disease and characteristic imaging findings of axial inflammatory disease, it is not clear-cut whether they should be diagnosed with PsA or AS with psoriasis. Such patients would commonly fulfil classification criteria for both AS and PsA. Most treatment recommendations for spinal involvement in PsA borrow from the AS literature since PsA studies generally enrol patients with peripheral disease and do not evaluate spinal outcomes [56]. Pragmatically, until intervention or natural history studies determine whether PsA axial disease behaves differently from AS, there seems to be more advantages in diagnosing such patients as AS, despite recognized differences in the way spinal disease may manifest in each condition.

Axial and peripheral spondyloarthritides classification criteria

The axial SpA disease concept arose from the recognition that the mNY criteria could not identify early AS. The Assessment of Axial Spondyloarthritis (ASAS) group correctly determined that the best way of addressing this issue would be new classification criteria, but (incorrectly) also decided that the criteria could not be for the identification of AS and that a new name was needed for the disease patients have before they develop radiographic sacroiliitis. The main reason for wanting to avoid the label AS was probably the view that radiographic sacroiliitis is required for the classification *and* diagnosis of AS [57] and therefore new criteria that identified early AS could not be labelled as such. Despite recent emphasis on the difference between diagnosis and classification, AS experts appear to make the diagnosis of AS mainly or always on the basis of the mNY criteria [58]. The result of that muddled thinking has been the creation of the disease concept axial SpA and its counterpart, peripheral SpA.

Another driver for the axial SpA concept was the recognition that some patients have back pain and other features suggestive of a SpA disorder, but do not have sufficient features to categorize more precisely. Such patients had traditionally been labelled as 'undifferentiated SpA' and two sets of classification criteria already existed to help identify such patients for clinical research. It is possible that some patients with this kind of axial SpA are never destined to develop radiographic sacroiliitis and might therefore be considered not to have AS. Amongst cohort studies of undifferentiated spondyloarthritis, only 11% of patients followed over time remain undifferentiated [59]. At this time, there is insufficient evidence to know how such patients should be diagnosed or managed, but there is definitely some evidence for heterogeneity in the broader group of patients who fulfil the axial SpA classification criteria.

The ASAS classification criteria for these entities suggest that it is quite easy to be classified as both axial and peripheral SpA. For axial SpA, patients need to have symptoms of back pain for more than 3 months before the age of 45 years and then one or more additional SpA features (including psoriasis and peripheral articular disease) depending on whether there are MRI features of sacroiliitis or presence of *HLA-B27*. For peripheral SpA, patients need to have peripheral articular disease and one or two SpA features (including prior IBP, sacroiliitis on imaging, and *HLA-B27*). Since peripheral and axial symptoms not uncommonly co-exist, it is difficult to see how these criteria should be applied.

Direct comparison of peripheral spondyloarthritides criteria and CASPAR criteria in psoriatic arthritis

There has been a single study that investigated the accuracy of the new ASAS SpA criteria amongst patients with early arthritis [53]. In this study, the high sensitivity of CASPAR (88.7%) for the identification of PsA was confirmed, compared with 52% for the ASAS peripheral SpA criteria and only 26% for the ESSG criteria. The peripheral SpA criteria had adequate specificity (89.8%) but poor sensitivity (48.7%) for identifying patients with SpA. For classification as PsA, CASPAR had a specificity of 94.7% amongst patients with non-PsA SpA and 95.6% amongst controls patients with non-SpA forms of inflammatory arthritis.

Therefore, there seems to be reasonable evidence that the CASPAR criteria remain best for classifying patients with PsA.

Subtypes of psoriatic arthritis

Classical subtypes proposed by Moll and Wright

PsA is well recognized as a heterogeneous disease with different patterns of musculoskeletal disease involvement. This led to the development of subtypes of disease in the initial reports of PsA by Moll and Wright. Initially, Wright proposed only three subtypes: DIP-predominant disease, RA-like disease, and severe

deforming arthritis which included patients with axial manifestations [60]. However in 1973, Moll and Wright proposed five subtypes which have become the most commonly recognized descriptions of PsA: monoarthritis, oligoarthritis, DIP-predominant disease, RA-like polyarticular disease, and arthritis mutilans [30].

Proposed modifications to subtypes

Various authors have proposed modifications to the original five subtypes proposed by Moll and Wright. Gladman was the first to propose modifications and expanded the subtypes to seven recognizing the additional involvement of the axial skeleton: distal disease (DIP joints only affected), oligoarthritis (four or fewer joints), polyarthritis, spondylitis only, distal plus spondylitis, oligoarthritis plus spondylitis, and polyarthritis plus spondylitis [33]. She removed the arthritis mutilans subgroup as a manifestation of severe disease rather than a specific subtype. Torre Alonso et al. retained the majority of the original Moll and Wright groups but did not believe that DIP disease was a subtype in its own right as it could occur within monoarthritis, oligoarthritis, or polyarthritis. Therefore the number of subgroups was decreased to four [18].

More drastic changes were proposed by Helliwell (and Wright) following scintigraphy studies identifying the specific variant of SAPHO syndrome (synovitis, acne, pustulosis, hyperostosis, osteitis). At that time, they proposed a split into just three subgroups: peripheral arthritis, spondarthritis, and SAPHO syndrome [61]. However, there was some concern that the peripheral arthritis category was too broad, encompassing phenotypically very different patients. Veale et al. proposed a different three groups splitting peripheral arthritis into asymmetrical oligoarthritis and symmetrical polyarthritis and removing the SAPHO group from the common subgroups [62].

Evolution in subtypes over time

One of the key issues with defining subtypes of disease is that many patients will show evolution in their disease over time. Many of the simplified subtypes proposed suggest a split into peripheral arthritis and spondyloarthritis but even this can evolve over time. One of the principle limitations in studies of axial PsA has been a poor agreement on how to classify this subtype.

Axial involvement in PsA has been shown to be a function of disease duration. The fact that classification relies on evidence of radiographic damage partially accounts for the increased prevalence of axial involvement seen with increasing disease duration. More recent studies in axial SpA have used MRI to show bone marrow oedema in the sacroiliac joints preceding radiographic changes, providing a possible identification of early disease. The ASAS classification criteria for axial SpA would potentially allow identification of early axial PsA with these MRI changes [57]. However, while the severity of bone marrow oedema has been shown to be a key predictor of future development of AS in a small study, only a third (n=13 patients) progressed to significant radiographic change in 10 years follow up [63].

Within the peripheral arthritis subgroups, many patients also evolve over time. Jones et al. showed that 64% of patients changed subgroup in a cohort of 100 patients. The DIP subgroup (only one patient) and spondyloarthritis subgroup remained stable over 2 years. However, in the majority of the cases with peripheral arthritis, there was increased joint involvement with mono and oligoarthritis patients frequently progressing to polyarthritis at

2 years [64]. Development of arthritis mutilans was also seen in four patients. This increase in the number of involved joints was also seen in a study by Marsal et al. where they concluded that dividing peripheral arthritis into polyarticular and oligoarticular disease was unhelpful as the majority of patients developed polyarticular disease over time [65].

Interestingly in the Dublin early arthritis clinic cohort, changes in subtypes were still seen but they reported a greater number of patients with reduction in joint counts. Although some patients with oligoarthritis did progress, the majority continued to have oligoarticular involvement or went into remission. A significant number of the polyarthritis group had also changed to have oligoarticular involvement (n=26) or remission (n=12), probably related to DMARD prescription.8 In an inception cohort in Toronto it was confirmed that the pattern of disease changed in the majority of patients (27/35 patients) over 5 years with more patients showing a reduction in disease activity over this time (13/27 reduced activity, 2/27 increased activity) [66]. The hope is that this highlights the potential impact of treatment on the natural history of the disease. More recent results from the Swedish PsA registry also showed considerable evolution in the first 2 years of the disease with only 8/60 patients progressing from mono or oligoarthritis to polyarthritis, but over half (35/64) of the polyarthritis patients showing decreasing joint involvement [67].

Future evolution of PsA classification criteria

GRAPPA project to define the inflammatory musculoskeletal stem of CASPAR

The majority of classification criteria have been developed by rheumatologists with the aim of identifying patients with PsA from a cohort of patients with confirmed arthritis. However, in other situations such as in primary care or dermatology clinics, the main limitation on the use of the CASPAR criteria is the definition of 'inflammatory musculoskeletal disease (joint, spine, or entheseal)' which is used as the stem for the criteria. Patients in psoriasis clinics will commonly fulfil the minimum of three points from the items within the CASPAR criteria, but the challenge facing the dermatologists and other non-rheumatologist physicians is identifying inflammatory musculoskeletal disease.

Recognizing this limitation, GRAPPA have started a project aiming to provide criteria to identify inflammatory musculoskeletal disease. Initial discussion focused on what sort of criteria should be assessed for inclusion [68]. Rheumatologists typically use clinical history and examination, laboratory results, and imaging findings to aid their diagnosis of inflammatory arthritis. However, requiring other specialties to perform and interpret laboratory and imaging tests would make them less practical in a busy clinical setting. In addition, a recent study in dermatology clinics found that in the majority of cases, the diagnosis of PsA could be made using history and clinical examination alone [69]. Therefore the research team decided to move forwards looking at only history and clinical examination items.

At the 2013 GRAPPA meeting, breakout groups including physicians, allied health professionals, and patient representatives brainstormed possible items that may identify inflammatory arthritis, enthesitis, dactylitis, and spondylitis [17]. The next step

in the project is to apply these individual items to a small cohort of patients with and without inflammatory arthritis to assess their sensitivity and specificity both individually and in combination for inflammatory arthritis including PsA. Finally, potential candidate criteria sets for inflammatory disease will need testing in large international cohorts to establish their accuracy in clinical practice.

References

1. Aggarwal R, Ringold S, Khanna D, et al. Distinctions between diagnostic and classification criteria? Arthritis Care Res. 2015; 67(7):891–7.
2. Taylor W J, Fransen, J. Distinctions between diagnostic and classification criteria: comment on the article by Aggarwal et al. [letter]. Arthritis Care Res. 2016; 68(1):149–50.
3. Miettinen OS. The modern scientific physician: 3. Scientific diagnosis. CMAJ. 2001;165(6):781–2.
4. Kane D, Pathare S. Early psoriatic arthritis. Rheum Dis Clin North Am. 2005;31(4):641–57.
5. Villani AP, Rouzaud M, Sevrain M, et al. Symptoms dermatologists should look for in daily practice to improve detection of psoriatic arthritis in psoriasis patients: an expert group consensus. J Eur Acad Dermatol Venereol. 2015;28 Suppl 5:27–32.
6. Bonifati C, Elia F, Francesconi F, et al. The diagnosis of early psoriatic arthritis in an outpatient dermatological centre for psoriasis. J Eur Acad Dermatol Venereol. 2012;26(5):627–33.
7. Coates LC, Conaghan PG, Emery P, et al. Sensitivity and specificity of the classification of psoriatic arthritis criteria in early psoriatic arthritis. Arthritis Rheum 2012;64(10): 3150–5.
8. Kane D, Stafford L, Bresnihan B, FitzGerald O. A prospective, clinical and radiological study of early psoriatic arthritis: an early synovitis clinic experience. Rheumatology. 2003;42(12):1460–8.
9. Reich K, Kruger K, Mossner R, Augustin, M. Epidemiology and clinical pattern of psoriatic arthritis in Germany: a prospective interdisciplinary epidemiological study of 1511 patients with plaque-type psoriasis. Br J Dermatol. 2009;160(5):1040–7.
10. Love T J, Gudbjornsson B, Gudjonsson JE, Valdimarsson, H. Psoriatic arthritis in Reykjavik, Iceland: prevalence, demographics, and disease course. J Rheumatol. 2007;34(10): 2082–8.
11. Moghaddassi M, Shahram F, Chams-Davatchi C, Najafizadeh SR., Davatchi F. Different aspects of psoriasis: analysis of 150 Iranian patients. Arch Iran Med. 2009;12(3): 279–83.
12. Niccoli L, Nannini C, Cassara E, et al. Frequency of iridocyclitis in patients with early psoriatic arthritis: a prospective, follow up study. Int J Rheum Dis. 2012;15(4):414–8.
13. Nossent JC, Gran JT. Epidemiological and clinical characteristics of psoriatic arthritis in northern Norway. Scand J Rheumatol. 2009;38(4):251–5.
14. Queiro, R., Alperi, M., Lopez, A., et al. Clinical expression, but not disease outcome, may vary according to age at disease onset in psoriatic spondylitis. Joint Bone Spine. 2008;75(5):544–7.
15. Scarpa R, Cuocolo A, Peluso R, et al. Early psoriatic arthritis: the clinical spectrum. J Rheumatol. 2008;35(1):137–41.
16. Yang Q, Qu L, Tian H, et al. Prevalence and characteristics of psoriatic arthritis in Chinese patients with psoriasis. J Eur Acad Dermatol Venereol. 2011;25(12):1409–14.
17. Mease PJ, Garg A, Helliwell PS, Park JJ, Gladman DD. Development of criteria to distinguish inflammatory from noninflammatory arthritis, enthesitis, dactylitis, and spondylitis: a report from the GRAPPA 2013 Annual Meeting. J Rheumatol. 2014;41(6):1249–51.
18. Torre Alonso JC, Rodriguez Perez A, Arribas Castrillo JM, Ballina Garcia J, Riestra Noriega JL, Lopez Larrea C. Psoriatic arthritis (PA): a clinical, immunological and radiological study of 180 patients. Br J Rheumatol. 1991;30(4):245–50.
19. Wilson FC, Icen M, Crowson CS, McEvoy MT, Gabriel SE, Kremers HM. Incidence and clinical predictors of psoriatic arthritis in

patients with psoriasis: A population-based study. Arthritis Rheum. 2009;61(2):233–9.

20. Eder L, Haddad A, Shen H, et al. The incidence and risk factors for PsA in patients with psoriasis—a prospective cohort study. Arthritis Rheum. 2014;66(S10);S814.

21. Helliwell PS, Porter G, Taylor WJ. Polyarticular psoriatic arthritis is more like oligoarticular psoriatic arthritis, than rheumatoid arthritis. Ann Rheum Dis. 2007;66(1):113–7.

22. Maejima H, Taniguchi T, Watarai A, Aki R, Katsuoka K. Analysis of clinical, radiological and laboratory variables in psoriatic arthritis with 25 Japanese patients. J Dermatol. 2010;37(7):647–56.

23. Alenius GM, Berglin E, Rantapaa Dahlqvist S. Antibodies against cyclic citrullinated peptide (CCP) in psoriatic patients with or without joint inflammation. Ann Rheum Dis. 2006;65(3): 398–400.

24. Bogliolo L, Alpini C, Caporali R, Scire CA, Moratti R, Montecucco C. Antibodies to cyclic citrullinated peptides in psoriatic arthritis. J Rheumatol. 2007;32(3):511–515.

25. Korendowych E, Owen P, Ravindran J, Carmichael C, McHugh N. The clinical and genetic associations of anti-cyclic citrullinated peptide antibodies in psoriatic arthritis. Rheumatology. 2005;44(8):1056–60.

26. Shibata S, Tada Y, Komine M, et al. Anti-cyclic citrullinated peptide antibodies and IL-23p19 in psoriatic arthritis. J Dermatol Sci. 2009;53(1):34–39.

27. Wright V. Psoriatic arthritis. A comparative radiographic study of rheumatoid arthritis and arthritis associated with psoriasis. Ann Rheum Dis. 1961;20:123–32.

28. Battistone MJ, Manaster BJ, Reda DJ, Clegg DO. The prevalence of sacroilitis in psoriatic arthritis: new perspectives from a large, multicenter cohort. A Department of Veterans Affairs Cooperative Study. Skeletal Radiol. 1999;28(4):196–201.

29. McEwen C, DiTata D, Lingg C, Porini A, Good A, Rankin T. Ankylosing spondylitis and spondylitis accompanying ulcerative colitis, regional enteritis, psoriasis and Reiter's disease. A comparative study. Arthritis Rheum. 1971;14(3):291–318.

30. Moll JM, Wright V. Psoriatic arthritis. Semin Arthritis Rheum. 1973;3:55–78.

31. Moll JMH, Haslock I, Macrae IF. Associations between ankylosing spondylitis, psoriatic arthritis, Reiter's disease, the intestinal arthropathies and Behçet's syndrome. Medicine (Baltimore). 1974;53:343–64.

32. Cats A. Is psoriatic arthritis an entity? Paper presented at the Rheumatology—85. Proceedings of the XVIth International Congress of Rheumatology, Sydney; 1985.

33. Gladman DD, Shuckett R, Russell ML, Thorne JC, Schachter, RK. Psoriatic arthritis (PSA)--an analysis of 220 patients. QJM. 1987; 62(238):127–41.

34. Bennett RM. Psoriatic arthritis. In D. J. McCarty (Ed.), Arthritis and Related Conditions (9th ed., pp. 645). Philadelphia: Lea and Febiger. 1979.

35. Vasey F, Espinoza LR. Psoriatic arthropathy. In A. Calin (Ed.), Spondyloarthropathies (pp. 151–85). Orlando, Florida: Grune and Stratton; 1984.

36. Dougados M, van der Linden S, Juhlin R, et al. The European Spondyloarthropathy Study Group preliminary criteria for the classification of spondyloarthropathy. Arthritis Rheum. 1991;34(10):1218–27.

37. McGonagle D, Conaghan PG, Emery P. Psoriatic arthritis: a unified concept twenty years on. Arthritis Rheum. 1999;42(6):1080–6.

38. Fournie B, Crognier L, Arnaud C, et al. Proposed classification criteria of psoriatic arthritis. A preliminary study in 260 patients. Revue Du Rhumatisme, English Edition, 1999;66(10):446–56.

39. Taylor WJ, Marchesoni A, Arreghini M, Sokoll K, Helliwell, PS. A comparison of the performance characteristics of classification criteria for the diagnosis of psoriatic arthritis. Semin Arthritis Rheum. 2004;34(3):575–84.

40. Taylor W, Gladman D, Helliwell P, Marchesoni A, Mease P, Mielants H. Classification criteria for psoriatic arthritis: development of new criteria from a large international study. Arthritis Rheum. 2005;54(8):2665–73.

41. Congi L, Roussou E. Clinical application of the CASPAR criteria for psoriatic arthritis compared to other existing criteria. Clin Exp Rheumatol. 2010;28(3):304–10.

42. Leung YY, Tam LS, Ho KW, et al. Evaluation of the CASPAR criteria for psoriatic arthritis in the Chinese population. Rheumatology. 2010;49(1):112–5.

43. Zlatkovic-Svenda M, Kerimovic-Morina D, Stojanovic RM. Psoriatic arthritis classification criteria: Moll and Wright, ESSG and CASPAR—a comparative study. Acta Reumatol Port. 2013;38(3):172–78.

44. Zlatkovic-Svenda MI, Kerimovic-Morina D, Stojanovic RM. Psoriatic arthritis criteria evaluation: CASPAR and Modified CASPAR. Clin Exp Rheumatol, 2011;29(5):899–900.

45. Gunal EK, Kamali S, Gul A, et al. Clinical evaluation and comparison of different criteria for classification in Turkish patients with psoriatic arthritis. Rheumatol Int. 2009;29(4):365–70.

46. Nas K, Karkucak M, Durmus B, et al. The performance of psoriatic arthritis classification criteria in Turkish patients with psoriatic arthritis. Int J Rheum Dis. 2017;20(8):985–9.

47. Chandran V, Schentag CT, Gladman DD. Sensitivity and specificity of the CASPAR criteria for psoriatic arthritis in a family medicine clinic setting. J Rheumatol. 2008;35(10); 2069–70; author reply 2070.

48. Tillett W, Costa L, Jadon D, et al. The ClASsification for Psoriatic ARthritis (CASPAR) criteria--a retrospective feasibility, sensitivity, and specificity study. J Rheumatol 2012;39(1):154–6.

49. Chandran V, Schentag CT, Gladman DD. Sensitivity of the classification of psoriatic arthritis criteria in early psoriatic arthritis. Arthritis Rheum. 2007;57(8):1560–3.

50. D'Angelo S, Mennillo GA, Cutro MS, et al. Sensitivity of the classification of psoriatic arthritis criteria in early psoriatic arthritis. J Rheumatol 2009;36(2):368–70.

51. D'Angelo S., Ferrante MC, Atteno M, et al. The performance of CASPAR criteria in early psoriatic arthritis: perliminary results from an italian prospective multicentre study. Ann Rheum Dis. 2008;67 (SII), 525 (abstract).

52. Ficco HM, Citera G, Cocco JA. Prevalence of psoriatic arthritis in psoriasis patients according to newer classification criteria. Clin Rheumatol. 2004;33(10):1489–93.

53. van den Berg R, van Gaalen F, van der Helm-van Mil A, Huizinga T, van der Heijde D. Performance of classification criteria for peripheral spondyloarthritis and psoriatic arthritis in the Leiden Early Arthritis cohort. Ann Rheum Dis, 2012;71(8):1366–9.

54. Pedersen OB, Junker P. On the applicability of the CASPAR criteria in psoriatic arthritis. Ann Rheum Dis. 2008;67(10):1495–6.

55. Williamson L, Dockerty JL, Dalbeth N, McNally E, Ostlere S, Wordsworth BP. Clinical assessment of sacroiliitis and HLA-B27 are poor predictors of sacroiliitis diagnosed by magnetic resonance imaging in psoriatic arthritis. Rheumatology. 2004;43(1):85–8.

56. Nash P, Lubrano E, Cauli A, Taylor W J, Olivieri I, Gladman DD. Updated guidelines for the management of axial disease in psoriatic arthritis. J Rheumatol. 2014;41(11):2286s–9.

57. Rudwaleit M, van der Heijde D, Landewe R., et al. The development of Assessment of SpondyloArthritis international Society classification criteria for axial spondyloarthritis (part II): validation and final selection. Ann Rheum Dis. 2009;68(6):777–83.

58. Deodhar A, Reveille JD, van den Bosch F et al. The concept of axial spondyloarthritis: Joint Statement of the Spondyloarthritis Research and Treatment Network and the Assessment of SpondyloArthritis International Society in Response to the US Food and Drug Administration's Comments and Concerns. Arthritis Rheumatol. 2014;66(10):2649–56.

59. Collantes E, Veroz R, Escudero A, et al. Can some cases of 'possible' spondyloarthropathy be classified as 'definite' or undifferentiated' spondyloarthropathy? Value of criteria for spondyloarthropathies. Joint Bone Spine. 2000;67:516–20.

60. Wright V. Rheumatism and psoriasis: a re-evaluation. Am J Med 1959;27:454–62.

61. Helliwell P, Marchesoni A, Peters M, Barker M., Wright V. A re-evaluation of the osteoarticular manifestations of psoriasis. Br J Rheumatol. 1991;30(5):339–45.

62. Veale D, Rogers S, Fitzgerald O. Classification of clinical subsets in psoriatic arthritis [see comment]. Br J Rheumatol. 1994;33(2):133–8.

63. Bennett AN, McGonagle D, O'Connor P, et al. Severity of baseline magnetic resonance imaging-evident sacroiliitis and HLA-B27 status in early inflammatory back pain predict radiographically evident ankylosing spondylitis at eight years. Arthritis Rheum. 2008;58(11):3413–8.

64. Jones SM, Armas JB, Cohen MG, Lovell CR., Evison G, McHugh NJ. Psoriatic arthritis: outcome of disease subsets and relationship of joint disease to nail and skin disease. Br J Rheumatol. 1994;33(9):834–9.

65. Marsal S, Armadans-Gil L, Martinez M, Gallardo D, Ribera A, Lience E. Clinical, radiographic and HLA associations as markers for different patterns of psoriatic arthritis. Rheumatology. 1999;38(4):332–7.

66. Khan M, Schentag C, Gladman DD. Clinical and radiological changes during psoriatic arthritis disease progression. J Rheumatol. 2003;30(5):1022–6.

67. Lindqvist UR, Alenius GM, Husmark T, Theander E, Holmstrom G, Larsson PT. The Swedish early psoriatic arthritis register—2-year followup: a comparison with early rheumatoid arthritis. J Rheumatol. 2008;35(4):668–73.

68. Mease PJ. Distinguishing inflammatory from noninflammatory arthritis, enthesitis, and dactylitis in psoriatic arthritis: a report from the GRAPPA 2010 annual meeting. J Rheumatol.2012;39(2):415–7.

69. Mease PJ, Garg A, Gladman DD, Helliwell PS. Development of simple clinical criteria for the definition of inflammatory arthritis, enthesitis, dactylitis, and spondylitis: a report from the GRAPPA 2012 annual meeting. J Rheumatol. 2013;40(8):1442–5.

Outcome and biomarkers

CHAPTER 21

The clinical course and outcome of psoriatic arthritis

Lihi Eder

Introduction

Verna Wright from Leeds provided the earliest detailed description of the clinical characteristics and natural history of psoriatic arthritis (PsA) [1]. In his series Wright found that oligoarthritis was the predominant pattern of joint involvement and that patients with PsA had fewer joint deformities than in rheumatoid arthritis (RA) patients. The notion that PsA has a benign course has since been challenged by other groups that showed a progressive joint damage accrual over time.

Longitudinal cohorts of PsA provided valuable information about the natural course of disease. The University of Toronto PsA cohort that was established by Dafna Gladman in 1978 provided large body of information about the natural history and outcomes in PsA [2]. Additional notable PsA cohorts are those from Bath (UK), Dublin (Ireland), and an early PsA cohort from Sweden [3, 4]. These cohorts are based on patients from secondary and tertiary centres, therefore, their population may be skewed towards a more severe spectrum of the disease. Recent population-based studies have used large administrative databases to investigate outcomes in PsA. The results of these studies may be more generalizable; however, they lack important clinical information about features of the disease that may have significant implications for outcome investigation. National registries that collect information on biologic therapies are another relatively new source of information particularly about predictors of treatment outcomes.

In this chapter, a review of the natural history and predictors of clinical outcomes in PsA is presented. Cohort rather than cross-sectional studies were preferred, as the latter study design is unable to determine a temporal relationship between potential predictors and outcomes and may provide a misleading picture. Investigating the natural course of PsA has become challenging as the clinical picture may be confounded by effective therapies that have emerged over the past decade. Therefore, information from older series from the pre-biologic era was synthesized as it provides a less biased picture of the natural course of the disease.

The emergence of the biological medications led to a revolution in the field of PsA. The ability to effectively control psoriasis and arthritis and the awareness of the importance of early intensive therapy have allowed many patients to achieve a state of clinical remission. This has likely improved long-term outcomes, such as the chances of developing structural joint damage, disability, and comorbidities. However, limited data are available about long-term outcomes in PsA from the post-biologic period.

Disease onset and pattern of presentation and progression

PsA is a heterogeneous disease, which complicates the description of the natural course of the disease. Five classical patterns of PsA were described by Moll and Wright in their seminal paper from 1973: asymetrical oligoarthritis, RA-like polyarthritis, spondylitis, arthritis mutilans, and distal predominant pattern [5]. These patterns were found to be less useful for prognostic purposes since they change over time. Patients who begin with polyarthritis are often reclassified as having oligoarthritis following effective treatment, while others who initially present with a few actively inflamed joints progress to the polyarticular pattern later in the course of their disease. Jones et al. found that 79% of patients with oligoarthritis and 20% of those with polyarthritis changed pattern [6]. In addition, patients with PsA tend to be less tender than RA patients, which may lead to underestimation of the extent of the actual number of actively inflamed joints [7]. Imaging studies have found a substantial prevalence of subclinical arthritis in patients with PsA. An ultrasound assessment of the joints in patients with early PsA led to re-classification of the majority of patients with oligoarthritis to polyarthritis [8]. These issues may decrease the predictive value of the traditional classification of peripheral patterns in PsA. Nevertheless, several clinical patterns, including polyarthritis vs oligoarthritis and dactylitis, can provide prognostic information [9].

Mild non-erosive PsA

Wright described in his early series a group of patients with a benign course who achieved a long-lasting remission after the initial presentation has subsided [10]. Indeed, there are patients who present with mild arthritis or enthesitis involving only a few sites that resolve completely with or without therapy and never reoccur. It should be noted, however, that oligoarthritis or enthesitis that affect large weight-bearing joint sites could have a significant impact on function and quality of life. The increasing awareness about the importance of early diagnosis and the growing collaboration between dermatologists and rheumatologists likely lead to an increase in the diagnosis of milder cases at earlier stages of the disease.

Approximately a third of patients with PsA present with oligoarthritis prior to the initiation of therapy. Kane et al. reported that only a minority of patients with early disease who presented with oligoarthritis progressed to polyarthritis and 21% achieved complete remission (11% disease modifying anti-rheumatic agents (DMARD)-free remission) at 2 years [11]. In the Toronto PsA cohort, a third of patients do not have any evidence of clinically damaged joints at presentation or follow-up in the clinic [12]. In addition, among 290 patients who were followed for at least 10 years, 12.4% were free of radiographic joint erosions [13]. This group tended to have a lower number of actively inflamed joints at presentation and almost a third of them were in clinical remission at their first clinic assessment. Furthermore, 28% of the patients in the clinic remained free of physical disability during the course of disease [14].

Thus, there appears to be a small group of PsA patients who have mild non-progressive form of arthritis. In some of them the arthritis may be transient. These patients are more likely to present with fewer involved joints at disease onset and to have improved long-term outcomes.

Progressive destructive PsA

In contrast to earlier reports suggesting a benign nature for PsA, later series showed that in the majority of patients, PsA runs a progressive course that can lead to structural joint damage and disability. In fact, PsA can lead to the same degree of structural joint damage and disability as RA [15, 16]. In most series, including those of early PsA, the most prevalent pattern of joint involvement is polyarthritis with or without axial involvement. Joint damage is a good surrogate of poor functional outcome and during the disease course the number of patients who develop deformities and radiographic damage increases over time. Fifty-five percent of the patients developed clinical damage in five or more joints and radiographic erosions were present in 87.6% of patients after 10 years of follow-up [13, 17]. Structural damage can develop very early in the course of disease. Kane et al. found that 26% of patients who were assessed within 2 years of the onset of PsA had radiographic erosions and 47% developed erosions after 2 years of follow-up despite treatment [18]. In the Swedish Early Psoriatic Arthritis Register, 20% and 32% of the patients with early PsA had radiographic erosive or proliferative joint damage at clinic entry and at 2 years, respectively [16]. In parallel, 34.5% of patients with long-standing disease have moderate to severe disability (Health Assessment Questionnaire (HAQ) score>1) [19]. In the Toronto PsA cohort, 72% of the patients had either persistent disability or had fluctuating disability state during the course of the disease [14]. Disability states correlated significantly with the number of actively inflamed joints and the degree of clinical joint damage.

A small subgroup of patients develops a rapidly progressive severe form of a destructive arthritis that was termed arthritis mutilans. The definition of arthritis mutilans is controversial, but it is generally accepted to include the extreme forms of radiographic phenotype including osteolysis and pencil-in-cup deformities manifested clinically as digital shortening [20]. In the CASPAR study that included 588 PsA patients from multiple international sites, 3.5% of patients had clinical features of arthritis mutilans [21]. These patients tended to have longer disease duration, spinal involvement, and polyarticular symmetric joint involvement, and they were also more likely to require joint surgeries. It is unclear, however, whether arthritis mutilans is a distinct subtype of PsA that is associated with distinct biological mechanisms.

Spondylitis

The occurrence of axial involvement in patients with PsA ranges from 15% to 43% depending on the definition used [22]. Many patients have asymptomatic spondylitis therefore studies that included routine spine radiographs tended to report higher proportion of spinal disease. Patients with PsA tend to have milder structural damage and better spinal mobility compared to patients with ankylosing spondylitis (AS) [23]. Furthermore, a pure axial involvement without peripheral arthritis is a rare pattern in PsA seen in 0–3.7% of the patients [4, 11, 24]. The progression of radiographic spinal damage and restriction of spine mobility was studied in 297 patients with axial PsA over a period of 10 years. At baseline, only 56% of the patients with axial spondylitis had back symptoms. At 10 years, up to 52% of the patients either developed new sacroiliitis or showed progression in sacroiliitis while only a minority showed a progression in syndesmophytes [25]. However, despite the improvement in spinal symptoms experienced by most patients, there was a significant decline in mobility of the lumbar and cervical spine. The presence of *HLA-B*27* was associated with the development of new lumbar syndesmophytes while therapy with DMARDs or the presence of syndesmophytes at baseline did not affect spinal structural damage progression [25].

Dactylitis and enthesitis

Limited information is available about the link between dactylitis and enthesitis, two important clinical characteristics of PsA, and long-term outcomes. Dactylitis presents clinically as a sausage-shaped digit, and affects up to 48% of patients with PsA at some point during the course of their disease. It is considered one of the key elements of the CASPAR criteria for classification of PsA [26]. Imaging studies of dactylitic digits have shown inflammation in articular and peri-articular structures (flexor tenosynovitis, pulley, bone oedema) in addition to soft tissue swelling [27]. Dactylitis is a marker of disease severity. Brockbank et al. found that among 185 patients with dactylitis-affected digits were more likely to exhibit progression of radiographic structural damage compared with unaffected digits (55% vs 27% in the hands and 29% vs 20% in the feet, respectively). In addition, digits with recurrent dactylitis were more likely to develop radiographic damage (45% vs 30%) [28].

Enthesitis is considered the hallmark clinical feature of spondyloarthritis (SpA). It has been suggested that enthesitis is the underlying lesion of the various musculoskeletal manifestations of PsA [29]. Symptomatic enthesitis affects 20–40% of patients with PsA [11, 30]. However, accurate clinical detection of enthesitis is challenging, as there is a high level of discordance between clinical-based and imaging-based assessment of the enethesis [31]. Although the importance of enthesitis in PsA is acknowledged, there is very limited information about its association with disease severity. Symptomatic enthesitis, particularly when affecting the lower limbs, can have significant implications for function and quality of life. In patients with AS a high number of tender entheseal sites was associated with increased levels of pain [32]. An analysis of 118 patients with SpA, including PsA patients, found a correlation between enthesitis and longer disease duration, prolonged morning stiffness, and higher tender joint count [33]. It is currently unknown whether the presence of enthesitis predicts long-term outcomes in PsA.

Outcomes of PsA

Remission and minimal disease activity state

Suppression of inflammation and achievement of minimal disease activity state is the primary goal in the treatment of PsA in order to prevent long-term complications including structural damage and disability. Remission has become a realistic target in the management of PsA with the advent of the various biologic medications. Currently there are no accepted criteria for remission in PsA. Minimal disease activity (MDA) is a validated composite outcome measure that was developed to encompass both remission and low disease activity in patients with PsA [34]. The achievement of sustained MDA is associated with less radiographic progression compared to patients who never achieve MDA [35]. Several cohort studies assessed predictors for remission and MDA in patients with PsA. Lindqvist et al. reported that 17% of the patients with early PsA achieved remission at 2 years. Lower tender joint count and psoriatic nail lesions at baseline predicted remission [16]. Similar rates of remission were reported by Gladman et al. and Cantini et al. in cohorts of patients with longstanding PsA (17.6% and 24%, respectively). Male gender, fewer actively inflamed and damaged joints, and better physical function at presentation predicted the achievement of remission [36, 37]. Predictors of MDA were studied in several independent cohorts. The probability of achieving MDA raged from 34% to 66%. Coates et al. reported that patients with polyarthritis and elevated erythrocyte sedimentation rate (ESR) were less likely to achieve MDA [38]. Theander et al. found that shorter delay between symptoms onset and diagnosis and low HAQ at inclusion were associated with higher chance of achieving MDA in patients with early PsA [39]. Higher HAQ scores at baseline were also associated with a lower probability of achieving persistent MDA during the 5 years extension phase of the GO-REVEAL trial of golimumab in PsA [35]. Obesity is a prevalent co-morbidity in patients with PsA and can also affect disease severity. Recent studies have found that overweight and obese patients with PsA are less likely to achieve MDA whereas patients who engage in a low-calorie diet that results in weight lose fare better [40–42]. Overall, remission and MDA are realistic treatment targets in PsA and correlate with improved long-term outcomes. Active inflammation and poor physical function reduce the chances of achieving these goals while early diagnosis and normal weight improve the outcome. The results of studies assessing predictors for remission and MDA in PsA are summarized in Table 21.1.

Table 21.1 Remission/minimal disease activity in PsA

Reference	Study population, country	No. of patients	Outcome	% achieving the outcome	Predictors of achieving the outcome
Lindqvist (16)	Early PsA, Sweden	135	Remission at 2 years	17%	• Low tender and swollen joint count • Psoriatic nail lesions
Gladman (36)	PsA cohort, Canada	391	Remission	18%	• Low tender and swollen joint count • Low damaged joint count • Male gender
Cantini (37)	PsA patients initiating DMARDs, Italy	236	Remission	24%	
Saber (43)	PsA patients initiating TNFα blockers, Ireland	152	EULAR DAS28 definition for remission at 12 months	58%	• Male gender • Low HAQ • Low patient global assessment score • Short duration of early morning stiffness
Coates (38)	PsA cohort, Canada	344	MDA for ≥12 months	34%	• Low joint count • Low ESR
Theander (44)	Early PsA, Sweden	197	MDA at 5 years	38%	• Short delay between symptoms onset to diagnosis • Low HAQ • Male gender
Kavanaugh (35)	PsA patients initiating golimumab (GO-REVEAL trial), International	395	MDA at 1 year	42% in the treatment arm	• Low HAQ
Haddad (45)	PsA patients initiating TNFα blockers, Canada	226	MDA for ≥12 months	64%	• Male gender • Low ESR
di Minno (40, 46)	PsA patients initiating treatment with anti TNFα agents, Italy	270	MDA at 1 year	36%	• Normal weight vs obese • Weight reduction in obese patients
Eder (42)	PsA cohort, Canada	557	MDA for ≥12 months	66%	• Normal weight vs overweight and obese

Peripheral joint damage

The development of structural joint damage is an important outcome in PsA. It is now well recognized that PsA can lead to the development of joint damage in a significant proportion of patients. Joint damage is a good surrogate of poor functional outcome [14] and prevention of joint damage is one of the main goals of treatment. Joint damage can be noted clinically as joint deformities, flail joints and fused joints, whereas radiographic joint damage identifies peri-articular erosions, joint space narrowing, subluxation, pencil-in-cup changes, and ankylosis. As mentioned above (see 'Progressive destructive PsA'), the majority of patients with PsA develop clinical and radiographic joint damage during the course of their disease and there is a good correlation between clinical and radiographic joint damage [47]. High swollen joint count, DMARD use, and elevated inflammatory markers predicted progression in clinical joint damage in general [48]. At the joint level, the presence of tenderness or swelling in a particular joint in the hands or feet predicted subsequent damage in the same joint [49]. In line with these findings, elevated ESR, high tender and swollen joint counts, the presence of joint damage at baseline, and dactylitis predicted the development of radiographic joint damage [12, 28, 50, 51]. A post hoc analysis of data from the Adalimumab Effectiveness in PsA Trial (ADEPT) showed that C-reactive protein was a strong predictor for radiographic progression [52]. Additionally, recent studies assessed the impact of delayed rheumatologic management of PsA on development of structural damage. Haroon et al. reported that a delay of more than 6 months from onset of symptoms to rheumatologic assessment was associated with a higher degree of radiographic joint damage after 10 years [53]. In accordance with these findings, Gladman et al. found that patients who were assessed in the clinic within the first 2 years of the onset of PsA developed less clinical joint damage [54]. The results of these studies highlight the strong link between active inflammation and subsequent development of joint damage and support the importance of early and aggressive suppression of musculoskeletal inflammation in patients with PsA.

HLA alleles and disease outcome

Psoriasis and PsA have substantive genetic determinants as indicated by their high familial aggregation. HLA class I alleles are the strongest susceptibility genes for psoriasis and PsA. HLA-C*06 confers the highest risk for psoriasis and also predisposes to earlier onset and more severe disease [55, 56]. HLA-B alleles are associated with musculoskeletal manifestations and HLA-B*27, *B38, B*39, and B*08 were reported as specific genetic markers for PsA among patients with psoriasis while HLA-C*06 has been associated with lower risk of developing PsA [57]. Additionally, HLA alleles have been implicated as markers of severity in patients with PsA. HLA-B*27 has been associated with a more severe sub-phenotype of PsA that presents with axial involvement, an earlier onset of arthritis, and progression of joint damage [58–60]. In an analysis of 282 patients with PsA, the presence of HLA-B*2705 was associated with enthesitis, dactylitis, and symmetric sacroiliitis whereas the haplotype HLA-B*0801-C*0701 was associated with joint fusion and deformities, asymmetric sacroiliitis, and dactylitis. In contrast, HLA-B*44 was associated with milder disease [61]. In line with these findings, an analysis of 649 patients with PsA found that the presence of HLA-B*27 was associated with more severe disease

phenotype including the development of clinical joint damage, dactylitis, and axial involvement [62, 63]. In addition, HLA-B*39 and A*02 were associated with higher risk of damage progression [60, 64]. Ho et al. reported that HLA-C*06 and DR*07 were associated with fewer damaged and involved joints. Unlike RA, the shared epitopes HLA-DR*04 and DR*03 did not predict damage progression in PsA [65]. Thus overall, HLA alleles serve as susceptibility markers for PsA among patients with psoriasis and several of these alleles are also markers of PsA severity. Despite their relation with disease outcome, it is unclear as yet whether these genetic markers provide an additional predictive value for risk stratification of PsA patients, independently of clinical variables.

Physical functioning and work disability

Physical function and work disability are important outcomes in patients with PsA. Physical functioning in patients with PsA is significantly decreased compared to non-psoriatic subjects and to patients with psoriasis alone [66, 67]. The degree of physical dysfunction in PsA is similar to that in RA patients [68–70]. The HAQ serves as the most widely used outcome measure for assessment of physical functioning in PsA in clinical trials and observational studies. Other outcome measures include the Medical Outcome Study Short Form Health Survey (SF-36) and the Disease Life Quality Index (DLQI). HAQ scores correlate with disease activity [71]. Predictors for disability were assessed in the Toronto PsA cohort by investigating transitions between pre-defined states of HAQ over the course of the disease. In this study, older age predicted slower improvement in HAQ and female gender predicted faster decline in disability. Longer disease duration was associated with reduced frequency of transition between the different physical functioning states while elevated damaged joint count reduced the likelihood of improvement and elevated active joint count predicted quicker deterioration [72]. Haroon et al. reported that delayed rheumatologic consultation (>6 months from the onset of symptoms) was associated with worse HAQ score in patients with long-standing PsA [53]. Similarly, a study from Bath, UK found that female gender, smoking, older age at the time of the diagnosis, and delay of more than a year from the onset of symptoms to the diagnosis predicted disability after 10 years of disease duration [19]. Leung et al. reported that older age, physical disability at baseline, and high number of damaged joints predicted physical disability at 4–6 years in a cohort of Chinese patients with PsA [66]. Data from clinical trials show that effective suppression of musculoskeletal inflammation by various biologic and non-biologic therapies is associated with improved short- and long-term physical function and reduced disability [73–75]. Therefore, these data highlight the importance of early and aggressive treatment in order to decrease the risk of developing structural damage and disability. Work disability has a significant impact on quality of life and financial status at the individual level and can also impose considerable economic burden at the society level. The prevalence of work disability in PsA varies widely from 20% to 67% depending on the population sampled, the method of assessment and the definition of work disability [76, 77]. The higher estimates were reported in studies sampling patients starting biologic therapy, which represent the most severe spectrum of the disease. In general, older age, female gender, severe arthritis, and poor response to treatment were associated with work disability. Roberts et al. reported that patients with 'deforming' arthritis were more likely to become work disabled (62%) compared to

Table 21.2 Predictors of disability

Reference	Study population, country	No. of patients	Outcome	Predictors of disability
Husted (14)	PsA cohort, Canada	341	HAQ	• Old age • Long disease duration • High damaged joint count • Female gender
Haroon (53)	Longstanding PsA, Ireland	283	HAQ	• Delayed rheumatologic consultation
Tillett (19)	Longstanding PsA, UK	267	HAQ	• Delayed rheumatologic consultation • Female gender • Smoking • Older age at diagnosis
Leung (66)	PsA cohort, China	97	HAQ	• Old age • Disability at baseline • High damaged joint count

those with DIP joint and RA-like patterns (3%) [78]. Kristensen et al. reported that being work disabled at baseline, poor response to therapy, older age, female gender, and longer disease duration at baseline predicted work disability at 3 years following the initiation of TNFα blockers [77]. The results of studies assessing predictors for disability in PsA are summarized in Table 21.2.

Economic considerations

PsA imposes a significant economic burden in addition to that related to psoriasis alone. Furthermore, both psoriasis and PsA are associated with other co-morbid conditions that are linked with increased healthcare utilization and high costs. The annual direct medical expenses for psoriasis in the United States were 5.17 billion dollars (US$ in 2006) [79]. Patients with PsA have more inpatient admission and outpatient consultations compared with those who have psoriasis alone [80]. An analysis of data from an US administrative claim database from the biologic medication era reported an annual incremental healthcare cost of $23,000 in patients with PsA compared to non-psoriatic patients, of which $18,000$ was attributed to pharmacy costs and $5000 to medical service costs [81]. Overall, PsA imposes a substantial economic burden even with the availability of the biologic treatments.

Mortality

Earlier studies from the Toronto PsA cohort about mortality in patients with PsA reported that standardized mortality rates were higher in these patients compared to the general population although a trend for a decline in mortality rate was observed in more recent cohorts [82, 83]. The overall standardized mortality ratio for the period of 1978 to 2004 was 1.36 with an estimated number of life-years lost by the PsA patient cohort was 2.99 years. The leading causes of death were cardiovascular diseases (24.6%), cancer (23.6%), and respiratory diseases (10.4%). In contrast, studies from Bath, UK and Rochester, Minnesota, USA did not find significant differences in mortality rate in patients with PsA compared with the general population [84, 85]. A recent population-based study that used data from a large medical records database suggested that mortality rates in PsA patients are similar to those in the general population [86]. Higher burden of disease activity including

elevated ESR and the presence of radiographic damage predicted mortality in PsA patients [87]. It is possible that the decline in mortality rates observed in PsA patients in recent decades reflects earlier diagnosis and improved therapies leading to a better control of inflammation.

Summary

In contrast to early reports, it is now appreciated that PsA can present as a destructive, progressive, and disabling arthritis with consequences as severe as those of RA. Longitudinal cohort studies identified predictors for improved outcomes including male gender and lower burden of inflammation at presentation while delayed diagnosis, disability, and joint damage are associated with worse long-term outcomes. These findings suggest that early diagnosis and aggressive control of inflammation are important as they may prevent the occurrence of subsequent joint damage. The latter is strongly correlated with long-term outcomes such as reduced physical function, work disability, and increased mortality. Further prognostic studies are needed as it is likely that with the advent of biologics era many of the outcomes have changed significantly. In addition, development of prediction models using clinical measures, laboratory biomarkers, and imaging is warranted to stratify patients with early disease into risk groups for long-term outcomes. Such models may direct the management of PsA patients in the future.

References

1. Wright V. Psoriatic arthritis; a comparative study of rheumatoid arthritis, psoriasis, and arthritis associated with psoriasis. AMA Arch Derm. 1959;80:27–35.
2. Gladman DD, Chandran V. Observational cohort studies: lessons learnt from the University of Toronto Psoriatic Arthritis Program. Rheumatology (Oxford). 2011;50:25–31.
3. Gladman DD, Ritchlin C, Helliwell PS. Psoriatic arthritis clinical registries and genomics. Ann Rheum Dis. 2005;64 Suppl 2:ii103–5.
4. Svensson B, Holmstrom G, Lindqvist U, Psoriatric Arthritis Register Group of the Swedish Society for R. Development and early experiences of a Swedish psoriatic arthritis register. Scand J Rheumatol. 2002;31:221–5.

5. Moll J, Wright V. Psoriatic arthritis. Semin Arthritis Rheum. 1973;3:55–78.

6. Jones SM, Armas JB, Cohen MG, Lovell CR, Evison G, Mchugh NJ. Psoriatic arthritis: outcome of disease subsets and relationship of joint disease to nail and skin disease. Brit J Rheum. 1994;33:834–9.

7. Buskila D, Langevitz P, Gladman DD, Urowitz S, Smythe HA. Patients with rheumatoid arthritis are more tender than those with psoriatic arthritis. J Rheumatol. 1992;19:1115–9.

8. Freeston JE, Coates LC, Nam JL, et al. Is there subclinical synovitis in early psoriatic arthritis? A clinical comparison with gray-scale and power Doppler ultrasound. Arthritis Care Res (Hoboken). 2014;66:432–9.

9. Khan M, Schentag C, Gladman DD. Clinical and radiological changes during psoriatic arthritis disease progression. J Rheumatol. 2003;30:1022–6.

10. Wright V. Psoriasis and arthritis. Ann Rheum Dis. 1956;15:348–56.

11. Kane D, Stafford L, Bresnihan B, FitzGerald O. A classification study of clinical subsets in an inception cohort of early psoriatic peripheral arthritis– 'DIP or not DIP revisited'. Rheumatology (Oxford). 2003;42:1469–76.

12. Bond SJ, Farewell VT, Schentag CT, Gladman DD. Predictors for radiological damage in psoriatic arthritis: results from a single centre. Ann Rheum Dis. 2007;66:370–6.

13. Touma Z, Thavaneswaran A, Chandran V, Gladman D. Predictors of erosion-free psoriatic arthritis. Arth Rheum. 2012;64 Supp:1371.

14. Husted JA, Tom BD, Farewell VT, Schentag CT, Gladman DD. A longitudinal study of the effect of disease activity and clinical damage on physical function over the course of psoriatic arthritis: Does the effect change over time? Arthritis Rheum. 2007;56:840–9.

15. Rahman P, Nguyen E, Cheung C, Schentag CT, Gladman DD. Comparison of radiological severity in psoriatic arthritis and rheumatoid arthritis. J Rheumatol. 2001;28:1041–4.

16. Lindqvist UR, Alenius GM, Husmark T, et al. The Swedish early psoriatic arthritis register–2-year followup: a comparison with early rheumatoid arthritis. J Rheumatol. 2008;35:668–73.

17. Gladman DD. Natural history of psoriatic arthritis. Baillieres Clin Rheumatol. 1994;8:379–94.

18. Kane D, Stafford L, Bresnihan B, FitzGerald O. A prospective, clinical and radiological study of early psoriatic arthritis: an early synovitis clinic experience. Rheumatology (Oxford). 2003;42:1460–8.

19. Tillett W, Jadon D, Shaddick G, et al. Smoking and delay to diagnosis are associated with poorer functional outcome in psoriatic arthritis. Ann Rheum Dis. 2013;72:1358–61.

20. Haddad A, Chandran V. Arthritis mutilans. Curr Rheumatol Rep. 2013;15:321.

21. Chandran V, Gladman DD, Helliwell PS, Gudbjornsson B. Arthritis mutilans: a report from the GRAPPA 2012 annual meeting. J Rheumatol. 2013;40:1419–22.

22. Gladman DD, Antoni C, Mease P, Clegg DO, Nash P. Psoriatic arthritis: epidemiology, clinical features, course, and outcome. Annals of the rheumatic diseases. 2005;64 Suppl 2:ii14–7.

23. Gladman DD, Brubacher B, Buskila D, Langevitz P, Farewell VT. Differences in the expression of spondyloarthropathy: a comparison between ankylosing spondylitis and psoriatic arthritis. Clin Invest Med. 1993;16:1–7.

24. Gladman DD, Shuckett R, Russell ML, Thorne JC, Schachter RK. Psoriatic arthritis (PSA)–an analysis of 220 patients. Q J Med. 1987;62:127–41.

25. Chandran V, Barrett J, Schentag CT, Farewell VT, Gladman DD. Axial psoriatic arthritis: update on a longterm prospective study. J Rheumatol. 2009;36:2744–50.

26. Taylor W, Gladman D, Helliwell P, et al. Classification criteria for psoriatic arthritis: development of new criteria from a large international study. Arthritis Rheum. 2006;54:2665–73.

27. Tan AL, Fukuba E, Halliday NA, Tanner SF, Emery P, McGonagle D. High-resolution MRI assessment of dactylitis in psoriatic arthritis shows flexor tendon pulley and sheath-related enthesitis. Ann Rheum Dis. 2015;74:185–9.

28. Brockbank JE, Stein M, Schentag CT, Gladman DD. Dactylitis in psoriatic arthritis: a marker for disease severity? Ann Rheum Dis. 2005;64:188–90.

29. McGonagle D. Enthesitis: an autoinflammatory lesion linking nail and joint involvement in psoriatic disease. J Eur Acad Dermatol Venereol. 2009;23 Suppl 1:9–13.

30. Scarpa R. Peripheral enthesopathies in psoriatic arthritis. J Rheumatol. 1998;25:2288–9.

31. Husic R, Gretler J, Felber A, et al. Disparity between ultrasound and clinical findings in psoriatic arthritis. Ann Rheum Dis. 2014;73:1529–36.

32. Mander M, Simpson JM, McLellan A, Walker D, Goodacre JA, Dick WC. Studies with an enthesis index as a method of clinical assessment in ankylosing spondylitis. Ann Rheum Dis. 1987;46:197–202.

33. Turan Y, Duruoz MT, Cerrahoglu L. Relationship between enthesitis, clinical parameters and quality of life in spondyloarthritis. Joint Bone Spine. 2009;76:642–7.

34. Coates LC, Helliwell PS. Validation of minimal disease activity criteria for psoriatic arthritis using interventional trial data. Arthritis Care Res (Hoboken). 2010;62:965–9.

35. Kavanaugh A, van der Heijde D, Beutler A, et al. Patients with psoriatic arthritis who achieve minimal disease activity in response to golimumab therapy demonstrate less radiographic progression: Results through 5 years of the randomized, placebo-controlled, GO-REVEAL study. Arthritis Care Res (Hoboken). 2015.

36. Gladman DD, Hing EN, Schentag CT, Cook RJ. Remission in psoriatic arthritis. J Rheumatol. 2001;28:1045–8.

37. Cantini F, Niccoli L, Nannini C, et al. Criteria, frequency, and duration of clinical remission in psoriatic arthritis patients with peripheral involvement requiring second-line drugs. J Rheumatol Suppl. 2009;83:78–80.

38. Coates LC, Cook R, Lee KA, Chandran V, Gladman DD. Frequency, predictors, and prognosis of sustained minimal disease activity in an observational psoriatic arthritis cohort. Arthritis Care Res (Hoboken). 2010;62:970–6.

39. Theander E, Husmark T, Alenius GM, et al. Early psoriatic arthritis: short symptom duration, male gender and preserved physical functioning at presentation predict favourable outcome at 5-year follow-up. Results from the Swedish Early Psoriatic Arthritis Register (SwePsA). Ann Rheum Dis. 2013;73(2):407–13.

40. di Minno MN, Peluso R, Iervolino S, Lupoli R, Russolillo A, Scarpa R, et al. Obesity and the prediction of minimal disease activity: a prospective study in psoriatic arthritis. Arthritis Care Res (Hoboken). 2013;65:141–7.

41. Di Minno MN, Peluso R, Iervolnjno S, Russolillo A, Lupoli R, Scarpa R. Weight loss and achievement of minimal disease activity in patients with psoriatic arthritis starting treatment with tumour necrosis factor alpha blockers. Ann Rheum Dis. 2014;73(6):1157–62.

42. Eder L, Thavaneswaran A, Chandran V, Cook R, Gladman D. Obesity is associated with lower probability of acheiving minimal disease activity state among patients with psoriatic arthritis. Ann Rheum Dis. 2013;74(5):813–7.

43. Saber TP, Ng CT, Renard G, , et al. Remission in psoriatic arthritis: is it possible and how can it be predicted? Arthritis Res Ther. 2010;12:R94.

44. Theander E, Husmark T, Alenius GM, et al. Early psoriatic arthritis: short symptom duration, male gender and preserved physical functioning at presentation predict favourable outcome at 5-year follow-up. Results from the Swedish Early Psoriatic Arthritis Register (SwePsA). Ann Rheum Dis. 2014;73:407–13.

45. Haddad A, Thavaneswaran A, Arruza IR, et al. Minimal disease activity and anti-TNF Therapy in psoriatic arthritis. Arthritis Care Res (Hoboken). 2015;67(6):842–7.

46. Di Minno MN, Peluso R, Iervolino S, et al. Weight loss and achievement of minimal disease activity in patients with psoriatic

arthritis starting treatment with tumour necrosis factor alpha blockers. Ann Rheum Dis. 2014;73:1157–62.

47. Siannis F, Farewell VT, Cook RJ, Schentag CT, Gladman DD. Clinical and radiological damage in psoriatic arthritis. Ann Rheum Dis. 2006;65:478–81.

48. Gladman DD, Farewell VT, Nadeau C. Clinical indicators of progression in psoriatic arthritis: multivariate relative risk model. J Rheumatol. 1995;22:675–9.

49. Cresswell L, Chandran V, Farewell VT, Gladman DD. Inflammation in an individual joint predicts damage to that joint in psoriatic arthritis. Ann Rheum Dis. 2011;70:305–8.

50. Queiro-Silva R, Torre-Alonso JC, Tinture-Eguren T, Lopez-Lagunas I. A polyarticular onset predicts erosive and deforming disease in psoriatic arthritis. Ann Rheum Dis. 2003;62:68–70.

51. Jones SM, Armas JB, Cohen MG, Lovell CR, Evison G, McHugh NJ. Psoriatic arthritis: outcome of disease subsets and relationship of joint disease to nail and skin disease. Br J Rheumatol. 1994;33:834–9.

52. Gladman DD, Mease PJ, Choy EH, Ritchlin CT, Perdok RJ, Sasso EH. Risk factors for radiographic progression in psoriatic arthritis: subanalysis of the randomized controlled trial ADEPT. Arthritis Res Ther. 2010;12:R113.

53. Haroon M, Gallagher P, FitzGerald O. Diagnostic delay of more than 6 months contributes to poor radiographic and functional outcome in psoriatic arthritis. Ann Rheum Dis. 2015;74:1045–50.

54. Gladman DD, Thavaneswaran A, Chandran V, Cook RJ. Do patients with psoriatic arthritis who present early fare better than those presenting later in the disease? Ann Rheum Dis. 2011;70:2152–4.

55. Nair RP, Stuart PE, Nistor I, et al. Sequence and haplotype analysis supports HLA-C as the psoriasis susceptibility 1 gene. Am J Hum Genet. 2006;78:827–51.

56. Gudjonsson JE, Karason A, Antonsdottir AA, et al. HLA-Cw6-positive and HLA-Cw6-negative patients with Psoriasis vulgaris have distinct clinical features. J Invest Dermatol. 2002;118:362–5.

57. Eder L, Chandran V, Pellet F, et al. Human leucocyte antigen risk alleles for psoriatic arthritis among patients with psoriasis. Ann Rheum Dis. 2012;71:50–5.

58. Chandran V, Tolusso DC, Cook RJ, Gladman DD. Risk factors for axial inflammatory arthritis in patients with psoriatic arthritis. J Rheumatol. 2010;37:809–15.

59. Queiro R, Torre JC, Gonzalez S, Lopez-Larrea C, Tinture T, Lopez-Lagunas I. HLA antigens may influence the age of onset of psoriasis and psoriatic arthritis. J Rheumatol. 2003;30:505–7.

60. Gladman DD, Farewell VT. The role of HLA antigens as indicators of disease progression in psoriatic arthritis. Multivariate relative risk model. Arthritis Rheum. 1995;38:845–50.

61. Haroon M, Winchester R, Giles JT, Heffernan E, FitzGerald O. Certain class I HLA alleles and haplotypes implicated in susceptibility play a role in determining specific features of the psoriatic arthritis phenotype. Ann Rheum Dis. 2016; 75(1):155–62.

62. Chandran V, Thavaneswaran A, Pellett F, Gladman D. The association between human leukocyte antigen and killer-cell immunoglobulin-like receptor gene variants and the development of arthritis mutilans in patients with psoriatic arthritis. Arth Rheum. 2011;63 Sup:1362.

63. Chandran V, Thavaneswaran A, Pellett F, Gladman D. The association between human leukocyte antigen and killer-cell immunoglobulin-like receptor gene variants and the development of axial arthritis among patients with psoriatic arthritis. Arth Rheum. 2011;63 Supp:1363.

64. Gladman DD, Farewell VT, Kopciuk KA, Cook RJ. HLA markers and progression in psoriatic arthritis. J Rheumatol. 1998;25:730–3.

65. Ho PY, Barton A, Worthington J, Thomson W, Silman AJ, Bruce IN. HLA-Cw6 and HLA-DRB1*07 together are associated with less severe joint disease in psoriatic arthritis. Ann Rheum Dis. 2007;66:807–11.

66. Leung YY, Ho KW, Li EK, et al. Predictors of functional deterioration in Chinese patients with psoriatic arthritis: a longitudinal study. BMC Musculoskelet Disord. 2014;15:284.

67. Rosen CF, Mussani F, Chandran V, Eder L, Thavaneswaran A, Gladman DD. Patients with psoriatic arthritis have worse quality of life than those with psoriasis alone. Rheumatology (Oxford). 2012;51:571–6.

68. Sokoll KB, Helliwell PS. Comparison of disability and quality of life in rheumatoid and psoriatic arthritis. J Rheumatol. 2001;28:1842–6.

69. Husted JA, Gladman DD, Farewell VT, Cook RJ. Health-related quality of life of patients with psoriatic arthritis: a comparison with patients with rheumatoid arthritis. Arthritis Rheum. 2001;45:151–8.

70. Husted JA, Gladman DD, Farewell VT, Long JA, Cook RJ. Validating the SF-36 health survey questionnaire in patients with psoriatic arthritis. J Rheumatol. 1997;24:511–7.

71. Blackmore MG, Gladman DD, Husted J, Long JA, Farewell VT. Measuring health status in psoriatic arthritis: the Health Assessment Questionnaire and its modification. The Journal of rheumatology. 1995;22:886–93.

72. Husted JA, Tom BD, Farewell VT, Schentag CT, Gladman DD. Description and prediction of physical functional disability in psoriatic arthritis: a longitudinal analysis using a Markov model approach. Arthritis Rheum. 2005;53:404–9.

73. Kavanaugh A, McInnes I, Mease P, et al. Golimumab, a new human tumor necrosis factor alpha antibody, administered every four weeks as a subcutaneous injection in psoriatic arthritis: Twenty-four-week efficacy and safety results of a randomized, placebo-controlled study. Arthritis Rheum. 2009;60:976–86.

74. Strand V, Schett G, Hu C, Stevens RM. Patient-reported Health-related Quality of Life with apremilast for psoriatic arthritis: a phase II, randomized, controlled study. J Rheumatol. 2013;40:1158–65.

75. Kavanaugh A, Menter A, Mendelsohn A, Shen YK, Lee S, Gottlieb AB. Effect of ustekinumab on physical function and health-related quality of life in patients with psoriatic arthritis: a randomized, placebo-controlled, phase II trial. Curr Med Res Opin. 2010;26:2385–92.

76. Tillett W, de-Vries C, McHugh NJ. Work disability in psoriatic arthritis: a systematic review. Rheumatology (Oxford). 2012;51:275–83.

77. Kristensen LE, Englund M, Neovius M, Askling J, Jacobsson LT, Petersson IF. Long-term work disability in patients with psoriatic arthritis treated with anti-tumour necrosis factor: a population-based regional Swedish cohort study. Ann Rheum Dis. 2013;72:1675–9.

78. Roberts ME, Wright V, Hill AG, Mehra AC. Psoriatic arthritis. Follow-up study. Ann Rheum Dis. 1976;35:206–12.

79. Gunnarsson C, Chen J, Rizzo JA, Ladapo JA, Naim A, Lofland JH. The direct healthcare insurer and out-of-pocket expenditures of psoriasis: evidence from a United States national survey. J Dermatolog Treat. 2012;23:240–54.

80. Kimball AB, Guerin A, Tsaneva M, et al. Economic burden of comorbidities in patients with psoriasis is substantial. J Eur Acad Dermatol Venereol. 2011;25:157–63.

81. Feldman SR, Zhao Y, Shi L, Tran MH, Lu J. Economic and comorbidity burden among moderate-to-severe psoriasis patients with comorbid psoriatic arthritis. Arthritis Care Res (Hoboken). 2015;67:708–17.

82. Wong K, Gladman DD, Husted J, Long JA, Farewell VT. Mortality studies in psoriatic arthritis: results from a single outpatient clinic. I. Causes and risk of death. Arthritis Rheum. 1997;40:1868–72.

83. Ali Y, Tom BD, Schentag CT, Farewell VT, Gladman DD. Improved survival in psoriatic arthritis with calendar time. Arthritis Rheum. 2007;56:2708–14.

84. Buckley C, Cavill C, Taylor G, et al. Mortality in psoriatic arthritis—a single-center study from the UK. J Rheumatol. 2010;37:2141–4.

85. Shbeeb M, Uramoto KM, Gibson LE, O'Fallon WM, Gabriel SE. The epidemiology of psoriatic arthritis in Olmsted County, Minnesota, USA, 1982-1991. J Rheumatol. 2000;27:1247–50.

86. Ogdie A, Haynes K, Troxel AB, et al. Risk of mortality in patients with psoriatic arthritis, rheumatoid arthritis and psoriasis: a longitudinal cohort study. Ann Rheum Dis. 2014;73(1):149–53.

87. Gladman DD, Farewell VT, Wong K, Husted J. Mortality studies in psoriatic arthritis: results from a single outpatient center. II. Prognostic indicators for death. Arthritis Rheum. 1998;41:1103–10.

CHAPTER 22

Biomarkers of psoriatic arthritis outcomes

Katerina Oikonomopoulou and Vinod Chandran

Introduction

Psoriatic arthritis (PsA) is defined as an inflammatory arthritis associated with psoriasis, usually seronegative for rheumatoid factor, and classified according to the CASPAR criteria [1]. Early diagnosis and appropriate treatment with systemic therapy to counter inflammation reduces disease activity and improves long-term outcomes [2–6]. However, the diagnosis and assessment of disease activity and severity is challenging due to the heterogeneous manifestations of PsA involving the skin, peripheral and axial joints, and periarticular structures, as well as the sometimes silent clinical presentation of the disease. Much of current research has, therefore, focused on the identification of clinical and routine laboratory markers associated with psoriasis and PsA that could help in the early diagnosis, risk stratification, and optimal management of the disease. In this chapter we present key concepts regarding the biomarkers of psoriatic arthritis, with a focus on soluble biomarkers and how these can be used to evaluate clinical outcomes in PsA, such as screening, diagnosis, prognosis, and monitoring of the disease and its progression. The challenges of bringing these biomarkers to clinical practice and to the development of therapeutics will also be briefly discussed.

Definition and biomarker categorization

A biomarker is defined by the US National Institute of Health (NIH) Biomarkers and Surrogate Endpoint Working Group as 'a characteristic that is objectively measured and evaluated as an indicator of normal biological processes, pathogenic processes, or pharmacologic responses to a therapeutic intervention' [7]. Based on this definition, in principle, any component identified via genomic, transcriptomic, proteomic, cellular, or imaging approaches that is associated with the pathophysiology, clinical course, or outcome of a specific disease can serve as a biological marker. With the revolution of the high-throughput '-omics' technologies in the recent decades, numerous proteomic, genomic, transcriptomic and metabolomic markers have attracted particular attention. Potential biomarkers derived from application of these technologies include gene expression products, enzymes, metabolites, polysaccharides, circulating nucleic acids, single nucleotide polymorphisms, and gene variants.

Biomarkers may be classified into the following categories; prognostic, predictive, pharmacodynamic biomarkers, and surrogate end-points [7–9] [http://www.fda.gov/downloads/drugs/ guidancecomplianceregulatoryinformation/guidances/ucm230597. pdf]. A prognostic biomarker is a baseline patient or disease characteristic that categorizes patients by the degree of risk for disease occurrence or progression and informs about the natural history of the disorder in that particular patient. A diagnostic biomarker is an attribute that characterizes the presence or absence of disease and is included under the prognostic biomarker category. A predictive biomarker is a baseline characteristic that categorizes patients by their likelihood of response to a particular treatment and may predict a favourable response or an unfavourable response (i.e. adverse event). A pharmacodynamic (or activity) biomarker is a dynamic assessment that shows that a biological response has occurred in a patient after having received a therapeutic intervention. A surrogate endpoint is a biomarker intended to substitute for a clinical efficacy endpoint and is expected to predict clinical benefit (or harm, or lack of benefit or harm). Surrogate endpoints are often considered to be a subset of pharmacodynamic biomarkers. Thus biomarkers can have valuable applications in screening, diagnosis, disease monitoring, risk stratification, prognosis, patient sub-classification, evaluation of drug toxicity, and prediction of clinical response to an intervention [7, 10]. More recently biomarkers have been discussed as a tool to be able to offer personalized treatment options to patients based on their profile of specific markers associated with a disease or its course [11].

Biomarkers of psoriatic arthritis

In rheumatic diseases, a number of biomarkers have an established role in diagnosis (e.g. rheumatoid factor, antinuclear and other antibodies, *HLA-B*27*), evaluation of disease activity [e.g. C-reactive protein (CRP), erythrocyte sedimentation rate (ESR), complement levels], and prognosis (e.g. ESR, CRP, *HLA-B*27*) of disease [12]. However, to date there are no validated biomarkers identified for PsA. Although progress is being made in identifying markers for PsA in patients with psoriasis, few studies have investigated biomarkers of disease activity, joint damage, treatment response, or comorbidities, especially atherosclerotic vascular disease [12].

In the context of psoriatic disease the clinical outcomes that biomarkers could identify may include:

1. Prognostic biomarker—e.g. marker that indicates development of PsA in patients with psoriasis, progression of joint damage in PsA, development of atherosclerotic vascular disease;

2. Predictive biomarker—e.g. a marker that predicts optimal effects of treatment in the skin and joints or predicts serious adverse reactions;

3. Pharmacodynamic biomarker—e.g. a marker that indicates whether a biologic response to a therapeutic agent has occurred;

4. Surrogate end-point biomarker—e.g. a marker that may be a surrogate for prevention of radiographic progression.

This is illustrated in Figure 22.1.

An overview of the type of markers identified for PsA thus far is given in the following sections.

Serum/plasma protein soluble biomarkers

Human blood contains the most comprehensive human proteome, a mixture of circulating components released during both physiological and pathological processes by proximal and distal cells/tissues [13, 14]. Blood plasma or serum can be obtained easily from patients using the non-invasive and minimally painful method of blood drawing. Furthermore, the medical laboratory infrastructure is widely available for serum/plasma analysis [13]. These factors contribute to the idea of blood remaining the most prevalent source for biomarker analysis in the foreseeable future.

Serum or plasma biomarkers may have diagnostic, prognostic, or predictive value for PsA patients (Table 22.1). CRP is an acute phase reactant that is a well-known marker of systemic inflammation. Traditional assays for CRP have performed poorly as a marker of disease activity in PsA. Highly sensitive CRP (hsCRP) assays have been developed to detect CRP levels less than 5 mg/L and may be a better marker of psoriatic inflammation. Retrospective analyses of data obtained in a randomized, double-blind, placebo-controlled study have shown that baseline hsCRP levels are elevated in patients with psoriasis with and without PsA [15]. Patients with PsA and patients with higher body mass index (BMI) had higher median baseline hsCRP values than patients with psoriasis without PsA and those with lower BMIs [15]. Serum interleukin (IL)-6 was also found to perform better as a marker of inflammation than inflammatory markers such as ESR and CRP in patients with PsA [16].

Investigations of the skin proteome of psoriasis patients with and without PsA, led to the identification of β_5 integrin and periostin as potential markers elevated in serum of PsA patients [17]. Another study also indicated CRP, MMP-3, and vascular endothelial growth factor (VEGF) as potential markers of PsA [18]. Antibodies against mutated citrullinated vimentin (anti-MCVs) [19] and plasma YKL-40 [20] were further reported to be higher in PsA compared to patients with psoriasis. Markers of bone and cartilage breakdown and repair released into the circulation, such as Dkk-1 and M-CSF, are also candidate markers for PsA [21]. The markers CRP, OPG, MMP-3, and the CPII:C2C ratio were found to discriminate patients with PsA from those with psoriasis without PsA [22]. Serum cartilage oligomeric matrix protein is also increased in patients with PsA [23]. These findings need to be validated in larger cross-sectional and prospective studies.

Soluble biomarkers have also been evaluated as predictors of therapeutic response and, by extension, disease activity. In a retrospective analysis of a randomized trial, etanercept reduced hsCRP levels in patients with psoriasis and PsA [15]. Etanercept had the greatest effect on decreasing CRP levels in overweight and obese patients with psoriasis without PsA, patients on statins, and in all patients with PsA. Thus, etanercept treatment may reduce future cardiovascular morbidity. A higher level of CRP was also found to be a predictor of an ACR50 response when treating PsA patients with adalimumab and infliximab [24, 25]. In the GO-REVEAL trial with golimumab, serum levels of apolipoprotein C III, ENRAGE, IL-16, myeloperoxidase, VEGF, pyridinoline, MMP-3, CRP, carcinoembryonic antigen, intercellular adhesion molecule 1 (ICAM1), and macrophage inflammatory protein 1α (MIP1α) at baseline or week 4 of therapy with golimumab [a TNF inhibitor (TNFi)] were strongly associated with ACR (American College of Rheumatology) 20 response and/or DAS28 (Disease Activity Score 28) at week 14. Interestingly, the power of the biomarker panel to predict clinical response to golimumab treatment was stronger than for CRP alone [26]. Another marker that was reported is

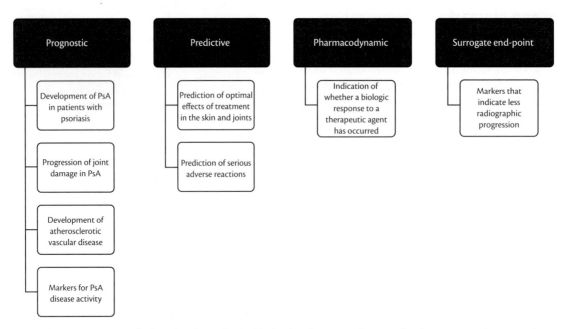

Figure 22.1 Examples of possible categories of biological markers with regard to the clinical outcomes they may identify in patients with psoriatic disease.

Table 22.1 Summary of recently published studies on soluble serum/plasma biomarkers for PsA

Marker	Function	Reference
hsCRP	Marker of inflammation; associated with PsA, high BMI; predictor of therapeutic response	15, 24, 25
IL-6	Marker of inflammation	16
ITGB5; POSTN	Elevated in serum of PsA patients	17
CRP; MMP-3; VEGF	Potential markers of PsA	18
anti-MCVs	Higher in PsA compared to patients with psoriasis	19
YKL-40	Higher in PsA compared to patients with psoriasis; decrease with TNFi	20
Dkk-1; M-CSF	Markers of PsA	21
M-CSF; RANKL	Correlated with radiographic erosion, joint-space narrowing, and osteolysis scores	21
CRP; OPG; MMP-3; CPII:C2C ratio	Markers of PsA	22
Serum cartilage oligomeric matrix protein	Increased in patients with PsA	23
Apolipoprotein C III; ENRAGE; IL-16; myeloperoxidase; VEGF; pyridinoline; MMP-3; CRP; carcinoembryonic antigen; ICAM1; MIP1α	Marker levels at baseline or week 4 of therapy with golimumab (a TNFi) were strongly associated with ACR20 response and/or DAS28 at week 14	26
IL-8; TNF-α; IL-6; MIP-1β; MCP-1; IL-23; IL-17; ferritin	Decreased with treatment with apremilast	27
MMP-3	Reduction associated with response to anti-TNF therapy in patients with PsA	28
IL-12p40; interferon alpha; IL-15; CCL3	Differentiated PsA patients with polyarticular disease from those with oligoarticular disease	30
S100A8/S100A9	Associated with disease severity and may predict increased joint damage in PsA	31,32

YKL-40, plasma levels of which are elevated in patients with PsA, and which decrease with treatment with TNFi [20]. It was also recently demonstrated that treatment with apremilast, a novel phosphodiesterase 4 inhibitor, was associated with significant reductions in circulating levels of IL-8, TNF-α, IL-6, MIP-1β, MCP-1, IL-23, IL-17, and ferritin [27]. In a longitudinal cohort setting, it was shown that baseline levels as well as a reduction in serum MMP-3 levels and an increase in serum COMP levels are associated with response to anti-TNF therapy in patients with PsA [28]. Decline in MMP-3 levels correlated with decline in hsCRP. Adipokine levels have also been shown to be disordered in PsA and associated with disease activity but these findings need further evaluation[29].

There are very few studies on biomarkers of joint damage in PsA. Circulating cytokines are potential markers for joint damage. Another study has suggested that increased levels of IL-12p40, interferon alpha, IL-15, and CCL3 could differentiate PsA patients with polyarticular disease from those with oligoarticular disease [30]. Since patients with polyarthritis have more severe joint involvement, proteins specifically associated with polyarthritis may be markers of disease progression. Similarly, serum calprotectin (S100A8/S100A9) is associated with disease severity and may predict increased joint damage in PsA [31, 32]. M-CSF and RANKL (but not Dkk-1) levels were shown to correlate with radiographic erosion, joint-space narrowing, and osteolysis scores in a small cross-sectional study [21]. Thus, a number of proteins are potential biomarkers for PsA disease activity and require further investigation.

Tissue protein biomarkers

Proteins are likely the most ubiquitously affected molecules during manifestations of disease, treatment response and recovery and, therefore, proteomics hold great promise for the discovery of novel biomarkers [13]. The concept has found some application in analysis of tissues from psoriasis/PsA patients (Table 22.2). Comparison of the proteome extracted from skin biopsies of psoriasis patients with and without PsA has pointed to 47 proteins that are overexpressed in PsA-derived skin as opposed to psoriasis alone [17]. Mass spectrometry-based multiple reaction monitoring (MRM) assays have confirmed eight of these proteins as potential markers of PsA: SRP14, ITGB5, POSTN, SRPX, FHL1, PPP2R4, CPN2, and GPS1 [17].

Table 22.2 Summary of recently published studies on tissue biomarkers for PsA

Marker	Function	Reference
SRP14; ITGB5; POSTN; SRPX; FHL1; PPP2R4; CPN2; GPS1	47 proteins were overexpressed in PsA-derived skin as opposed to psoriasis alone; MRM confirmed 8 of these markers as potential markers of PsA	17
Albumin; apolipoprotein AI; serum amyloid P; haptoglobin	119 proteins were differentially expressed in response to anti-TNF-α treatment and 25 proteins were differentially expressed between 'good responders' and 'poor responders'; MRM confirmed expression of 4 of these markers	33
S100-A8; S100-A10; Ig kappa chain C fibrinogen-α and γ; haptoglobin; annexin A1 and A2; collagen alpha-2; vitronectin; alpha-1 acid glycoprotein; cofilin; prolargin; 14-3-3ε; clusterin isoform 1	A panel of 57 proteins predicted response of PsA patients to treatment with an area under the curve of 0.76	34

Protein expression differences in response to anti-TNF-α treatment were also investigated in synovial tissue proteomes of PsA patients [33]. A total of 119 proteins were differentially expressed in response to anti-TNF-α treatment and 25 proteins were differentially expressed between 'good responders' and 'poor responders'. Expression of four of these markers, albumin, apolipoprotein AI, serum amyloid P, and haptoglobin was confirmed by MRM [33]. Another study using a tissue proteomics approach investigated the predictive value of 57 synovial tissue proteins in PsA patients under biologic treatment [34]. The panel included S100-A8, S100-A10, Ig kappa chain C fibrinogen-α and γ, haptoglobin, annexin A1 and A2, collagen alpha-2, vitronectin, alpha-1 acid glycoprotein, cofilin, prolargin, 14-3-3ε, and clusterin isoform 1. The multimarker panel was predictive of response to treatment with an area under the curve of 0.76 [34].

Biomarkers from synovial fluid

Given the inherent complexity of human serum/plasma due to the presence of high abundance proteins and by-products of metabolism that may be irrelevant to the disease, biomarker discovery may prove easier to accomplish using proximal fluids related to the disease. In an arthritic joint, proteomic components can be shed by cells of the synovial fluid (SF), synovial membrane (SM), and articular cartilage [35]. SF is an ultra-filtrate of plasma but contains a number of specific additions made from proximal joint tissues including SM and articular cartilage [35]. Many of the constituents of SF present in active disease states, including cytokines, proteinases, and antibodies, are produced locally. Thus, the SF is the proximate body fluid that reflects the pathogenetic events occurring in the arthritic joint and thus biomarker analysis of SF provides the opportunity to understand disease processes and identify potential biomarkers in arthritides like PsA [36, 37].

SF markers have been studied as indicators of therapeutic response (Table 22.3). SF white blood cell (WBC) counts, cytokine and chemokine levels, and synovial tissue markers before and after intra-articular etanercept injections have been reported [38]. CRP and/or ESR were significantly correlated with SF cytokines IL-1β, IL-1Ra, IL-6, and IL-8 and the chemokine CCL3 prior to injections, while there was a significant reduction in SF WBC and in IL-1β, IL-1Ra, IL-6, and IL-22 post treatment. Significant

correlations between synovial tissue markers and SF cytokines, namely IL-1β with CD45, IL-1β and IL-6 with CD31, and between the SF chemokines CCL4 and CCL3 with CD3 were identified independently of treatment. There was also a significant reduction in disease activity indices as well as in the synovial tissue markers CD45 and CD3 [38].

Mass-spectrometry based proteomic analysis of SF has shown that 137 proteins are differentially expressed between PsA and control SF, 44 being upregulated [39]. The elevated expression of 12 of these proteins, namely EPO, M2BP, DEFA1, H4, H2AFX, ORM1, CD5L, PFN1, C4BP, MMP3, S100A9, and CRP was confirmed using targeted MRM assays and has led to current investigations of their utility in serum in serum as potential biomarkers for PsA [39]. SF IL-1 may be a marker of disease severity. As mentioned previously, increased levels of IL-1 have been detected in the synovial fluid of PsA patients and has been associated with polyarthritis rather than monoarthritis [29].

Genomic biomarkers

There is considerable interest in identifying genomic markers that distinguish patients with PsA from those with psoriasis alone (Table 22.4). The primary risk locus for both PsA and cutaneous-only psoriasis (PsC) lies within the major histocompatibility complex region on chromosome 6p [40]. Fine mapping of this region revealed that the heterogeneity between PsA and PsC might be driven by HLA-B amino acid position 45, indicating that different genetic factors underlie the overall risk of psoriasis and the risk of specific psoriasis subphenotype and psoriasis with PsA [40]. Recent

Table 22.3 Summary of recently published studies on synovial fluid biomarkers for PsA

Marker	Function	Reference
WBC; CRP and/or ESR; IL-1β; IL-1Ra; IL-6; and IL-8; IL-22; CCL3; CD45; CD3	Differential marker expression before and after intra-articular etanercept injections; correlation with inflammatory markers	38
EPO; M2BP; DEFA1; H4; H2AFX; ORM1; CD5L; PFN1; C4BP; MMP3; S100A9; CRP	137 proteins were differentially expressed between PsA and control SF, 44 being upregulated; SRM confirmed the differential expression of 12 of these proteins	39
IL-1	Detected in synovial fluid of patients and has been associated with polyarthritis rather than monoarthritis	29

Table 22.4 Summary of recently published studies on genomic and transcriptomic biomarkers for PsA

Marker	Function	Reference
HLA-B amino acid position 45; HLA-C*06; IL-12B; IL-23R; IL-23A; TNIP1; TNFAIP3; LCE3B-LCE3C; TRAF3IP2; NFkBIA; FBXL19; TYK2; IFIH1; REL; ERAP1	Associated with psoriasis	40, 41
HLA-B/C; HLA-B; IL-12B; IL-23R; TNIP1; TRAF3IP2; FBXL19; REL	Associated with PsA	41
HLA-B*27:05:02; HLA-B*08:01:01-C*07:01:01; HLA-B*27:05:02-C*02:02:02; HLA-B*08:01:01- C*07:01:01; HLA-B*37:01:01-C*06:02:01; HLA-B*44	Associated with increased risk of enthesitis, dactylitis and symmetric sacroiliitis; associated with joint fusion and deformities, asymmetrical sacroiliitis, and dactylitis; associated with disease severity	42
FCGR2A/CD32A; TNFAIP3 variants	Associated with response to TNFi in PsA	43, 44
NOTCH2NL; HAT1; CXCL10; SETD2	494 genes were differentially expressed between PsA and PsC patients (Agilent 44k Human Oligo microarrays; 24% upregulated and 76% downregulated)	45

GWAS have revealed that *HLA-C*06, IL-12B, IL-23R, IL-23A, TNIP1, TNFAIP3, LCE3B-LCE3C, TRAF3IP2, NFkBIA, FBXL19, TYK2, IFIH1, REL,* and *ERAP1* are associated with psoriasis [41]. Genes identified in PsA studies include *HLA-B/C, HLA-B, IL-12B, IL-23R, TNIP1, TRAF3IP2, FBXL19,* and *REL* [41].

The lack of robust genetic susceptibility loci for PsA (except HLA-B) is largely attributed to the much smaller number of PsA patients studied and the greater clinical heterogeneity of PsA. These markers may be useful in predicting PsA in patients with psoriasis in addition to helping us understand the aetiology of PsA in patients with psoriasis.

HLA alleles could also contribute to the phenotypic heterogeneity and severity of PsA. It has been shown that *HLA-B*27:05:02* is associated with increased risk of enthesitis, dactylitis, and symmetric sacroiliitis, whereas the *HLA-B*08:01:01-C*07:01:01* haplotype is associated with joint fusion and deformities, asymmetrical sacroiliitis, and dactylitis [42]. Patients with severe PsA were more likely to have *HLA-B*27:05:02-C*02:02:02, HLA-B*08:01:01-C*07:01:01,* and *HLA-B*37:01:01-C*06:02:01,* but not the *HLA-B*27:05:02-C*01:01:01,* or *HLA-B*57:01:01-C*06:02:01* haplotypes [42]. *HLA-B*44* haplotypes were associated with presence of milder disease [42]. Studies that have investigated markers for response to therapy to TNF inhibitors (TNFi) have indicated that *FCGR2A/CD32A* and *TNFAIP3* variants are associated with response to TNFi in PsA [43, 44]. Thus genetic markers may have a role in stratifying patients with PsA in to those with severe disease or those likely to respond to therapy.

Transcriptomic biomarkers

Transcriptomic studies from easily accessible peripheral blood samples obtained from patients with psoriasis without PsA and those with PsA have shown significant differences in gene expression profiles (Table 22.4). In a recent study conducted on 20 PsA, 20 PsC, and 12 healthy controls using the Agilent 44k Human Oligo microarrays 494 genes were differentially expressed between PsA and PsC patients (24% upregulated and 76% downregulated) at a false discovery rate adjusted q<0.05 [45]. Potential biomarkers of PsA in PsC patients indicated by this study included *NOTCH2NL, HAT1, CXCL10,* and *SETD2*. Further validation of these findings is required.

A comprehensive analysis of cytokine and chemokine activation and genes representative of the inflammatory processes in the synovium and skin biopsies obtained from patients with PsA showed that gene expression in PsA synovium was more closely related to gene expression in PsA skin than to gene expression in synovium in other forms of arthritis [46]. However, PsA gene expression patterns in skin and synovium were clearly distinct, showing a stronger *IL-17* gene signature in skin than in synovium and more equivalent *TNF* and *IFN-γ* gene signatures in both tissues. These findings may explain the observation that skin and joint manifestations are similarly responsive to TNF inhibitors, while inhibitors of the Th17 pathway and IL-17 inhibitors have better results in PsA skin than in PsA joints [46]. Similar methods may be used to determine personalized approaches to therapy in patients with severe or resistant disease.

Cellular biomarkers

The hypothesis that specific cell populations act as markers of PsA has been investigated (Table 22.5). Circulating osteoclast precursors (OCPs) have been suggested as potential cell markers of

Table 22.5 Summary of recently published studies on cellular biomarkers for PsA

Marker	Function	Reference
Circulating osteoclast precursors	Associated with PsA presence and increased severity; predicted response to therapy	47, 48
DC-STAMP	Potential OCP-associated marker in inflammatory arthritis; declined during osteoclastogenesis	49
CD3; CD68	Association with greater response to anakinra or etanercept therapy as opposed to the non-responders; CD3 change correlated with change in DAS28	50, 51

PsA presence and increased severity [47, 48]. They may also have value as biomarkers predictive of response to therapy. Nevertheless, using the number and types of cells as disease marker(s) may technically prove laborious and expensive for clinical usage. The identification of cell-specific surface markers may instead prove of higher value for clinical practice. In this regard, the dendritic cell-specific transmembrane protein (DC-STAMP), a seven-pass transmembrane receptor-like protein known to be essential for cell-to-cell fusion during osteoclastogenesis, has been indicated as a potential OCP-associated marker in inflammatory arthritis [49]. Work in isolated monocytes, has identified a DC-STAMP positive cell population termed high and another population termed low, differentiated by their capability of producing osteoclasts when in culture [49]. It was shown that the cell surface expression of DC-STAMP gradually declined during osteoclastogenesis.

Other potential cellular biomarkers come from studies on synovial biopsies. In previous work, arthroscopic synovial biopsies and magnetic resonance imaging (MRI) scans of an inflamed knee joint were taken at baseline and 12 weeks after starting treatment with either anakinra or etanercept [50]. Changes in CD3 and CD68 expression in the synovial sublining layer was significantly greater in the patients that responded to therapy as opposed to the non-responders. The CD3 change correlated with change in DAS28 [50]. Similar results showing reduction in CD3-positive cells after treatment were also previously reported with adalimumab [51].

Imaging biomarkers

Imaging tools, especially MRI, can serve as biomarkers for disease activity and therapeutic response (Table 22.6). MRI bone oedema, proliferation, and erosion scores are higher in PsA patients with arthritis mutilans [52]. Therapy with TNF inhibitors improves bone oedema [48, 53, 54]. Treatment with abatacept is accompanied by a dose-dependent and improved MRI score [55]. Treatment with zoledronic acid was also shown to reduce the progression of bone oedema as detected by MRI, indicating probable suppression of osteitis [56]. Changes in MRI synovitis scores in parallel with changes in DAS28, CD3, CD68, and Factor VIII in synovial biopsies obtained prior to and after treatment with anakinra or etanercept have also been reported [50]. This work has indicated that a change in CD3, but not CD68 or FVIII, is associated with change in both DAS28 and MRI findings [50]. Whole-body MRI

Table 22.6 Imaging biomarkers for PsA

Marker	Function	Reference
MRI bone oedema, proliferation and erosion scores	Higher in PsA patients with arthritis mutilans; TNFi and zoledronic acid improved bone oedema (probable suppression of osteitis)	48, 52–54, 56
Whole-body MRI	Marker of enthesitis in patients with PsA and axial SpA	57
MRI score	Treatment with abatacept was accompanied by a dose-dependent and improved MRI score	55
MRI synovitis score	Changed in parallel with changes in DAS28, CD3, CD68, and factor VIII in synovial biopsies obtained prior to and after treatment with anakinra or etanercept; change in CD3 was associated with both DAS28 and MRI findings	50
Sonographic entheseal abnormalities	Increased in PsA patients as compared to patients with psoriasis but without PsA and healthy controls	58

is a promising new imaging tool under investigation for its clinical usage as a marker for the evaluation of enthesitis in patients with PsA and axial SpA [57].

More recent work has indicated that ultrasonography may find additional usage in screening and stratification of PsA. As PsA can present with enthesitis early in the course of disease, the entheseal indices have been investigated. A recent study showed that the severity of sonographic entheseal abnormalities is increased in PsA patients as opposed to patients with psoriasis without PsA and healthy controls [58]. The sensitivity of the MAdrid Sonographic Enthesitis Index (MASEI) score of ≥20 to correctly identify PsA patients was 30% and the specificity was 95% and 89% when compared to healthy controls and psoriasis patients, respectively [58].

Challenges in bringing biological markers to clinical practice

The high-throughput '-omics' technologies have led to a wealth of information about potential genomic/transcriptomic/proteomic/metabolomic markers derived from even a single experiment. The development of novel biomarker panels subsequent to the phase of discovery includes the qualification, verification, and validation of the markers followed by a clinical assay development [13]. A complete biomarker development pipeline for PsA patients must carefully regulate all aspects of this process [13]. An ideal biomarker coming out of this pipeline would have to be specific for PsA, allow sensitive detection of its levels in biological fluids early in the course of a disease, and be able to be offered to the patient at low cost [59]. However, out of the multiple promising markers that enter the biomarker pipeline very few ultimately stand the test of time and clinical validation by having the ability to transform clinical practice. Many promising biomarkers fail to perform when tested at large scale in the clinic for the following reasons. The analytical together with the clinical validity of potential biomarkers

must first be demonstrated early in the stages of the biomarker pipelines using relevant clinical samples to assure performance and utility in clinical practice [60]. A quality test should also be available for following the suggested biomarker. Analytical validation will guarantee the consistency of the test in being able to measure the specific biomarker [8, 10]. Clinical validation will ensure that the biomarker test can accurately predict the clinical target or outcome claimed, and that the test is exhibiting the high sensitivity and specificity for the targeted analyte in order to offer a satisfactory positive predictive value for the disease or the outcome under question. Clinical utility evaluation will provide evidence that the test can improve the benefit/risk of an associated screening or treatment plan and thus help physicians in clinical decision making [8, 10].

In addition to addressing the aforementioned analytical and clinical bottlenecks to ensure that a single biomarker can find a place in clinical practice for PsA patients, complementary approaches that utilize multiple biomarkers have proven useful in highlighting a biomarker's 'hidden' clinical value. There are several examples that take advantage of the combinatorial power of putting together different biomarkers that even though alone are not characterized by clinically sufficient specificity or sensitivity, together can have value for routine clinical practice [10]. Such an example is the human epididymis protein 4 (HE4) and the CA125 and their utility as markers for diagnosis of ovarian carcinoma. A combination algorithm of these two markers is now a US Food and Drug Administration approved tool for the differentiation of the malignant vs benign pelvic tumours [61]. Similar combinatorial efforts have been conducted in rheumatoid arthritis biomarker research to assess disease activity [62, 63]. In one of these reports, a panel of 12 biomarkers that represent the pathophysiologic spectrum of rheumatoid arthritis, termed Vectra-DA, has successfully been evaluated as a marker of disease activity in rheumatoid arthritis. The Vectra-DA multimarker panel has been shown to have a higher clinical value than conventional measures to predict risk for joint damage and assist in decision making [63].

Conclusions and future directions

Biomarkers can potentially transform the evaluation and management of PsA. Over the last few decades we have witnessed breakthrough developments in high-throughput technologies that have led to an explosion of information in biomarker discovery. In addition to thorough analytical/clinical validation approaches, there is an additional need to associate the potential biomarkers with the molecular basis of the disease. A number of markers from genomic, proteomic, cellular, and imaging studies that may indicate the presence of PsA, its severity, and response to therapy, have been identified over the last few years by many research groups working independently on various aspects of biomarkers in PsA. However, to date, none of these markers have been validated and remain outside of routine clinical use. The Group for Research and Assessment of Psoriasis and Psoriatic Arthritis (GRAPPA) has identified two key areas for biomarker development: 1) biomarkers of PsA in patients presenting with psoriasis; and 2) biomarkers of joint damage in PsA [64]. GRAPPA and the Outcome Measures in Rheumatology Clinical Trials (OMERACT) Soluble Biomarkers Working Group have developed a longitudinal study for identifying biomarkers of joint damage in PsA. GRAPPA in collaboration with industry partners is now spearheading a joint effort in identifying bio-markers, especially markers indicating structural damage in PsA.

References

1. Taylor W, Gladman D, Helliwell P, Marchesoni A, Mease P, Mielants H. Classification criteria for psoriatic arthritis: development of new criteria from a large international study. Arthritis Rheum 2006;54(8):2665–73.
2. Gladman DD, Thavaneswaran A, Chandran V, Cook RJ. Do patients with psoriatic arthritis who present early fare better than those presenting later in the disease? Ann Rheum Dis 2011;70(12):2152–4.
3. Theander E, Husmark T, Alenius GM et al. Early psoriatic arthritis: short symptom duration, male gender and preserved physical functioning at presentation predict favourable outcome at 5-year follow-up. Results from the Swedish Early Psoriatic Arthritis Register (SwePsA). Ann Rheum Dis 2014;73(2):407–13.
4. Tillett W, Jadon D, Shaddick G et al. Smoking and delay to diagnosis are associated with poorer functional outcome in psoriatic arthritis. Ann Rheum Dis 2013;72(8):1358–61.
5. Haroon M, Gallagher P, Fitzgerald O. Diagnostic delay of more than 6 months contributes to poor radiographic and functional outcome in psoriatic arthritis. Ann Rheum Dis 2015;74(6):1045–50.
6. Kirkham B, de Vlam K, Li W et al. Early treatment of psoriatic arthritis is associated with improved patient-reported outcomes: findings from the etanercept PRESTA trial. Clin Exp Rheumatol 2015;33(1):11–19.
7. Biomarkers Definitions Working Group. Biomarkers and surrogate endpoints: preferred definitions and conceptual framework. Clin Pharmacol Ther 2001;69(3):89–95.
8. Drucker E, Krapfenbauer K. Pitfalls and limitations in translation from biomarker discovery to clinical utility in predictive and personalised medicine. EPMA J 2013;4(1):7.
9. Strimbu K, Tavel JA. What are biomarkers? Curr Opin HIV AIDS 2010;5(6):463–6.
10. Diamandis EP. The failure of protein cancer biomarkers to reach the clinic: why, and what can be done to address the problem? BMC Med 2012;10:87.
11. Duffy MJ, Crown J. Companion biomarkers: paving the pathway to personalized treatment for cancer. Clin Chem 2013;59(10):1447–56.
12. Chandran V, Scher JU. Biomarkers in psoriatic arthritis: recent progress. Curr Rheumatol Rep 2014;16(11):453.
13. Rifai N, Gillette MA, Carr SA. Protein biomarker discovery and validation: the long and uncertain path to clinical utility. Nat Biotechnol 2006;24(8):971–83.
14. Anderson NL, Anderson NG. The human plasma proteome: history, character, and diagnostic prospects. Mol Cell Proteomics 2002;1(11):845–67.
15. Strober B, Teller C, Yamauchi P et al. Effects of etanercept on C-reactive protein levels in psoriasis and psoriatic arthritis. Br J Dermatol 2008;159(2):322–30.
16. Alenius GM, Eriksson C, Rantapaa DS. Interleukin-6 and soluble interleukin-2 receptor alpha-markers of inflammation in patients with psoriatic arthritis? Clin Exp Rheumatol 2009;27(1):120–3.
17. Cretu D, Liang K, Saraon P, Batruch I, Diamandis EP, Chandran V. Quantitative tandem mass-spectrometry of skin tissue reveals putative psoriatic arthritis biomarkers. Clin Proteomics 2015;12(1):1.
18. Ramonda R, Modesti V, Ortolan A et al. Serological markers in psoriatic arthritis: promising tools. Exp Biol Med (Maywood) 2013;238(12):1431–6.
19. Dalmady S, Kiss M, Kepiro L et al. Higher levels of autoantibodies targeting mutated citrullinated vimentin in patients with psoriatic arthritis than in patients with psoriasis vulgaris. Clin Dev Immunol 2013;2013:474028.
20. Jensen P, Wiell C, Milting K et al. Plasma YKL-40: a potential biomarker for psoriatic arthritis? J Eur Acad Dermatol Venereol 2013;277):815–9.
21. Dalbeth N, Pool B, Smith T et al. Circulating mediators of bone remodeling in psoriatic arthritis: implications for disordered osteoclastogenesis and bone erosion. Arthritis Res Ther 2010;12(4):R164.
22. Chandran V, Cook RJ, Edwin J et al. Soluble biomarkers differentiate patients with psoriatic arthritis from those with psoriasis without arthritis. Rheumatology (Oxford) 2010;49(7):1399–405.
23. Skoumal M, Haberhauer G, Fink A et al. Increased serum levels of cartilage oligomeric matrix protein in patients with psoriasis vulgaris: a marker for unknown peripheral joint involvement? Clin Exp Rheumatol 2008;26(6):1087–90.
24. Van den Bosch F, Manger B, Goupille P et al. Effectiveness of adalimumab in treating patients with active psoriatic arthritis and predictors of good clinical responses for arthritis, skin and nail lesions. Ann Rheum Dis 2010;69(2):394–9.
25. Gratacos J, Casado E, Real J, Torre-Alonso JC. Prediction of major clinical response (ACR50) to infliximab in psoriatic arthritis refractory to methotrexate. Ann Rheum Dis 2007;66(4):493–7.
26. Wagner CL, Visvanathan S, Elashoff M et al. Markers of inflammation and bone remodelling associated with improvement in clinical response measures in psoriatic arthritis patients treated with golimumab. Ann Rheum Dis 2013;72(1):83–8.
27. Schafer PH, Chen P, Fang L, Wang A, Chopra R. The pharmacodynamic impact of apremilast, an oral phosphodiesterase 4 inhibitor, on circulating levels of inflammatory biomarkers in patients with psoriatic arthritis: substudy results from a phase III, randomized, placebo-controlled trial (PALACE 1). J Immunol Res 2015;2015:906349.
28. Chandran V, Shen H, Pollock RA et al. Soluble biomarkers associated with response to treatment with tumor necrosis factor inhibitors in psoriatic arthritis. J Rheumatol 2013;40(6):866–71.
29. Eder L, Jayakar J, Pollock R, et al. Serum adipokines in patients with psoriatic arthritis and psoriasis alone and their correlation with disease activity. Ann Rheum Dis 2013;72(12):1956–61.
30. Szodoray P, Alex P, Chappell-Woodward CM et al. Circulating cytokines in Norwegian patients with psoriatic arthritis determined by a multiplex cytokine array system. Rheumatology (Oxford) 2007;46(3):417–25.
31. Kane D, Roth J, Frosch M, Vogl T, Bresnihan B, Fitzgerald O. Increased perivascular synovial membrane expression of myeloid-related proteins in psoriatic arthritis. Arthritis Rheum 2003;48(6):1676–85.
32. Aochi S, Tsuji K, Sakaguchi M et al. Markedly elevated serum levels of calcium-binding S100A8/A9 proteins in psoriatic arthritis are due to activated monocytes/macrophages. J Am Acad Dermatol 2011;64(5):879–87.
33. Collins ES, Butt AQ, Gibson DS et al. A clinically based protein discovery strategy to identify potential biomarkers of response to anti-tnf-alpha treatment of psoriatic arthritis. Proteomics Clin Appl 2016;10(6):645–62.
34. Ademowo OS, Hernandez B, Collins E et al. Discovery and confirmation of a protein biomarker panel with potential to predict response to biological therapy in psoriatic arthritis. Ann Rheum Dis 2016; 75(1):234–41.
35. Gibson DS, Rooney ME. The human synovial fluid proteome: A key factor in the pathology of joint disease. Proteomics Clin Appl 2007;1(8):889–99.
36. Cretu D, Diamandis EP, Chandran V. Delineating the synovial fluid proteome: recent advancements and ongoing challenges in biomarker research. Crit Rev Clin Lab Sci 2013;50(2):51–63.
37. Hui AY, McCarty WJ, Masuda K, Firestein GS, Sah RL. A systems biology approach to synovial joint lubrication in health, injury, and disease. Wiley Interdiscip Rev Syst Biol Med 2012;4(1):15–37.
38. Fiocco U, Sfriso P, Oliviero F et al. Synovial effusion and synovial fluid biomarkers in psoriatic arthritis to assess intraarticular tumor necrosis factor-alpha blockade in the knee joint. Arthritis Res Ther 2010;12(4):R148.

39. Cretu D, Prassas I, Saraon P et al. Identification of psoriatic arthritis mediators in synovial fluid by quantitative mass spectrometry. Clin Proteomics 2014;11(1):27.

40. Okada Y, Han B, Tsoi LC et al. Fine mapping major histocompatibility complex associations in psoriasis and its clinical subtypes. Am J Hum Genet 2014;95(2):162–72.

41. O'Rielly DD, Rahman P. Genetics of psoriatic arthritis. Best Pract Res Clin Rheumatol 2014;28(5):673–85.

42. Haroon M, Winchester R, Giles JT, Heffernan E, Fitzgerald O. Certain class I HLA alleles and haplotypes implicated in susceptibility play a role in determining specific features of the psoriatic arthritis phenotype. Ann Rheum Dis 2016; 75(1):155–62.

43. Ramirez J, Fernandez-Sueiro JL, Lopez-Mejias R et al. FCGR2A/CD32A and FCGR3A/CD16A variants and EULAR response to tumor necrosis factor-alpha blockers in psoriatic arthritis: a longitudinal study with 6 months of followup. J Rheumatol 2012;39(5):1035–41.

44. Tejasvi T, Stuart PE, Chandran V et al. TNFAIP3 gene polymorphisms are associated with response to TNF blockade in psoriasis. J Invest Dermatol 2012;132(3 Pt 1):593–600.

45. Pollock RA, Abji F, Liang K et al. Gene expression differences between psoriasis patients with and without inflammatory arthritis. J Invest Dermatol 2015;135(2):620–3.

46. Belasco J, Louie JS, Gulati N et al. Comparative genomic profiling of synovium versus skin lesions in psoriatic arthritis. Arthritis Rheumatol 2015;67(4):934–44.

47. Ritchlin CT, Haas-Smith SA, Li P, et al. Mechanisms of TNF-alpha- and RANKL-mediated osteoclastogenesis and bone resorption in psoriatic arthritis. J Clin Invest 2003;111:821–31.

48. Anandarajah AP, Schwarz EM, Totterman S et al. The effect of etanercept on osteoclast precursor frequency and enhancing bone marrow oedema in patients with psoriatic arthritis. Ann Rheum Dis 2008;67(3):296–301.

49. Chiu YH, Mensah KA, Schwarz EM et al. Regulation of human osteoclast development by dendritic cell-specific transmembrane protein (DC-STAMP). J Bone Miner Res 2012;27(1):79–92.

50. Pontifex EK, Gerlag DM, Gogarty M et al. Change in CD3 positive T-cell expression in psoriatic arthritis synovium correlates with change in DAS28 and magnetic resonance imaging synovitis scores following initiation of biologic therapy–a single centre, open-label study. Arthritis Res Ther 2011;13(1):R7.

51. van Kuijk AW, Gerlag DM, Vos K et al. A prospective, randomised, placebo-controlled study to identify biomarkers associated with active treatment in psoriatic arthritis: effects of adalimumab treatment on synovial tissue. Ann Rheum Dis 2009;68(8):1303–309.

52. Tan YM, Ostergaard M, Doyle A et al. MRI bone oedema scores are higher in the arthritis mutilans form of psoriatic arthritis and correlate with high radiographic scores for joint damage. Arthritis Res Ther 2009;11(1):R2.

53. Marzo-Ortega H, McGonagle D, Rhodes LA et al. Efficacy of infliximab on MRI-determined bone oedema in psoriatic arthritis. Ann Rheum Dis 2007;66(6):778–81.

54. Anandarajah AP, Ory P, Salonen D, Feng C, Wong RL, Ritchlin CT. Effect of adalimumab on joint disease: features of patients with psoriatic arthritis detected by magnetic resonance imaging. Ann Rheum Dis 2010;69(1):206–209.

55. Mease P, Genovese MC, Gladstein G et al. Abatacept in the treatment of patients with psoriatic arthritis: results of a six-month, multicenter, randomized, double-blind, placebo-controlled, phase II trial. Arthritis Rheum 2011;63(4):939–48.

56. McQueen F, Lloyd R, Doyle A et al. Zoledronic acid does not reduce MRI erosive progression in PsA but may suppress bone oedema: the Zoledronic Acid in Psoriatic Arthritis (ZAPA) Study. Ann Rheum Dis 2011;70(6):1091–4.

57. Poggenborg RP, Eshed I, Ostergaard M et al. Enthesitis in patients with psoriatic arthritis, axial spondyloarthritis and healthy subjects assessed by 'head-to-toe' whole-body MRI and clinical examination. Ann Rheum Dis 2015;74(5):823–9.

58. Eder L, Jayakar J, Thavaneswaran A et al. Is the MAdrid Sonographic Enthesitis Index useful for differentiating psoriatic arthritis from psoriasis alone and healthy controls? J Rheumatol 2014;41(3):466–72.

59. Witkowska HE, Hall SC, Fisher SJ. Breaking the bottleneck in the protein biomarker pipeline. Clin Chem 2012;58(2):321–3.

60. Amur S, Frueh FW, Lesko LJ, Huang SM. Integration and use of biomarkers in drug development, regulation and clinical practice: a US regulatory perspective. Biomark Med 2008;2(3):305–11.

61. Molina R, Escudero JM, Auge JM et al. HE4 a novel tumour marker for ovarian cancer: comparison with CA 125 and ROMA algorithm in patients with gynaecological diseases. Tumour Biol 2011;32(6):1087–95.

62. Bakker MF, Cavet G, Jacobs JW et al. Performance of a multi-biomarker score measuring rheumatoid arthritis disease activity in the CAMERA tight control study. Ann Rheum Dis 2012;71(10):1692–7.

63. Segurado OG, Sasso EH. Vectra DA for the objective measurement of disease activity in patients with rheumatoid arthritis. Clin Exp Rheumatol 2014;32(5 Suppl 85):S-34.

64. Ritchlin CT, Qureshi AA, de VK et al. Biomarkers in psoriasis and psoriatic arthritis: GRAPPA 2008. J Rheumatol 2010;37(2):462–7.

Domains, instruments, and composite scores

CHAPTER 23

Domains and instruments

Alberto Cauli

Introduction

Psoriatic arthritis (PsA) is a systemic inflammatory disease characterized by arthritis, usually seronegative for rheumatoid factor, associated with cutaneous psoriasis (PsO). The PsA clinical picture is generally dominated by peripheral joint involvement with or without inflammatory spinal disease, as well as enthesitis, tendonitis, dactylitis, and possibly by the other extra-articular features that are frequently observed in the spectrum of the spondyloarthropathies (i.e. uveitis and gut inflammation) [1]. Historically, because of its heterogeneous clinical spectrum, PsA has been difficult to assess and has largely borrowed evaluating tools from other diseases, as evidenced by the therapeutic clinical trials performed in the past.

In order to define and validate standardized outcome measurement tools both for therapeutic trials and for real life clinics, the need to precisely identify the relevant domains of psoriasis and psoriatic arthritis has lead to the 'rassemblement' of PsA and PSO 'aficionados' in the Group for Research and Assessment of Psoriasis and Psoriatic Arthritis (GRAPPA), founded in 2003 [2]. This group is characterized by the inclusion of both rheumatologists and dermatologists, as well as patients and other investigators. The first goal of GRAPPA is to define the key domains for assessment of response in PsA and PsO in randomized controlled trials (RCT) and longitudinal observational studies (LOS). They were identified through a multi-step process, starting with initial literature review [3], a Delphi exercise [4], and consensus meetings [5]. The breakthrough occurred in a dedicated workshop during OMERACT 7, where all possible domains were considered; 11 domains received more than 60% of the consensus of the delegates and therefore they were initially considered the 'core set' to be recommended in RCT and/or LOS in PsA (Table 23.1). Some domains were not included in the core set but were considered relevant from a clinical and research perspective; a research agenda was therefore established in order to study the domains, and to identify and/or develop appropriate tools for assessment. Of note was the recommendation that peripheral and axial joint involvement should be evaluated separately. Participation was considered an independent domain, different from health-related quality of life (HRQOL) or ability to work. Furthermore, it was recommended that patient global assessment of disease activity should include perception of skin and joint involvement together, but also two separate assessments (skin and joint global assessments evaluated individually).

In detail, the current updated core set of domains for the assessment of patients with PsA, and the search to select and/or develop the appropriate instruments which reflected activity in the individual domains, found momentum at the PsA module during OMERACT 8. Three main objectives were fulfilled: (a) achieve consensus on the core set of domains to be assessed in research trials in PsA; (b) review and endorse outcome measures to evaluate these domains on the basis of evidence; (c) set up a new research agenda to identify and/or develop new instruments in PsA evaluation. The selection of domains and instruments was based on evidence and discussions by experts.

Musculoskeletal domains

The peripheral arthritis issue was supported by data from phase 2 trials with etanercept and infliximab, which showed that in PsA, tender and swollen joint counts, American College of Rheumatology 20/50/70 responses, and Disease Activity Score 28 (DAS28), as well as the EULAR response criteria using the DAS score all distinguished active treatment from placebo, as did the Psoriatic Arthritis Response Criteria (PsARC) [6]. Given the frequent involvement of the interphalangeal joints in the fingers and toes, it was recommended that the 68 tender/66 swollen joint count should be performed as the preferred instrument, as confirmed later by data from Coates et al. [7].

Discussions about the spinal assessment were deeply influenced by the INSPIRE (International Spondyloarthritis Inter-rater Reliability Exercise) study, which found that classical measurements of spinal mobility developed for ankylosing spondylitis (AS) were also good performers in PsA [8].

To assess the dactylitis domain, a number of measures exist, ranging from a simple counting of swollen digits to a new instrument that measures the circumference of the affected digit and also assesses the degree of tenderness, the Leeds Dactylitis Index [9]. The new Leeds index is the only measure with reliability data and was thought to be the best option for clinical trials since it provides the best approximation to 'truth', although the simple counting of digits with dactylitis is also able to identify improvement after treatment [10].

To assess the enthesitis domain several instruments have been proposed, previously used in AS. These instruments partially meet the requirement of the OMERACT filter; ultrasonographic enthesitis does not always correlate with tenderness at the insertion of the enthesis, therefore the 'truth' aspect of the OMERACT filter is not fully satisfied. Among the several instruments proposed for this domain: the Mander, Maastricht AS Enthesitis Score (MASES) and Spondyloarthritis Research Consortium Canada (SPARCC) enthesitis indices were developed in AS while a more recent index, the Leeds enthesitis index (LEI), has been specifically derived from patients with PsA and it also appears to be feasible in daily use [10].

Table 23.1 Domains considered for inclusion in PsA patients evaluation at OMERACT 7

Position	Domain	Grade of support (% of votes)
1	Joint activity	99
2	Patient global	96
3	Pain assessment	94
4	Physical function	91
5	Skin disease	86
6	Quality of life	78
7	Structural damage	66
8	Acute phase reactant	64
9	Axial involvement	61
10	Participation	61
11	Enthesitis	60
12	Physician global	51
13	Dactylitis	48
14	Fatigue	48
15	Tissue histology	38
16	MRI	34
17	Morning stiffness	25
18	Damage joint count	20

Skin and nail domains

Instruments to assess the skin domain were compared, including the Psoriasis Activity and Severity Index (PASI), the target lesion score, and the Dermatologist Static Global Assessment [11]. The degree of skin involvement was considered critical when selecting the proper instrument of evaluation. For the nails domain a single instrument was proposed: the Nail Psoriasis Severity Index (NAPSI).

Patient reported outcome and imaging domains

Domains of PsA and PSO assessment which were considered relevant and discussed in details included the concept of pain, HRQOL and physical function; data presented in the GRAPPA process suggested that Medical Outcomes Study Short Form-36 Health Survey Physical Function (SF-36 PF) subscore could better summarize generic physical function compared to the Health Assessment Questionnaire-Disability Index (HAQ-DI) in PsA patients. Other strictly Patient Reported Outcomes (PRO) such as the patient global assessment (PGA), and participation were considered domains of great importance, although with different priorities.

Imaging-related domains were considered and data resulting from comparison of different methods of radiographs scoring, derived from anti TNF-alpha drugs RCT, were evaluated, although it was not possible to identify a preferred method. It is important to note that radiographs of hands and feet are mainly used to score bone damage. Current scoring methods are limited in PsA by the fact that they mainly score periarticular erosions, while there is

demand for new instruments to better grade the effect of the new biologic drugs on new bone formation lesions. In this regard, a new scoring method for axial involvement in PsA patients has been developed [12], which also takes into account the PsA spondylitis specificities. Magnetic resonance imaging (MRI) has great potential both in specific cases as well as in research studies, while ultrasound is increasingly important in particular for the assessment of enthesitis; computed tomography (CT) was also included for joint damage assessment. All imaging domains, except traditional radiology, have been included in the research agenda. Data from tissue analyses in PsA was also presented and, of note, also evidence that C-reactive protein may not clearly distinguish the active treatment arm from the placebo-treated patients in therapeutic RCTs.

Physician Global Assessment (PGA) was also considered a domain of importance due to its ability to summarize the different features of the disease. It is also noteworthy that PsA patients from different countries were invited to participate in this process in order to represent 'the patient's perspective'.

Following the long and multistep process previously summarized, the GRAPPA/OMERACT initiative proposed a final frame for the long list of domains discussed, having in mind that there were no available validated instruments for some of the domains. Three categories were considered: 'inner core,' 'outer core', and 'research agenda'. The domains included in the inner core must be assessed in all RCTs and LOS; other relevant domains recommended but not mandatory are considered in the outer core. Furthermore, a group of items requiring further investigations were included in an outer circle as the research agenda. In summary, peripheral joint activity, skin activity, pain, PGA, physical function, and HRQOL are part of the core set. Spinal disease, dactylitis, enthesitis, fatigue, nail disease, radiography, PGA, and acute phase reactants are in the middle core set. Imaging techniques such as MRI and ultrasound of joints and entheses, tissue analysis, and participation are important but still need further research [13] (Figure 23.1).

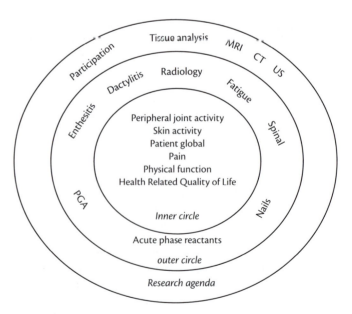

Figure 23.1 The OMERACT Core Set of outcome measures for PsA
Reproduced from Gladman DD, Mease PJ, Strand V, et al. Consensus on a core set of domains for psoriatic arthritis. J Rheumatol 2007;34(5):1167–70 with permission from The Journal of Rheumatology, all rights reserved.

Present and future directions

The need to revise the existing PsA core set has emerged over recent years, primarily to integrate the extensive research work done from 2005, and also to increase patient involvement in domain and instrument selection. Revision of the core set will also provide the opportunity to rethink the most appropriate position for domains important to patients such as fatigue, dactylitis, and participation (both work and leisure activities) that were not previously included in the core set [14–15]. At the OMERACT 12 PsA workshop, held in 2014, the need to update the PsA core set was unanimously endorsed.

The updating process of the actual core set is an opportunity to ameliorate the possible redundancy within the core area of pathophysiology. An umbrella term has been suggested for arthritis, enthesitis, dactylitis, and axial disease: 'inflammatory musculoskeletal disease'. Skin and nail disease may be summarized as 'psoriasis activity' and 'biomarkers' for acute-phase reactants. Life impact including domains such as pain, HRQOL, physical function, and patient global assessment [17] are still ranked in the core set, with the proposal to add fatigue which has also been ranked high in the EULAR PsAID study [16]. The potential overlap of domains including the patient global assessment [17] and the option to move domains such as dactylitis and enthesitis from the second circle to the inner circle, are all matters for future discussion.

It seems logical and practical to embrace all PsA clinical domains in a disease activity and responder index [18]. It is still controversial whether patient or physician global scores are able and sufficient to encompass the assessment of all the clinical domains such as joints (peripheral and axial), skin, enthesitis, and dactylitis; for this reason the need for a composite measure in PsA is still strong although detailed information on specific domains should be recorded at least in RCTs.

Instruments

To assess the applicability of a proposed instrument in the evaluation of a disease, the original OMERACT filter classically requires the fulfilment of its components that can be summarized in three words: truth, discrimination, and feasibility [19] (Table 23.2).

Three main developments have suggested a rethink and review of the OMERACT filter. Firstly, experience derived by OMERACT members in the application of the filter in an increasing range of rheumatological conditions; secondly, the increasing number of professionals that have become involved; and thirdly, the increasing role of the patients in these processes in the attempt to incorporate the patient perspective in developing and validating patient-reported outcomes (PRO) [20].

In order to develop a core set of widely accepted outcome measurements, consensus must be reached both on which domains should be measured, as well as on how to measure them, in other words which instruments to apply (if already available). A framework is therefore needed to ensure comprehensiveness of the domains chosen for measurement of the whole spectrum of disease. The proposed new framework includes four core 'areas', as follows: death, life impact (the way disease affect patient life, his/her feelings and function), resource use (all costs caused by the disease), and pathophysiological manifestations (disease-specific signs and symptoms, biomarkers and potential surrogate outcome

Table 23.2 The original OMERACT filter to assess applicability of a measurement instrument in a setting

Truth	Is the measure truthful? Does it measures what is intended? Is the result unbiased and relevant? The word captures issues of face, content, construct and criterion validity.
Discrimination	Does the measure discriminate between situation of interest? The situation can be determined at one time (for classification or prognosis) or at different times (to measure changes) (reliability and sensitivity to change).
Feasibility	Can the measure be applied easily, given constraints of time, money and interpretability?

Reprinted from Boers M et al. (1998) The OMERACT filter for Outcome Measures in Rheumatology. The Journal of Rheumatology 25:198–9 with permission from the Journal of Rheumatology.

measures); some of the key concepts included in the framework are summarized in Table 23.3 [21].

According to the new 'OMERACT Filter 2.0', all core sets (including PsA core set) should contain at least one measurement instrument from the three core areas Death, Life Impact, and Pathophysiological Manifestations; it is also recommended to include one from the area Resource Use [22].

The process to develop a core set for a disease such as PsA should start by selecting core domains within the areas ('core domain set'). The first step of this process generally is a detailed literature search, involvement of experts in PsA as well as patients, and consensus processes (Delphi and/or meetings). Then, at least one applicable measurement instrument for each core domain

Table 23.3 Some of the key concepts used in the OMERACT Filter2.0 framework

Health	A state of complete physical, mental and social well-being and not merely the absence of disease or infirmity (WHO 1948).
Core area	An aspect of health or a health condition that needs to be measured to appropriately assess the effects of a health intervention. Core Areas are broad concepts consisting of a number of more specific concepts called Domains.
Domain	A concept to be measured, a further specification of an aspect of health categorized within a Core Area.
Outcome	Any identified result in a domain arising from exposure to a casual factor or a health intervention.
Instrument	A tool to measure a quality or quantity of a variable.
Core domain set	For studies of health interventions, the minimum set of Domains necessary to adequately cover all Core Areas.
Core outcome measurement set	The minimum set of outcome measurement instruments that must be administered in each intervention study of a certain health condition to adequately cover a corresponding Core Domain Set.

Adapted from Boers M et al. (2014) The OMERACT filter for Outcome Measures in Rheumatology. The Journal of Rheumatology 41:978–85 with permission from the Journal of Rheumatology.

should be selected (if available). Applicability must take into account the original OMERACT filter and therefore requires that the assessing tool must be truthful (face—is the instrument credible?; content—the instrument sufficiently sample the core domain addressed; and construct validity—does the instrument agree with the expected results from other instruments measuring the same construct or concept?; Table 23.4), discriminative (between situations of interest), and feasible (easy to understand and acceptable in terms of time and monetary costs).

In this section are detailed the most popular instruments developed in the assessment of the 'Pathophysiological Manifestations' of PsA; PRO instruments, composite indices, imaging and laboratory assessment tools will be detailed elsewhere in this book (Table 23.4).

Peripheral joints

Moll and Wright described four clinical patterns of peripheral joint involvement: oligoarticular (equal or less than 4 joints involved), polyarticular, distal interphalangeal and mutilans. The fifth subset was spinal involvement [1]. At present articular involvement of PsA patients is generally classified simply as peripheral or axial, because of a different therapeutic approach, although the fine clinical differences described by Moll and Wright are still observed and are undoubtedly of interest. Assessment of peripheral joint involvement in PsA is actually widely performed by means of the 66/68 American College for Rheumatology (ACR) joint count [23]. The ACR joint count was developed for the evaluation of patients with rheumatoid arthritis (RA) and reports the number of joints with tenderness and/or swelling. This instrument includes the evaluation the following joints: temporomandibular, sternoclavicular, acromioclavicular, shoulder, elbow, wrist (considering the carpometacarpal and intercarpal joints as one single joint), metacarpophalangeal, proximal and distal interphalangeal, hip, knee, ankle, mid-tarsal, metatarsal, and interphalangeal joints of the toes (considering proximal and distal of each toe as one single joint). The total separate joint counts, tender or swollen joints, are generally considered and this instrument was found to be reliable in RA, both in terms of reproducibility and sensitivity to change over time. Later on Gladman and collaborators demonstrated that the number of inflamed joints is also a reliable measure of articular disease activity in PsA [24]. Another study, performed by the SPondyloArthritis Research Consortium of Canada (SPARCC), confirmed the validity of the 66/68 ACR joint count in PsA. Although they demonstrated an excellent agreement among the involved clinicians, they suggested common training to reduce observer variability [25].

A restricted joint count evaluation which considers only 28 joints (shoulders, elbows, wrists, metacarpophalangeals , proximal interphalangeals of hands and knees) has been developed for RA [26]. It is generally considered not appropriate in PsA because foot involvement, often with dactylitis, is a frequent occurrence clinical manifestation in PsA, and therefore excluding the foot from the assessment of peripheral joints would compromise the reliability of the evaluation. For these reasons, the use of DAS28, a Disease Activity composite Score developed for RA which evaluates only 28 joints [27], does not appear to be a suitable instrument for PsA joint evaluation [7], even if it has been proved to be discriminant and responsive in trials with anti TNF-alpha drugs [28]. Similarly to the ACR joint count, the Ritchie index was also developed to evaluate peripheral joint disease in patients with RA [29]. In its original

Table 23.4 Domains of PsA and main instruments in the assessment

Core set domains	Instruments
Peripheral joints	Tender and swollen joint counts (68/66)
Skin	Psoriasis Activity and Severity Index (PASI)
	Physician Global Assessment (static/dynamic)
	Target lesion assessment
	Body Surface Area (BSA)
	PGA of skin activity (VAS skin)
	Psoriasis Symptom Inventory (PSI)
Patient global	Patient Global Assessment (VAS skin + joint)
Pain	VAS pain
Physical function	Health Assessment Questionnaire (HAQ or modified HAQ)
	Short Form-36 (SF-36)
Health related quality of life	PsA Quality of Life (PsAQoL)
	Dermatology Life Quality Index (DLQI)
Outer circle domains	
Spinal	Schober test, finger to floor, spine lateral flexion, chest expansion, tragus to wall, cervical rotation.
	BASMI (summary of five measurements)
	BASFI
	BASDAI
Dactylitis	Count of dactylitis digits
	Leeds Dactylitis Index (LDI)
Enthesitis	Mander Enthesitis Index (MEI)
	Spondyloarthritis Research Consortium of Canada (SPARCC)
	Maastricht Ankylosing Spondylitis Enthesitis Score (MASES)
	Leeds Enthesitis Index (LEI)
Nails	Nail Psoriasis Severity Index (NAPSI)
Fatigue	Functional Assessment of Chronic Illness Therapy (FACIT)
Physician global	Physician Global assessment (VAS skin + joint)
Radiology	Sharp/Van der Heijde score of hand and feet
	PASRI
Acute phase reactants	Erythrocyte sedimentation rate (ESR)
	C-reactive protein (CRP)
Research agenda domains	
Participation	To be determined
Tissue analysis	To be determined
Imaging (MRI, US, CT)	PsA Magnetic Resonance Image Scoring System (PsAMRIS)
	Glasgow Ultrasound Enthesitis Scoring System (GUESS)

version the Ritchie index did not considered single joints of hands or feet, but all were considered as a single unit. Its main strength or limit was that it considered a severity measure for tenderness and swelling on a 0–3 scale. A modified version was then developed which evaluated single joints according to the ACR joint count and considered the degree of tenderness and swelling for each single joint on a 0–3 scale. The Ritchie index over time has demonstrated greater observer-related variation compared to the ACR joint count in RA [30], and it does not appear to be an appropriate instrument for the assessment of patients with PsA, especially since patients with PsA are not as tender as patients with RA.

The GRAPPA study group strongly suggests to perform the full 68 tender joint and 66 swollen joint count in the assessment of PsA peripheral articular involvement [7, 31].

Spine

Axial involvement in patients with PsA has been reported in half of cases, and furthermore sacroiliitis has been detected in up to 25% in several cohort of PsA patients [32]. Spondylitis in PsA tends to be less severe and heterogeneous, showing a more asymmetric pattern and radiological differences. Nevertheless, so far the assessment instruments for axial involvement in PsA have been borrowed from tools validated for ankylosing spondylitis (AS), although some specific PsA radiological scores have been developed and validated [12, 33].

Axial clinical assessment includes reporting the degree of sacroiliac joint tenderness and measurement of the spinal range of movements.

Sacroiliac joint assessment

Sacroiliac joints are not mobile and not directly accessible, and for this reason their clinical assessment is challenging if not unreliable. Clinical manoeuvres to produce stress pain, proposed in the past in the assessment of AS, have not proven to be sufficiently sensitive and specific [34]. Furthermore in a study in PsA patients, there was not good agreement among clinicians regarding the assessment of sacroiliac tenderness [25]. Therefore clinical testing of sacroiliac joint tenderness is not routinely performed in daily clinical setting or in PsA clinical trials and they are not recommended.

Back movements

Clinical evaluation of spinal movement has been extensively studied for AS. In this regard a study performed in Toronto [8] aimed to determine whether the axial measures used in primary AS were reproducible for both AS and PsA with axial disease. A group of rheumatologists with expertise in spondyloarthritis met for a combined physical examination exercise to assess patients with both diseases. Measures included: occiput to wall, tragus to wall, cervical rotation, chest expansion, lateral spinal bending, modified Schober, and hip mobility. The majority of the variance was due to the patients. Observer effect was noted especially for chest expansion for both AS and PsA patients, and for the modified Schober in PsA. The study showed very good to excellent agreement for most measures for both AS and PsA, with the exception of chest expansion. The authors concluded that measures of spinal mobility used in primary AS perform well with respect to inter-observer reliability and are similarly reproducible when applied to PsA patients with spinal involvement. These results support the general clinical practice of borrowing from AS instruments to use as the main assessment tools for PsA spinal evaluation. Nevertheless, for the majority of them, it is still to be determined whether these measurements will change over time and following new drug treatment in patients with PsA.

The main evaluations of spinal mobility are summarized as follows.

Finger to floor distance

The measurement of the distance between the tip of the third fingers of the hands and the floor, after inviting the patient to bend down keeping his/her knees straight, has been historically used to determine spinal mobility in AS [35]. This measurement tool was also tested in PsA with a good concordance rate between clinicians [25]. This instrument is therefore widely accepted and in use in routine clinics, both in AS and PsA patients.

Schober test

The original version of the Schober test measured the increase in length from an initial 10 cm segment placed over the lumbar spine of a standing patient after inviting him/her to bend forward. In a healthy individual the distance would increase to 16 cm [36]. The Schober test was soon modified because without an anchor point it would be unreliable even for the same clinician on repeat measurements. In the modified Schober test the clinician places a mark at the L5-S1 vertebral space (dimples of Venus) and then at 10 cm above and 5 cm below with the patient standing upright [37]. In a healthy subject, the marked 15 cm segment should increase to 21 cm after inviting the patient to bend forward. The main limitation of the Schober test is that it measures only the movement of the lumbar spine, whereas early changes in the spine may occur at the thoracolumbar junction. This version is actually widely used in clinical practice and trials and is recommended.

The modified Schober test was further modified by Miller and colleagues when they included higher levels of the spine [38]. According to this modified new version, a mark is placed at the level of the dimples of Venus and three 10-cm segments are then marked on the skin at different spine levels, with the patient bending forward and knees straight. The reduction of these three 10-cm segments is then reported with the patient invited to stand in full extension. This measurement has not been tested for sensitivity to change over time and has not gained popularity among rheumatologists.

Spine lateral flexion

Spine lateral flexion is determined by measuring, on the right and left sides, the distance between the third fingers and the floor, after inviting the patient to bend laterally. In order to avoid bending forward or flexion of the knees, this exercise can be done back to the wall [35]. In this modality, lateral flexion is measured by the difference between the distance of the third finger and the floor along a rule on the wall inviting the patient to stand erect, and then inviting the patient to bend laterally as much as he/she can [8, 39].

Cervical flexion–extension and rotation

The distance measured from the tip of the chin to the chest surface, with the head completely bent forward, has been proposed and used to evaluate cervical flexion. On the other hand, the tragus or occiput to wall distance has been proposed as a surrogate for cervical extension and has achieved general consensus among rheumatologists and good agreement in patients with PsA. These measurements are applied in symptomatic patients and are not generally employed in clinical trials; none of them is strongly recommended. The assessment of cervical spinal range of motion include also cervical rotation, generally by means of goniometer or tape-based methods and is particularly important in axial PsA patients because cervical involvement may determine severe functional impairment and disability [40].

Other measurements related to spondylitis

It is questionable if hip mobility belongs to axial or peripheral joint assessment. Historically intermalleolar distance has been used to measures the ability of the patient to abduct his/her legs while keeping the knees straight. This measurement is strongly influenced by the stature of the patients and it is hard to interpret the result; nevertheless it is generally well reproducible. As for AS, its usefulness in the assessment of the axial involvement in patients with PsA remains controversial, although measurement of intra-maleollar distance was highly reliable in the INSPIRE study. The Bath Ankylosing Spondylitis Metrology Index (BASMI) is a composite index which include five different metrology assessments [39]; together with the Bath Ankylosing Spondylitis Disease Activity Index (BASDAI) [41] and the Bath Ankylosing Spondylitis Functional Index (BASFI) [42] which are composite PRO instruments, they have been developed and validated for AS and are of wide use both in routine clinics and in RCTs in axial SpA. These tools have not been validated in PsA but BASDAI has been applied in patients with axial disease in PSUMMIT trials showing ability to differentiate active drug arms compared to placebo [43].

Enthesitis

The first enthesitis index was proposed by Mander and colleagues based on the assessment of all the entheseal sites accessible to clinical examination. The instrument included 66 entheseal sites evaluated on a semi-quantitative score from 0 to 3 (0=no pain, 1=mild tenderness, 2=moderate tenderness, and 3=wince or withdraw) [44]. The Mander Enthesitis Index (MEI) was shown to correlate with pain and stiffness VAS scales and to decrease following NSAID treatment, although the main pitfall was the variability between different examiners applying the score [44]. This index has not become popular among rheumatologists and researchers in clinical trials because of the difficulties in scoring all the entheseal sites and concerns relating to possible overlap with fibromyalgia tender points.

A second simplified score was then proposed. The Maastrict Ankylosing Spondylitis Enthesitis Score (MASES) was developed selecting the 13 most specific and sensitive MEI sites with a dichotomous 0/1 score for tenderness. A correlation between the enthesitis scores and disease activity measures was reported [45]. Data from the golimumab PsA trials suggest that MASES demonstrates discrimination and responsiveness [46].

Another instrument to assess enthesitis was proposed by the Spondyloarthritis Research Consortium of Canada (SPARCC) for patients with SpA [47]. The 16 most frequently affected and accessible entheseal sites were defined. Inter-observer reliability as well as correlation between the enthesitis score and disease activity measures were satisfactory. It is noteworthy that the SPARCC score failed to improve following anti-TNF treatment after 12 weeks of therapy [47] in AS patients, although it did work in many studies in PsA.

While the previous instruments have been validated in AS, the Leeds Enthesitis Index (LEI) is the only tool developed specifically in PsA patients. Notably, the LEI assess only the six most frequently affected entheseal sites and has showed close correlation with other PsA disease activity scores as well as the ability to identify the majority of patients with enthesitis, resulting therefore in the more feasible tool [48]. Furthermore, the LEI has been initially validated in a RCT with certolizumab in PsA showing significant improvements in the treatment arms compared to the placebo arm, indicating the ability of LEI to detect response to treatment [49]. It is also noteworthy that both LEI and SPARCC has showed excellent agreement in the INSPIRE study when applied to patients with PsA [50], furthermore the MASES is excellent for AS but not as good for PsA because it concentrates on axial enthesitis points, whereas the SPARCC and LEI have more peripheral points which are more common in PsA.

The main limitation of these scores is the difficulty in detecting specific tenderness in these entheseal areas. Many of the entheseal points are close to joints and fibromyalgia tender points; it is therefore easy to misjudge and/or to detect tenderness due to other causes. The possible solutions lie in adequate training and clinical practice of the examiners. A second option is to rely on imaging techniques such as ultrasound scanning (US) or MRI. MRI scan is able to detect bone marrow oedema at tendon insertions as well as abnormal signal around the enthesis [51]. US, by means of grey scale and power Doppler for increased vascularization, can detect abnormal findings in symptomatic and asymptomatic enthuses [52]. The reported US and MRI alterations have been correlated in other rheumatic conditions with inflammation; it is therefore conceivable that at entheseal sites they may also provide confirmatory evidence of 'enthesitis', thereby acting as gold standard [53]. It is noteworthy that correlation of US or MRI imaging abnormalities with clinical tenderness is not very strong. Clinical and imaging data needs therefore to be considered with caution, and this also has implications for the validation of instruments for enthesitis assessment [54]. These issues will be expanded in the specific sections.

Dactylitis

Dactylitis is defined as uniform swelling of a digit secondary to inflammation, with the appearance of the so called 'sausage digit'. It is a very characteristic feature of PsA and for this reason it is one of the classification criteria identified by the CASPAR study. Dactylitis can present as acute/tender, often erythematous and warm, or as chronic/sub-acute/non-tender. For this reason in clinical practice, it is conceivable to find variation in assessment between observers, with low agreement particularly in mild cases when digits are only slightly swollen. These difficulties in assessing mild cases is confirmed by a reliability study performed in Canada showing only moderate agreement between experienced rheumatologists for number of digits with dactylitis [25].

In view of the above, Philip Helliwell and colleagues developed the Leeds Dactylitis Instrument, which aimed to provide a clinical, objective, and validated outcome measure for dactylitis. The proposed tool is based on the evaluation of the difference in digital circumference between the inflamed digits and control digits of the other hand/feet. Dactylitis was therefore defined as an increase in circumference of more than 10% compared to the contralateral non-inflamed digit [55]. The aim of the Leeds Dactylitis Index (LDI) is to quantify both the size and tenderness by means of a 0–3 score (LDI scoring) or a simplified dichotomous score of 0 for non-tender and 1 for tender digits (LDI basic) [55]. Although the LDI and LDI basic measures are more time consuming compared to the simple count of inflamed digits, particularly if multiple digits are involved, these instruments perform better in terms of both truth and discrimination in the context of the OMERACT filter [56]. The Leeds index represents therefore the most validated clinical outcome measure available for dactylitis. In an RCT where the effect of treatment on dactylitis was a secondary outcome, the LDI was able to detect clinical improvements of inflamed digits in the treatment groups compared to the placebo arm [49].

Skin

The Psoriasis Area and Severity Index (PASI) is the most used instrument for assessing disease severity in chronic plaque psoriasis in RCTs, as well as skin involvement in PsA [57]. PASI should be used in patients with at least 3% of the skin area involved, being poorly sensitive in patients with limited skin involvement. The most commonly used method to estimate skin surface area is the palmar method, where palmar surface area is assumed to be around 1% of body surface area (BSA). Calculation of BSA involvement in psoriasis, as well as in other dermatological diseases, is also frequently used to simply measure disease severity and treatment responses. To assess the PASI dermatologists have to estimate the proportion of involved area for each body district: head and neck (H) (10% of body skin), trunk (T) (30%), upper (U) (20%), and lower extremities (L) (40%). The area of psoriatic skin involved for each of the four areas is calculated and scored as follows: 1=less than 10% of area; 2=10–29%; 3=30–49%; 4=50–69%; 5=70–89%; 6 >90%. For each region erythema (E), desquamation (D), and induration (I) of the plaques are rated according to a 0 to 4 severity scale. PASI scores are then calculated by means of electronic devices or spreadsheets to implement the following formula: PASI=0.1 (EH+IH+DH) AH+0.2 (EU+IU+DU) AU+0.3 (ET+IT+DT) AT+0.4 (EL+IL+DL) AL [57]. The PASI score can range from 0 (no involvement) to 72 (hypothetical maximum score). It has been proposed that PASI <7.0 correspond to mild plaque psoriasis, PASI 7.0–12.0 corresponds to moderate skin disease, and PASI >12.0 corresponds to severe disease [58]. Although it is used widely, the PASI has some limitations mainly due to its high inter-observer variability, and because it is not applicable to the less common clinical subsets of psoriasis, such as pustular psoriasis. Furthermore it does not consider patient's subjective symptoms, such as itching or pain, which may be disabling.

A second option in the evaluation of psoriasis skin response to a therapeutic intervention is represented by the target lesion score which has been used in RCT, and is a measurement of the degree of erythema, induration and scale of a 2-cm psoriatic lesion selected as a target reference for response to the treatment [59]. This instrument may be particularly useful in patients with PsA who are characterized frequently by limited skin involvement, quite often with less than 3% of BSA affected by psoriasis.

Finally, a more simplified approach is represented by the Dermatologist Static Global Assessment, which evaluates global psoriasis involvement on a 0–5 scale from 'clear' to 'very severe'

disease [59]. This instrument is clearly less precise and detailed compared to the PASI score, but because of its 'feasibility', this scoring instrument is very popular in particular in the dermatology community. Another instrument which is becoming popular is the Psoriasis Symptom Inventory (PSI) developed as a simple tool to allow patients to self-score psoriasis severity. It has been shown to be reliable and discriminative, and it correlated with PASI in a psoriasis clinical trial; it has been also validated in PsA [60].

Nails

The various clinical signs of nail psoriasis can be measured by means of the NAPSI instrument [61]. This tool has been designed and tested in order to provide a simple evaluation score of both nail bed and nail matrix psoriasis for each nail. The nail plate is divided into quadrants which are evaluated for the presence of pitting, leukonychia, nail plate crumbling in the nail matrix, and oil drop discoloration, onycholysis, hyperkeratosis, and splinter haemorrhages in the nail bed [61]. The possible highest score for each fingernail is 8, therefore 80 is the theoretical higher total score in hand finger nails. If toenails are also considered then the maximum total score is 160. The National Institute for Health and Care Excellence in UK (NICE) has suggested the use of NAPSI in the evaluation of nail disease in specialist settings when a major functional or cosmetic impact is present and when evaluating a specific treatment for nail disease (www.nice.com). Among the limitations of NAPSI, it must be underlined that some nail signs as leukonychia are not specific features for psoriasis [62]. Furthermore when NAPSI is applied by rheumatologists with no experience in using this tool, the results show that NAPSI is not very reliable. In order to overcome the interobserver variability in nail scores, a modified version was developed and validated, which showed good interrater reliability and construct validity [63].

In this chapter, the process of defining Domains of interest in PsA, as well as the process of developing and selecting the Instruments of assessment in PsA, have been reviewed. The PRO instrument and the composite indices will be extensively detailed in Chapters 24 and 25. Although great advancements have been achieved in the last ten years in the approach to PsA assessment, nevertheless a great amount of work (to be done by physicians and patients together) is still needed to develop new instruments to score 'inflammatory musculoskeletal disease', 'psoriasis activity', and in the search of effective 'biomarkers'.

References

1. Wright V, Moll JMH. Seronegative polyarthritis. Amsterdam: North Holland Publishing Co.; 1976.
2. Mease PJ, Gladman DD, Krueger GG. Prologue: Group for Research and Assessment of Psoriasis and Psoriatic Arthritis (GRAPPA). Ann Rheum Dis 2005;64:ii1-ii2.
3. Gladman DD, Helliwell P, Mease PJ, Nash P, Ritchlin C, Taylor W. Assessment of patients with psoriatic arthritis. A review of currently available measures. Arthritis Rheum 2004;50:24–35.
4. Taylor WJ. Preliminary identification of core domains for outcome studies in psoriatic arthritis using Delphi methods. Ann Rheum Dis 2005;64 Suppl 2:ii110-2.
5. Gladman DD. Consensus exercise on domains in psoriatic arthritis. Ann Rheum Dis 2005;64 Suppl 2:ii113-4.
6. Fransen J, Antoni C, Mease P, et al. Performance of response criteria for assessing peripheral arthritis in patients with psoriatic

arthritis: analysis of data from randomised controlled trials of two tumour necrosis factor inhibitors. Ann Rheum Dis 2006;65:1373–8.

7. Coates LC, FitzGerald O, Gladman DD, et al. Reduced joint counts misclassify patients with oligoarticular psoriatic arthritis and miss significant numbers of patients with active disease. Arthritis Rheum 2013;65:1504–9.

8. Gladman DD, Inman RD, Cook RJ, et al. International spondyloarthritis interobserver reliability exercise the INSPIRE study: I. Assessment of spinal measures. J Rheumatol. 2007;34:1733–9.

9. Helliwell PS, Firth J, Ibrahim GH, Melsom RD, Shah I, Turner DE. Development of an assessment tool for dactylitis in psoriatic arthritis. J Rheumatol 2005;32:1745–50.

10. Ferguson EG, Coates LC. Optimization of rheumatology indices: dactylitis and enthesitis in psoriatic arthritis. Clin Exp Rheumatol 2014;32(Suppl 85):S113–S117.

11. Chalmers RJ. Assessing psoriasis severity and outcomes for clinical trials and routine clinical practice. Dermatol Clin. 2015;33:57–71.

12. Lubrano E. Marchesoni A. Olivieri I. et al. Psoriatic arthritis spondylitis radiology index: a modified index for radiologic assessment of axial involvement in psoriatic arthritis. J Rheumatol 2009;36:1006–11.

13. Gladman DD, Mease P, Krueger G, et al. Outcome measures in psoriatic arthritis. OMERACT 7 Workshop. J Rheumatol 2005;32:2262–9.

14. Tillett W, Adebajo A, Brooke M, et al. Patient involvement in outcome measures for psoriatic arthritis. Curr Rheumatol Rep 2014;16:418.

15. de Wit M, Campbell W, FitzGerald O, et al. Patient participation in psoriasis and psoriatic arthritis outcome research: a report from the GRAPPA 2013 annual meeting. J Rheumatol 2014;41:1206–11.

16. Gossec L, de Wit M, Kiltz U, et al. A patient-derived and patient-reported outcome measure for assessing psoriatic arthritis: elaboration and preliminary validation of the Psoriatic Arthritis Impact of Disease (PsAID) questionnaire, a 13-country EULAR initiative. Ann Rheum Dis 2014;73:1012–9.

17. Cauli A, Gladman DD, Mathieu A, et al. GRAPPA 3PPsA Study Group. Patient global assessment in psoriatic arthritis: a multicenter GRAPPA and OMERACT study. J Rheumatol. 2011;38:898–903.

18. Coates LC, Fitzgerald O, Mease PJ, et al. Development of a disease activity and responder index for psoriatic arthritis—report of the psoriatic arthritis module at OMERACT 11. J Rheumatol 2014;41:782–91.

19. Boers M, Brooks P, Strand V, Tugwell P. The OMERACT Filter for outcome measures in rheumatology. J Rheumatol 1998;25:198–9.

20. Kirwan J, Newman S, Tugwell P, Wells G. Patient perspective on outcomes in rheumatology—a position paper for OMERACT 9. J Rheumatol 2009;36:2067–70.

21. Boers M, Idzerda L, Kirwan JR, et al. Toward a generalized framework of core measurement areas in clinical trials: a position paper for OMERACT 11. J Rheumatol. 2014;41:978–85.

22. Boers M, Kirwan JR, Wells G, et al. Developing core outcome measurement sets for clinical trials: OMERACT filter 2.0. J Clin Epidemiol 2014;67:745–53.

23. Cooperating Clinics Committee of the American Rheumatism Association. A seven-day variability study of 488 patients with peripheral rheumatoid arthritis. Arthritis Rheum 1965;8:302–34.

24. Gladman DD, Farewell V, Buskila D, et al: Reliability of measurements of active and damaged joints in psoriatic arthritis. J Rheumatol 1990;17:62–4.

25. Gladman DD, Cook RJ, Schentag C, et al. The clinical assessment of patients with psoriatic arthritis: results of a reliability study of the spondyloarthritis research consortium of Canada. J Rheumatol. 2004;31:112631.

26. Fuchs HA, Pincus T. Reduced joint counts in controlled clinical trials in rheumatoid arthritis. Arthritis Rheum 1994;37:470–5.

27. van der Heijde DM, van 't Hof MA, van Riel PL, et al. Judging disease activity in clinical practice in rheumatoid arthritis: first step in the development of a disease activity score. Ann Rheum Dis. 1990;49:916–20.

28. Antoni CE, Kavanaugh A, Kirkham B, Tutuncu Z, Burmester GR, Schneider U, et al. Sustained benefits of infliximab therapy for dermatologic and articular manifestations of psoriatic arthritis: results from the infliximab multinational psoriatic arthritis controlled trial (IMPACT). Arthritis Rheum. 2005;52:1227–36. Erratum in: Arthritis Rheum. 2005;52:2951.

29. Ritchie DM, Boyle JA, McKinnes JM, et al. Clinical studies with an articular index for the assessment of joint tenderness in patients with rheumatoid arthritis. Q J Med 1968;37:393–406.

30. Thompson PW, Hart LE, Goldsmith CH, Spector TD, Bell MJ, Ramsden MF. Comparison of four articular indices for use in clinical trails in RA: patient, order and observer variation. J Rheumatol 1991;18:661–5.

31. Gladman DD. Mease PJ. Healy P. et al. Strand V. Outcome measures in psoriatic arthritis. J Rheumatol. 2007;34:1159–66.

32. Veale D, Rogers S, Fitzgerald O. Classification of clinical subsets in psoriatic arthritis. Br J Rheumatol 1994;33:133–8.

33. Lubrano E, Marchesoni A, Olivieri I, et al. The radiological assessment of axial involvement in psoriatic arthritis: a validation study of the BASRI total and the modified SASSS scoring methods. Clin Exp Rheumatol. 2009; 27:977–80.

34. Gladman DD, Shuckett R, Russell ML, Thorne JC, Schachter RK. Psoriatic arthritis (PSA)—an analysis of 220 patients. Q J Med 1987;62:127–41.

35. Pile KD, Laurent MR, Salmond CE, Best MJ, Pyle EA, Moloney RO. Clinical assessment of ankylosing spondylitis: a study of observer variation in spinal measurements. Br J Rheumatol 1991;30:29–34.

36. Schober P. The lumbar vertebral column and the backache. MMW 1937;84:336–8.

37. Macrae IF, Wright V. Measurement of back movement. Ann Rheum Dis 1969;28:584–9.

38. Miller MH, Lee P, Smythe HA, Goldsmith CH. Measurements of spinal mobility in the sagittal plane: new skin contraction technique compared with established methods. J Rheumatol 1984;11:507–11.

39. Jenkinson TR, Mallorie PA, Whitelock HC, Kennedy LG, Garrett SL, Calin A. Defining spinal mobility in ankylosing spondylitis (AS). The Bath AS Metrology Index. J Rheumatol. 1994;21:1694–8.

40. Maksymowych WP, Mallon C, Richardson R, et al. Development and Validation of a Simple Tape-based Measurement Tool for Recording Cervical Rotation in Patients with Ankylosing Spondylitis: Comparison with a Goniometer-based Approach. J Rheumatol 2006;33:2242–8.

41. Garrett S, Jenkinson T, Kennedy LG, Whitelock H, Gaisford P, Calin A. A new approach to defining disease status in ankylosing spondylitis: the Bath Ankylosing Spondylitis Disease Activity Index. J Rheumatol. 1994;21:2286–91.

42. Calin A, Garrett S, Whitelock H, et al. A new approach to defining functional ability in ankylosing spondylitis: the development of the Bath Ankylosing Spondylitis Functional Index. J Rheumatol. 1994;21:2281–5.

43. McInnes IB, Kavanaugh A, Gottlieb AB, et al. Efficacy and safety of ustekinumab in patients with active psoriatic arthritis: 1 year results of the phase 3, multicentre, double-blind, placebo-controlled PSUMMIT 1 trial. Lancet. 2013 31;382:780–9.

44. Mander M, Simpson JM, McLellan A, Walker D, Goodacre JA, Dick WC. Studies with an enthesis index as a method of clinical assessment in ankylosing spondylitis. Ann Rheum Dis 1987;46:197–202.

45. Heuft-Dorenbosch L, Spoorenberg A, Van Tubergen A, et al. Assessment of enthesitis in ankylosing spondylitis. Ann Rheum Dis 2003;62:127–32.

46. Kavanaugh A, McInnes I, Mease P, et al.: Golimumab, a new human tumor necrosis factor alpha antibody, administered every four weeks as a subcutaneous injection in psoriatic arthritis: Twenty-four-week efficacy and safety results of a randomized, placebo-controlled study. Arthritis Rheum 2009;60:976–86.

47. Maksymowych WP, Mallon C, Morrow S, et al. Development and validation of the Spondyloarthritis Research Consortium of Canada (SPARCC) Enthesitis Index. Ann Rheum Dis 2009;68:948–53.

48. Healy PJ, Helliwell PS: Measuring clinical enthesitis in psoriatic arthritis: assessment of existing measures and development of an instrument specific to psoriatic arthritis. Arthritis Rheum 2008; 59: 686–91.

49. Mease PJ, Fleischmann R, Deodhar AA, et al. Effect of certolizumab pegol on signs and symptoms in patients with psoriatic arthritis: 24-week results of a Phase 3 double-blind randomised placebo-controlled study (RAPID-PsA). Ann Rheum Dis 2014;73:48–55.

50. Gladman DD, Inman RD, Cook RJ, et al. International spondyloarthritis interobserver reliability exercise—the INSPIRE study: II. Assessment of peripheral joints, enthesitis, and dactylitis. *J Rheumatol* 2007;34:1740–5.

51. Marzo-Ortega H, McGonagle D, O'Connor P, Emery P. Efficacy of etanercept in the treatment of the entheseal pathology in resistant spondylarthropathy: a clinical and magnetic resonance imaging study. Arthritis Rheum 2001;44: 2112–7.

52. D'Agostino MA, Said-Nahal R, Hacquard-Bouder C, Brasseur JL, Dougados M, Breban M. Assessment of peripheral enthesis in the spondylarthropathies by ultrasonography combined with power Doppler: a cross-sectional study. Arthritis Rheum 2003; 48: 523–33.

53. McQueen FM, Gao A, Ostergaard M, et al. High-grade MRI bone oedema is common within the surgical field in rheumatoid arthritis patients undergoing joint replacement and is associated with osteitis in subchondral bone. Ann Rheum Dis 2007;66:1581–7.

54. Eder L, Jayakar J, Thavaneswaran A, et al. Is the MAdrid Sonographic Enthesitis Index useful for differentiating psoriatic arthritis from psoriasis alone and healthy controls? J Rheumatol 2014;41:466–72.

55. Helliwell PS, Firth J, Ibrahim GH, Melsom RD, Shah I, Turner DE. Development of an assessment tool for dactylitis in patients with psoriatic arthritis. J Rheumatol 2005;32: 1745–50.

56. Healy PJ, Helliwell PS. Measuring dactylitis in clinical trials: which is the best instrument to use? J Rheumatol 2007;34:1302–6.

57. Fredriksson T, Pettersson U. Severe psoriasis—oral therapy with a new retinoid. Dermatologica 1978;157:238–44.

58. Schmitt J, Wozel G. The psoriasis area and severity index is the adequate criterion to define severity in chronic plaque-type psoriasis. Dermatology. 2005;210:194–9.

59. Feldman SR, Krueger GG. Psoriasis assessment tools in clinical trias. Ann Rheum Dis 2005; 64(Suppl 2):ii65–8.

60. Mease PJ The psoriasis Symptom Inventory: an effective patient-reported outcome measure of psoriasis severity. J Rheumatol 2015;42:1034–36.

61. Rich P, Scher RK. Nail Psoriasis Index: a useful tool for evaluation of nail psoriasis. J Am Acad Dermatol 2003;49:206–12.

62. Garzitto A, Ricceri F, Tripo L, Pescitelli L, Prignano F. Possible reconsideration of the Nail Psoriasis Severity Index (NAPSI) score. J Am Acad Dermatol 2013;69:1053–4.

63. Cassell SE, Bieber JD, Rich P, et al. The modified Nail Psoriasis Severity Index: validation of an instrument to assess psoriatic nail involvement in patients with psoriatic arthritis. J Rheumatol. 2007;34:123–9.

CHAPTER 24

Patient-reported outcome measures in psoriatic arthritis

Laure Gossec, Tania Gudu, and Maarten de Wit

Introduction

Patient reported outcomes (PROs) are measurements coming directly from patients about how they feel or function in relation to a health condition and its therapy without interpretation by healthcare professionals. PROs can relate to symptoms, signs, functional status, perceptions, or other aspects such as convenience and tolerability [1]. To understand how patients are doing, and how psoriatic arthritis (PsA) is affecting not only physical outcomes such as pain and itching, but also mobility and activities of daily life, it is logical to ask the patient directly, using PROs [2–4]. The patient perspective plays a important role particularly in rheumatology because musculoskeletal diseases often lead to a considerable burden of disease for patients, including symptoms such as pain, functional disability, and fatigue. Since the final objective of treatment is to improve health-related quality of life [5], monitoring patients' symptoms and the impact they have on the patient's life is necessary if we want to be able to assess the efficacy of our treatments [6]. Indeed, there is a growing interest in PROs in rheumatology, in trials, observational studies, and routine clinical practice. This interest coincides with a global trend for more 'patient-centred care' and for better shared decision making [5, 7–11]. PROs can serve two purposes: first to capture aspects of the disease that might be inadvertently omitted or ignored by professionals who lack the experience of living with a condition; and second to provide a way of communicating with patients about the outcomes of their disease and the treatment options in a way which is meaningful to patients.

There is also a growing interest in actively engaging with patients in the context of scientific research [12, 13]. Involving patients in the development of outcome measures, and in particular PROs, ensures their relevance, acceptability, and quality [13–17, 18]. As we will see, this principle has recently been applied in the field of PsA [19].

There are many PROs available for use either in clinical practice or in clinical studies and trials. Some are generic and others have been developed specifically for PsA [20–22]. Collectively, they provide a wide spectrum of PROs that covers many of the possible outcomes, including direct (e.g. pain) and indirect (e.g. sleep disturbance) outcomes related to the pathogenesis of PsA.

In the present chapter, we will discuss PROs firstly in rheumatology, then in the context of PsA and we will present the most widely-used disease-specific and generic PROs for PsA.

Importance of PROs in rheumatology and their advantages as outcome measures

PRO assessment historically in rheumatology

For over 20 years, pain and functional assessment have been taken into account in chronic, symptomatic inflammatory rheumatic disorders such as rheumatoid arthritis (RA) or PsA [23]. But over the last 10 years, it has become apparent that a wider assessment of (other) PROs may be needed.

OMERACT (Outcome Measures in Rheumatology) is an international organization which plays a leading role in developing Core Outcome Sets and outcome measures in the field of rheumatology. For more than a decade OMERACT has been a pioneer in organizing long-term involvement of patients as collaborating partners in its bi-annual, worldwide conferences [24–28]. Initially through OMERACT, then through other expert groups and studies, the importance of PROs has been put increasingly forward.

In RA, there is now a wealth of qualitative studies allowing us to better understand the impact of the disease on patients' lives. Several publications issued from patient surveys, interviews, or patient focus groups indicate that some domains or areas of health which are important for patients are little recognized in RA, both in trials and in clinical practice [29–31]. These domains include fatigue, well-being, sleep, psychological distress, ability to cope, and the final consequences of the disease impact, including ability to work and to have a family and social life [29–32].

In the context of shared decision making, it is important to measure what is important for patients, so that these assessments can be shared with patients. This is where PROs become all-important. But are they valid outcome measures?

PROs as valid outcomes

PROs can be used to measure a range of different outcomes in clinical trials. These should be viewed as bringing additional information that is complementary to the physician-derived measures such as joint counts or physician global assessment. PROs are the only way to assess some of the aspects related to PsA that, when combined with physician reported or more objective measurements such as imaging or biology results, ensure a more comprehensive evaluation of disease activity and disease impact. Thus, PROs do not replace physician reported outcomes but complement these outcomes [33].

An outcome measure should reflect the current status of the disease including pathophysiological signs, but also may reflect life impact outcomes, i.e. the impact on the quality of life of the patient [34]. When discussing PROs as outcome measures, we need to recognize that treatment objectives in chronic inflammatory rheumatisms are dual: the first one is symptom resolution, i.e. to improve the current symptomatic condition as soon as possible; the second objective ('the preventative approach') aims to prevent subsequent structural deterioration. PROs are clearly valuable in assessing symptoms, but their role in assessing inflammation and/or damage is less clear [35]. Outcome measures need to be able to assess change, whether it is an improvement or a worsening (flare) [36].

PROs have strong points from a psychometric point of view.

- *They reflect the patient's perspective.* PROs bring unique information, i.e. that cannot be collected from a physician, and useful information, in particular on symptoms.

- *PROs have good psychometric properties.* They have face and construct validity, and are as reproducible as joint counts [22, 34, 37, 38].

- *PROs have high feasibility.* They are often at no cost (unless copyrighted), they are non-invasive, are not painful, and do not require costly equipment [39]. However, sometimes it may not be easy to have access to cross-culturally validated questionnaires. This is why European League Against Rheumatism (EULAR) developed an Outcome Measures Library where validated translations are freely available [22, 39].

- *PROs are sensitive to change.* That is, they improve when the patient's status improves [40].

Thus, PROs are important outcomes to consider in the assessment of chronic, symptomatic diseases such as PsA.

Domains of health assessed by PROs in PsA

The PsA OMERACT core set

Several years ago, the international group OMERACT and the Group for Research and Assessment of Psoriasis and Psoriatic Arthritis (GRAPPA) decided through consensus on a Core Set of variables to be collected in clinical trials of PsA [41]. These experts have proposed six core domains to be measured in clinical trials and observational studies of PsA: peripheral joint activity, skin activity, pain, patient global assessment (PGA), physical function, and health-related quality of life (Figure 24.1). These domains represent the 'inner circle' of Figure 24.1. The 'outer circle' corresponds to domains which are not necessary to assess in PsA trials or domains which are still under evaluation.

Over recent years, and based in particular on input from patient research partners, the Core Set is being revisited. A systematic literature review has shown that existing, frequently used outcome measures have been devised with little or no involvement of patients [42]. Another study showed that none of these instruments capture the full experience of PsA from the perspective of patients [43]. Therefore, patients and physicians have been working together since 2012 to identify domains that are important to patients and to review outcome measures that reflect the perspective of patients. One of the domains that is increasingly considered as important is fatigue, as will be discussed later in this chapter. In PsA, fatigue

should be taken into consideration when assessing disease impact. In fact, there is growing consensus about the importance of fatigue in PsA: it was recently recognized as a core domain to be assessed in clinical trials in PsA [44], but further research is needed to determine the best instrument to assess it.

Other outcomes that were brought forward for consideration in the new Core Set are dactylitis, enthesitis, and work participation [45].

Domains of health reported in recently published studies of PsA

A systematic literature review was performed regarding clinical outcomes in PsA analysing 58 articles published on PsA in 2006–2010 [46]. Of these studies, around half reported functional disability, pain, and patient global assessment; other domains of health were less frequently reported, e.g. fatigue reported in only 15% of the studies (see Table 24.1) [46].

Domains of health important for PsA patients—qualitative aspects

Qualitative methodology (such as focus groups or individual in-depth interviews) provide the opportunity to explore the perspective of those who experience the disease, i.e. the patient's perspective in detail. Such studies have yielded a wealth of information in RA. In PsA, however, there have been few published qualitative studies to date, although several are ongoing [42, 43, 47].

A systematic literature review reported on 11 studies assessing impact of PsA from the patient's perspective [43, 48]. Impact of PsA was shown to be wide-reaching, covering various aspects of life, as reflected in Figure 24.2. The most frequently reported dimensions of health were mainly related to the consequences and societal aspects of the disease, i.e. ability to work, social participation, and

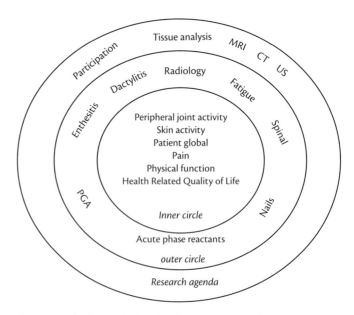

Figure 24.1 The OMERACT Core Set of outcome measures for PsA
Reproduced from Gladman DD, Mease PJ, Strand V, et al. Consensus on a core set of domains for psoriatic arthritis. J Rheumatol 2007;34(5):1167-70 with permission from The Journal of Rheumatology, all rights reserved.

Table 24.1 Domains of health reported in 58 publications of PsA published 2006–2010

Patient-reported domain of health	Articles reporting the domain N (% of 58 articles)
Function/Disability	28 (48.0)
Pain	27 (46.6)
Patient's Global Assessment	23 (39.6)
Quality of life	22 (37.9)
Skin	2 (3.4)
Fatigue	9 (15.5)
Composite scores	6 (10.3)
Morning stiffness	6 (10.3)
Utility/Productivity	4 (6.9)
Other	2 (3.4)
Coping/Self Efficacy	1 (1.7)

Reproduced from Palominos, P. E., Gaujoux-Viala, C., Fautrel, B., Dougados, M. and Gossec, L. (2012), Clinical outcomes in psoriatic arthritis: A systematic literature review. Arthritis Care Res, 64: 397–406. doi:10.1002/acr.21552 with permission from Wiley.

leisure followed by physical aspects, i.e. functional capacity, pain, and emotional aspects, i.e. embarrassment due to appearance.

Two questionnaires have been developed specifically for PsA and used qualitative methods in their elaboration. In the elaboration of the PsA Impact of Disease (PsAID) [49], 16 domains of

health that were considered important by patients were identified (Table 24.2). Similarly, the development of the PsA Quality of Life (PsAQoL) questionnaire yielded domains of health that could be categorized into four main experiences: reaction to diagnosis, life changes, adaptation and acceptance, and concerns for the future (Table 24.2). These included as expected pain or skin disease, but also other domains, such as fatigue, coping, and emotional and social problems.

The domains of impact identified through qualitative studies bring to light aspects that were not previously reported as important in PsA, such as fatigue, social and sexual life, coping mechanisms, emotional problems, such as anger, anxiety, fear, and embarrassment, and shame due to appearance.

The perspective of patients is crucial when assessing quality of life or impact of disease; corresponding instruments should be based on information derived directly from patients, ensuring that respondents find the instrument acceptable and relevant to their condition. This should be taken into consideration particularly in PsA where quality of life instruments should reflect both rheumatic and dermatological impact on patients [42].

Specific PROs for PsA

Patient reported outcome measures used in studies of PsA (e.g. the Health Assessment Questionnaire, the Arthritis Impact Measurement Scale and the Short Form—36) may be inadequate when evaluating the impact of the disease from the patient's perspective, as they are generic instruments and do not capture the duality of the disease, i.e. rheumatic and dermatological. There are very few questionnaires which have been developed specifically for PsA; we will review here two of them.

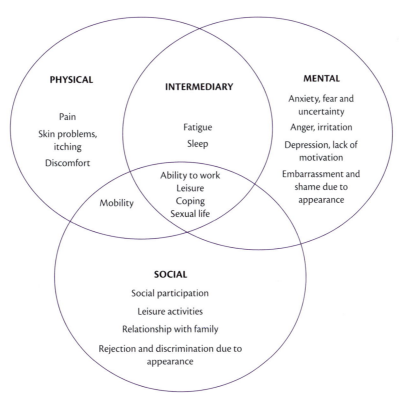

Figure 24.2 Domains of health important for patients with PsA.

Table 24.2 Domains of health important for patients with PsA as reflected in two patient-derived questionnaires assessing impact of PsA

Domains of health	16 domains identified in the PsAID development process (Gossec et al.)	20 domains of health included in the PsAQoL (McKenna et al.)
Pain	X	
Skin problems	X	
Fatigue	X	X
Ability to work/ leisure	X	
Functional capacity (capacity to perform daily physical activities, loss of independence)	X	X
Feeling of discomfort	X	
Mobility		X
Morning stiffness		X
Sleep disturbance	X	
Anxiety, fear and uncertainty	X	
Anger, irritation		X
Coping	X	X
Embarrassment and/ or shame due to appearance	X	
Social participation	X	X
Depression	X	X
Relationship with family	X	X
Concentration difficulties	X	
Rejection and discrimination due to appearance	X	
Sexual life	X	

PsA: psoriatic arthritis; PsAID: Psoriatic Arthritis Impact of Disease; PsAQoL: Psoriatic Arthritis Quality of Life
Data sourced from Gossec L, de Wit M, Kiltz U, et al. A patient-derived and patient-reported outcome measure for assessing psoriatic arthritis: elaboration and preliminary validation of the Psoriatic Arthritis Impact of Disease (PsAID) questionnaire, a 13-country EULAR initiative. Ann Rheum Dis 2014;73(6): 1012–19 and McKenna SP, Doward LC, Whalley D, et al. Development of the PsAQoL: a quality of life instrument specific to psoriatic arthritis. Ann Rheum Dis 2004;63(2):162–9.

The PsAQoL questionnaire

The Psoriatic Arthritis Quality of Life (PsAQoL) [50] assesses quality of life defined as the extent to which needs are fulfilled and reflects impact from the perspective of the patient. Its content was derived from unstructured, qualitative interviews conducted with patients with PsA, which generated a 51-item questionnaire. Face and content validity were assessed by field test interviews with

another sample of PsA patients. Then a postal survey was conducted and the resulting analysis led to a 35-item version of the questionnaire. Finally a test—retest postal survey was conducted to improve the scaling properties, reliability, internal consistency, and validity. Rasch analysis of data from this postal survey identified a 20-item version with good item fit and excellent psychometric properties (internal consistency 0.91, test–retest reliability 0.89 and good external construct validity). The final 20 items of the questionnaire consisted, as far as possible, of wording taken from the transcripts. They cover various domains of impact such as physical problems, fatigue, and emotional and social problems (Table 24.2).

Sensitivity and responsiveness to change have been further assessed in 28 PsA patients [51], demonstrating significant change at 3 and 6 months after change of disease modifying therapy ($P<0.01$ and $P<0.05$, respectively). Standardized response mean was large at 3 months (0.71) and small at 6 months (0.41). The PsAQoL has been translated and validated in Dutch and Swedish [52, 53].

In summary, the PsAQoL is a disease-specific instrument which is derived directly from qualitative interviews, has good psychometric properties, and is quick and easy to complete, making it suitable for use in both research and clinical settings. However, the PsAQoL has been little used to date [54–58]. Furthermore, it is subject to copyright.

The PsAID questionnaire

EULAR recently developed the PsAID (Psoriatic Arthritis Impact of Disease) questionnaire, a multi-dimensional patient-reported questionnaire to assess the impact of PsA from the patient's perspective [19, 49].

The objective was to develop a questionnaire which can be used to calculate a score, reflecting the impact of PsA based on the patients' perspective. The questionnaire has been developed by a mixed group of rheumatologists/researchers, patient research partners, and health professionals, including an International Classification of Health and Functioning expert, and a nurse practitioner/researcher. Compared to existing instruments, the PsAID-score is unique because it has been developed with the active involvement of 11 patient research partners from 11 European countries. Therefore the instrument is fully based on the patient perspective of the illness [19].

First, the 11 patient research partners identified 16 domains (areas of health) important for patients with PsA; then 139 patients prioritized the 16 domains according to importance and the lowest priority 4 domains were excluded from the next steps. Numeric rating scale (NRS) questions were developed, one for each of the 12 domains of health. To combine the domains into a single score, relative weights were determined for each domain, based on relative importance as reported by 474 PsA patients from across Europe. At the same time, an international cross-sectional and longitudinal validation study was performed in 13 countries (474 patients) to validate the PsAID in terms of psychometric properties, regarding cross-sectional relation with other well-known outcome measures, and longitudinal validation for reliability and sensitivity to change in smaller samples (N = 80 and 71 respectively). The measures performed well; reliability was high (intra-class correlation coefficient, 0.95, 95% confidence interval (CI) 0.92–0.96) and so was sensitivity to change (standardized response mean 0.90) [49].

There are two versions of the PsAID. For clinical practice the 12-item version is recommended. This version covers: pain, skin problems, fatigue, work and/or leisure activities, functional capacity, discomfort, sleep disturbance, anxiety/fear and uncertainty, coping, embarrassment and/or shame, social participation, and depression (Table 24.2). For clinical research (clinical trials and longitudinal observational studies) the 9-item version (which is shorter and does not contain the last three items embarrassment and/or shame, social participation. and depression) is recommended. The PsAID-score provides information on each individual item as well as one overall score. The PsAID-score gives a number between 0 and 10. A higher score on the PsAID indicates more impact of the disease. A score below 4 out of 10 is considered a patient-acceptable status. A change of 3 or more points is considered a relevant absolute change [59].

In summary, the PsAID is a disease-specific instrument which has the advantages of being patient-derived with very active involvement of patient research partners at several levels throughout [19], and it is a short and simple questionnaire with good psychometric properties and is suitable for use in both research and clinical settings. However, currently there is a lack of data regarding validation in other cohorts or studies than the one used for the validation of the PsAID. The PsAID questionnaires are available online free of charge with their available translations [59].

Widely-used PROs in PsA

Although as stated above, generic questionnaires (i.e. questionnaires not developed specifically for PsA) present disadvantages in terms of face validity, they also have strong points including experience of use, wide validation in other diseases, and comparisons across diseases.

We will review here some of the generic PROs most frequently-used in the context of PsA, in particular in PsA clinical trials [46].

Single questions used in PsA

Single questions are usually in the format of visual analogue scales (VAS) or NRSs. Both of these are reported with a figure from 0 to 10 or 0 to 100 where 0 is usually perfect status, and 10 or 100 usually the worse status [60].

Patient global assessment

PGA is one of the most widely used PROs in PsA [46, 61], and is usually assessed by the following question: *'Considering all the ways psoriatic arthritis has affected you during the last week, circle the number that best describes how you have been doing'* [49, 60].

PGA is an overall measure of the patient status, and is included in several composite measures of disease activity such as the PASDAS or the definition of Minimal Disease Activity (see Chapter 25).

Recently GRAPPA has also suggested using other 'patient global' questions, specific to joints and skin: the joint and skin patient assessments [61], respectively by the following questions: *'Considering all the ways your joints have affected you during the last week, circle the number that best describes how you have been doing'* and *'Considering all the ways psoriasis (skin disease) has affected you during the last week, circle the number that best describes how you have been doing'* [49].

In an initial study, PGA appeared to be related to both of these patient assessments [61].

We have recently shown in 223 PsA patients that intra-class correlations between PGA and joint or skin patient assessment were respectively 0.71 [95% CI 0.64–0.77] and 0.52 [95% CI 0.42–0.60] [62]. This indicates the joint global assessment proposed by GRAPPA may be redundant with regard to PGA whereas the skin global assessment may bring additional and different information. Furthermore, in multivariate analysis PGA was explained (R^2 of model 0.75) by coping ($\beta = 0.287$); pain ($\beta = 0.240$); work and/or leisure activities ($\beta = 0.141$); and anxiety ($\beta = 0.109$) [62]. Thus PGA in PsA is explained by physical aspects of impact such as pain and activities, but also psychological aspects: coping and anxiety. In this study, skin impact was not an additional explanatory factor of PGA, perhaps because many of the patients had limited skin involvement [49].

Pain

Pain is a widely assessed outcome in PsA, often using a single question VAS or NRS though the wording may vary slightly.

One validated formulation of the pain question is the following:

Circle the number that best describes the pain you felt due to your psoriatic arthritis during the last week with anchors going from 'none' to 'extreme'.

Pain is a major component of the impact of PsA and is reported by patients as the most important domain of health in this disease, as is also the case in RA [32, 49, 63].

The interpretation of improvement in pain in PsA rests on the minimally clinical important difference (MCID) cutoff which has been validated as an improvement from baseline of at least 10 points on a 0–100 scale [64].

Assessment of functional capacity

Health Assessment Questionnaire

The Stanford Health Assessment Questionnaire Disability Index (HAQ-DI) is currently the most widely used measure of functioning and disability across rheumatic diseases [16, 46]. Although the HAQ was originally developed for RA and is validated in a variety of rheumatic diseases (including PsA), it should be considered a generic rather than a disease-specific instrument.

The HAQ is a self-administered questionnaire and measures impairment of functioning [65]. It contains 20 items that deal with difficulties experienced with eight categories of daily living: dressing, arising, hygiene, eating, reaching, gripping, walking, and activities. There are also items about the assistance used to perform these activities. The HAQ can be completed by the patient in approximately 5 minutes and is scored in less than 1 minute. The HAQ results in a total score between 0 (no disability) and 3 (severe disability).

Other versions of the HAQ, such as the shorter 'modified HAQ' which contains only one item for each of the eight categories, have been proposed but have not been specifically validated in PsA [66]. Work is currently ongoing to develop a modification of the HAQ using computerized adaptive testing methods, but this modified version of the HAQ should also be further validated [67].

The HAQ has good psychometric properties. In different contexts, this measure is sensitive to change and is a good predictor of future disability and costs [68]. It has demonstrated reliability: test–retest correlations range from 0.87 to 0.99. Face and content validity have been demonstrated in many studies: correlations between questionnaire or interview scores and task performance range from

0.71 to 0.95 demonstrating criterion validity [68]. The construct/convergent validity based on the pattern of correlations with other clinical and laboratory measures, predictive validity, and sensitivity to change have also been established in numerous studies and clinical trials [68]. Specifically in PsA, the HAQ has been shown to be reliable, valid [69] and sensitive to change in several PsA trials [70, 71]. The interpretation of the HAQ is slightly different in PsA than in RA. Whereas in RA, the cut-off for a minimally important difference is 0.25, in PsA it is higher and has been suggested to be 0.35 [70].

The HAQ has been translated and validated in many languages [39]. The HAQ-DI is copyrighted to ensure that it will be used unmodified to preserve the validity of results and contribute to standardization of assessment across studies. However, it is considered to be in the public domain [68].

Dermatological Life Qquality Index

The Dermatological Life Quality Index (DLQI) is not a generic questionnaire but nor was it developed for PsA: it is a psoriasis and dermatology questionnaire. The DLQI is a 10-item questionnaire assessing the effect of psoriasis on daily activities and level of disability over the previous 7 days [72]. The DLQI questions are grouped into six subcategories: symptoms and feelings; daily activities; leisure; work/school; personal relationships; and treatment. The DLQI is a validated questionnaire with scores ranging from 0–30, with higher scores indicating more impairment, and although it is not *per se* a function tool, it has been used in some studies as a measure of dermatological-related functional limitations [71].

The MCID for the DLQI has not been established for PsA, but in psoriasis patients it has been estimated as a 5-point improvement [73].

Generic quality of life measured by the Medical Outcomes Study Short Form-36 (SF36)

The SF-36 is a generic questionnaire to measure quality of life [74]. It has been developed with the aim to compare various aspects of health status across a general and broad patient population. The instrument is widely used, also in the field of rheumatology. The SF-36 has 36 items that are divided into eight subdomains: Physical functioning (PF), role limitations due to physical problems (RP), bodily pain (BP), general health (GH), vitality (VT), social functioning (SF), role limitations due to emotional problems (RE), and mental problems (MH). The total score of the SF-36 is the sum of the eight weighted subscales, transformed into a scale from 0 (worst possible health state) to 100 (best possible health state). Two subscores can be calculated for the physical health (PCS) and mental health (MCS) components. A shorter version is available in the SF-12. Through the use of the Short-Form 6-Dimension (SF-6D) it is possible to use SF-36 or SF-12 data to calculate a preference based single index measure for economic evaluations. By using the SF-6D it is even possible to obtain quality adjusted life years (QALYs) for use in cost utility analysis [74, 75].

The SF-36 has been validated in PsA [76] and is often used in clinical trials to assess the domain of health-related quality of life in PsA populations [46]. A comparative study of quality of life in patients with PsA versus RA or psoriasis indicated significant alteration of quality of life in particular in RA and PsA, with great alterations in the mental components for patients with RA, as illustrated in Figure 24.3 [77].

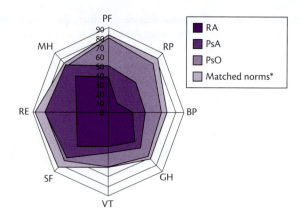

Figure 24.3 Relative alterations in quality of life in a comparative study of patients with PsA, RA and psoriasis starting a biologic treatment.
Adapted from Strand, V et al. 'Use of 'spydergrams' to Present and Interpret SF-36 Health-Related Quality of Life Data across Rheumatic Diseases.' Annals of the rheumatic diseases 68.12 (2009): 1800–1804 with permission from BMJ publishing group.

MCIDs have been established for the SF-36 summary scores and are different for improvement and deterioration: 5.0 points and -2,5 points, respectively. The SF-12 and SF-6D have different cutoffs [55, 78].

The SF-36 is copyrighted which may limit its use [39, 76].

Fatigue

Fatigue is a subjective experience that can be described as an overwhelming, sustained sense of exhaustion and decreased capacity for physical and mental work. It is an important symptom in PsA and provides additional information to the PsA Core Set. Levels of fatigue in PsA are elevated: in a large cross-sectional cohort almost 50% of PsA patients reported moderate fatigue and 29% experienced severe fatigue [79]. The importance attributed to fatigue is also high: in a priority exercise of 474 patients with PsA from 13 countries [49], patients ranked fatigue as the second most important domain after pain and before skin problems (Figure 24.4).

Data regarding causes of fatigue in PsA are sparse [46, 79, 84]: fatigue is reported to be mostly related to physical disability, and psychological distress in PsA. Recently, we showed in a study of 246 patients with PsA from 13 countries [80] that high fatigue was explained mainly by disease-related factors (current skin psoriasis, tender joint count, and enthesitis), but also patient-related characteristics (years of education and female gender) [80]; this indicates that fatigue in PsA is multifactorial, but may be more strongly related to the disease process in PsA than in RA.

There is no consensus regarding which instrument should be used to assess fatigue in PsA. In a systematic literature review on clinical outcomes in PsA [46] most frequently used tools were VAS and NRS single questions. Fatigue assessed with NRS was shown to be an independent outcome measure and sensitive to change in patients with PsA [81]. Fatigue can also be assessed using more complex scales which were adapted and validated for patients with PsA, namely the modified Fatigue Severity Scale (mFSS) [82] and the Functional Assessment of Chronic Illness Therapy—Fatigue (FACIT—Fatigue) [83]. The SF-36 vitality subscale has a high correlation (r=−0.76) with fatigue measures such as the FSS [84]. FACIT—Fatigue demonstrated good reliability and validity and has

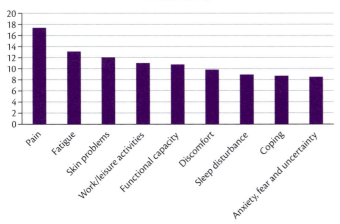

Relative importance of domains of impact in
Psoriatic arthritis

Figure 24.4 Fatigue had high relative importance among domains of impact in PsA in a priority exercise of 474 PsA patients.

Data sourced from Gossec L, de Wit M, Kiltz U, et al. A patient-derived and patient-reported outcome measure for assessing psoriatic arthritis: elaboration and preliminary validation of the Psoriatic Arthritis Impact of Disease (PsAID) questionnaire, a 13-country EULAR initiative Annals of the Rheumatic Diseases 2014;73:1012-1019.

the advantage of covering a broader concept of fatigue. However, good correlations have been shown between the fatigue NRS and more complex scales [85] and the fatigue VAS is reported to perform as well as or better than longer scales [86].

Conclusions

The field of PROs in PsA is of great interest, and is clearly relevant in these days of patient-centred care. In PsA trials, PROs are important because they reflect the patient's perspective, and they bring additional and different information. Pain, function, patient global assessment, and skin are the domains most frequently assessed in trials; however, they may not render a complete picture of patients' lives with PsA. Other aspects of importance for patients such as fatigue, sleep, or psychological well-being are rarely assessed. Using patient-reported composite scores such as the EULAR-developed PsAID might be of use in PsA trials [46].

Assessing PROs more completely and more systematically in PsA clinical care is also an objective. This should improve the doctor–patient relationship because it requires the active involvement of the patient in the evaluation and management of the disease. PROs provide information that is well understood by patients and offers a meaningful agenda for the conversation about issues that matter to the patient. Implementing the use of PROs in daily care may enhance opportunities for shared decision making and stimulate patients to take responsibility for their own health. Such an increased involvement of patients may ultimately lead to improved adherence, more self-management and hopefully better health outcomes.

As future years see research advancing in PROs, we will certainly learn more about these aspects, thus helping us to give better care to people with PsA.

References

1. http://handbook.cochrane.org/chapter_17/17_patient_reported_outcomes.htm, accessed Feb 16, 2015.
2. Kirwan JR, Heiberg T, Hewlett SA. Outcomes from the Patient Perspective Workshop at OMERACT 6. J Rheumatol 2003;30:868–72.
3. Kirwan JR, Bartlett SJ, Beaton DE, et al. Updating the OMERACT filter: implications for patient-reported outcomes. J Rheumatol. 2014;41(5):1011–5.
4. Anderson J, Caplan L, Yazdany J, et al. Rheumatoid arthritis disease activity measures: American College of Rheumatology recommendations for use in clinical practice. Arthritis Care Res (Hoboken). 2012;64(5):640–7.
5. Gossec L, Smolen JS, Ramiro S, et al. European League Against Rheumatism (EULAR) recommendations for the management of psoriatic arthritis with pharmacological therapies: 2015 update. Ann Rheum Dis. 2016;75:499–510.
6. Sanderson T, Hewlett S, Richards P, et al. Utilizing qualitative data from nominal groups: exploring the influences on treatment outcome prioritization with rheumatoid arthritis patients. J Health Psychol. 2012;17(1):132–42.
7. Stoffer MA, Smolen JS, Woolf A, et al. Development of patient-centred standards of care for rheumatoid arthritis in Europe: the eumusc.net project. Ann Rheum Dis. 2014;73(5):902–5.
8. http://www.pcori.org/ accessed Feb 16, 2015.
9. Smolen JS, Landewé R, Breedveld FC, et al. EULAR recommendations for the management of rheumatoid arthritis with synthetic and biological disease-modifying antirheumatic drugs: 2013 update. Ann Rheum Dis. 2014;73(3):492–509.
10. http://www.fda.gov/downloads/Drugs/Guidances/UCM193282.pdf accessed Feb 16, 2015
11. Sanderson TC, Hewlett SE, Flurey C, et al. The impact triad (severity, importance, self-management) as a method of enhancing measurement of personal life impact of rheumatic diseases. J Rheumatol. 2011;38(2):191–4.
12. Broerse JEW, Elberse JE, Caron-Flinterman JFW, Zweekhorst MBM. Enhancing a transition towards a needs-oriented health research system. In: Broerse JEW, Bunders JFG, editors. Transitions in Health Systems: Dealing with persistent problems. Amsterdam: VU University Press, 2010:181–205.
13. Staley K. Summary Exploring Impact: Public involvement in NHS. Eastleigh: public health and social care research INVOLVE, 2009.
14. Tugwell P, Boers M, Baker P, et al. Endpoints in rheumatoid arthritis. J Rheumatol Suppl 1994;42:2–8.
15. Staniszewska S, Haywood KL, Brett J, et al. Patient and public involvement in patient-reported outcome measures: evolution not revolution. Patient 2012;5(2):79–87.
16. Oliver SR, Rees RW, Clarke-Jones L, et al. A multidimensional conceptual framework for analysing public involvement in health services research. Health Expect. 2008;11(1):72–84.
17. van der Heijde D, Calin A, Dougados M, et al. Selection of instruments in the core set for DC-ART, SMARD, physical therapy, and clinical record keeping in ankylosing spondylitis. Progress report of the ASAS Working Group. Assessments in Ankylosing Spondylitis. J Rheumatol 1999;26(4):951–4.
18. Cheung PP, de Wit M, Bingham CO 3rd, et al. Recommendations for the Involvement of Patient Research Partners (PRP) in OMERACT Working Groups. A Report from the OMERACT 2014 Working Group on PRP. J Rheumatol 2016 43(1):187–93.
19. De Wit M, Kvien T, Gossec L. Patient participation as an integral part of patient reported outcomes development guarantees the representativeness of the patient voice—A case-study from the field of rheumatology. RMD Open 2015;1:1 e000129.
20. http://www.proqolid.org/ accessed Feb 16, 2015.
21. http://Olga-QoL.com accessed Feb 16, 2015.
22. http://oml.eular.org/ accessed Feb 16, 2015.
23. Felson DT, Anderson JJ, Boers M, et al. The American College of Rheumatology preliminary core set of disease activity measures for rheumatoid arthritis clinical trials. The Committee on Outcome Measures in Rheumatoid Arthritis Clinical Trials. Arthritis Rheum. 1993;36:729–40.

24. Hewlett S, Wit M, Richards P, et al. Patients and professionals as research partners: challenges, practicalities, and benefits. Arthritis Rheum 2006;55(4):676–80.

25. de Wit MPT, Berlo SE, Aanerud GJ, et al. European League Against Rheumatism recommendations for the inclusion of patient representatives in scientific projects. Ann Rheum Dis 2011;70(5):722–6.

26. Bingham CO, 3rd, Alten R, de Wit MP. The importance of patient participation in measuring rheumatoid arthritis flares. Ann Rheum Dis 2012;71(7):1107–9.

27. Shea B, Santesso N, Qualman A, et al. Consumer-driven health care: building partnerships in research. Health Expect 2005;8(4):352–9.

28. Gossec L, Kirwan J, de Wit MPT. Patient perspective in outcome measures developed by OMERACT. Indian J Rheumatol 2013;8(Supplement 1):17–22.

29. Kirwan J.R, Hewlett S.E, Heiberg T, et al. Incorporating the patient perspective into outcome assessment in rheumatoid arthritis–progress at OMERACT 7. J Rheumatol. 2005;32:2250–6.

30. Ahlmen M, Nordenskiöld U, Archenholtz B, et al. Rheumatology outcomes: the patient's perspective. A multicentre focus group interview study of Swedish rheumatoid arthritis patients. Rheumatology 2005;44:105–10.

31. Carr A, Hewlett S, Hughes R, et al. Rheumatology outcomes: the patient's perspective. J Rheumatol. 2003;30:880–3.

32. Gossec L, Dougados M, Rincheval N, et al. Elaboration of the preliminary Rheumatoid Arthritis Impact of Disease (RAID) score: A EULAR initiative. Ann Rheum Dis 2009;68:1680–5.

33. Doward LC, Gnanasakthy A, Baker MG. Patient reported outcomes: looking beyond the label claim. Health Qual Life Outcomes 2010;8:89.

34. Boers M, Kirwan JR, Wells G, et al. Developing core outcome measurement sets for clinical trials: OMERACT filter 2.0. J Clin Epidemiol. 2014;67(7):745–53.

35. Gossec L, Dougados M, Dixon W. Patient-reported outcomes as endpoints in clinical trials in rheumatoid arthritis. Review. RMD Open 2015;1:e000019 doi:10.1136/rmdopen-2014-000019.

36. Bartlett SJ, Hewlett S, Bingham CO 3rd, et al. OMERACT RA Flare Working Group. Identifying core domains to assess flare in rheumatoid arthritis: an OMERACT international patient and provider combined Delphi consensus. Ann Rheum Dis. 2012;71(11):1855–60.

37. Boers M, Kirwan JR, Gossec L, et al. How to choose core outcome measurement sets for clinical trials: OMERACT 11 approves filter 2.0. J Rheumatol. 2014;41(5):1025–30.

38. Tugwell P, Wells G, Strand V, et al. Clinical improvement as reflected in measures of function and health-related quality of life following treatment with leflunomide compared with methotrexate in patients with rheumatoid arthritis: sensitivity and relative efficiency to detect a treatment effect in a twelve-month, placebo-controlled trial. Leflunomide Rheumatoid Arthritis Investigators Group. Arthritis Rheum. 2000;43(3):506–14.

39. Castrejón I, Gossec L, Carmona L. The EULAR Outcome Measures Library: an evolutional database of validated patient-reported instruments. Ann Rheum Dis. 2015;74(2):475–6.

40. Wells G, Li T, Maxwell L, et al. Responsiveness of patient reported outcomes including fatigue, sleep quality, activity limitation, and quality of life following treatment with abatacept for rheumatoid arthritis. Ann Rheum Dis. 2008;67(2):260–5.

41. Gladman DD, Mease PJ, Strand V, et al. Consensus on a core set of domains for psoriatic arthritis. J Rheumatol 2007;34(5):1167–70.

42. Tillett W, Adebajo A, Brooke M, et al. Patient involvement in outcome measures for psoriatic arthritis. Curr Rheumatol Rep 2014;16(5):418.

43. Stamm TA, Nell V, Mathis M, et al. Concepts important to patients with psoriatic arthritis are not adequately covered by standard measures of functioning. Arthritis Rheum 2007;57(3):487–94.

44. Tillett W, Eder L, Goel N, et al. Enhanced patient involvement and the need to revise the core set- report from the Psoriatic Arthritis working group at OMERACT 2014. J Rheumatol. 2015; 42(11):2198–203.

45. Orbai AM, Mease P, de Wit M, et al. The GRAPPA OMERACT Psoriatic Arthritis Working Group Report from the GRAPPA 2015 Annual Meeting. 2016; 43(5):965–9.

46. Palominos PE, Gaujoux-Viala C, Fautrel B, et al. Clinical outcomes in psoriatic arthritis: A systematic literature review. Arthritis Care Res (Hoboken) 2012;64(3):397–406.

47. Moverley AR, Vinall-Collier KA, Helliwell PS. It's not just the joints, it's the whole thing: qualitative analysis of patients' experience of flare in psoriatic arthritis. Rheumatology 2015;54(8):1448–53.

48. Gudu T, Kiltz U, de Wit M, et al. Mapping the effect of psoriatic arthritis using the International Classification of Functioning, Disability and Health J Rheumatol. 2017;44(2):193–200. doi:10.3899/jrheum.160180. Epub 2016 Dec 15. PubMed PMID: 27980011.

49. Gossec L, de Wit M, Kiltz U, et al. A patient-derived and patient-reported outcome measure for assessing psoriatic arthritis: elaboration and preliminary validation of the Psoriatic Arthritis Impact of Disease (PsAID) questionnaire, a 13-country EULAR initiative. Ann Rheum Dis 2014;73(6): 1012–19.

50. McKenna SP, Doward LC, Whalley D, et al. Development of the PsAQoL: a quality of life instrument specific to psoriatic arthritis. Ann Rheum Dis 2004;63(2):162–9.

51. Healy PJ, Helliwell PS. Psoriatic arthritis quality of life instrument: an assessment of sensitivity and response to change. J Rheumatol. 2008;35(7):1359–61.

52. Wink F, Arends S, McKenna SP, et al. Validity and reliability of the Dutch adaptation of the Psoriatic Arthritis Quality of Life (PsAQoL) Questionnaire. PLoS One. 2013;8(2).

53. Billing E, McKenna SP, Staun M, et al. Adaptation of the Psoriatic Arthritis Quality of Life (PsAQoL) instrument for Sweden. Scand J Rheumatol. 2010;39(3).

54. Marzo-Ortega H, McGonagle D, Rhodes LA, et al. Efficacy of infliximab on MRI-determined bone oedema in psoriatic arthritis. Ann Rheum Dis. 2007;66(6):778–81.

55. Gladman D, Fleischmann R, Coteur G, et al. Effect of certolizumab pegol on multiple facets of psoriatic arthritis as reported by patients: 24-week patient-reported outcome results of a phase III, multicenter study. Arthritis Care Res (Hoboken). 2014;66(7):1085–92.

56. Tezel N, Yilmaz Tasdelen O, Bodur H, et al. Is the health-related quality of life and functional status of patients with psoriatic arthritis worse than that of patients with psoriasis alone? Int J Rheum Dis. 2015;18(1):63–9.

57. Osterhaus JT, Purcaru O. Discriminant validity, responsiveness and reliability of the arthritis-specific Work Productivity Survey assessing workplace and household productivity in patients with psoriatic arthritis. Arthritis Res Ther. 2014;16(4):R140.

58. Gezer O, Batmaz I, Sariyildiz MA, et al. Sleep quality in patients with psoriatic arthritis. Int J Rheum Dis. 2017; 20(9):1212–18.

59. http://www.eular.org/tools_products_.cfm accessed Aug 21, 2015.

60. Katz PP. Introduction to special issue: patient outcomes in rheumatology, 2011. Arthritis Care Res (Hoboken). 2011;63 Suppl 11:S1–3.

61. Cauli A, Gladman D, Mathieu A, et al. Patient global assessment in psoriatic arthritis: a multicenter GRAPPA and OMERACT study. J Rheumatol 2011; 38:5.

62. Talli S, Etcheto A, Fautrel B, et al. Patient global assessment in psoriatic arthritis—what does it mean? An Analysis of 223 Patients from the Psoriatic Arthritis Impact of Disease (PsAID) Study. Joint Bone Spine 2016; 83(3):335–405.

63. Gossec L, Paternotte S, Aanerud G, et al. Finalisation and validation of the Rheumatoid Arthritis Impact of Disease (RAID) score: a patient-derived composite measure of impact of RA. A EULAR initiative. Ann Rheum Dis 2011;70:935–42.

64. Dworkin RH, Turk DC, Wyrwich KW, et al. Interpreting the clinical importance of treatment outcomes in chronic pain clinical trials: IMMPACT recommendations. J Pain. 2008;9(2):105–21.

65. Bruce B, Fries JF. The Stanford Health Assessment Questionnaire HAQ): a review of its history, issues, progress, and documentation. J Rheumatol 2003;30:167–78.

66. Bruce B, Fries JF. The Health Assessment Questionnaire (HAQ). Clin Exp Rheumatol. 2005;23(5 Suppl 39):S14–8.

67. Fries JF, Krishnan E, Rose M, et al. Improved responsiveness and reduced sample size requirements of PROMIS physical function scales with item response theory. Arthritis Res Ther. 2011;13(5):R147.

68. http://aramis.stanford.edu/downloads/HAQ%20Instructions%20 %28ARAMIS%29%206-30-09.pdf accessed Aug 21, 2015.

69. Blackmore MG, Gladman DD, Husted J, Long JA, Farewell VT. Measuring health status in psoriatic arthritis: the Health Assessment Questionnaire and its modification. J Rheumatol. 1995;22(5):886–93.

70. Mease PJ, Woolley JM, Bitman B, et al. Minimally important difference of Health Assessment Questionnaire in psoriatic arthritis: relating thresholds of improvement in functional ability to patient-rated importance and satisfaction. J Rheumatol. 2011;38(11):2461–5.

71. Gladman DD, Mease PJ, Cifaldi MA, et al. Adalimumab improves joint-related and skin-related functional impairment in patients with psoriatic arthritis: patient-reported outcomes of the Adalimumab Effectiveness in Psoriatic Arthritis Trial. Ann Rheum Dis. 2007;66(2):163–8.

72. Finlay AY, Khan GK. Dermatology Life Quality Index (DLQI)-a simple practical measure for routine clinical use. Clin Exp Dermatol. 1994;19(3):210–6.

73. Feldman SR, Kimball AB, Krueger GG, et al. Etanercept improves the health-related quality of life of patients with psoriasis: results of a phase III randomized clinical trial. J Am Acad Dermatol. 2005;53(5):887–9.

74. Ware JE, Sherbourne CD. The RAND 36 Short-form Health Status Survey: 1.Conceptual framework and item selection. Med Care 1992; 30:473–81.

75. http://www.sf-36.org/, accessed Aug 21, 2015.

76. Husted JA, Gladman DD, Farewell VT, et al. Validating the SF-36 health survey questionnaire in patients with psoriatic arthritis. J Rheumatol 1997;24(3):511–7.

77. Strand V, Sharp V, Koenig AS, et al. Comparison of health-related quality of life in rheumatoid arthritis, psoriatic arthritis and psoriasis and effects of etanercept treatment. Ann Rheum Dis 2012;71(7):1143–50.

78. Strand V, Schett G, Hu C, et al. Patient-reported Health-related Quality of Life with apremilast for psoriatic arthritis: a phase II, randomized, controlled study. J Rheumatol. 2013;40(7):1158–65.

79. Husted JA, Tom BD, Schentag CT, et al. Occurrence and correlates of fatigue in psoriatic arthritis. Ann Rheum Dis 2009; 68(10): 1553–8.

80. Gudu T, Etcheto A, de Wit M, Heiberg, et al. Fatigue in psoriatic arthritis—a cross-sectional study of 246 patients from 13 countries. Joint Bone Spine 2016; l;83(4):439–43.

81. Minnock P, Kirwan J, Veale D, et al. Fatigue is an independent outcome measure and is sensitive to change in patients with psoriatic arthritis. Clin Exp Rheumatol 2010;28(3):401–4.

82. Schentag CT, Cichon J, MacKinnon A, et al. Validation and normative data for the 0–10 point scale version of the fatigue severity scale (FSS). Arthritis Rheum 2000;43:S177.

83. Chandran V, Bhella S, Schentag C, et al. Functional assessment of chronic illness therapy-fatigue scale is valid in patients with psoriatic arthritis. Ann Rheum Dis. 2007;66(7):936–9.

84. Husted JA, Tom BD, Farewell VT, et al. Longitudinal analysis of fatigue in psoriatic arthritis. J Rheumatol 2010;37(9):1878–84.

85. van Tubergen A, Coenen J, Landewé R, et al. Assessment of fatigue in patients with ankylosing spondylitis: a psychometric analysis. Arthritis Rheum 2002;47(1):8–16.

86. Wolfe F. Fatigue assessments in rheumatoid arthritis: comparative performance of visual analog scales and longer fatigue questionnaires in 7760 patients. J Rheumatol. 2004;31(10):1896–902.

CHAPTER 25

Composite scores in psoriatic arthritis

Philip S. Helliwell

Introduction

What are composite scores?

Composite scores are assessment tools that combine a number of separate evaluations into one score. The composite score generally has more statistical power than the individual items, is more responsive, and has a greater effect size. A composite score allows synthesis of several elements into one score which can then, if psychometrically appropriate, allow the determination of disease activity (both low and high) cut offs, and response criteria.

In general, each element of the score should represent the same underlying concept of disease activity. In the case of psoriatic arthritis (PsA) the elements may not always combine in this way. An example of this might be discordance in skin and joint activity. Thus, as a general principle, whatever composite measure is used, it is recommended that the individual scores which make up the composite are always recorded separately.

History of composite scores in psoriatic arthritis clinical trials

The first trial to use a composite score was the Veterans Administration study, published in 1996 [1]. For this study an empirical score was developed (the Psoriatic arthritis response criteria, or PsARC) which was, essentially, a 30% response measure (Box 25.1). Subsequently, with the advent of tumour necrosis factor inhibitors (TNFi) investigators 'borrowed' composite measures from rheumatoid arthritis (RA)—the American College of Rheumatology (ACR) response criteria (ACR20) and the disease activity score for 28 joints (DAS28). As new biologic agents have appeared, further studies have continued to use these criteria, not only to allow comparative efficacy of different agents but because, until recently, nothing else was available. However, a number of new composite measures are now available for PsA. These include the Composite Psoriatic Disease Activity Index (CPDAI), the GRAPPA Composite Index (GRACE), the Psoriatic Arthritis Disease Activity Index (PASDAS), the Disease Activity for Psoriatic Arthritis (DAPSA), the Psoriatic Arthritis Joint Activity Index (PsAJAI) and the minimal disease activity criteria (MDA).

Utility of composite scores

Composite indices are more 'efficient' thus permitting, in clinical trials, a smaller sample size to demonstrate efficacy. By putting different assessments together into one index the sum performs better than the individual parts. With larger effect sizes, sample sizes become smaller. In a disease such as PsA, where disease manifestations are heterogeneous, the challenge is not only conceptual but practical. What, for example, if one aspect of the disease, for example the skin, responds differently to another, such as the joints? The net effect might be no change in the index. This scenario is actually less likely than one in which one domain changes and the other does not, thus somewhat negating the purpose of a composite index. There may also be methodological problems—combining assessments of disease using, for example, in one domain a visual analogue scale score, and in another domain a self-completed questionnaire with multiple questions. In actual fact, the latter approach may not be incorrect if an appropriate statistical approach is made in the development phase.

The GRAPPA composite index study

In 2008 GRAPPA initiated a study to develop new composite measures for PsA. This was partly in response to an OMERACT module in which domains and instruments for clinical trials in PsA were established [2].

Thirty-one centres, all members of GRAPPA, participated in this study [3]. Centres were asked to provide data on a minimum of 10 and a maximum of 40 patients. All patients granted informed consent, with ethical committee approval at each site. Data were collected at baseline (the first assessment), and 3, 6, and 12 months but the new composite indices were developed using baseline data only. It was agreed that the 'gold standard' metric for active disease was a decision to change treatment at that clinic visit. In the development of a new composite measure two approaches were used. The first simulated methods used in development of the Ankylosing Spondylitis Disease Activity Score (ASDAS) [4]. Initially, principal component analysis was used to manage and reduce the variables into related components. Components with an eigenvalue of >1 were accepted. Factor loadings were then used to inform a discriminant function analysis. Finally, forward stepwise multiple linear regression analysis used the discriminant function as the dependent variable, and original variables as independent variables. The resulting index was called the PASDAS with a score range from 0–10 (see Box 25.2) The second approach was akin to that suggested by Fransen et al., where desirability functions were developed for variables deemed important in assessing disease activity, based on core domains selected for PsA randomized clinical trials (RCTs) at OMERACT 8 [5]. Cut-offs were determined and used to transform each variable into linear functions ranging from 0 (totally unacceptable state) to 1 (normal). The

Box 25.1 PsARC: The psoriatic arthritis response criteria of Clegg et al.

A responder is defined as someone in whom 2/4 domains improve (at least one of these being domains A or B), with deterioration in 0/4 domains.

Domains

A Swollen joint count (76 joints) (improvement or worsening: change by ≥30%)

B Tender joint count (78 joints) (improvement or worsening: change by ≥30%)

C Patient global assessment* (improvement > or = to 1 unit; deterioration > or = 1 unit)

D Physician global assessment* (improvement > or = to I unit; deterioration > or = 1 unit)

* as measured by a 5 point Likert scale.
Data sourced from Clegg et al. (1996), Comparison of sulfasalazine and placebo in the treatment of psoriatic arthritis. A department of veterans' affairs cooperative study. Arthritis & Rheumatism, 39: 2013–2020.

Box 25.3 The Arithmetic Mean of the Desirability Function (AMDF) or GRACE measure

The AMDF is a composite score comprising assessments of joints, skin, pain, function, and health-related quality of life. Each domain is transformed into a 0 to 1 scale where 0 is a completely unacceptable state and 1 is normal. The variables transformed were:

◆ 68 tender joint count

◆ 66 swollen joint count

◆ Health assessment questionnaire (HAQ)

◆ Patient global assessment of disease activity by VAS

◆ Patient VAS for skin

◆ Patient VAS for joints

◆ Psoriasis area and severity index (PASI)

◆ Psoriatic arthritis quality of life index (PsAQoL)

The 8 transformed variables were combined using the arithmetic mean. For simplification, and to simplify and improve interpretation of this index, the AMDF was transformed and renamed, as follows:

GRACE index = $(1 - AMDF) \times 10$

Data sourced from Helliwell, FitzGerald, Fransen et al. The development of candidate composite disease activity and responder indices for psoriatic arthritis (GRACE project) Annals of the Rheumatic Diseases 2013;72:986–991.

eight transformed variables were then combined using the arithmetic mean, and represented as a score range from 0–10, called the GRACE index (Box 25.3). The data collected in the GRACE study not only enabled the development of two new indices but also permitted the comparison of the new indices with established measures, and compare their performance over time.

Response measures

American College of Rheumatology response criteria

The ACR criteria were developed in the 1990s for the purpose of assessing response in therapeutic clinical trials in RA. They represent

the point at which standardization was introduced to assessment in rheumatology clinical trials and herald the arrival of OMERACT. The ACR criteria use joint counts as the prime measure of improvement but add further dimensions with the addition of other outcomes: an assessment of function represented by the Health Assessment Questionnaire, a patient and physician global score, an acute phase response and a patient pain score. For response (20%, 50%, or 70%) that percentage of improvement must be demonstrated in the tender and swollen joint counts, and three of the five other domains (Box 25.4).

Box 25.2 The Psoriatic arthritis disease activity score (PASDAS)

PASDAS = $(((0.18 \times \sqrt{\text{Physician global VAS}}) + (0.159 \times \sqrt{\text{Patient global VAS}}) - (0.253 \times \sqrt{\text{SF36} - \text{PCS}}) + (0.101 \times \text{LN (Swollen joint count} + 1)) + (0.048 \times \text{LN (Tender joint count} + 1)) + (0.23 \times \text{LN (Leeds Enthesitis Count} + 1)) + (0.377 \text{ LN (Dactylitis count} + 1)) + (0.102 \times \text{LN (CRP} + 1)) + 2)*1.5$.

Where 'Physician global VAS' is the physicians' global opinion of the skin and joints recorded on a 0–100 mm scale; 'Patient global VAS is the patients' global opinion of the skin and joints recorded on a 0–100mm scale; 'SF36-PCS' is the physical component scale of the short form 36; 'Swollen joint count' is a 66 joint count; 'Tender joint count' is a 68 joint count; 'Leeds Enthesitis Count' ranges from 0–6; 'Dactylitis count' is the tender dactylitis count with a score range of 0–20; 'CRP' is the C-reactive protein level in mg/l). The score range of the PASDAS is 0–10.

Data sourced from Helliwell PS, FitzGerald O, Fransen J, et al. The development of candidate composite disease activity and responder indices for psoriatic arthritis (GRACE project). Ann Rheum Dis 2013;72(6):986–91.

Box 25.4 The American College of Rheumatology response criteria

ACR measures improvement (20%, 50% or 70%) in tender and swollen joint counts (which traditionally in psoriatic arthritis are 66 swollen and 68 tender joints) and similar percentage improvement in at least 3 of the following 5 measures:

◆ acute phase reactant, CRP or ESR

◆ patient global VAS score

◆ physician global VAS score

◆ patient pain VAS score

◆ disability/function by Health Assessment Questionnaire

Data sourced from Felson et al. American College of Rheumatology preliminary definition of improvement in rheumatoid arthritis (1995) 38(6):727–735.

The ACR20 criteria have become the benchmark in clinical trials in RA and PsA. In the latter , they were introduced because of the lack of an alternative, at a time when the first biological drugs were introduced [6]. The criteria were modified for PsA by the use of a 66 tender and 68 swollen joint count (in contrast to the 44 tender and swollen joint count in the original). Nonetheless, the ACR criteria do not incorporate any of the other elements of disease that are traditionally found in PsA: dactylitis, enthesitis, axial disease, and the skin/nail component, although a patient global assessment is included.

In fact, the ACR20 criteria have worked well in PsA clinical trials, demonstrating a clear difference between active drug and placebo [7]. However, it must be noted that most of the cases enrolled in PsA trials have polyarthritis. The ACR20 criteria give differential responses according to joint count and cases of oligoarthritis are less likely to achieve an ACR20 response: patients are more likely to achieve an ACR20 response in cases of polyarthritis [8]. At the current time, it is difficult to see alternative primary outcomes being adopted for PsA clinical trials. This will be driven by the appropriate authorities of course (US Food and Drug Administration, and the European Medicines Agency) but more validation work will be necessary before alternative composites are introduced.

Psoriatic arthritis response criteria, PsARC

See Box 25.1

The PsARC criteria were developed specifically for a trial of sulfasalazine in PsA, in the 1990s [1]. Their development was determined by the need for a composite measure to use in PsA, at a time when the ACR response criteria had been introduced for RA. With the PsARC, to achieve response patients must have a 30% improvement in tender and swollen joint count and improvement of at least one point on a Likert scale of patient and physician global score. To achieve response, there must be no deterioration in any of the dimensions. Similar to the ACR criteria, important other aspects of disease in PsA are not included.

The PsARC criteria have been used extensively as secondary outcome measures, and as the primary outcome measure in the only fully powered RCT of methotrexate in PsA—the MIPA trial [9]. Of interest, the PsARC is also used to determine treatment response according to the UK NICE guidelines for the use of anti-TNF biologic drugs in PsA [10]. The criteria are able to distinguish active drug from placebo but there is a high placebo response rate with these criteria: 39% in the MIPA study.

Psoriatic arthritis Joint Activity Index, PsAJAI

See Box 25.5)To develop an alternative to the ACR response criteria, the group from Toronto set out to derive a data driven set of response criteria using data from a number of interventional studies [11, 12]. This resulted in the PsA joint activity index, PsAJAI (Box 25.5). Interestingly, the skin component of the disease did not appear in the final model which is essentially a weighted 30% response measure, with components similar to the ACR response criteria.

Despite the rigorous methodology employed in this study, the criteria have not been used as the primary outcome in any of the subsequently published interventional studies. Why is this? The PsAJAI probably does not represent a significant advance over the ACR criteria, and with the ACR criteria already in use it is likely that investigators, and the approving authorities, wished to

---

Box 25.5 The Psoriatic arthritis Joint Activity Index (PsAJAI)

- Weighted sum of 30% improvement in core measures: joint count, CRP and physician global

- Pain, patient global and Health Asssessment Questionnaire (HAQ) weighted differently

PsAJAI = 2 (if a 30% decrease in either tender or swollen joint count) + 2 (if a 30% decrease in CRP) + 2 (if a 30% decrease in physician global) + 1 (if a 30% decrease in patient global) + 1 (if a 30% decrease in pain) + 1 (if a 30% decrease in HAQ),

Score range 0–9.

Proposed cut-off for response: 5 or more

Data sourced from Gladman et al. Informing Response Criteria for Psoriatic Arthritis (PsA). II: Further considerations and a proposal—the PsA joint activity index. J. Rheum (2010) 37(12):2559–2565.

---

continue with what had been used before, to enable appropriate comparison between drugs.

Minimal disease activity, MDA

See Box 25.6

MDA was a GRAPPA supported endeavour developed for use in the first treat-to-target strategy trial in PsA [13–15]. The criteria were developed using a 'paper patient' exercise. The cases were derived from a real patient database and cases of both high and low disease activity were included. Data were extracted to reflect the core domains identified at OMERACT with the addition of data on enthesitis [16]. For each case, a summary of assessments across different domains was presented to the reviewers in a web-based exercise. Each reviewer was asked to judge if the patient was in minimal disease activity. With many different profiles generated receiver operating curves were used to select the criteria with the optimal performance.

The MDA criteria have been validated in a number of databases [17–19]. Patients achieving MDA are less likely to have radiographic progression in interventional studies and, achievement of MDA on more than three occasions was associated with better

---

Box 25.6 The minimal disease activity criteria

A patient is classified as in MDA when they meet 5 of 7 of the following criteria:

- tender joint count ≤1
- swollen joint count ≤1
- PASI ≤1 or BSA ≤3%
- patient pain VAS ≤15/100
- patient global activity VAS ≤20/100
- HAQ ≤0.5
- tender entheseal points ≤1

Data sourced from Coates LC, Fransen J, Helliwell PS Defining minimal disease activity in psoriatic arthritis: a proposed objective target for treatment Annals of the Rheumatic Diseases 2010;69:48–53.

outcomes in a longitudinal database. In addition, the criteria have been used in a treat-to-target strategy trial where better skin and joint outcomes were found in the group specifically treated to the MDA target [15]. In addition, the MDA criteria have been used in a treatment withdrawal study, in this case 'not being in MDA' (i.e. relapse) was the primary outcome measure [20].

Although the physician must make assessment of enthesitis, skin and joints, and the patient must complete two VAS scores and the 8 domain Health Assessment Questionnaire (HAQ) [21] in practice these criteria are quick and easy to complete, taking no more than 10 minutes. The MDA criteria represent a low disease activity target, but they are not equivalent to remission, and they assess the level of disease activity slightly more stringently than physicians 'global' assessment and patients' assessment of satisfactory disease control [22]. Further, since only five of seven criteria must be met, it is possible to be classified as in MDA with a high tender and swollen joint count. In practice, the latter scenario does not seem to occur: in the TICOPA study approximately 30% of people in MDA met 5/7 criteria, 30% 6/7, and 30% 7/7. Of the people meeting 5/7 criteria the most frequently 'missed' items were the skin item and the tender joint item (Coates and Helliwell, unpublished data).

Composite disease activity measures

Disease activity score for 28 joints (DAS28)

Measurement of disease activity in RA is most often represented by the disease activity score for 28 joints (DAS28) [23]. Although initially used only in the clinical trial environment, the DAS28 has gained widespread use in many routine clinics. The necessity for a concurrent acute phase response has limited its 'real time' use [24] but familiarity, ease of calculation (with hand held or on-line devices), availability of response criteria and cut-offs have all strengthened the use of the measure. In fact, owing to the lack of a true specific measure for PsA, and its performance in RA clinical trials, the DAS28 has been used as a disease activity measure in PsA clinical trials, in registries, and in day to day clinics. Although Fransen et al. have demonstrated that the DAS28 works well as a disease activity measure in PsA, it should be noted that the data on which this conclusion was based were taken from clinical trials where most of the patients had polyarticular disease [25]. The DAS28 may not function as well in oligoarticular disease, which can be seen in up to a third of patients presenting with PsA. Indeed it has been shown that in this scenario up to 20% of patients may be misclassified in terms of disease activity [26]. In addition, no specific measures of skin, enthesitis, dactylitis, or axial disease are made, although the patient global may of course reflect disease activity in these other domains.

Disease activity for psoriatic arthritis, DAPSA

The DAPSA was derived from a measure initially used to assess disease activity in reactive arthritis, the Disease Activity in ReactivE Arthritis (DAREA) [27]. This measure was adopted because it specifically used a 66swollen/68tender joint count and the items matched those previously selected in a principal component analysis of patient measures in PsA (Box 25.7). The DAPSA underwent some validation using interventional trial data and data from a longitudinal cohort. Subsequently cut-offs for disease activity have been developed [28].

The DAPSA is simple and quick to perform in clinic making it feasible for use in clinical practice but, like the DAS28, there are

---

> **Box 25.7 The disease activity for psoriatic arthritis (DAPSA) measure**
>
> The index measures disease activity in peripheral arthritis using:
>
> - 68 tender and 66 swollen peripheral joint count
> - Patient global VAS, 1–10 scale
> - Patient pain VAS, 1–10 scale
> - CRP, mg/dL.
>
> The composite score is a simple sum of the scores
>
> Data sourced from Aletaha, Alasti, and Smolen, Disease activity states of the DAPSA, a psoriatic arthritis specific instrument, are valid against functional status and structural progression Annals of the Rheumatic Diseases Published Online First: 25 July 2016. 76(2):418–421.

concerns about the limitations of just assessing the joints in such a heterogeneous condition. Of the six key outcomes designated by the GRAPPA/OMERACT group, the DAPSA covers just three.

This is particularly concerning when developing definitions of low disease activity and remission for potential use in a treat to target strategy. Interestingly, the definitions of low disease state differ according to different methodologies: with patient and physician input into defining low disease activity the cut-off is 18.5 [29], with just physician input the cut-off was found to be 14.

Composite psoriatic disease activity index, CPDAI

See Table 25.1.

The CPDAI was conceived and designed to match the domains originally targeted by the GRAPPA treatment recommendations [30]. The five domains, joints, skin, dactylitis, enthesitis, and axial were subdivided according to the level of disease activity. The definitions of mild, moderate, and severe disease were somewhat arbitrary but a modified version of the CPDAI (excluding the axial component) was able to distinguish between two different doses of etanercept, whereas the DAPSA, in the same dataset, despite showing improvement, did not differentiate between the two doses [31]. The CPDAI has been further validated in an interventional trial dataset and is available as an online application where patients and physicians can add data and the application will automatically compute both the CPDAI value and whether patient is in MDA (https://mopsa.ie) .

In comparison to some of the other measures, the CPDAI can be calculated at the time of assessing the patient, as there is no need for a laboratory measure. However, there are a number of patient reported outcomes to complete, and clinical assessment of the joints, skin, entheses, and dactylitis. The absence of a patient assessment of pain, and a global patient assessment, as recommended by the GRAPPA/OMERACT group is a disadvantage but a simple modification of the instrument could be made by the addition of a 'patient VAS' domain (O. FitzGerald, personal communication).

GRAPPA composite score, GRACE

See Box 25.3.

The GRACE index, originally described as the Arithmetic Mean of the Desirability Function (AMDF), was one of the composite indices developed as a result of the GRAPPA Composite Exercise (GRACE)

Table 25.1 The Composite Psoriatic Disease Activity Index (CPDAI). The score range is 0–15

	None (0)	Mild (1)	Moderate (2)	Severe (3)
Peripheral arthritis	–	≤ 4 joints; normal function (HAQ <0.5)	≤ 4 joints but function impaired; or > 4 joints, normal function	> 4 joints *and* function impaired
Skin disease	–	PASI ≤ 10 and DLQI ≤ 10	PASI ≤ 10 but DLQI >10; or PASI > 10 but DLQI ≤ 10	PASI > 10 *and* DLQI > 10
Enthesitis	–	≤ 3 sites; normal function (HAQ <0.5)	≤ 3 sites but function impaired; or >3 sites but normal function	>3 sites *and* function impaired
Dactylitis	–	≤ 3 digits; normal function (HAQ <0.5)	≤ 3 digits but function impaired; or >3 digits but normal function	>3 digits *and* has function impaired
Spinal disease	–	BASDAI ≤4; normal function (ASQol ≤ 6)	BASDAI >4 but normal function; BASDAI ≤4 but function impaired	BASDAI >4 *and* function impaired

Data sourced from Mumtaz A, Gallagher P, Kirby B, et al. Development of a preliminary composite disease activity index in psoriatic arthritis Annals of the Rheumatic Diseases 2011;70:272–277.

The joint count is a 66 swollen, 68 tender count.

HAQ, health assessment questionnaire; PASI, psoriasis area and severity index; DLQI, dermatology life quality index.

Enthesitis score is based on the 6 sites of the Leeds enthesitis index.

Dactylitis is a simple count of tender dactylitic digits.

ASQoL, ankylosing spondylitis quality of life measure; BASDAI, Bath Ankylosing spondylitis disease activity index.

study. The AMDF is a composite score designed to reflect the core items of the GRAPPA/OMERACT domains and comprises assessments of joints, skin, pain, function, and health-related quality of life (QOL). Each domain went through a process of transformation to a 'desirability' scale in order to be able to combine all the items. Items thus transformed were combined and the arithmetic mean obtained giving a 0–1 scale where 0 is a completely unacceptable state and 1 is normal (Table 25.1). To make the scale more comparable with other disease activity indices, and after agreement at the GRAPPA meeting in Washington, DC November 2012, the AMDF was transformed, and renamed, as follows: GRACE index = (1–AMDF) × 10, which provides a score range of 0–10 with worse disease activity represented by higher scores.

Further validation of the AMDF has been undertaken in interventional trial datasets where it has been found to have an effect size comparable to other composite disease measures (see below). However, despite its performance and conceptual pedigree, it is regarded with some reluctance by trialists as being too complex and inherently difficult to comprehend (P. Helliwell, unpublished data).

Psoriatic arthritis Disease Activity Score, PASDAS

See Box 25.2.

The other disease activity index developed in the GRACE study was the PASDAS. The PASDAS was developed by a purely data-driven technique, as indicated in Box 25.2. The PASDAS is a weighted index comprising assessments of joints, dactylitis, enthesitis, acute phase response, QOL, and patient and physician global disease activity by VAS. The score range of the PASDAS is 0–10, with worse disease activity represented by higher scores.

The data manipulation necessary to develop the PASDAS was undertaken in a manner similar to that developed for the Ankylosing Spondylitis Disease activity Score (ASDAS [4]) and was so designed to give a score of 0 to 10, with higher disease activity represented by increasing scores. The score range was designed to be analogous to the DAS28, as this has been adopted widely in RA clinical trials. Further, having a normal distribution the measure can be treated as a parametric function and used to develop cut-offs for disease activity and response. With the DAS28 cut-offs for disease activity have been endorsed by organizations such as the National Institute for Health and Care Excellence (NICE) in the UK, and are in daily use to establish eligibility for TNF inhibitors in RA [32]. The score range of the PASDAS was so developed that use and interpretation of cut-offs could occur in a similar way.

The PASDAS has been validated in interventional trial datasets and cut-offs for disease activity and response have been developed [29]. In the Golimumab interventional study effect sizes at 24 weeks for the 50 mg (100 mg) golimumab doses were 2.18 (2.36), 2.08 (2.36), 1.09 (1.41), and 1.13 (1.18) for PASDAS, GRACE, a modified version of the CPDAI, and the DAPSA, respectively. Comparison of 24-week values across the three treatment groups (placebo, golimumab 50 mg and 100 mg) by an analysis of covariance using the baseline values as covariates gave the following F statistics for the PASDAS (F=18.3), GRACE (F=19.6), modified CPDAI (F=9.4), and DAPSA (F=7.9), all of which were highly significant [33]. In the same dataset achieving a poor, moderate, or good response, as measured by the PASDAS, was associated with significant difference in radiographic progression (Figure 25.1) [34]. In the certolizumab interventional study, the largest effect size for treatment at 12 weeks was seen for the PASDAS (Effect size, ES, 1.0), compared to a modified CPDAI (ES 0.8) and the DAS28 (ES 0.95) [35].

As mentioned above, cut-offs for disease activity and response have been developed for the PASDAS, GRACE, CPDAI, DAS28, and DAPSA, and these are given in Table 25.2. It should be noted that the cut-offs for the DAS28 are different to those developed for RA, and similarly the cut-offs for the DAPSA are different to those developed in an independent study [28]. The cut-offs in Table 25.2 were developed by a consensus process and incorporate the judgement of both physician and patient. More recent analysis suggests that these may be less stringent than other

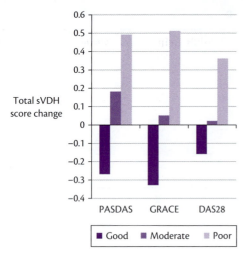

Figure 25.1 Radiographic progression, as measured by the total Sharp/van der Heidje method, for all groups in the GO-REVEAL study at week 24. Outcome at week 24 measured by the PASDAS, GRACE and DAS28 according to response criteria (see Table 25.2) The differences between the response categories for each measure were highly significant.

Data sourced from Helliwell PS, Kavanaugh A. Comparison of Composite Measures of Disease Activity in Psoriatic Arthritis Using Data From an Interventional Study With Golimumab. Arthritis Care & Research. 2014;66(5):749–56 and Helliwell PS, Kavanaugh A. Radiographic progression is less in psoriatic arthritis achieving a good response to treatment: data using newer composite indices of disease activity. Arthritis Care Res (Hoboken) 2018;70(5):797–800.

which assess multiple domains have been criticized on the basis that some therapies may work well for one domain of disease but not for others, and that these subtleties may be lost in a single measure. Whilst this has not been a common experience with any of the recently tested therapies in PsA (TNF inhibitors [36], IL-12/23 inhibitors [37], and IL-17 inhibitors [38]), it is clear that the individual components of a composite score such as the CPDAI or PASDAS could be reported as part of the score documentation thus identifying any potential differential responses across domains of disease. It does seem, from comparative studies, that there is more 'power' in the composites that assess the complete spectrum of the disease with larger comparative statistics, as noted above [31, 33, 35]. The other key question is whether these new composite measures can have prognostic impact. Initial, albeit post hoc analyses, suggest that may be the case for the PASDAS, GRACE, and MDA [18].

Overall, the performance of the composite measures which assess the complete spectrum of disease has been better, statistically. However, there is a question of feasibility. Measures such as the PASDAS, GRACE, and CPDAI are unlikely to be used in the routine clinic situation, despite the likely introduction of computerized programs for their calculation. However, as health professionals making decisions on disease activity, and by inference treatment choice, we have to be cognizant of all aspects of the disease. In some way, therefore, we have to link these necessary clinical assessments with a composite measure of disease activity. This will be discussed further in the next section.

judgements of low disease activity, such as the physician opinion of minimal disease activity and the patient opinion of good disease control [22].

Comparative studies and overall assessment

There is always a difficult balance between comprehensive assessment of a heterogeneous disease and feasibility of outcome measures, particularly in clinical practice. A comparison of each of the domains/components measured by each of the composite measures is given in Table 25.3.

A measure such as the DAPSA performs well in studies where patients have significant articular disease but it does not cover important manifestations such as the skin, enthesitis, and the axial component. It has been suggested that these aspects can be captured by additional measures, recorded separately, but such 'add-ons' might as well be captured in a more comprehensive measure such as the PASDAS or CPDAI. Composite measures

Conclusions and future considerations

The challenges of assessing disease activity in such an heterogeneous disease as PsA are legion but in the last 10 years GRAPPA has developed new outcome measures across the disease spectrum. There remains the problem of utilizing composite scores that function efficiently. In this scenario the skin component is most problematic. For most cases of PsA seen in routine rheumatology clinics skin involvement is minimal, and the skin may not always respond synchronously with the musculoskeletal manifestations. Conversely, the paradox of early skin response to some therapies, such as methotrexate, can lead the observing physician into a false impression that all components of disease are improving. Only by systematically, and objectively, measuring individual components of the disease can an accurate appraisal of overall disease activity be made. Putting all the assessments together in a composite index

Table 25.2 Cut-offs for disease activity and response for five composite measures of disease activity

Measure	Low cut-off	High cut-off	Good improvement*	Moderate improvement*	Poor improvement*
PASDAS	3.2	5.4	≥ 1.6	> 0.8, < 1.6	≤ 0.8
GRACE	2.3	4.7	≥ 2	> 1, < 2	≤ 1
CPDAI	4	8	≥ 4	> 2, < 4	≤ 2
DAS28-CRP	2.8	4.2	≥ 1.6	> 0.8, < 1.6	≤ 0.8
DAPSA	18.5	45.1	≥ 28.4	> 14.2, < 28.4	≤ 14.2

* measures of improvement depend on initial and final value of disease activity measure—see Helliwell PS, FitzGerald O, Fransen J. Composite disease activity and responder indices for psoriatic arthritis: a report from the GRAPPA 2013 Meeting on Development of Cutoffs for Both Disease Activity States and Response. J Rheumatol 2014;41(6):1212–7.

Table 25.3 Clinical domains included in composite measures in psoriatic arthritis

	Peripheral arthritis	Pain	Patient global	Physician global	Skin	Enthesitis	Dactylitis	Spine disease	Function	HRQoL	CRP
PsARC	Yes	No	Yes	Yes	No	No	No	No	No	No	No
PASDAS	Yes	No	Yes	Yes	No	Yes	Yes	No	No	Yes	Yes
GRACE	Yes	No	Yes	Yes	Yes	No	No	No	Yes	Yes	No
ACR20	Yes	Yes	Yes	Yes	No	No	No	No	Yes	No	Yes
PsAJAI	Yes	Yes	Yes	Yes	No	No	No	No	Yes	No	Yes
MDA	Yes	Yes	Yes	No	Yes	Yes	No	No	Yes	No	No
DAPSA	Yes	Yes	Yes	No	No	No	No	No	No	No	Yes
CPDAI	Yes	No	No	No	Yes	Yes	Yes	Yes	Yes	Yes	No

DAPSA: Disease Activity for Psoriatic Arthritis; PsAJAI: Psoriatic Arthritis Joint Activity Index; CPDAI: Composite Psoriatic Disease Activity Index; HAQ: Health Assessment Questionnaire; CRP: C-reactive protein.

is, for now, probably only done in the context of clinical trials, but trends may change. MDA as a suitable target for treatment outcome has been used in a strategy trial [15], and a trial of treatment withdrawal [20], and may be a feasible outcome in the routine clinic situation. At a GRAPPA/OMERACT consensus meeting, held in London, in February 2017, a weighted vote was cast for composite measures: for RCTs, most popular measures were PASDAS [40 votes] and GRACE [28 votes]; for clinical practice, most popular were the use of a three VAS score (patient and physician global and a patient VAS for skin) [45 votes], DAPSA [26 votes]). After discussion there was no overall consensus. The group unanimously agreed that remission should be the ideal target with minimal/low disease activity a feasible alternative. The target should include assessment of musculoskeletal disease, skin, and health-related QOL (Coates et al. unpublished data).

Despite the need to assess all the potential manifestations of this disease, there is no doubt that practitioners will continue to seek efficient, and possibly shorthand measures of disease activity. This was seen with the development of the DAS28, where a reduced 28 joint count was found optimal. In the case of the DAS28, the composite index performed equally well, irrespective of including important joints in the foot and ankle [39]. In a similar manner, it might be that a reduced component composite measure for assessing disease activity in PsA would function equally well. The CPDAI and GRACE are so designed that disease components can be omitted without loss of score range, and a reduced CPDAI has been used in an analysis of a clinical trial dataset, where the axial disease was not part of the assessments [35]. The PASDAS, on the other hand, cannot be used in this way, given the nature of the formula by which it is calculated. However, it is instructive to examine the contribution of the various terms to the total score. The PASDAS is a weighted index yet the contribution of the various terms may not be accurately reflected by this weighting. Table 25.4 gives a breakdown of the relative contribution of the terms to the total score, using data taken from the GRACE data set. It can be seen that consistently across all the time assessments, three terms make up almost 90% of the score: physician and patient global, and the SF36-physical component summary score. The SF36-PCS is, of course, derived from a composite patient-reported outcome and each of the domains are

weighted in the calculation of the summary score. Nevertheless, it is of interest to carry out the same exercise with the domains of the SF36. Accordingly, the overall contribution of the domains to the total summary score was as follows: physical function, 22.3%; role physical, 20.5%; bodily pain, 17.5%; general health, 15.5%; vitality, 1.6%; social functioning, 0.4%; role emotional 10.9%; and mental health, 11.4%. It is of interest that the component of the SF36 most related to fatigue, the vitality component, only contributes 1.6% to the total score in this analysis. It could also be argued that the SF36 reflects the impact of the disease, rather than the disease activity, and as such is conceptually incongruous in this score. In defence of the SF36 summary scale, it should be remembered that the physical component scale component was included not by external selection but as a result of the regression analysis employed in the GRACE study. Further work is needed on the PASDAS, perhaps incorporating new data concerning the updated core set (see below).

For the future, the development of a new core set of domains, under the auspices of the OMERACT group, will necessitate a reappraisal of the current composite measures. The challenge will be to strike the correct balance between comprehensiveness and

Table 25.4 Relative contribution of each of the terms in the PASDAS formula to the total score

Term	Baseline	3 months	6 months	12 months
Patient global	25.3	24.1	24.3	23.4
Physician global	21.8	19.6	18.2	18.7
Swollen joint count	1.9	1.6	1.3	1.4
Tender Joint count	1.6	1.2	1.2	1.2
Enthesitis	1.3	0.8	0.9	1.1
Dactylitis	0.8	0.7	0.5	0.3
SF36 - PCS	41.6	45.7	46.2	47.4
CRP	4.8	4.5	5.0	4.9

Figures are percentages. Column time indicators represent each of the assessment time points in the GRACE study.

Box 25.8 The updated 2016 core domains for psoriatic arthritis. Inner circle: recommended to be used in all randomized controlled trials and longitudinal observational studies

MSK disease activity (includes peripheral joints, dactylitis, enthesitis, axial disease)

Skin disease activity (includes both skin and nails)

Pain

Patient global

Physical function

Health-related quality of life

Fatigue

Systemic inflammation

Data sourced from Orbai A-M et al. International patient and physician consensus on a psoriatic arthritis core outcome set for clinical trials. Ann Rheum Dis. 2017;76(4):673–80.

feasibility. At OMERACT 12, held in Budapest, Hungary in 2014, a workshop was held to review the existing core set of outcomes and to review the need for an update, using the Filter 2.0 framework. Significantly, at this workshop acknowledgement was made of work done in the Patient Involvement in Outcome Measures for Psoriatic Arthritis (PIOMPSA) group [40], and a noticeable proportion of group members were patient partners. At the meeting OMERACT participants endorsed the need to update the PsA core set, the workshop breakout group discussions identifying opportunities the core set revision would allow, including the potential of consolidating existing redundancy within the core set, improved incorporation of the patient perspective, and the possibility of including disease impact, such as fatigue, in the inner circle [41]. At OMERACT-13, May 2016, the meeting approved a revised core set based on the updated OMERACT filter 2 (Box 25.8) [42] and work within GRAPPA is ongoing to match existing composite measures with this revised core set.

References

1. Clegg DO, Reda DJ, Mejias E, et al. Comparison of sulfasalazine and placebo in the treatment of psoriatic arthritis: a Department of Veterans Affairs cooperative study. Arthritis Rheum 1996;39(12):2013–20.
2. Gladman DD, Mease PJ, Strand V, et al. Consensus on a core set of domains for psoriatic arthritis. J Rheumatol 2007;34(5):1167–70.
3. Helliwell PS, FitzGerald O, Fransen J, et al. The development of candidate composite disease activity and responder indices for psoriatic arthritis (GRACE project). Ann Rheum Dis 2013;72(6):986–91.
4. Lukas C, Landewe R, Sieper J, et al. Development of an ASAS-endorsed disease activity score (ASDAS) in patients with ankylosing spondylitis. Ann Rheum Dis 2009;68(1):18–24.
5. Fransen J, Kavanaugh A, Borm GF. Desirability scores for assessing multiple outcomes in systemic rheumatic diseases. Commun Stats Theory Methods. 2009;38:3461–71.
6. Mease PJ, Goffe BS, Metz J, VanderStoep A, Finck B, Burge DJ. Etanercept in the treatment of psoriatic arthritis and psoriasis: a randomised trial. Lancet. 2000;356(9227):385–90.
7. Antoni C, Krueger GG, de Vlam K, et al. Infliximab improves signs and symptoms of psoriatic arthritis: results of the IMPACT 2 trial. Ann Rheum Dis 2005;64(8):1150–7.
8. Coates L, Caperon A, Helliwell PS. Are arthritis outcome measures responsive in oligoarticular PsA? EULAR; 2011; London, UK: Abstract 0385.
9. Kingsley GH, Kowalczyk A, Taylor H, et al. A randomized placebo-controlled trial of methotrexate in psoriatic arthritis. Rheumatology. 2012;51(8):1368–77.
10. NICE (National Institute for Clinical Excellence). Etanercept, infliximab and adalimumab for the treatment of psoriatic arthritis. 2010.
11. Gladman DD, Tom BDM, Mease PJ, Farewell VT. Informing response criteria for psoriatic arthritis. i: discrimination models based on data from 3 anti-tumor necrosis factor randomized studies. J Rheumatol 2010;37(9):1892–7.
12. Gladman DD, Tom BDM, Mease PJ, Farewell VT. Informing response criteria for psoriatic arthritis (PsA). II: Further considerations and a proposal–the PsA joint activity index. J Rheumatol 2010;37(12):2559–65.
13. Coates LC, Fransen J, Helliwell PS. Defining minimal disease activity in psoriatic arthritis: a proposed objective target for treatment. Ann Rheum Dis 2010;69(1):48–53.
14. Coates LC, Navarro-Coy N, Brown SR, et al. The TICOPA protocol (TIght COntrol of Psoriatic Arthritis): a randomised controlled trial to compare intensive management versus standard care in early psoriatic arthritis. BMC Musculoskelet Disord. 2013;14:101.
15. Coates LC, Moverley AR, McParland L, et al. Effect of tight control of inflammation in early psoriatic arthritis (TICOPA): a UK multicentre, open-label, randomised controlled trial. Lancet. 2015; 386(10012):2489–98.
16. Gladman DD, Mease PJ, Strand V, et al. Consensus on a core set of domains for psoriatic arthritis. J Rheumatol 2007;34(5):1167–70.
17. Coates LC, Cook R, Lee KA, Chandran V, Gladman DD. Frequency, predictors, and prognosis of sustained minimal disease activity in an observational psoriatic arthritis cohort. Arthr Care Res. 2010;62(7):970–6.
18. Coates LC, Helliwell PS. Validation of minimal disease activity criteria for psoriatic arthritis using interventional trial data. Arthritis Care Res (Hoboken). 2010;62(7):965–9.
19. Coates L, Fitzgerald O, Gladman D, et al. MDA criteria for PsA show good correlation with physician and patient opinion and proposed composite measures. Ann Rheum Dis 2012;71(Suppl3):575. 2012.
20. Moverley A, Coates L, Marzo-Ortega H, et al. A feasibility study for a randomised controlled trial of treatment withdrawal in psoriatic arthritis (REmoval of treatment for patients in REmission in psoriatic ArThritis (RETREAT (F)). Clin Rheumatol 2015; 34(8):1407–12.
21. Kirwan JR, Reeback JS. Stanford Health Assessment Questionnaire modified to assess disability in British patients with rheumatoid arthritis. Br J Rheumatol 1986;25:206–9.
22. Coates L, Helliwell PS. Defining low disease activity states in psoriatic arthritis using novel composite disease instruments. J Rheum. 2016;43(2):371–5.
23. van Gestel A, Prevoo M, van 'T Hof M, van Rijswijk M, van der Putte L, van Riel P. Development and validation of the European League against rheumatism response criteria for rheumatoid arthritis. Arthr Rheum. 1996;39(1):34–40.
24. Lindsay K, Ibrahim G, Sokoll K, Tripathi M, Melsom RD, Helliwell PS. The composite DAS Score is impractical to use in daily practice: evidence that physicians use the objective component of the DAS in decision making. J Clin Rheumatol. 2009;15(5):223–5.
25. Fransen J, Antoni C, Mease PJ, et al. Performance of response criteria for assessing peripheral arthritis in patients with psoriatic arthritis: analysis of data from randomised controlled trials of two tumour necrosis factor inhibitors. Ann Rheum Dis 2006;65(10):1373–8.

26. Coates LC, Fitzgerald O, Gladman DD, et al. Reduced joint counts misclassify patients with oligoarticular psoriatic arthritis and miss significant numbers of patients with active disease. Arthr Rheum 2013;65(6):1504–9.

27. Schoels M, Aletaha D, Funovits J, Kavanaugh A, Baker D, Smolen JS. Application of the DAREA/DAPSA score for assessment of disease activity in psoriatic arthritis. Ann Rheum Dis 2010;69(8):1441–7.

28. Schoels M, Aletaha D, Alasti F, Smolen JS. Disease activity in psoriatic arthritis (PsA): defining remission and treatment success using the DAPSA score. Ann Rheum Dis 2016; 75(5):811–8.

29. Helliwell PS, FitzGerald O, Fransen J. Composite disease activity and responder indices for psoriatic arthritis: a report from the GRAPPA 2013 Meeting on Development of Cutoffs for Both Disease Activity States and Response. J Rheumatol 2014;41(6):1212–7.

30. Ritchlin CT, Kavanaugh A, Gladman DD, Mease PJ, Helliwell P, Boehncke WH, et al. Treatment recommendations for psoriatic arthritis. Ann Rheum Dis 2009;68(9):1387–94.

31. FitzGerald O, Mumtaz A, Helliwell P, et al. Application of composite disease activity scores in psoriatic arthritis to the PRESTA data set. Ann Rheum Dis 2012;71(3):358–62.

32. NICE (National Institute of Clinical Excellence) Adalimumab, etanercept and infliximab for the treatment of rheumatoid arthritis. 2007.

33. Helliwell PS, Kavanaugh A. Comparison of composite measures of disease activity in psoriatic arthritis using data from an interventional study with golimumab. Arthritis Care Res (Hoboken). 2014;66(5):749–56.

34. Helliwell PS, Kavanaugh A. Radiographic progression is less in psoriatic arthritis achieving a good response to treatment: data using newer composite indices of disease activity. Arthritis Care Res (Hoboken) 2018;70(5):797–800.

35. Helliwell PS, Mease P, Nurminen T, Fitzgerald O. Further analysis of psoriatic arthritis disease activity score (PASDAS) and composie psoriatic disease activity index (CPDAI) using data from a placebo controlled trial of certolizumab pegol in psoriatic arthritis. Ann Rheum Dis. 2014;Presented at EULAR 2014:EULAR14-SCIE-1654.

36. Kavanaugh A, McInnes I, Mease P, et al. Clinical efficacy, radiographic and safety findings through 2 years of golimumab treatment in patients with active psoriatic arthritis: results form a long-term extension of the randomised, placebo controlled GO-REVEAL study. AnnRheumDis. 2013;72(11):1777–85.

37. McInnes IB, Kavanaugh A, Gottlieb AB, . Efficacy and safety of ustekinumab in patients with active psoriatic arthritis: 1 year results of the phase 3, multicentre, double blind, placebo-controlled PSUMMIT 1 trial. Lancet. 2013;382:780–9.

38. McInnes IB, Mease P, Kirkham B, et al. Secukinumab, a human anti-interleukin-17A monoclonal antibody, in patients with psoriatic arthritis (FUTURE 2): a randomised, double-blind, placebo-controlled, phase 3 trial. Lancet. 2015;386(9999):1137–46.

39. Kapral T, Dernoschnig F, Machold K, et al. Remission by composite scores in rheumatoid arthritis: are ankles and feet important? Arthr Res Ther 2007;9:R72.

40. Tillett W, Adebajo A, Brooke M, et al. Patient Involvement in Outcome Measures for Psoriatic Arthritis. Curr Rheum Rep. 2014;16(5):1–10.

41. Tillett W, Eder L, Goel N, et al. Enhanced Patient Involvement and the Need to Revise the Core Set—Report from the Psoriatic Arthritis Working Group at OMERACT 2014 J Rheum. 2015; 42(11):2198–203.

42. Orbai A-M, de Wit M, Mease P, et al. International patient and physician consensus on a psoriatic arthritis core outcome set for clinical trials. Ann Rheum Dis. 2017;76(4):673–80.

Treatment

CHAPTER 26

Psoriasis treatment

Ami Saraiya, Deep Joshipura, and Alice Gottlieb

Introduction

Psoriasis is a chronic, immune-mediated skin condition composed of varying types. Chronic plaque psoriasis, the most common type, is distinguished by erythematous plaques with fine, silvery scale. Psoriasis is caused by multiple factors including immune system dysregulation, genetic predisposition, and environmental triggers. Psoriasis affects 2–3% of the population [1–2]. The prevalence of psoriatic arthritis among patients with psoriasis in the United States population was reported to be 11% [3], and up to 40% of patients with psoriasis may develop psoriatic arthritis [4]. Psoriatic skin disease occurs through keratinocyte activation, leukocyte migration with Th1 and Th17 cell signalling, and vascularization [5]. Other types of psoriatic skin disease include guttate, pustular, inverse, and erythrodermic psoriasis. This chapter is an evidence-based review of the treatment of plaque psoriasis in the outpatient clinical setting.

Multiple treatment options exist for psoriasis including topical agents, phototherapy, oral systemic agents, and biologic agents. In order to determine the appropriate therapy, a clinician must consider the extent of the involved skin, severity of disease, presence of psoriatic arthritis, as well as consider a comprehensive approach taking into account patient comorbidities, adherence, quality of life, finances, efficacy of different agents, and patient preferences [6].

Various psoriasis assessment tools exist. In clinical trials, the Psoriasis Area Severity Index (PASI), originally developed by Fredricksson and Pettersson in 1978, is the gold standard [7–8]. The PASI measures the body surface area (BSA) and erythema, induration, and scaling of psoriatic plaques. In addition to the PASI, the physician's global assessment (PGA) and determination of BSA are other important assessment tools. The simple measure for assessing psoriasis activity (S-MAPA) has been validated against the PASI and is calculated by multiplying BSA and PGA [9–11].

In the outpatient clinical setting, psoriatic skin disease severity is evaluated by extent of BSA, location of involved areas, thickness, and consideration of the impact of the disease on the patient [12]. A panel of experts including Board members of the National Psoriasis Foundation and clinicians participating in clinical research trials on psoriasis has recommended distinguishing mild, moderate, and severe psoriatic skin disease by considering a quality of life approach taking into account the impact of the disease in a patient's life rather than considering solely BSA [13]. The 2002 American Academy of Dermatology's consensus statement also recommended categorizing psoriasis into mild, moderate, or severe types by taking into consideration the overall disease, as well as recognizing factors such as activity of disease, resistance to prior treatments, and psychosocial factors [14].

In 2007, a task force of the Medical Advisory Board of the National Psoriasis Foundation proposed a two-tier system for psoriatic treatment differentiating patients as candidates for localized therapy, or systemic, and/or phototherapy. Patients in the former group usually have BSA<5%, whereas patients who are candidates for systemic therapy and/or phototherapy have BSA >5%, or BSA <5% but in vulnerable body locations, or inadequately controlled disease, or different forms of psoriasis, or presence of psoriatic arthritis [12]. An important consideration for the clinician is to gauge the patient's expectations and goals of treatment [15]. Clearance is more likely to be achieved using systemic and combination therapy, and it is necessary to determine if patients are willing to undergo treatments with potential side-effects or adverse reactions in order to achieve clearance [16].

Topical therapy

For patients with mild psoriasis, topical monotherapy is often the foundation of therapy for psoriatic skin disease. These treatments are relatively safe, but compliance may be reduced due to the time and patience required for treatment application [6]. For patients with moderate to severe psoriasis, topical agents can be used in combination with phototherapy and/or systemic therapy. In addition to combination therapy, topical treatments may be used in rotation with other agents or sequentially, where a stronger agent is used first to clear psoriasis and then a weaker agent is used for maintenance [14].

Topical corticosteroids are classified by potency, with class I topical steroids being the most potent and class VII the least potent. A 2002 systematic review has shown that potent and very potent topical steroids have more efficacy than lower potency topical psoriatic treatments [17].

In addition to potency, a clinician should consider various factors when prescribing topical steroids such as vehicle, potential side-effects, and frequency and duration of treatment application. Adverse reactions with topical corticosteroids include potential systemic absorption, exacerbation of coexisting dermatoses, contact dermatitis, and cutaneous side-effects such as skin atrophy, striae distensae, acne, folliculitis, and purpura [18]. Rebound disease is also a concern, where psoriasis is worse after the topical corticosteroid is discontinued than the pretreatment baseline [18].

Other topical treatments include the topical retinoid tazarotene, which is available as a 0.05% or 0.1% cream or gel and the topical Vitamin D3 analogue calcipotriene. A 2013 Cochrane Review of topical treatments for chronic plaque psoriasis studied 177 studies which included 34,808 people and found that potent corticosteroids perform at least as well as Vitamin D analogues and are less likely to cause skin irritation or burning for body and scalp psoriasis, but there was a lack of evidence regarding the risk of skin atrophy from topical steroids [19] The topical calcineurin inhibitors, tacrolimus and pimecrolimus, are not approved by the US Food and Drug Administration (FDA), but they may be used off label for facial and intertriginous psoriasis [18].

Coal tar shampoo has been used for many years for psoriasis, but it is associated with potential carcinogenicity, odour, and weak efficacy [20]. Anthralin has been used since the early 1900s, but side-effects include skin irritation and discoloration [21]. Salicylic acid is a topical keratolytic agent that can be used to soften scaling [18]. Furthermore, many non-medicated moisturizers are available over the counter and are beneficial to maintain skin hydration and include occlusive agents, emollients, and humectants.

Phototherapy and photochemotherapy

Ultraviolet B (UVB) and ultraviolet A (UVA) light directly act on Langerhans cells, indirectly act on cytokines to suppress the immune system, as well as inhibit epidermal hyperproliferation and angiogenesis, and decrease T lymphocytes in psoriatic skin [22]. UVB and UVA radiation induce apoptosis of T cells [23–24]. Interestingly, the effect of climatotherapy in the Dead Sea on psoriasis clearance is likely attributable to the UVA component of Dead Sea sunlight [25].

UVB therapy consists of narrowband (NB-UVB) and broadband UVB (BB-UVB). NB-UVB delivers 311 nm radiation, while BB-UVB is further separated into selective BB-UVB: 305 to 325 nm radiation and conventional BB-UVB: 280 to 320 nm radiation. NB-UVB is more effective than BB-UVB, safer than psoralen and UVA treatment (PUVA), and is typically dosed three times per week for at least 3 months [26].

PUVA treatment involves the combined use of psoralen and long-wave UVA radiation. PUVA can be divided into oral, bath, and topical PUVA according to the route of psoralen. Adverse reactions associated with phototherapy include erythema, pruritus, burning or blisters, and nausea with PUVA therapy [22]. Photoaging, lentigines, and telangiectasias are common with phototherapy and photocarcinogenesis is associated with PUVA therapy [22]. A 1998 meta-analysis showed that long-term high-dose exposure to PUVA in psoriatic patients has been consistently observed to significantly increase the risk of squamous cell carcinoma [27].

With regards to efficacy, a 2013 Cochrane review found that NB-UVB seemed to be equal to selective BB-UVB for clearing chronic plaque psoriasis, but evidence regarding NB-UVB and conventional BB-UVB was found to be lacking [28].

Systemic therapy

Methotrexate

Traditional systemic therapies for psoriasis include methotrexate, acitretin, and cyclosporine. Another systemic agent, apremilast, was approved in the United States for moderate to severe plaque psoriasis and psoriatic arthritis in 2014.

Methotrexate is typically taken at 10–25 mg weekly with folic acid supplementation. The main risks of therapy are myelosuppression, hepatotoxicity/hepatic fibrosis, and pulmonary fibrosis, and while on treatment frequent monitoring of complete blood cell count, platelet count, renal function studies, liver chemistries, and pregnancy test

in women of childbearing potential is important [29]. A 2011 systematic review recommended the starting dose of methotrexate to be between 5 and 10 mg per week for the first week with escalation to reach a target dose of 15–25 mg per week, as well as oral dosing over subcutaneous dosing and folic acid supplementation [30].

In a randomized controlled trial comparing the efficacy of methotrexate vs cyclosporine, no significant differences in efficacy were found [31]. In a randomized double-blind placebo-controlled trial of methotrexate vs adalimumab vs placebo for psoriasis, adalimumab demonstrated significantly superior efficacy (79.6% of patients reaching PASI 75 by week 16) compared with 35.5% of patients for methotrexate and 18.9% for placebo [32].

Furthermore, in a 2012 randomized double-blind placebo-controlled trial for patients with moderate to severe plaque psoriasis, combination therapy with etanercept plus methotrexate had acceptable tolerability and increased efficacy compared with etanercept monotherapy [33].

Acitretin

Acitretin is a systemic retinoid that was approved for psoriasis in 1997. Risks of therapy include mucocutaneous side-effects, teratogenicity, hyperlipidemia, and increased liver function tests [34].

One study looking at acitretin for patients with plaque psoriasis who were on continuous treatment for 12 months found the mean effective dose to be 41 mg [35].

Acitretin may be used as monotherapy for pustular or erythrodermic psoriasis [34]. Patients may have increased efficacy in combination with phototherapy. Studies have shown that acitretin and UVB combination are more efficacious and require lower UVB radiation [36–37].

Cyclosporine

Cyclosporine, another systemic medication for psoriasis, is typically dosed 2.5–4 mg/kg/day. The major risks of therapy include nephrotoxicity and hypertension. Blood pressure measurement and baseline laboratory testing should be done including renal function tests, liver chemistries, complete blood cell count, lipid panel, and serum magnesium, potassium, and uric acid [38].

Cyclosporine is not effective as monotherapy for plaque psoriasis but may be used in combination with phototherapy for plaque psoriasis [39]. However, one study found that patients treated with cyclosporine A plus PUVA required higher cumulative UVA doses for clearance, and they had significantly higher incidence of severe and early relapse compared to the retinoid etretinate plus PUVA group [40]. Etretinate has since been removed from the market.

In 2011, a systematic review recommended cyclosporine for patients with plaque psoriasis, pustular psoriasis, and erythrodermic psoriasis, a cumulative treatment duration of 2 years or less, and determined that a starting dose of 5 mg/kg is associated with a higher degree of clearance [41].

A Cochrane review found that cyclosporine significantly increases blood pressure compared to placebo in a dose-related fashion and recommended that prescribers try to find the lowest effective dose in all patients receiving cyclosporine [42].

Apremilast

Apremilast, a phosphodiesterase type 4 (PDE4) inhibitor approved in 2014, elevates intracellular cAMP levels, decreases pro-inflammatory cytokines such as interleukin-23 and TNF alpha, and enhances anti-inflammatory cytokines such as nterleukin-10 [43].

ESTEEM 1 and 2 are current phase III randomized, double-blind, placebo-controlled trials comparing apremilast 30 mg twice a day to placebo in patients with moderate-to-severe plaque psoriasis.

In a phase II, open-label study of apremilast in recalcitrant plaque psoriasis, 67% of patients had a ≥1-point improvement in static Physician's Global Assessment at week 12, and mean percent decrease from baseline was -59% for PASI score [44]. In a phase IIb trial, PASI 75 at week 16 was reached in 10 (11%) of patients in the apremilast 10 mg group, 25 (29%) in the 20 mg group, 36 (41%) in the 30 mg group, and 5 (6%) in the placebo group [45]. In a phase III randomized controlled trial (ESTEEM 1) in patients with moderate-to-severe plaque psoriasis, 33% of patients on apremilast 30 mg twice daily achieved PASI-75 at week 16 compared to 5.3% of placebo group [46]. In a phase III randomized placebo-controlled trial (PALACE 1) looking at apremilast in patients with active psoriatic arthritis, significantly more patients in the apremilast 20 mg twice daily group (31%) and 30 mg twice daily group (40%) reached ACR20 vs placebo (19%) [47].

The most frequently reported adverse events were diarrhoea, nausea, and headaches [44].

Second-tier systemic agents that are not FDA approved for psoriasis treatment are azathioprine, fumaric acid esters, hydroxyurea, leflunomide, mycophenolate mofetil, sulfasalazine, tacrolimus, and 6-thioguanine [48].

Biological therapy

TNF inhibitors

The advent of biological therapy has revolutionized the understanding of the pathogenesis and treatment of psoriasis. TNFα blockers bind to the inflammatory cytokine tumour necrosis factor alpha (TNFα), which is produced by antigen presenting cells and T cells, and increase the production of the proinflammatory cytokines IL-1, IL-6, IL-8, the adhesion molecules ICAM-1, P-selectin, and E-selectin, and the transcription factor NFκB [49–51]. TNF inhibition has been demonstrated to suppress Th17 cell products and effector molecules [52].

The TNF inhibitors have shown therapeutic efficacy for the treatment of psoriasis. In a randomized controlled trial of infliximab monotherapy for patients with plaque psoriasis, 9 of 11 patients in the infliximab 5 mg/kg group were responders and 10 of 11 patients in the infliximab 10 mg/kg group were responders, compared with two of 11 patients in the placebo group [53]. In a multicentre, double-blind, placebo-controlled trial of infliximab induction therapy for patients with severe psoriasis, 72–88% of patients treated with infliximab reached PASI 75 [54]. Infusion reactions were reported in 18% and 22% of patients in the infliximab (3 and 5 mg/kg) groups vs 2% in the placebo group and mostly were mild reactions [54]. In a phase III trial of infliximab induction and maintenance therapy for moderate-to-severe psoriasis, 80–82% of patients treated with infliximab reached PASI 75 by week 24 [55]. The most common adverse events were upper respiratory infection, headache, fatigue, increased hepatic enzymes, infections, and three patients in the infliximab-treated group had delayed hypersensitivity reactions [55].

In a randomized trial of etanercept monotherapy for psoriasis, 44% of patients in the medium dose group and 59% of patients in the high dose group reached PASI 75 by week 24 [56]. In another randomized study of etanercept monotherapy in psoriasis, 56% of patients treated with etanercept reached PASI 75 [57]. In a multicentre phase III study of etanercept for patients with psoriasis, PASI 75 was achieved by 49% of patients in the etanercept 50 mg twice weekly group and by 34% of patients in the 25 mg twice weekly group [58]. The most common adverse events were injection site reactions, upper respiratory infection, headache, injection site ecchymosis, accidental injury, and flu syndrome [58]. In another clinical trial, 47% of patients treated with etanercept achieved PASI 75 at week 12 [59]. In this trial, injection site reactions were the most commonly reported adverse event, and 87 patients (27.9%) in the etanercept group vs 3 patients (1%) in the placebo group had at least 1 infection, with no reported tuberculosis cases or opportunistic infections [59].

In a multicentre study looking at adalimumab therapy for psoriasis, 53% of patients taking adalimumab every other week and 80% of patients taking adalimumab weekly reached PASI 75 at week 12 [60]. In a phase III multicentre randomized controlled trial of adalimumab therapy for plaque psoriasis, 71% of patients treated with adalimumab achieved at least PASI 75 by week 16 [61]. Infections and injection site reactions were the most common adverse events in all patients who received at least one dose of adalimumab in the study, and infections were the most common serious adverse events [61]. In this study, one patient had oral candidiasis that was treated with fluconazole, another patient who had a normal chest X-ray and positive PPD at baseline developed tuberculosis, and it was also found that this patient discontinued prophylaxis with isoniazid due to gastrointestinal upset without informing his physician [61].

Ustekinumab

Ustekinumab, a human monoclonal antibody targeting the p40 subunit shared by both interleukin-12 and interleukin-23 and thereby inhibiting them, has shown therapeutic efficacy for the treatment of psoriasis.

In phase III clinical trials studying the efficacy and safety of ustekinumab for patients with moderate-severe plaque psoriasis, results showed that 67–76% of patients reached PASI 75 [62–63]. The most commonly reported adverse events with ustekinumab therapy were upper respiratory tract infection, nasopharyngitis, headache, and arthralgia, and two patients who received ustekinumab 90 mg had serious infections; bilateral lower extremity cellulitis and herpes zoster which resolved with therapy [62].

In a clinical trial comparing the efficacy of ustekinumab and etanercept for moderate-to-severe psoriasis, 67.5% of patients who received 45 mg of ustekinumab and 73.8% of patients who received 90 mg reached PASI 75 at week 12 vs 56.8% of those who received etanercept, and among patients who did not respond to etanercept, 48.9% reached PASI 75 within 12 weeks after crossover to ustekinumab [64].

In a retrospective study comparing the efficacy of biologics vs conventional systemic therapies at a tertiary care centre, biologics showed superior efficacy with 70.2% improvement at week 24 of S-MAPA compared to baseline, vs 40.4% improvement at week 24 of S-MAPA compared to baseline for patients on systemic therapy [9].

Combination therapy

Combination therapy can include a systemic and topical agent, or a systemic agent and phototherapy, or two systemic agents [65]. Synergism is seen with paired combinations of acitretin, phototherapy, cyclosporine, and methotrexate [66]. However, it is necessary to remain cognizant of the increased risk of cancer with combination therapy involving PUVA.

A systematic review of eight studies looking at combination therapy of a biologic and methotrexate found that combination therapy had higher efficacy than biologic monotherapy, but determined that there was not sufficient evidence to propose guidelines [67]. This finding of superior efficacy with combination biologic and methotrexate has also been seen in the rheumatoid arthritis literature [68–70].

New biological therapies

New biological therapies are interleukin-17 (IL-17) and interleukin-23 (IL-23) inhibitors.

IL-17 inhibitors

The IL-17 inhibitors include secukinumab and ixekizumab, which both inhibit IL-17A, and brodalumab, an IL-17-receptor blocker [71].

Secukinumab demonstrates excellent efficacy and obtained FDA approval on 21 January 21 2015 for the treatment of moderate-to-severe plaque psoriasis at a recommended dose of 300 mg subcutaneously at weeks 0, 1, 2, 3, 4, and then every 4 weeks. Clinical trial data demonstrated that the PASI 75 rates at week 12 for secukinumab in the phase III ERASURE study (secukinumab's time to response on patient-reported psoriasis symptoms) were 81.6% with 300 mg of secukinumab, 71.6% with 150 mg of secukinumab, and 4.5% with placebo [72]. In the phase III FIXTURE study (safety and efficacy of secukinumab compared to etanercept in subjects with moderate-to-severe, chronic plaque-type psoriasis), PASI 75 rates were 77.1% with 300 mg of secukinumab, 67.0% with 150 mg of secukinumab, 44.0% with etanercept, and 4.9% with placebo [72]. The most common adverse events included infections, infestations,

nasopharyngitis, headache, upper respiratory tract infection, and diarrhoea [72].

In a phase II trial of secukinumab vs placebo for patients with psoriatic arthritis, ACR 20 responses at week 6 were 39% for secukinumab vs 23% for placebo; ACR 20 responses at week 12 were 39% for secukinumab vs 15% for placebo; and ACR 20 responses at week 24 were 43% for secukinumab vs 18% for placebo [73].

In a randomized, double-blind, placebo-controlled phase II dose-ranging study of secukinumab for psoriasis, after 12 weeks of treatment secukinumab 3 × 150 mg (82%) and 3 × 75 mg (57%) resulted in significantly higher PASI 75 response rates vs. placebo (9%) [74].

In another phase II, randomized, double-blind, placebo-controlled regimen-finding study on secukinumab induction and maintenance therapy in moderate-to-severe plaque psoriasis, at week 12 early (weeks 0, 1, 2, 4) and monthly (weeks 0, 4, 8) induction regimens resulted in higher PASI 75 response rates vs placebo; 54.5% and 42%, respectively, vs 1.5% [75].

In a phase II, double-blind, placebo-controlled trial looking at ixekizumab for patients with chronic plaque psoriasis, PASI 75 rates at 12 weeks were significantly greater with ixekizumab at doses of 150 mg (82.1%), 75 mg (82.8%), and 25 mg (76.7%) compared with placebo, and the most common adverse events were nasopharyngitis, upper respiratory infection, injection site reaction, and headache [76]. In a phase II, randomized, double-blind, placebo-controlled study of brodalumab for moderate-to-severe plaque psoriasis, the mean percentage improvements in PASI at week 12 were 45% in the 70 mg group, 85.9% in the 140 mg group, 86.3% in the 210 mg group, 76.0% in the 280 mg group, and 16% in the placebo group (P<0.001 for all comparisons with placebo) [77]. The most common adverse events in the brodalumab groups were nasopharyngitis, upper respiratory tract infection, and injection-site erythema [77].

In a phase II, randomized, double-blind study looking at brodalumab for patients with psoriatic arthritis, week 12 ACR 20 response rates were 37% in the brodalumab 140 mg group, 39% in the 280 mg group, and 18% in the placebo group, and ACR 50

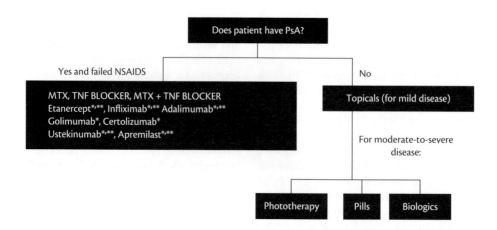

*FDA approved for the treatment of psoriatic arthritis, **FDA approved for psoriasis.

Figure 26.1 Choosing a therapy for psoriasis patients.

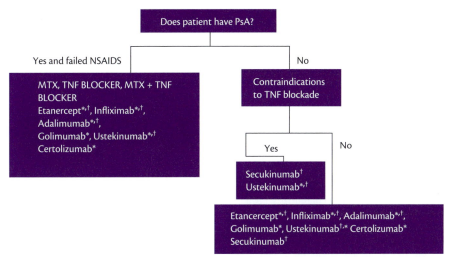

*FDA approved for the treatment of psoriatic arthritis, †FDA approved for the treatment of plaque psoriasis.

Figure 26.2 Treatment algorithm for choosing a biologic therapy for psoriasis patients.

response rates were 14% in both brodalumab groups and 4% in placebo [78].

IL-23 inhibitors

The IL-23 inhibitors include tildrakizumab and guselkumab. In a randomized, double-blind, placebo-controlled trial studying guselkumab for patients with moderate-to-severe plaque psoriasis, at week 12 50% of the 10 mg guselkumab group, 60% of the 30 mg and 100 mg groups, and 100% of the 300 mg group reached PASI 75 vs 0% of patients in the placebo group [79].

The oral therapies under investigation include fumaric acid esters and Janus kinase (JAK) inhibitors. Fumaric acid esters are chemical compounds derived from the unsaturated dicarbonic acid fumaric acid, and Fumaderm is an enteric-coated tablet containing dimethyl fumarate that was approved for the treatment of psoriasis in Germany in 1994 [80].

In March 2013, dimethyl fumarate was approved in the United States for adults with relapsing forms of multiple sclerosis. Dimethyl fumarate improves both multiple sclerosis and psoriasis by interacting with nuclear factor kappa B (NFκB) and interfering with IL-12 and IL-23 expression [81]. In one study, six patients treated with dimethyl fumarate 720 mg daily for 16 weeks demonstrated significant decreases in PASI scores at week 16 [82].

Side-effects include gastrointestinal complaints and flushing, as well as laboratory abnormalities such as lymphocytopenia and transient eosinophilia [83].

The JAK inhibitor tofacitinib is a JAK1 and JAK3 inhibitor that has been studied for psoriasis [84]. In a phase II randomized controlled trial comparing tofacitinib to placebo, PASI 75 response rates at week 12 were significantly higher for all tofacitinib-dosing groups [85]. PASI 75 response rates were 25% in the 2 mg twice-daily group, 40.8% in the 5 mg twice-daily group, and 66.7% in the 15 mg twice-daily group [85]. The most common adverse events were upper respiratory infection, nasopharyngitis, and headache, and dosing with tofacitinib was associated with laboratory abnormalities such as a mild decrease in haemoglobin, hypercholesterolaemia, and hyperlipidaemia [85].

Conclusion

Several treatment algorithms exist for psoriatic treatment (see Figures 26.1 and 26.2), as well as other examples in the literature [1, 65, 86]. When considering the choice of therapy many factors must be considered, and a clinician should evaluate and discuss a patient's expectations, goals of treatment, severity and extent of disease, presence of psoriatic arthritis, risks of therapy, comorbidities, cost, and efficacy of different therapeutic options. When treatment becomes difficult, referral to a dermatologist is often necessary.

References

1. Menter A, Gottlieb A, Feldman SR, et al. Guidelines of care for the management of psoriasis and psoriatic arthritis: Section 1. Overview of psoriasis and guidelines of care for the treatment of psoriasis with biologics. J Am Acad Dermatol. 2008;58(5):826–50.
2. Kurd SK, Gelfand JM. The prevalence of previously diagnosed and undiagnosed psoriasis in US adults: results from NHANES 2003-2004. J Am Acad Dermatol. 2009;60(2):218–24.
3. Gelfand JM, Gladman DD, Mease PJ, et al. Epidemiology of psoriatic arthritis in the population of the United States. J Am Acad Dermatol. 2005;53(4):573.
4. Winterfield LS, Menter A, Gordon K, Gottlieb A. Psoriasis treatment: current and emerging directed therapies. Ann Rheum Dis. 2005;64 Suppl 2:ii87–90.
5. Nestle FO, Kaplan DH, Barker J. Psoriasis. N Engl J Med. 2009 Jul 30;361(5):496–509.
6. Menter A, Griffiths CE. Current and future management of psoriasis. Lancet. 2007 Jul 21;370(9583):272–84.
7. Puzenat E, Bronsard V, Prey S, et al. What are the best outcome measures for assessing plaque psoriasis severity? A systematic review of the literature. J Eur Acad Dermatol Venereol. 2010;24 Suppl 2:10–6.
8. Fredriksson T, Pettersson U. Severe psoriasis–oral therapy with a new retinoid. Dermatologica. 1978;157(4):238–44.
9. Au SC, Madani A, Alhaddad M, Alkofide M, Gottlieb AB. Comparison of the efficacy of biologics versus conventional systemic therapies in the treatment of psoriasis at a comprehensive psoriasis care center. J Drugs Dermatol. 2013;12(8):861–6.
10. Levin AA, Gottlieb AB, Au SC. A comparison of psoriasis drug failure rates and reasons for discontinuation in biologics vs conventional systemic therapies. J Drugs Dermatol. 2014;13(7):848–53.

11. Walsh JA, McFadden M, Woodcock J, et al. Product of the Physician Global Assessment and body surface area: a simple static measure of psoriasis severity in a longitudinal cohort. J Am Acad Dermatol. 2013;69(6):931–7.

12. Pariser DM, Bagel J, Gelfand JM, et al. National Psoriasis Foundation clinical consensus on disease severity. Arch Dermatol. 2007;143(2):239–42.

13. Krueger GG, Feldman SR, Camisa C, et al. Two considerations for patients with psoriasis and their clinicians: what defines mild, moderate, and severe psoriasis? What constitutes a clinically significant improvement when treating psoriasis? J Am Acad Dermatol. 2000;43(2 Pt 1):281–5.

14. Callen JP, Krueger GG, Lebwohl M, et al. AAD consensus statement on psoraisis therapies. J Am Acad Dermatol 2003;49:897–9.

15. Lebwohl M. A clinician's paradigm in the treatment of psoriasis. J Am Acad Dermatol. 2005;53(1 Suppl 1): S59–69.

16. Al-Suwaidan SN, Feldman SR. Clearance is not a realistic expectation of psoriasis treatment. J Am Acad Dermatol. 2000;42(5 Pt 1):796–802.

17. Mason J, Mason AR, Cork MJ. Topical preparations for the treatment of psoriasis: a systematic review. Br J Dermatol. 2002;146(3): 351–64.

18. Menter A, Korman NJ, Elmets CA, et al. Guidelines of care for the management of psoriasis and psoriatic arthritis. Section 3. Guidelines of care for the management and treatment of psoriasis with topical therapies. J Am Acad Dermatol. 2009;60(4):643–59.

19. Mason AR, Mason J, Cork M, Dooley G, Hancock H. Topical treatments for chronic plaque psoriasis. Cochrane Database Syst Rev. 2013 Mar 28;3:CD005028.

20. Griffiths CE, Finlay AY, Fleming CJ, Barker JN, Mizzi F, Arsonnaud S. A randomized, investigator-masked clinical evaluation of the efficacy and safety of clobetasol propionate 0.05% shampoo and tar blend 1% shampoo in the treatment of moderate to severe scalp psoriasis. J Dermatolog Treat. 2006;17(2):90–5.

21. Sehgal VN, Verma P, Khurana A. Anthralin/dithranol in dermatology. Int J Dermatol. 2014;53(10):e449–60.

22. Menter A, Korman NJ, Elmets CA, et al. Guidelines of care for the management of psoriasis and psoriatic arthritis: Section 5. Guidelines of care for the treatment of psoriasis with phototherapy and photochemotherapy. J Am Acad Dermatol. 2010;62(1):114–35.

23. Krueger JG, Wolfe JT, Nabeya RT, et al. Successful ultraviolet B treatment of psoriasis is accompanied by a reversal of keratinocyte pathology and by selective depletion of intraepidermal T cells. J Exp Med. 1995 Dec 1;182(6):2057–68.

24. Morita A, Werfel T, Stege H, et al. Evidence that singlet oxygen-induced human T helper cell apoptosis is the basic mechanism of ultraviolet-A radiation phototherapy. J Exp Med. 1997 Nov 17; 186(10):1763–8.

25. Hodak E, Gottlieb AB, Segal T, et al. Climatotherapy at the Dead Sea is a remittive therapy for psoriasis: combined effects on epidermal and immunologic activation. J Am Acad Dermatol. 2003;49(3):451–7.

26. Lapolla W, Yentzer BA, Bagel J, Halvorson CR, Feldman SR. A review of phototherapy protocols for psoriasis treatment. J Am Acad Dermatol. 2011;64(5):936–49.

27. Stern RS, Lunder EJ. Risk of squamous cell carcinoma and methoxsalen (psoralen) and UV-A radiation (PUVA). A meta-analysis. Arch Dermatol. 1998;134(12):1582–5.

28. Chen X, Yang M, Cheng Y, Liu GJ, Zhang M. Narrow-band ultraviolet B phototherapy versus broad-band ultraviolet B or psoralen-ultraviolet A photochemotherapy for psoriasis. Cochrane Database Syst Rev. 2013 Oct 23;10:CD009481.

29. Kalb RE, Strober B, Weinstein G, Lebwohl M. Methotrexate and psoriasis: 2009 National Psoriasis Foundation Consensus Conference. J Am Acad Dermatol. 2009;60(5):824–37.

30. Montaudié H, Sbidian E, Paul C, et al. Methotrexate in psoriasis: a systematic review of treatment modalities, incidence, risk factors and monitoring of liver toxicity. J Eur Acad Dermatol Venereol. 2011;25 Suppl 2:12–8.

31. Heydendael VM, Spuls PI, Opmeer BC, et al. Methotrexate versus cyclosporine in moderate-to-severe chronic plaque psoriasis. N Engl J Med. 2003 Aug 14;349(7):658–65.

32. Saurat JH, Stingl G, Dubertret L, et al. Efficacy and safety results from the randomized controlled comparative study of adalimumab vs. methotrexate vs. placebo in patients with psoriasis (CHAMPION). Br J Dermatol. 2008;158(3):558–66.

33. Gottlieb AB, Langley RG, Strober BE, et al. A randomized, double-blind, placebo-controlled study to evaluate the addition of methotrexate to etanercept in patients with moderate to severe plaque psoriasis. Br J Dermatol. 2012;167(3): 649–57.

34. Lee CS, Koo J. A review of acitretin, a systemic retinoid for the treatment of psoriasis. Expert Opin Pharmacother. 2005; 6(10):1725–34.

35. Murray HE, Anhalt AW, Lessard R, et al. A 12-month treatment of severe psoriasis with acitretin: results of a Canadian open multicenter study. J Am Acad Dermatol. 1991;24(4):598–602.

36. Ruzicka T, Sommerburg C, Braun-Falco O, et al. Efficiency of acitretin in combination with UV-B in the treatment of severe psoriasis. Arch Dermatol. 1990;126(4):482–6.

37. Lowe NJ, Prystowsky JH, Bourget T, Edelstein J, Nychay S, Armstrong R. Acitretin plus UVB therapy for psoriasis. Comparisons with placebo plus UVB and acitretin alone. J Am Acad Dermatol. 1991;24(4):591–4.

38. Rosmarin DM, Lebwohl M, Elewski BE, Gottlieb AB; National Psoriasis Foundation. Cyclosporine and psoriasis: 2008 National Psoriasis Foundation Consensus Conference. J Am Acad Dermatol. 2010;62(5):838–53.

39. Korstanje MJ, Hulsmans RF. Combination therapy cyclosporin A–PUVA in psoriasis. Acta Derm Venereol. 1990;70(1):89–90.

40. Petzelbauer P, Hönigsmann H, Langer K, et al. Cyclosporin A in combination with photochemotherapy (PUVA) in the treatment of psoriasis. Br J Dermatol. 1990;123(5):641–7.

41. Maza A, Montaudié H, Sbidian E, et al. Oral cyclosporin in psoriasis: a systematic review on treatment modalities, risk of kidney toxicity and evidence for use in non-plaque psoriasis. J Eur Acad Dermatol Venereol. 2011;25 Suppl 2:19–27.

42. Robert N, Wong GW, Wright JM. Effect of cyclosporine on blood pressure. Cochrane Database Syst Rev. 2010 Jan 20;(1):CD007893.

43. Schafer P. Apremilast mechanism of action and application to psoriasis and psoriatic arthritis. Biochem Pharmacol. 2012 Jun 15;83(12):1583–90.

44. Gottlieb AB, Matheson RT, Menter A, et al. Efficacy, tolerability, and pharmacodynamics of apremilast in recalcitrant plaque psoriasis: a phase II open-label study. J Drugs Dermatol. 2013;12(8):888–97.

45. Papp K, Cather JC, Rosoph L, et al. Efficacy of apremilast in the treatment of moderate to severe psoriasis: a randomised controlled trial. Lancet. 2012;380(9843): 738–46.

46. Papp K, Reich K, Leonardi CL, et al. Apremilast, an oral phosphodiesterase 4 (PDE4) inhibitor, in patients with moderate to severe plaque psoriasis: Results of a phase III, randomized, controlled trial (Efficacy and Safety Trial Evaluating the Effects of Apremilast in Psoriasis [ESTEEM] 1). J Am Acad Dermatol. 2015;73(1):37–49.

47. Kavanaugh A, Mease PJ, Gomez-Reino JJ, et al. Treatment of psoriatic arthritis in a phase 3 randomised, placebo-controlled trial with apremilast, an oral phosphodiesterase 4 inhibitor. Ann Rheum Dis. 2014;73(6):1020–6.

48. Menter A, Korman NJ, Elmets CA, Gordon KB, et al. Guidelines of care for the management of psoriasis and psoriatic arthritis: section 4. Guidelines of care for the management and treatment of psoriasis with traditional systemic agents. J Am Acad Dermatol. 2009;61(3):451–85.

49. Goldminz AM, Au SC, Kim N, Gottlieb AB, Lizzul PF. NF-κB: an essential transcription factor in psoriasis. J Dermatol Sci. 2013;69(2):89–94.

50. Victor FC, Gottlieb AB. TNF-alpha and apoptosis: implications for the pathogenesis and treatment of psoriasis. J Drugs Dermatol. 2002;1(3):264–75.

51. Gottlieb AB, Chamian F, Masud S, et al. TNF inhibition rapidly down-regulates multiple proinflammatory pathways in psoriasis plaques. J Immunol. 2005 Aug 15;175(4):2721–9.

52. Zaba LC, Cardinale I, Gilleaudeau P, et al. Amelioration of epidermal hyperplasia by TNF inhibition is associated with reduced Th17 responses. J Exp Med. 2007 Dec 24;204(13):3183–94.

53. Chaudhari U, Romano P, Mulcahy LD, Dooley LT, Baker DG, Gottlieb AB. Efficacy and safety of infliximab monotherapy for plaque-type psoriasis: a randomised trial. Lancet. 2001 Jun 9;357(9271):1842–7.

54. Gottlieb AB, Evans R, Li S, et al. Infliximab induction therapy for patients with severe plaque-type psoriasis: a randomized, double-blind, placebo-controlled trial. J Am Acad Dermatol. 2004;51(4):534–42.

55. Reich K, Nestle FO, Papp K, et al. Infliximab induction and maintenance therapy for moderate-to-severe psoriasis: a phase III, multicentre, double-blind trial. Lancet. 2005;366(9494):1367–74.

56. Leonardi CL, Powers JL, Matheson RT, et al. Etanercept as monotherapy in patients with psoriasis. N Engl J Med. 2003;349(21):2014–22.

57. Gottlieb AB, Matheson RT, Lowe N, et al. A randomized trial of etanercept as monotherapy for psoriasis. Arch Dermatol. 2003;139(12):1627–32.

58. Papp KA, Tyring S, Lahfa M, et al. A global phase III randomized controlled trial of etanercept in psoriasis: safety, efficacy, and effect of dose reduction. Br J Dermatol. 2005;152(6):1304–12.

59. Tyring S, Gottlieb A, Papp K, et al. Etanercept and clinical outcomes, fatigue, and depression in psoriasis: double-blind placebo-controlled randomised phase III trial. Lancet. 2006;367(9504):29–35.

60. Gordon KB, Langley RG, Leonardi C, et al. Clinical response to adalimumab treatment in patients with moderate to severe psoriasis: double-blind, randomized controlled trial and open-label extension study. J Am Acad Dermatol. 2006;55(4):598–606.

61. Menter A, Tyring SK, Gordon K, et al. Adalimumab therapy for moderate to severe psoriasis: A randomized, controlled phase III trial. J Am Acad Dermatol. 2008; 58(1):106–15.

62. Leonardi CL, Kimball AB, Papp KA, et al. Efficacy and safety of ustekinumab, a human interleukin-12/23 monoclonal antibody, in patients with psoriasis: 76-week results from a randomised, double-blind, placebo-controlled trial (PHOENIX 1). Lancet. 2008;371(9625):1665–74.

63. Papp KA, Langley RG, Lebwohl M, et al. Efficacy and safety of ustekinumab, a human interleukin-12/23 monoclonal antibody, in patients with psoriasis: 52-week results from a randomised, double-blind, placebo-controlled trial (PHOENIX 2). Lancet. 2008;371(9625):1675–84.

64. Griffiths CE, Strober BE, van de Kerkhof P, et al. Comparison of ustekinumab and etanercept for moderate-to-severe psoriasis. N Engl J Med. 2010 Jan 14;362(2):118–28.

65. Lebwohl M, Menter A, Koo J, Feldman S. Case studies in severe psoriasis: A clinical strategy. J Dermatolog Treat. 2003;14 Suppl 2:26–46.

66. Lebwohl M, Menter A, Koo J, Feldman SR. Combination therapy to treat moderate to severe psoriasis. J Am Acad Dermatol. 2004;50(3):416–30.

67. van Bezooijen JS, Prens EP, Pradeepti MS, et al. Combining biologics with methotrexate in psoriasis: a systematic review. Br J Dermatol. 2015; 172(6):1676-8.

68. Klareskog L, van der Heijde D, de Jager JP, et al. Therapeutic effect of the combination of etanercept and methotrexate compared with each treatment alone in patients with rheumatoid arthritis: double-blind randomised controlled trial. Lancet. 2004;363(9410):675–81.

69. Keystone EC, van der Heijde D, Kavanaugh A, et al. Clinical, functional, and radiographic benefits of longterm adalimumab plus methotrexate: final 10-year data in longstanding rheumatoid arthritis. J Rheumatol. 2013;40(9):1487–97.

70. St Clair EW, van der Heijde DM, Smolen JS, et al. Combination of infliximab and methotrexate therapy for early rheumatoid arthritis: a randomized, controlled trial. Arthritis Rheum. 2004;50(11):3432–43.

71. Belge K, Brück J, Ghoreschi K. Advances in treating psoriasis. F1000Prime Rep. 2014 Jan 2;6:4.

72. Langley RG, Elewski BE, Lebwohl M, et al. Secukinumab in plaque psoriasis--results of two phase 3 trials. N Engl J Med. 2014;371(4):326–38.

73. McInnes IB, Sieper J, Braun J, et al. Efficacy and safety of secukinumab, a fully human anti-interleukin-17A monoclonal antibody, in patients with moderate-to-severe psoriatic arthritis: a 24-week, randomised, double-blind, placebo-controlled, phase II proof-of-concept trial. Ann Rheum Dis. 2014;73(2):349–56.

74. Papp KA, Langley RG, Sigurgeirsson B, et al. Efficacy and safety of secukinumab in the treatment of moderate-to-severe plaque psoriasis: a randomized, double-blind, placebo-controlled phase II dose-ranging study. Br J Dermatol. 2013;168(2):412–21.

75. Rich P, Sigurgeirsson B, Thaci D, et al. Secukinumab induction and maintenance therapy in moderate-to-severe plaque psoriasis: a randomized, double-blind, placebo-controlled, phase II regimen-finding study. Br J Dermatol. 2013;168(2):402–11.

76. Leonardi C, Matheson R, Zachariae C, et al. Anti-interleukin-17 monoclonal antibody ixekizumab in chronic plaque psoriasis. N Engl J Med. 2012;366(13):1190–9.

77. Papp KA, Leonardi C, Menter A, et al. Brodalumab, an anti-interleukin-17-receptor antibody for psoriasis. N Engl J Med. 2012;366(13):1181–9.

78. Mease PJ, Genovese MC, Greenwald MW, et al. Brodalumab, an anti-IL17RA monoclonal antibody, in psoriatic arthritis. N Engl J Med. 2014;12;370(24):2295–306.

79. Sofen H, Smith S, Matheson RT, et al. Guselkumab (an IL-23-specific mAb) demonstrates clinical and molecular response in patients with moderate-to-severe psoriasis. J Allergy Clin Immunol. 2014;133(4):1032–40.

80. Roll A, Reich K, Boer A. Use of fumaric acid esters in psoriasis. Indian J Dermatol Venereol Leprol. 2007;73(2):133–7.

81. Ghoreschi K, Brück J, Kellerer C, Deng C, Peng H, Rothfuss O, et al. Fumarates improve psoriasis and multiple sclerosis by inducing type II dendritic cells. J Exp Med. 2011;208(11):2291–303.

82. Bovenschen HJ, Langewouters AM, van de Kerkhof PC. Dimethylfumarate for psoriasis: Pronounced effects on lesional T-cell subsets, epidermal proliferation and differentiation, but not on natural killer T cells in immunohistochemical study. Am J Clin Dermatol. 2010;11(5):343–50.

83. Mrowietz U, Christophers E, Altmeyer P. Treatment of psoriasis with fumaric acid esters: results of a prospective multicentre study. German Multicentre Study. Br J Dermatol. 1998;138(3):456–60.

84. Meyer DM, Jesson MI, Li X, et al. Anti-inflammatory activity and neutrophil reductions mediated by the JAK1/JAK3 inhibitor, CP-690,550, in rat adjuvant-induced arthritis. J Inflamm (Lond). 2010;11:7:41.

85. Papp KA, Menter A, Strober B, et al. Efficacy and safety of tofacitinib, an oral Janus kinase inhibitor, in the treatment of psoriasis: a Phase 2b randomized placebo-controlled dose-ranging study. Br J Dermatol. 2012;167(3):668–77.

86. Feldman SR, Koo JY, Menter A, Bagel J. Decision points for the initiation of systemic treatment for psoriasis. J Am Acad Dermatol. 2005;53(1):101–7.

CHAPTER 27

Approach to management and symptomatic (including non-pharmacologic) management of psoriatic arthritis

Laura Acosta Felquer and Enrique R. Soriano

General approach to the management of psoriatic arthritis

Since the recognition of psoriatic arthritis (PsA) as a distinct entity, but especially in the last decade, research and knowledge about the disease have grown exponentially. In a similar way to rheumatoid arthritis, new paradigms in the management of PsA have emerged that are gaining great acceptance within the rheumatology community. These include early identification and treatment [1], remission, or minimal disease activity as a treatment objective [2, 3], assessment of all domains involved within this heterogeneous disease [4–6], frequent measuring of disease activity and adjusting therapy accordingly (treat to target) [7–9], and last but not least, something that has always been present in the patient—physician relationship, but that lately has been much more obvious, verbalized and registered: patient preferences [10, 11].

As patients preferences do not always match with physicians' beliefs [12], this movement that now involves patients even in the classical evidence-based treatment recommendations [13] is switching from disease progression as the main focus for treatment to more emphasis on symptom alleviation.

Due to the heterogeneous manifestations of the disease, collaborative management with other specialists is more and more frequent nowadays. Although shared management has been common practice for a long time in referral centres, it is not the general approach among most rheumatologists and dermatologists or in most rheumatology and dermatology units around the world. Combined management is driven by the increased knowledge of different disease manifestations, the presence of comorbidities, and by the use of expensive treatments that requires coordination among the different specialists seeing the patient.

All these issues should be taken into account for the effective treatment of this complex disease.

In this chapter we focus on the symptomatic management of PsA, including non-pharmacological treatment.

Symptoms in psoriatic arthritis

Physical symptoms are a significant burden in patients with PsA. Pain, heat, stiffness, swelling, and psoriasis were the major symptoms mentioned by patients in a recent study looking at patients' definition of flare [14]. In a study where PsA patients were asked for an evaluation of the absolute and relative impact of general and specific rheumatic symptoms, half of the global burden of disease was attributed to rheumatic symptoms with peripheral arthritis as the leading component, whereas the other half was equally distributed between psoriatic and additional common symptoms such as fatigue [12]. Fatigue is a frequent symptom that is usually disregarded by physicians. In the study defining flare, patients complained of feeling tired, 'battery gone', and having flu-like symptoms [14]. Patients also experienced other related symptoms, such as lack of motivation and loss of appetite, linked to fatigue [14]. Thus, even in a PsA population with predominant musculoskeletal involvement, almost half of the burden of disease is due to non-rheumatic specific symptoms, which becomes even more important if all symptom clusters are present [12].

Among the rheumatic symptoms, the relative impact of arthritis was highest (37%), followed by axial disease (26%), whereas the relative contribution of enthesitis and dactylitis were both below 20% [12]. Within the psoriatic cluster, the contribution of skin involvement was perceived to be more severe than the involvement of the nails (52% vs 23%) [12]. Patients also complained of a significant loss of normal function. In addition to loss of independence and increased dependence on others, patients noted loss of movement and loss of hobbies [14].

Psychological symptoms included frustration, depression, embarrassment, and fear [14]. Fatigue and loss of normal function were cited by patients as contributing to some of the psychological symptoms they described, highlighting the impact of these themes upon the patient [14].

In a study where 'willingness-to-pay' was used to measure the relative impact of PsA in 8 domains of HR-QOL (physical, emotional, sleep, work, social, self-care, intimacy, and concentration), median willingness-to-pay values were highest in the physical, work, sleep, and self-care domains [15].

Recently in a cross-sectional study, disease burden in rheumatoid arthritis (RA), PsA and axial spondyloarthritis (ax-SpA) were compared [16]. The reported pain, joint pain, patient global assessment, and fatigue were similar in PsA and ax-SpA, but significantly lower in RA after adjusting for sex and age, disease duration, and current use of biologic disease-modifying anti-rheumatic drugs (DMARDs) [16]. The reasons for the differences were not clear but were explained, in part, by the suggestion that pain mechanisms in RA and PsA may be different as the inflammatory process in PsA frequently involves entheses and the spine [16]. Depression and anxiety are common among patients with PsA, and contribute substantially to quality of life and have effects on pain scores [17]. Depression and anxiety was found in 36.6% and 22.2%, respectively of patients with PsA, compared with 24.4% and 9.6% in patients with psoriasis alone in a recent study [18]. While treating PsA might improve depression and anxiety, recognizing depression and anxiety and subsequent referral for treatment are important in patients with PsA [17]. In the recently published Evidence-based Recommendations for the Management of Comorbidities in Rheumatoid Arthritis, Psoriasis, and Psoriatic Arthritis: Expert Opinion of the Canadian Dermatology-Rheumatology Comorbidity Initiative, it was recommended that PsA and PsO patients should be screened for depression, and managed appropriately (Grade of Recommendation: C) [19]. Treatment with apremilast has been associated with worsening depression and perhaps should be avoided in patients with depressive symptoms [20].

Sleep quality has been reported to be diminished in patients with PsA. In a study comparing PsA patients with healthy controls, subjective sleep quality, sleep latency, sleep duration, habitual sleep efficiency, sleep disturbance, daytime dysfunction and total Pittsburgh Sleep Quality Index (PSQI) scores were significantly higher in patients with PsA [21]. Sleep disturbance was particularly associated with generalized pain, anxiety, enthesitis and levels of C-reactive protein and erythrocyte sedimentation ratio (ESR) [21].

Nonsteroidal anti-inflammatory drugs

Nonsteroidal anti-inflammatory drugs (NSAIDs) are the most common drugs used for pain alleviation in musculoskeletal complains [22]. They are recommended as first-line therapy in almost all clinical guidelines for the treatment of PsA, including different manifestations, such as peripheral arthritis, axial disease, enthesitis, and dactylitis [23–26]. Good quality evidence of their efficacy is, however, scarce [27]. Only two randomized controlled trials (RCTs) have been published so far [28, 29]. In the first one, a 4-week study, patients were randomized to nimesulide (NIM; 100, 200, or 400 mg/day) or placebo. NIM doses of 200 mg or 400 mg, but not 100 mg/day, were significantly better ($P = 0.03$) than placebo for reducing the number of tender and swollen joints, and improving physician and patient global assessment of efficacy [28]. The second study was a 12-week parallel-group study comparing celecoxib 400 mg (n=201) or celecoxib 200 mg (n=213) once daily with placebo (n=194) in PsA in flare [29]. At week 12, no statistically significant differences in ACR20 response criteria between treatment groups were observed.

NSAIDs are not free of risks. It is currently considered that all NSAIDs (Cox2 selective and non-selective) in varying degrees are associated with increased gastrointestinal (GI) and cardiovascular (CV) risk [30].

The administration of NSAIDs is associated with an increased risk of developing acute coronary syndrome or other atherothrombotic CV events (stroke and peripheral arterial problems), so CV risk estimation should be performed systematically in all patients who chronically use NSAIDs at least once a year [30]. NSAID use is associated with increased risk of injury and complications of the upper and lower GI tract. In all patients that are going to receive NSAIDs, a baseline assessment of GI risk should be performed using stablished risk assessments tools and accepted concomitant risk factors (such as age, history of peptic ulcer) [30].

Although the continued long-term use of NSAIDs may be justified in certain conditions, such as axial involvement in PsA, in general NSAIDs should be prescribed at the lowest effective dose and for the shortest possible time, and, one should consider other treatment options before prescribing NSAIDs [30]. If NSAIDs are prescribed GI and CV risk assessment should be performed. Several useful algorithms for the use of NSAIDs have been published [30, 31] (Figure 27.1).

Intra-articular and soft tissue injections of steroids

Corticosteroid joint injections are based on theoretical arguments and clinical experience, more than on clinical trials, and their use is less standardized compared to other therapies.

Glucocorticoid injections may be a useful adjunctive therapy in localized disease (oligoarticular forms, enthesitis or dactylitis) [32], mono/oligoarthritis or single joint flares, in otherwise well-controlled polyarthritis [33]. Glucocorticoid injections may also be performed in dactylitis (tendon sheath/peritendinous injections) and in entheseal areas, for example, elbow, or retrocalcaneal bursa in Achilles enthesitis [25].

In one large prospective observational study [32], 133 patients were evaluated, most of them with polyarthritis; 79 received one injection, and 54 received more than one. Clinical response (absence of tenderness or effusion) at 3 months was obtained in 41.6% of injected joints and was associated with the use of DMARDs. The relapse rate after 12 months was 25.5% and was associated with large-joint involvement and elevated ESR [32].

Rehabilitation and physical therapy

Rehabilitation and physical therapy in rheumatology focus on prevention of functional disorders of the musculoskeletal system, maintenance of working ability, prevention of muscle weakness, maintaining range of motion (ROM), and prevention of care dependency. Rehabilitative measures must be integrated into rheumatic care. Rehabilitative therapy in rheumatology includes physiotherapy, patient education, and occupational therapy [34]. Physical therapy is also one of the most useful ways to restore function and health status.

Since the pre-biologic era, physical therapy has been part of non-pharmacological treatment in patients with rheumatic disease. Unfortunately there is little evidence of the efficacy of rehabilitation in PsA with no study with grade of evidence 1 A in a systematic literature review [35]: only minor studies on the role of physical therapies were found [35], such as interferential current [36], effects of

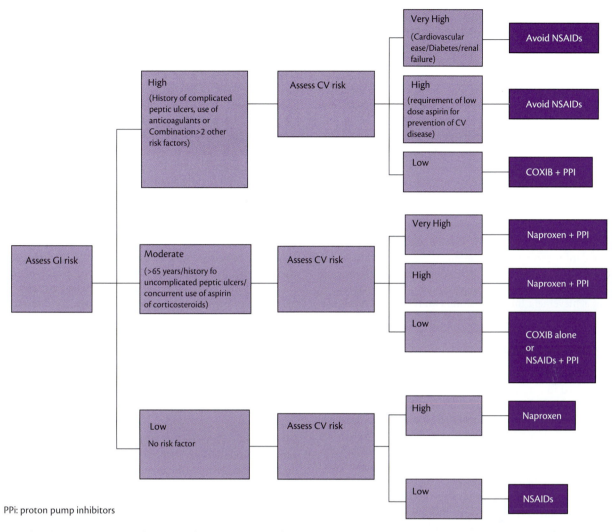

PPi: proton pump inhibitors

Figure 27.1 Algorithm recommendations for the use of non-steroidal anti-inflammatory drugs (NSAIDs) according to the cardiovascular and gastrointestinal risk.
Published with permission from the Publisher. Original source: Lanas, A. et al. Safe Prescription Recommendations for Non Steroidal Anti-inflammatory Drugs: Consensus Document Elaborated by Nominated Experts of Three Scientific Associations (SER-SEC-AEG) Reumatol Clin 2014;10:68-84, © Copyright 2017. Sociedad Española de Reumatologíay el Colegio Mexicano de Reumatología.

climatic therapy at Tiberias Hot Springs [37], and effect of balneo-therapy in the Dead Sea area for patients with PsA and concomitant fibromyalgia [38]. In a self-administered questionnaire, Lubrano et al. found that patients considered exercise as an important part of the treatment plan and a good approach to reduce the chance of joint deformity [39], indicating that, in general, physical therapy and exercise are well accepted by patients. The authors proposed a rehabilitation programme for patients with PsA that is shown in Table 27.1 [35].

As in ankylosing spondylitis, in PsA patients with axial involvement, rehabilitation plays an important role in the management of the disease. Due to very little evidence being available for PsA, data has been borrowed from ankylosing spondylitis; rehabilitation was considered by the GRAPPA Group (Group for Research and Assessment of Psoriasis and Psoriatic Arthritis), as part of treatment of axial PsA [40].

As many of the techniques and methods are difficult to implement until inflammation and pain are under medical control, some degree of disease control, in general, is needed before physical therapy can be started [41]. A properly designed programme

Table 27.1 Proposal for a rehabilitation program for patients with psoriatic arthritis

Predominant peripheral disease	Predominant axial involvement
Muscle-strengthening exercises	Muscle-strengthening exercises
General fitness exercises	General fitness exercises
Stretching exercises	Stretching exercises
Physical therapy (when necessary)	Physical therapy (when necessary)
Occupational therapy	Occupational therapy
Patient education	Patient education
	Postural exercises
	Breathing exercises

Reprinted from Lubrano E, Spadaro A, Parsons WJ, Atteno M, Ferrara N (2009) Rehabilitation in psoriatic arthritis. The Journal of Rheumatology Supplement 83:81–8 with permission from the Journal of Rheumatology.

of physical activity should be planned for each patient, combining flexibility (ROM), strengthening, and aerobic exercises.

In a recent study aimed at evaluating the benefits of home-based exercise programmes on disease activity and quality of life in minimum disease activity-PsA patients treated with an anti-tumour necrosis factor and disease-modifying anti-rheumatic drug therapy, a self-reported adherence rate to home-based exercise of 76.6% was reported [42]. Data also showed the impact of the exercise programme on self-reported health and mental assessment, and that a positive relationship between patient and therapist was crucial, influencing the quality of the performance, the emotional support, and increasing motivation in PsA patients [42].

The main results of rehabilitation in PsA could be summarized as follows: 1) very little evidence is available to evaluate the efficacy of rehabilitation; 2) most data have been borrowed from studies on ankylosing spondylitis; and 3) covering aspects of the disease by the standard measures of functioning presents difficulties [35]. At the OMERACT 8 meeting, consensus was obtained to measure physical function as a core domain, which could be considered an important achievement for future studies on the role of rehabilitation in PsA [6].

Surgical management

As with rehabilitation, there are a limited number of studies in the literature related to surgical procedures in patients with PsA, and most of them included small number of patients or are retrospectives studies. The objective of musculoskeletal surgery is to alleviate pain and improve physical function.

In a retrospective study of 444 PsA patients, 7% needed surgical management after an average of 14 years of the disease onset [43]. Extended radiological damage and a high active joints count at initial assessment were predictors of the need of future surgical treatment [43]. Other reports indicate that 23.8% of PsA patients required hand surgery, 1.8% required hip arthroplasty, 1.4% underwent total knee replacement, and 1.2% needed foot or ankle surgery [44]. Surgical management is dependent on the pattern and severity of joint involvement. Surgical procedures include total joint arthroplasty, arthrodesis, and arthroscopic synovectomy [44].

In a cohort of patients with PsA in Rochester, Minnesota, United States, among 66 patients with newly diagnosed PsA, after 7.2 years of follow up, six orthopedic procedures were performed: three synovectomies, one arthroplasty, and two reconstructive surgeries [45].

In the 10-year results of 71 orthopedic surgical procedures performed in 43 PsA patients, it was concluded that outcomes were similar to those of surgical management of other forms of arthritis [46]. Patients were categorized as having either distal PsA, oligoarticular PsA, or polyarticular disease. Those with distal disease (10%) underwent proximal interphalangeal (PIP) and distal interphalangeal (DIP) fusions. Patients with oligoarticular disease (25%) were treated with large joint surgery as hip replacement, knee replacement, or knee synovectomy. Those with polyarticular disease (65%) underwent a variety of upper and lower extremity surgeries, most of them were reconstructive procedures [46].

Arthroscopic knee synovectomy is another surgical procedure that has been explored in patients with PsA. Knee synovectomy was performed in 32 patients (17 with PsA, 15 with RA) in a prospective study [47]. The patients were followed for 36 months, and local signs of inflammation and ROM were scored. Patients have 73% definite improvement and 61% of clinical remission, which was higher in PsA than RA knees (86.3% vs 45.7%, respectively) [47].

Joint replacement is an uncommon procedure in PsA patients. In a cohort study of hip disease in PsA patients that included 504 patients only 32 (6%) developed symptomatic hip arthropathy [48]. After a mean follow up of 5.7 years (range 1–45 years) data were available for 17 of these 32 patients. Nine (53%) underwent hip arthroplasty within 5 years after onset of hip pain [48]. In this cohort, mean age at time of arthroplasty was 41 years (range, 25–63 years). In a previous publication Zagger et al., found that disease onset before 30 years of age and evidence of axial involvement, appeared to be risk factors for developing symptomatic hip joint arthropathy [43].

Hand and wrist surgery procedures include total wrist fusion, distal ulna resection, arthroplasty, manipulation, arthrodesis, and synovectomy. A retrospective study reviewed 25 PsA patients who underwent hand and wrist surgery [49]. Eight patients received wrist surgery because of persistent wrist pain, joint erosion, and / or deformity at that level. Three were managed with arthroplasty, three with distal ulna resections, and two with fusions. Although all eight patients reported improvement in relief of wrist pain, ROM in the arthroplasty cases was limited. Seventeen of the 25 patients in that cohort underwent surgical intervention for PIP joint disease [49]. Fifty PIP fusions, 11 arthroplasties, and 10 joint manipulations were performed during the study period. Every arthrodesis cases achieved union without incident. Overall ROM after PIP arthroplasty was limited to 20°. Malposition of spontaneous DIP joint ankylosis was treated with realignment and arthrodesis in eight patients, each of whom experienced pain relief and improved function [49, 50].

Buryanov et al. analysed 14 metacarpophalangeal joint silicone arthroplasty in nine PsA patients over 3 to 6 years and concluded that is an effective method because patients experienced improvement in pain and ROM [51].

Before surgery procedures in PsA patients, special considerations should be given to the prevention of site infections, and awareness of the chance of a Koebner phenomenon (exacerbation of psoriatic skin lesions) occurring at the surgical site [52].

Summary

Symptom alleviation is important in PsA. While pain is still one of the major symptoms, other symptoms such as fatigue, those related to skin involvement, and psychological symptoms including, frustration, depression, embarrassment, and fear should be taken into account. Most of the evidence for symptom relieving treatments is of low quality, borrowed from other diseases, or non-existent. NSAIDs and local glucocorticosteroid injections remain important treatment options that should be used, although with caution, in the appropriate patient. There is little evidence for the benefit of rehabilitation, which goes against the more widespread use of probably a very useful treatment. Surgery, although very effective, should be reserved for advanced cases as the new paradigms in the treatment of PsA (early diagnosis and treatment, remission as an objective, and treat to target), would very probably reduce the already low number of patients that need this last treatment option.

References

1. Gladman DD Early psoriatic arthritis. RheumDis Clin North Am 2012;38 (2):373–86.

2. Gladman DD, Hing EN, Schentag CT, Cook RJ. Remission in psoriatic arthritis. J Rheumatol. 2001;28 (5):1045–8.

3. Acosta Felquer ML, Ferreyra Garrott L, Marin J, et al. Remission criteria and activity indices in psoriatic arthritis. Clin Rheumatol. 2014;33 (9):1323–30.

4. Gladman DD, Landewe R, McHugh NJ, et al. Composite measures in psoriatic arthritis: GRAPPA 2008. J Rheumatol. 2010;37 (2):453–61.

5. Gladman DD, Mease PJ, Healy P, et al. Outcome measures in psoriatic arthritis. J Rheumatol. 2007;34 (5):1159–66.

6. Gladman DD, Mease PJ, Strand V, et al. Consensus on a core set of domains for psoriatic arthritis. J Rheumatol. 2007;34 (5):1167–70.

7. Coates LC, Navarro-Coy N, Brown SR, et al. The TICOPA protocol (TIght COntrol of Psoriatic Arthritis): a randomised controlled trial to compare intensive management versus standard care in early psoriatic arthritis. BMC musculoskeletal disorders 2013;14:101.

8. Schoels MM, Braun J, Dougados M, et al. Treating axial and peripheral spondyloarthritis, including psoriatic arthritis, to target: results of a systematic literature search to support an international treat-to-target recommendation in spondyloarthritis. Ann Rheumatic Dis. 2014;73(1):238–42.

9. Coates LC, Moverley AR, McParland L, et al. Effect of tight control of inflammation in early psoriatic arthritis (TICOPA): a UK multicentre, open-label, randomised controlled trial. Lancet 2015;386 (10012):2489–98.

10. Helliwell P, Coates L, Chandran V, et al. Qualifying unmet needs and improving standards of care in psoriatic arthritis. Arthritis care Res. 2014;66 (12):1759–66.

11. Smolen JS, Braun J, Dougados M, et al. Treating spondyloarthritis, including ankylosing spondylitis and psoriatic arthritis, to target: recommendations of an international task force. Ann Rheum Dis. 2014;73 (1):6–16.

12. Dandorfer SW, Rech J, Manger B, Schett G, Englbrecht M. Differences in the patient's and the physician's perspective of disease in psoriatic arthritis. Sem Arthritis Rheum. 2012;42 (1):32–41.

13. Agree Collaboration. Development and validation of an international appraisal instrument for assessing the quality of clinical practice guidelines: the AGREE project. Qual Saf Health care 2003;12 (1):18–23.

14. Moverley AR, Vinall-Collier KA, Helliwell PS. It's not just the joints, it's the whole thing: qualitative analysis of patients' experience of flare in psoriatic arthritis. Rheumatology. 2015;54(8):1448–53.

15. Hu SW, Holt EW, Husni ME, Qureshi AA. Willingness-to-pay stated preferences for 8 health-related quality-of-life domains in psoriatic arthritis: a pilot study. Semin Arthritis Rheum. 2010;39 (5):384–97.

16. Michelsen B, Fiane R, Diamantopoulos AP, et al. A comparison of disease burden in rheumatoid arthritis, psoriatic arthritis and axial spondyloarthritis. PloS One 2015;10 (4):e0123582.

17. Ogdie A, Schwartzman S, Husni ME. Recognizing and managing comorbidities in psoriatic arthritis. Curr Opinion Rheumatol. 2015;27 (2):118–26.

18. McDonough E, Ayearst R, Eder L, et al. Depression and anxiety in psoriatic disease: prevalence and associated factors. J Rheumatol. 2014;41 (5):887–96.

19. Roubille C, Richer V, Starnino T, et al. Evidence-based recommendations for the management of comorbidities in rheumatoid arthritis, psoriasis, and psoriatic arthritis: Expert opinion of the Canadian Dermatology-Rheumatology Comorbidity Initiative. J Rheumatol. 2015;42(10):1767–80.

20. Mease P, Kavanaugh A, Gladman, DD, et al. Long-term safety and tolerability of apremilast, an oral phospho- diesterase 4 inhibitor, in patients with psoriatic arthritis: pooled safety analysis of three Phase 3, randomized, controlled trials. Arthritis Rheum. 2013;65(Suppl):S131.

21. Gezer O, Batmaz I, Sariyildiz MA, et al. Sleep quality in patients with psoriatic arthritis. Int J Rheum Dis. 2017;20(9):1212–18.

22. Koffeman AR, Valkhoff VE, Jong GW, et al. Ischaemic cardiovascular risk and prescription of non-steroidal anti-inflammatory drugs for musculoskeletal complaints. Scand J Prim Health Care 2014;32 (2):90–98.

23. Soriano ER. Treatment guidelines for psoriatic arthritis. Int J Clin Rheumatol 2009;4:329–42.

24. Gossec L, Smolen JS, Gaujoux-Viala C, et al. European League Against Rheumatism recommendations for the management of psoriatic arthritis with pharmacological therapies. Ann Rheum Dis. 2012;71 (1):4–12.

25. Ritchlin CT, Kavanaugh A, Gladman DD, et al. Treatment recommendations for psoriatic arthritis. Ann Rheum Dis. 2009;68 (9):1387–94.

26. Sevrain M, Villani AP, Rouzaud M, et al. Treatment (biotherapy excluded) of psoriatic arthritis: an appraisal of methodological quality of international guidelines. J Eur Acad Dermatol Venereol. 2014;28 Suppl 5:33–9.

27. Acosta Felquer ML, Coates LC, Soriano ER, et al. Drug therapies for peripheral joint disease in psoriatic arthritis: a systematic review. J Rheumatol. 2014;41 (11):2277–85.

28. Sarzi-Puttini P, Santandrea S, Boccassini L, Panni B, Caruso I. The role of NSAIDs in psoriatic arthritis: evidence from a controlled study with nimesulide. Clin Exp Rheumatol 2001:9 (1 Suppl 22):S17–20.

29. Kivitz AJ, Espinoza LR, Sherrer YR, Liu-Dumaw M, West CR. A comparison of the efficacy and safety of celecoxib 200 mg and celecoxib 400 mg once daily in treating the signs and symptoms of psoriatic arthritis. Sem Arthritis Rheum. 2007;37 (3):164–73.

30. Lanas A, Benito P, Alonso J, Hernandez-Cruz B, et al. Safe prescription recommendations for non steroidal anti-inflammatory drugs: consensus document ellaborated by nominated experts of three scientific associations (SER-SEC-AEG). Reumatol Clin 2014;10 (2):68–84.

31. Lanza FL, Chan FK, Quigley EM, Practice Parameters Committee of the American College of Gastroenterologists. Guidelines for prevention of NSAID-related ulcer complications. Am J Gastroenterol. 2009;104 (3):728–38.

32. Eder L, Chandran V, Ueng J, Bhella S, et al. Predictors of response to intra-articular steroid injection in psoriatic arthritis. Rheumatology 2010;49(7):1367–73.

33. Ash Z, Gaujoux-Viala C, Gossec L, et al. A systematic literature review of drug therapies for the treatment of psoriatic arthritis: current evidence and meta-analysis informing the EULAR recommendations for the management of psoriatic arthritis. Ann Rheum Dis. 2012;71 (3):319–26.

34. Luttosch F, Baerwald C. [Rehabilitation in rheumatology]. Internist (Berl) 2010;51 (10):1239–45.

35. Lubrano E, Spadaro A, Parsons WJ, Atteno M, Ferrara N. Rehabilitation in psoriatic arthritis. J Rheumatol Suppl 2998;83:81–82.

36. Walker UA, Uhl M, Weiner SM, et al. Analgesic and disease modifying effects of interferential current in psoriatic arthritis. Rheumatol Int. 2006:26(10):904–907.

37. Hashkes PJ. Beneficial effect of climatic therapy on inflammatory arthritis at Tiberias Hot Springs. Scand J Rheumatol. 2002;31 (3):172–7.

38. Sukenik S, Baradin R, Codish S, et al. Balneotherapy at the Dead Sea area for patients with psoriatic arthritis and concomitant fibromyalgia. IMAJ 2001:3 (2):147–50.

39. Lubrano E, Helliwell P, Parsons W, Emery P, Veale D. Patient education in psoriatic arthritis: a cross sectional study on knowledge by a validated self-administered questionnaire. J Rheumatol. 1998;25 (8):1560–5.

40. Nash P. Therapies for axial disease in psoriatic arthritis. A systematic review. J Rheumatol. 2006;33 (1):1431–4.

41. Dougados M, Revel M, Khan MA. Spondylarthropathy treatment: progress in medical treatment, physical therapy and rehabilitation. Bailliere's Clinical Rheumatol. 1998;12 (4):717–36.

42. Chimenti MS, Triggianese P, Conigliaro P, Santoro M, Lucchetti R, Perricone R. Self-reported adherence to a home-based exercise

program among patients affected by psoriatic arthritis with minimal disease activity. Drug Dev Res 2014;75 Suppl 1:S57–9.

43. Zangger P, Gladman DD, Bogoch ER. Musculoskeletal surgery in psoriatic arthritis. J Rheumatol. 1998;25 (4):725–9.

44. Day MS, Nam D, Goodman S, Su EP, Figgie M. Psoriatic arthritis. J Am Acad Orthop Surg 2012;20 (1):28–37.

45. Shbeeb M, Uramoto KM, Gibson LE, O'Fallon WM, Gabriel SE. The epidemiology of psoriatic arthritis in Olmsted County, Minnesota, USA, 1982-1991. J Rheumatol. 2000;27 (5):1247–50.

46. Zangger P, Esufali ZH, Gladman DD, Bogoch ER. Type and outcome of reconstructive surgery for different patterns of psoriatic arthritis. J Rheumatol. 2000;27 (4):967–74.

47. Fiocco U, Cozzi L, Rigon C, et al. Arthroscopic synovectomy in rheumatoid and psoriatic knee joint synovitis: long-term outcome. Br J Rheumatol. 1996;35 (5):463–70.

48. Michet CJ, Mason TG, Mazlumzadeh M. Hip joint disease in psoriatic arthritis: risk factors and natural history. Ann Rheum Dis. 2005;64 (7):1068–70.

49. Belsky MR, Feldon P, Millender LH, Nalebuff EA, Phillips C. Hand involvement in psoriatic arthritis. J Hand Surg Am 1982;7 (2):203–7.

50. Rose JH, Belsky MR. Psoriatic arthritis in the hand. Hand Clin. 1989;5 (2):137–44.

51. Buryanov A, Kotiuk V, Kvasha V, Samokhin A. Three- to six-year results of metacarpophalangeal joints arthroplasty in psoriatic arthritis. J Long Term Eff Med Implants 2013;23 (4):285–92.

52. Iofin I, Levine B, Badlani N, Klein GR, Jaffe WL. Psoriatic arthritis and arthroplasty: a review of the literature. Bull NYU Hospital Joint Dis. 2008;66 (1):41–8.

CHAPTER 28

Synthetic DMARDs

Frank Behrens, Michaela Koehm,
and Michael J. Parnham

Introduction

Conventional synthetic disease modifying anti-rheumatic drugs (sDMARDs) represent the first line therapeutic option both in patients with active psoriatic arthritis (PsA) after failure of non-steroidal anti-inflammatory drug (NSAID) treatment and in established PsA. This in view of the fact that NSAID treatment is only indicated in monoarticular or modest polyarticular diseases for a limited period of time. The performance of PsA-specific clinical studies has been limited, due to the lack of specific validated outcome criteria for PsA. Since for some time, a similar aetiopathological relationship with rheumatoid arthritis (RA) has been considered, sDMARD therapies for PsA treatment have been based mainly on evidence originally derived from clinical studies in RA. Only for sulfasalazine (SSZ) has sufficient evidence been generated using randomized clinical studies specifically designed for PsA, but with only mild responses [1].

Despite all these limitations, it has been recommended that patients with active disease should receive sDMARDs for control of signs and symptoms [2]. In addition, the heterogeneous phenotypes of PsA (peripheral arthritis, skin psoriasis, enthesitis, dactylitis, and axial disease) and the limited data on efficacy of treatment options for these specific manifestations are issues that need consideration for each individual patient. In general, methotrexate (MTX), leflunomide (LEF), sulfasalazine (SSZ), and cyclosporin (CsA) are recommended and used in active PsA as sDMARD therapy. Unfortunately, no head-to-head studies on these treatments have been carried out to provide direct comparison of levels of efficacy. Recently, apremilast (APR) was launched as a targeted, oral sDMARD treatment option and licenced in the United States, Canada, and Europe. In general, all the products demonstrate reasonable safety profiles, but adherence to CsA treatment is low and it is often used for only a limited time period. Most frequent adverse events are infections, as a class effect, and gastrointestinal adverse reactions.

The main goals of systemic treatment of PsA are the control of signs and symptoms of (all) musculoskeletal manifestations and skin involvement, as well as normalization of impaired life quality, prevention of structural damage, and preservation of functionality. Bearing this definition in mind, clinical studies with sDMARD therapy have not demonstrated clear inhibition of radiographic progression in PsA. This is one of the major weaknesses of sDMARD therapy and must be taken adequately into account when therapeutic response is monitored.

sDMARDs as a treatment option for peripheral arthritis

The clinical feature of PsA with the best level of evidence for sDMARD treatment is peripheral arthritis. This is because most of the clinical studies conducted in PsA included polyarticular PsA patients. Characteristics of sDMARDs are displayed in Figure 28.1.

Methotrexate

MTX is the most frequently used sDMARD in PsA treatment, although only two randomized clinical trials (RCTs) have been published since 2003 [3, 4]. Scarpa et al. [3] conducted a 6-month, randomized, open-label trial including patients with early PsA (oligoarthritis <12 weeks duration). The study population was randomized to NSAID alone or NSAIDs plus MTX for 3 months, before all patients were treated with the combined therapy of MTX plus NSAID. Outcome measures were assessed after 3 and 6 months. Patients using MTX-treatment had significantly ($P < 0.05$) better joint count responses after 3 months compared with the patients on NSAID alone. Nevertheless, the results after 6 months were similar when both groups took the MTX-NSAID combination. In the MIPA (Methotrexate In Psoriatic Arthritis) study [4], 221 patients were included. In this RCT, with an observational period of 6 months, patients were randomized to MTX (15 mg per week) or placebo. Only 65% and 69% of patients in the active and placebo groups completed the trial. After 6 months, the Psoriatic Arthritis Response Criterion (PsARC) showed improvement in both groups in comparison to baseline. No significant differences were observed between MTX and placebo for PsARC, ACR response or Disease Activity Score (DAS28), Tender Joint Count (TJC), Swollen Joint Count (SJC) or ESR. However, the dose of MTX administered in the trial was lower than that usually used in clinical practice (15 mg/week) and MTX was only given orally. It is possible that a dose of 20–25 mg per week given by parenteral administration could enhance the response to MTX [5]. Therefore, when using MTX, it is important to select an appropriate dose (15–25 mg once weekly) and because of the wide range of bioavailability, parenteral application may help to increase efficacy and reduce side-effects.

Leflunomide

LEF was one of the first drugs to be developed specifically for the treatment of PsA, following its licensing for RA. LEF has a well-defined target and a clearly described mode of action. Evidence for

Agent/Dosage	Structure	Mode of Action	Bioavailability	Half-Life	Elimination	Interactions	Administration	Potential side-effects
Leflunomide 10 to 20 mg/ once daily	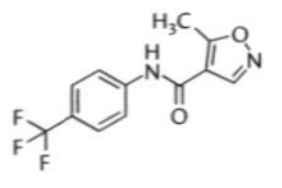	Prodrug, Inhibition of dehydroorotate-dehydrogenase: de-novo pyrimidine synthesis ↘ T-lymphocytes ↘ cytokine production ↘	82–95%	Approx. 15 days	43% renal 48% faeces	Rifampicine: Leflunomide ↑ Leflunomide: Phenytoin ↑, Warfarin ↑, Phenprocoumon ↑	p.o.	Nausea, vomiting, rush/ skin reactions, elevated blood pressure, elevation of transaminases
Methotrexate 15–25mg once weekly	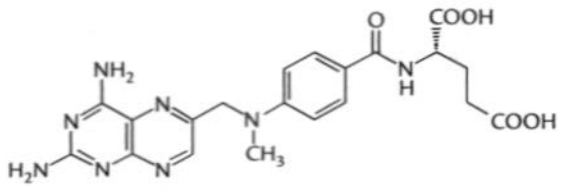	Inhibition of dehydrofolate reductase: de-novo purine synthesis ↘ ↘ T-lymphocytes ↘ cytokine production ↘	Mean 70% (range 25–100%)	3-17 hours	Renal	NSAID/Penicillin: Elimination ↘ Plasma level ↑ Tetracyclines, Phenytoin, Salyzilates: Replacement from plasma binding, Serum level ↑	p.o. s.c i.m.	Nausea, vomiting, dermatitis, stomatitis, alveolitis, pneumonitis, elevation of transaminases
Sulfasalazine 1000mg twice daily	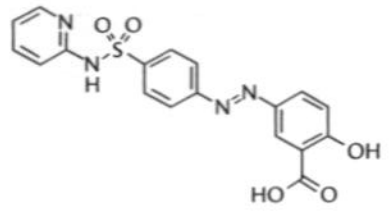	Prodrug, mechanism unclear, assumed inhibition NFκB activation	Less than 15%	5 to 10 hours	Prodrug is metabolised in the GI-tract and liver, renal elimination	Reduced absorption of folid acid (anaemia) and digoxin, serum level of MTX ↑	p.o.	Nausea, vomiting, rush/ skin reactions, elevation of transaminases, hypospermie, in rare cases agranulocytosis
Cyclosporin 3-5mg/kg body weight daily	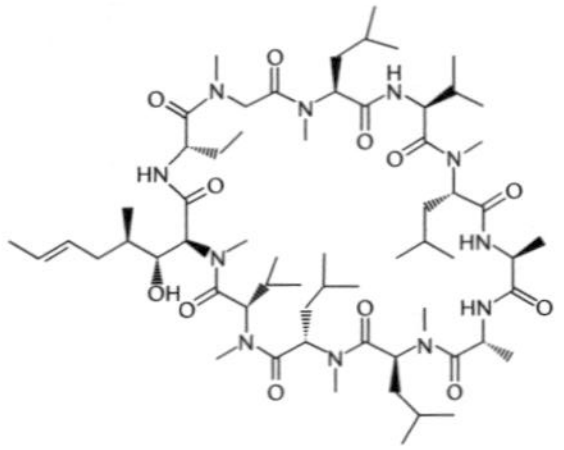	Calcineurin inhibition, T-cell activity ↘ ↘ IL-2 synthesis ↘	Mean 35% (20–50%)	Between 6 and 16 hours, low therapeutic index	Renal, faeces, Fast metabolization of the drug	Cyp3a4 Inhibitors (e.g. ketoconazole, grapefruit juice): Elimination in liver ↘, level of CsA ↑	p.o.	Nephro-, cardio-, livertoxicity, Hyperlipidaemia Tremor Gingiva hyperplasia Hypertonia Oedema Hypertrichiosis
Apremilast 30mg twice daily	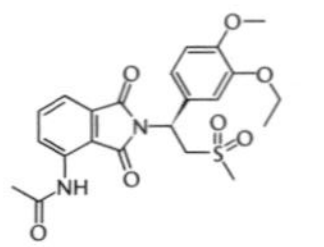	Phosphordiesterase 4 inhibition: cAMP ↑ ↘ pro-inflammatory cytokines ↘ anti-inflammatory cytokines ↖	Approx. 73%	6-9 hours	Metabolites are eliminated renal (58%) and faeces (39%)	Level of ketonidazol ↑, level of rifampine ↘	p.o.	Nausea, vomiting, diarrhoea, urine tract infection, nasopharyngitis

Figure 28.1 Characteristics of sDMARD therapies.

efficacy (PsARC, ACR 20 response respectively) in peripheral arthritis in PsA was demonstrated mainly in a single placebo-controlled RCT, including more than 90 patients per arm [6]. Additional information was provided by a prospective study with more than 400 patients. A significant effect (PsARC) was demonstrated, compared with placebo; the effect size in general was moderate [7]. The dosage used was that licensed for LEF in RA, entailing a 100 mg loading dose for three days, followed by maintenance therapy with 20 mg per day. In daily clinical practice, most of the treating physicians skip the loading dose due to the strong association of gastrointestinal side-effects, which reduces adherence and the compliance of the patients.

Sulfasalazine

SSZ is the sDMARD which has been most extensively studied in PsA as a result of specific development for PsA. SSZ demonstrated limited efficacy that was, nevertheless, superior to placebo in an RCT. In addition, SSZ provided some improvement in functional outcome. However, in a small case-controlled study, it was shown that SSZ is not able to prevent radiographic progression [8].

Cyclosporin

CsA has been shown to be effective in peripheral PsA, not only in monotherapy, but also in combination with MTX and anti-TNF. A double blind RCT was conducted in which CsA was combined with MTX and outcome measures for efficacy and safety were compared to MTX in combination with placebo. In the combinational group containing CsA and MTX, significant improvements in peripheral arthritis and C-reactive protein were detected, compared with MTX and placebo therapy. In daily practice, the use of CsA is limited due to the tight monitoring needed to control safety issues, especially in relation to the high doses of CsA required and its low therapeutic index. CsA is often used as sequential therapy; more than 40% of the treated patients in an RCT, though, stopped CsA within the first year of treatment [9]. Importantly, CsA is only approved for severe arthritis, not specifically for PsA.

Apremilast

APR is a specific phosphodiesterase 4 inhibitor, with an immunomodulating effect, that leads to an increase in cAMP, which results in the reduction of the release of pro-inflammatory and an increase in the release of anti-inflammatory cytokines. In a large development programme which included four RCTs in PsA (three in patients failing previous therapy, one in naive patients [10]) and one for skin psoriasis alone, APR was associated with a significant response on skin and in PsA with moderate efficacy [11]. In the PALACE 3 trial, a change in ACR20 response was seen in 28% (20 mg twice daily) and 41% (30 mg twice daily) compared to placebo (18%) at week 16 and 56% (20 mg twice daily) and 63% (30 mg twice daily) at week 52, demonstrating sustained efficacy [11]. In addition, APR demonstrated tolerable safety. The most common adverse events were gastrointestinal side-effects (diarrhoea, nausea) which occurred during the induction phase of the treatment in 15% and 11% of the patients, respectively, independent of the dosage [12]. Since this programme was conducted recently with a large cohort of PsA patients, the current evidence for efficacy of APR for the treatment of active PsA is very good. The drug is licensed by the EMA (European Medical Agency) in patients who cannot take

or who have not responded well enough to other DMARDs. APR is the only DMARD to be licensed as monotherapy and in combination therapy with other sDMARDs.

Responses to treatment of additional musculoskeletal manifestations

Enthesitis

Enthesitis is defined as inflammation at sites where ligaments, tendons, and joint capsules are fixed to bone. It is prevalent in 25–78% of PsA patients and is thought to be one of the initial inflammatory manifestations of the disease [13], but the clinical detection of active disease and observations on changes during therapy are limited. Outcome measures of enthesitis have been developed and become key instruments in clinical trials [14]. A number of clinical measurements for the outcome of enthesitis are available and demonstrate excellent inter-reader reliability in the group of patients with axial spondyloarthritis [15]. Only one (Leeds Enthesitis Index) has been developed and validated specifically for PsA and shows excellent agreement [16]. Additionally, power Doppler ultrasound and MRI are used for discrimination of inflammatory changes from chronic abnormalities.

Evidence for efficacy of sDMARD therapy on enthesitis is limited. In a study comparing SSZ treatment in PsA with placebo [1], the modified Mander Enthesitis Index was used for the enthesitis outcome measurement [17]. No statistically significant improvement in enthesitis could be detected, either for the SSZ or the placebo group.

In the APR trial [11], the MASES (Maastricht AS Enthesitis Score [18]) score was used. The mean enthesitis change score (MASES index) at week 24 was statistically significantly for the APR 30 mg (twice daily) treatment vs placebo. Unfortunately, no studies detecting changes in enthesitis during sDMARD therapy have been performed for LEF, MTX, and CsA.

Dactylitis

Dactylitis is one of the typical clinical manifestations of PsA [19, 20]. Its diagnosis is challenging for clinicians who are not familiar with it because of the appearance of mild dactylitis or of inactive swelling of a digit or toe. Discriminative diagnosis of dactylitis can be supported by ultrasound or MRI [21]. Because of the various measurement strategies employed for the differentiation and improvement of clinical dactylitis, its treatment, for a long time, was exclusively empirical. For clinical trials, among other variables, the number of dactylitic digits (max. 20 digits; either tender and/or not tender on 0–3 scale), the percentage of patients with dactylitis, the Leeds Dactylitis Index and its simplified version (LDI, LDI basic), as well as MRI dactylitis scores have proved useful [22].

Unfortunately, in the studies that focused on efficacy of sDMARD therapy, including LEF [6] and SSZ [1], no statistically significant benefit could be demonstrated on dactylitis. However, in a prospective, uncontrolled, observational study [7], reduction of dactylitis was detected when patients were treated with LEF.

Moreover, in an RCT in which infliximab in combination with MTX was compared with MTX alone, the combination treatment group (infliximab/MTX) provided significant improvement in

Table 28.1 Overview of efficacy of sDMARDs on different manifestations of psoriatic disease

	Peripheral arthritis	Enthesitis	Dactylitis	Axial	Psoriasis	Radiographic progression
LEF	+	0	(+)	−	+	0
MTX	(+)	0	0	−	+	0
SSZ	+	0	0	−	(+)	−
CsA	(+)	0	0	−	+	0
APR	+	+	(+)	(+)	+	0

+ Proven efficacy with robust evidence (data RCTs)

(+) Weak evidence of efficacy

0 Uncertain efficacy

− Proven inefficacy

dactylitis compared to the exclusive MTX treatment [23]. It is suggested that sDMARD therapy alone may be mildly effective, but this has not actually been demonstrated in RCTs, as the studies that have been performed have not been powered for efficacy against dactylitis.

APR demonstrated a clear trend towards a beneficial response on dactylitis, in the PALACE study programme, but did not achieve statistically significance compared with placebo in terms of the dactylitis severity index [11].

An overview on efficacy of sDMARD therapy is shown in Table 28.1. Moreover, suggestions from the authors on sDMARD treatment strategies on different disease pattern including arthritis, enthesitis, dactylitis and skin are displayed in Figure 28.2.

sDMARDs in axial PsA

Evidence of effectiveness of sDMARDs for axial PsA is limited due to the fact that no clinical studies were designed and powered for this specific disease involvement. In addition, the presence of axial PsA disease in clinical trials is mostly only decided upon by the opinion of the investigator and not examined systematically. Treatment goals for axial PsA include relief of signs and symptoms (pain, stiffness, and restriction in spinal mobility), improvements in physical function and quality of life, inhibition of progression of structural damage, and the prevention of disability. No new studies on sDMARD treatment of axial PsA have been published since 2006.

In the MIPA study [4], comparing MTX therapy with placebo treatment in PsA, no attempt was made to analyse the data on efficacy in axial PsA. Moreover, with the exception of infliximab, DMARD co-therapy (MTX) does not appear to improve maintenance anti-TNF-treatment [24].

In general, axial PsA should be treated according to the guidelines for ankylosing spondylitis or axial spondyloarthritis, including adequate dosing with NSAIDs, followed by anti-TNF treatment in cases of inadequate response to NSAIDs [25].

At present, only APR has been shown to have some effect on outcome measures of axial disease, based on a small number of patients in a study with ankylosing spondylitis, although it did not meet its primary endpoint of change in Bath Ankylosing Spondylitis Disease Activity Index (BASDAI) compared to placebo at week 12 [26]. In the PALACE study (PsA), 37% of the patients were affected by axial involvement [11]. This subgroup showed a significant improvement in BASDAI.

Effects of sDMARDs on skin psoriasis in PsA patients

The guidelines and recommendations for the treatment of psoriasis are numerous and are based on a large number of clinical trials [27]. Most of the guidelines focus on plaque-type psoriasis, as the most common form of psoriasis. In addition, in most of the guidelines patients are stratified for severity of skin involvement (mild vs moderate to severe), as assessed by the Psoriasis Area and Severity Index (PASI), the affected body surface area (BSA), and the burden of disease measured by the Dermatology Life Quality Index (DLQI) questionnaire [28]. The regulatory status of sDMARD therapy as regards licensing for psoriasis and/or PsA treatment is shown in Table 28.2.

Plaque psoriasis in PsA patients

In general, measurement of response in skin disease in patients with PsA is often limited due to low PASI and BSA involvement at baseline and therefore, limited sensitivity to change in skin response measures. Several studies have been performed to detect efficacy on psoriasis and safety of MTX in PsA patients. In total, 410 patients have been assessed. Kingsley et al. treated 109 patients with PsA using MTX in a placebo-controlled setting [4]. In the patients with active psoriasis, mean PASI decreased from 3.76 at baseline to 2.2 at month 6. Mease et al. demonstrated, in a study using alefacept and MTX treatment in PsA patients, a PASI 50 response of 31% and a PASI 75 response of 24% in the patients who were exclusively treated with MTX [29]. In an RCT conducted by Fraser et al. [9], the combination therapy of MTX and CsA was compared with MTX plus placebo therapy. Thirty-four patients received MTX alone at a dose of 15 mg/week. At month 12, the mean PASI decreased from 2.2 to 1.9. In the treatment group using the combination therapy of MTX and CsA, PASI was reduced from 2.0 (baseline) to 0.8. A longitudinal observational study demonstrated a PASI 50 response in patients using MTX (mean dose, 16.2 mg/week) of 57% after 24 weeks [26]. In a study by Baranauskaite et al., exclusive MTX treatment was compared with its combination with infliximab [23]. After 4 months of treatment, 54% of the patients who were previously naive to MTX treatment, reached a PASI 75 response.

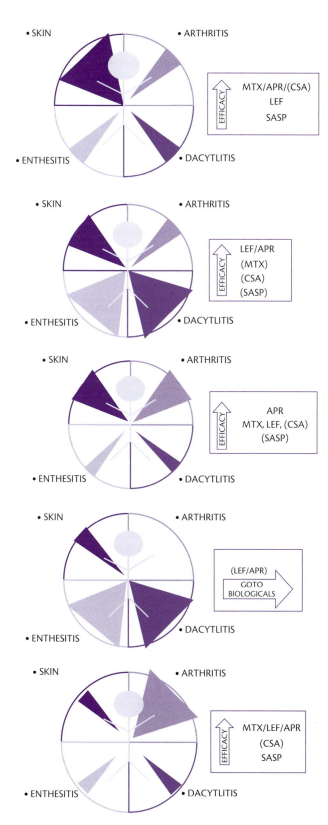

Figure 28.2 Treatment options with synthetic DMARDs based on potential phenotypic patterns of disease activity (size of triangle represents severity of involvement of the different PsA manifestations).

Table 28.2 sDMARD characteristics on regulatory approval

	US		EU	
	PsA	Pso	PsA	Pso
LEF	-	-	x	-
MTX	x	x	x	x
SSZ	-	-	-	-
CsA	-	x	-	x
APR*	x	x	x	x

*Approved after failure/contraindication of previous sDMARD therapy

The TOPAS study, investigating efficacy of LEF in PsA, included 92 patients with skin involvement assessed by PASI. After the loading dose of 100mg/day for 3 days, a maintenance dose of 20 mg/day was administered for another 6 months, according to summary of product characteristics. A PASI50 response was reached by 30.4% (vs 18% for placebo response), whereas a PASI 75 response was reached by 17.4% (vs 7.8% in the placebo group) of the PsA patients [6].

Karanikolas et al. [30] conducted a study on CsA as monotherapy or in combination with adalimumab. The treatment group with CsA alone included 56 patients. Sixty-five percent of these patients achieved a PASI50 response, whereas 45% reached PASI75 and 27.5% a PASI90 response after 12 months of treatment. Spadaro et al. [31] included, in a smaller prospective study, 10 patients receiving CsA treatment over a 12-month observational period. A mean PASI reduction of 7.6 was reported in the treatment group. Additionally, in another study using CsA as treatment in PsA patients, a CsA dosage of 3 mg/kg/day was administered to 60 patients over 24 months. A mean reduction of PASI of 15.1 to 5.2 was observed [32].

APR was developed through clinical testing in patients with active PsA and psoriasis. In three clinical studies in active PsA (PALACE 1-3), not only was the response assessed in terms of musculoskeletal manifestations, but the effect on skin psoriasis was also investigated. At the primary endpoint of the study (week 16), 50% of the patients achieved a PASI 50 reduction [11]. At week 24, a 75% reduction in PASI was seen in 20–30% of the patients (compared to 4.6% in the placebo group). In addition, RCTs in skin psoriasis were performed and a significant effect was demonstrated.

SSZ did not lead to a significant response in skin psoriasis and is, therefore, not indicated for the treatment of PsA patients with significant skin manifestations, unless the skin disease is treated additionally with another agent.

Nail psoriasis

Systemic therapies for treatment of nail psoriasis have never been systematically tested. However, it is suggested that oral CsA, as an immunosuppressant drug that interferes with activity and growth of T cells, has modest effects on nail psoriasis [30, 33].

Oral MTX, which was tested more strictly than CsA in clinical studies, did not provide any significant improvement in nail disease, as shown in a number of studies [4, 34, 35].

For patients with significant skin and nail disease, a recently published review, based on data of the ESTEEM study, recommends the use of APR. Within this study, a mean decrease from baseline in the Nail Psoriasis Severity Index (NAPSI) of 60.2% was observed at week 52 [36]. Unfortunately, studies focused on sDMARD therapy that were statistically powered for detection of changes in nail psoriasis have not been performed with LEF and SSZ.

Effects on extra-musculoskeletal manifestations and comorbidities in PsA patients

PsA patients have a higher risk for development of cardiovascular disease. This is clear from the higher prevalence of ischaemic heart disease, cerebrovascular disease, diastolic dysfunction, left ventricular dysfunction, abnormal carotid intimal thickness, and cardiovascular death [37, 38, 39]. Furthermore, an increased prevalence has been observed of risk factors such as hypertension, obesity, diabetes, and dyslipidaemia [40, 41]. Patients with PsA also have a higher incidence of inflammatory bowel disease (including Crohn's disease and ulcerative colitis) [42]. Moreover, the prevalence of fatty liver disease [43] and kidney disease [44] is higher in patients with moderate to severe PsA.

To date, no prospective studies have been performed in patients with active PsA treated with sDMARDs that address outcome on cardiovascular events. With regard to inflammatory bowel disease, treatment choices should be taken carefully in the light of the systemic disease and its dermal, musculoskeletal, and gastro-intestinal manifestations [45]. Liver disease may be the result of the disease itself, but the medication used can be a risk factor as well. Furthermore, the presence of liver disease has an impact on the treatment options for PsA.

In a cross-sectional study, it was shown that combination therapy with a TNF inhibitor and MTX was associated with a lower risk of liver fibrosis than in patients treated with MTX alone [46]. MTX and LEF have been associated with elevated liver function tests as well as with the development of non-alcoholic steatohepatitis and/or cirrhosis [47]. Therapy options for chronic kidney disease in the

PsA patient present another challenge to the treatment of active immune-mediated disease. Thus, the elimination pathways of the drugs have to be taken into consideration; for instance, elimination of LEF via the faeces could be an option in this comorbid condition, while CSA and MTX are contraindicated. Moreover, evidence for the use of immunosuppressive agents under these conditions is limited and treatment strategies in patients requiring haemodialysis are challenging. One study demonstrated that LEF might be used in RA patients on haemodialysis [48], whereas the use of MTX is restricted because the risk of pancytopenia is increased [49]. Nephrotoxicity is another challenge with immunosuppressive treatments. In a study by Maza et al., it was shown that nephrotoxicity in patients with psoriasis treated with CsA was associated with longer use, a higher cumulative dose, and higher daily dose [50]. Hierarchical order of sDMARD use in skin and arthritis is displayed in Figure 28.3 based on evidence and effect size of each substance.

Combination therapy with other sDMARDs or with biologicals

In RA, combinations of two or more sDMARDs are well-established treatment options to optimize therapeutic outcome. Add-on of sDMARDs in RA has also clearly shown synergistic effects in biological-treated patients. Unfortunately, in PsA, this clear evidence for combination therapy is not available. In an open-label prospective study, combination therapy with MTX and LEF was compared with that of LEF alone and no superiority of the combined therapy over monotherapy was seen in this non-randomized setting [7]. In one randomized clinical study, the combination of MTX and CsA demonstrated superiority to MTX monotherapy [9], but in this study, only the add-on of CsA in MTX failure patients was addressed in the chosen study design.

For the add-on of sDMARD to anti-TNF (or any biological therapy), there is a lack of robust data. It is known that biological therapy demonstrates the same effect in patients who are treated with ongoing DMARD therapy as in those naive to sDMARD therapy when biological therapy is initiated. Data from prospective observational studies have not provided strong evidence for enhanced efficacy of these combination therapies versus treatment with biological therapies alone. However, some data from registries suggest that adherence, especially to anti-TNF antibody therapy, might be

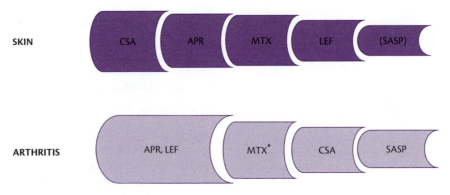

Figure 28.3 Hierarchical order of sDMARD therapies for skin disease and arthritis in PsA patients based on the size of their effects (ACR Response, PASI) and level of evidence.

*The place of MTX within the order is mainly driven by lack of evidence of effectiveness due to missing data from well-designed RCTs.

prolonged when adding MTX, possibly due to an influence on the production of neutralizing anti-drug antibodies [24, 51].

Other findings suggest that combination therapy with CsA and TNF inhibitors is associated with an acceptable safety profile and good therapeutic responses in skin psoriasis that may be slightly superior to combination of CsA with MTX in psoriasis patients. Furthermore, addition of MTX to infliximab, in the treatment of skin psoriasis, demonstrated superiority in terms of outcome measures [52].

sDMARD treatment in patients planning to have children

The treatment of patients with immune-mediated chronic diseases who are pregnant or plan to have children represents a challenge in clinical routine care. Options to treat pregnant patients are limited. Both MTX and LEF have a clear teratogenic potential.

The United States Food and Drug Administration has classified SSZ as a category B treatment. However, the effect of SSZ on the development of the unborn child has not been studied extensively. There are strict restrictions on the use of SSZ during pregnancy: it should only be used when clearly indicated. SSZ is detectable in breast milk and could affect the nursing infant.

Data on CsA as a therapeutic option in pregnant patients is limited to case reports and data from registries. Thus, data on its risk profile only refer to exposure to the drug alone or to pre-existing maternal comorbidities. Therapy with CsA during pregnancy should therefore, be considered carefully by the treating physician [53].

References

1. Clegg DO, Reda DJ, Mejias E, et al. Comparison of sulfasalazine and placebo in the treatment of psoriatic arthritis. A Department of Veterans Affairs Cooperative Study. Arthritis Rheum. 1996;39(12):2013–20.
2. Coates LC, Ritchlin CT, Kavanaugh AF. GRAPPA treatment recommendations: an update from the GRAPPA 2013 Annual Meeting. J Rheumatol. 2014;41(6):1237–9.
3. Scarpa R, Peluso R, Atteno M, et al. The effectiveness of a traditional therapeutical approach in early psoriatic arthritis: results of a pilot randomised 6-month trial with methotrexate. Clin Rheumatol. 2008;27(7):823–6.
4. Kingsley GH, Kowalczyk A, Taylor H, et al. A randomized placebo-controlled trial of methotrexate in psoriatic arthritis. Rheumatology (Oxford). 2012;51(8):1368–77.
5. Chandran V, Schentag CT, Gladman DD. Reappraisal of the effectiveness of methotrexate in psoriatic arthritis. Results from a longitudinal observational cohort. J Rheumatol 2008;35:469–71.
6. Kaltwasser JP, Nash P, Gladman D, et al. Efficacy and safety of leflunomide in the treatment of psoriatic arthritis and psoriasis: a multinational, double-blind, randomized, placebo-controlled clinical trial. Arthritis Rheum. 2004;50(6):1939–50.
7. Behrens F, Finkenwirth C, Pavelka K, et al. Leflunomide in psoriatic arthritis: results from a large European prospective observational study. Arthritis Care Res (Hoboken). 2013;65(3):464–70.
8. Gupta AK, Grober JS, Hamilton TA, et al. Sulfasalazine therapy for psoriatic arthritis: a double blind, placebo controlled trial. J Rheumatol. 1995;22(5):894–8.
9. Fraser AD, van Kuijk AW, Westhovens R, et al. A randomised, double blind, placebo controlled, multicentre trial of combination therapy with methotrexate plus cyclosporin in patients with active psoriatic arthritis. Ann Rheum Dis 2005;64:859–64.
10. Bissonnette R, Pariser DM, Wasel NR, et al. Apremilast, an oral phosphodiesterase-4 inhibitor, in the treatment of palmoplantar psoriasis: Results of a pooled analysis from phase II PSOR-005 and phase III Efficacy and Safety Trial Evaluating the Effects of Apremilast in Psoriasis (ESTEEM) clinical trials in patients with moderate to severe psoriasis. J Am Acad Dermatol. 2016;75(1):99–105.
11. Kavanaugh A, Mease PJ, Gomez-Reino JJ, et al. Treatment of psoriatic arthritis in a phase 3 randomised, placebo-controlled trial with apremilast, an oral phosphodiesterase 4 inhibitor. Ann Rheum Dis. 2014;73(6):1020–6.
12. Edwards CJ, Blanco FJ, Crowley J, et al. Apremilast, an oral phosphodiesterase 4 inhibitor, in patients with psoriatic arthritis and current skin involvement: a phase III, randomised, controlled trial (PALACE 3). Ann Rheum Dis. 2016;75(6):1065–73.
13. Sakkas LI, Alexiou I, Simpopoulou T, Vlychou M. Enthesitis in psoriatic arthritis. Semin Arthritis Rheum 2013;43:325–34.
14. Smolen JS, Braun J, Dougados M, et al. Treating spondyloarthritis, including ankylosing spondylitis and psoriatic arthritis, to target: recommendations of an international task force. Ann Rheum Dis. 2014 ;73(1):6–16.
15. Gladman DD, Inman R, Cook R, et al. International Spondyloarthritis Inter-Observer Reliability Exercise—The INSPIRE Study: II. Assessment of peripheral joints, enthesitis and dactylitis. J Rheumatol 2007;34:1740–5.
16. Healy PJ, Helliwell PS. Measuring clinical enthesitis in psoriatic arthritis: Assessment of existing measures and development of an instrument specific to psoriatic arthritis. Arthritis Rheum 2008;59:686–91.
17. Mander M, Simpson JM, McLellan A, et al. Studies with an enthesis index as method of clinical assessment in ankylosing spondylitis. Ann Rheum Dis 1987;46:197–202.
18. Heuft-Dorenbosch L, Spoorenberg A, van Tubergen A, et al. Assessment of enthesitis in ankylosing spondylitis. Ann Rheum Dis 2003;62:127–32.
19. Moll JM, Wright V. Psoriatic arthritis. Semin Arthritis Rheum. 1973;3:55–78.
20. Brockbank J, Stein M, Schentag CT, Gladman DD. Dactylitis in psoriatic arthritis (PsA): a marker for disease severity? Ann Rheum Dis 2005;62:188–90.
21. Blakewell CJ, Oliveiri I, Aydin SZ, et al. Ultrasound and magnetic resonance imaging in the evaluation of psoriatic dactylitis: Status and perspectives. J Rheumatol 2013;40:1951–7.
22. Helliwell PS, Kavanaugh A. Comparison of composite measures of disease activity in psoriatic arthritis using data from an interventional study with golimumab. Arthritis Care Res (Hoboken). 2014;66(5):749–56.
23. Baranauskaite A, Raffayová H, Kungurov NV, et al. Infliximab plus methotrexate is superior to methotrexate alone in the treatment of psoriatic arthritis in methotrexate-naive patients: the RESPOND study. Ann Rheum Dis. 2012;71(4):541–8.
24. Fagerli KM1, Lie E, van der Heijde D, et al. The role of methotrexate co-medication in TNF-inhibitor treatment in patients with psoriatic arthritis: results from 440 patients included in the NOR-DMARD study. Ann Rheum Dis. 2014;73(1):132–7.
25. Nash P, Lubrano E, Cauli A, Taylor WJ, Olivieri I, Gladman DD. Updated guidelines for the management of axial disease in psoriatic arthritis. J Rheumatol. 2014;41(11):2286–9.
26. Pathan E, Abraham S, Van Rossen E, et al. Efficacy and safety of apremilast, an oral phosphodiesterase 4 inhibitor, in ankylosing spondylitis. Ann Rheum Dis. 2013;72(9):1475–80.
27. Nast A, Boehncke WH, Mrowietz U, et al. Guidelines on the treatment of psoriasis vulgaris. Update. J Dtsch Dermatol Ges 2012;10 Suppl 2: S1–95.
28. Boehncke WH, Alvarez Martinez D, Solomon JA, Gottlieb AB. Safety and efficacy of therapies for skin symptoms of psoriasis in patients with psoriatic arthritis: a systematic review. J Rheumatol. 2014;41(11):2301–5.

29. Mease PJ, Gladman DD, Keystone EC. Alefacept in combination with methotrexate for the treatment of psoriatic arthritis: Results of a randomised, double-blind, placebo-controlled study. Arthritis Rheum 2006;54:1638–45.

30. Karanikolas GN, Koukli EM, Katsalira A, et al. Adalimumab or cyclosporin as monotherapy and in combination in severe psoriatic arthritis: results from a prospective 12-month nonrandomized unblinded clinical trial. J Rheumatol. 2011;38(11):2466–74.

31. Spadaro A, Riccieri V, Sili-Scavalli A, Sensi F, Taccari E, Zoppini A. Comparison of cyclosporin A and methotrexate in the treatment of psoriatic arthritis: a one-year prospective study. Clin Exp Rheumatol. 1995;13(5):589–93.

32. Sarzi-Puttini P, Cazzola M, Panni B, et al. Long-term safety and efficacy of low-dose cyclosporin A in severe psoriatic arthritis. Rheumatol Int. 2002;21(6):234–8.

33. Cassell S, Kavanaugh AF. Therapies for psoriatic nail disease. A systematic review. J Rheumatol. 2006;33(7):1452–6.

34. Gümüşel M, Özdemir M, Mevlitoğlu I, Bodur S. Evaluation of the efficacy of methotrexate and cyclosporin therapies on psoriatic nails: a one-blind, randomized study. J Eur Acad Dermatol Venereol. 2011;25(9):1080–4.

35. Demirsoy EO, Kıran R, Salman S, Cağlayan C, et al. Effectiveness of systemic treatment agents on psoriatic nails: a comparative study. J Drugs Dermatol. 2013;12(9):1039–43.

36. Crowley JJ, Weinberg JM, Wu JJ, Robertson AD, Van Voorhees AS. Treatment of nail psoriasis best practice recommendations from the Medical Board of the National Psoriasis Foundation JAMA Dermatol. 2015;151.

37. Shang Q, Tam LS, Sanderson JE, Sun JP, Li EK, Yu CM. Increase in ventricular-arterial stiffness in patients with psoriatic arthritis. Rheumatology (Oxford). 2012;51(12):2215–23.

38. Shang Q, Tam LS, Yip GW, et al. High prevalence of subclinical left ventricular dysfunction in patients with psoriatic arthritis. J Rheumatol. 2011;38(7):1363–70.

39. Jamnitski A, Symmons D, Peters MJ, Sattar N, McInnes I, Nurmohamed MT. Cardiovascular comorbidities in patients with psoriatic arthritis: a systematic review. Ann Rheum Dis. 2013;72(2):211–6.

40. Husted JA, Thavaneswaran A, Chandran V, et al. Cardiovascular and other comorbidities in patients with psoriatic arthritis: a comparison with patients with psoriasis. Arthritis Care Res (Hoboken). 2011;63(12):1729–35.

41. Armstrong AW, Harskamp CT, Armstrong EJ. The association between psoriasis and hypertension: a systematic review and meta-analysis of observational studies. J Hypertens. 2013;31(3):433–42; discussion 442–3.

42. Scarpa R, Manguso F, D'Arienzo A, D'Armiento FP, Astarita C, Mazzacca G, Ayala F. Microscopic inflammatory changes in colon of patients with both active psoriasis and psoriatic arthritis without bowel symptoms. J Rheumatol. 2000;27(5):1241–6.

43. Madanagobalane S, Anandan S. The increased prevalence of non-alcoholic fatty liver disease in psoriatic patients: a study from South India. Austral J Dermatol. 2012;53(3):190–7.

44. Wan J, Wang S, Haynes K, Denburg MR, Shin DB, Gelfand JM. Risk of moderate to advanced kidney disease in patients with psoriasis: population based cohort study. BMJ. 2013 Oct 15;347:f5961.

45. Talley NJ, Abreu MT, Achkar JP, et al. An evidence-based systemic review on medical therapies for inflammatory bowel disease. Am J Gastroenterol 2011;106 Suppl 1:S2-25; quiz S6.

46. Seitz M, Reichenbach S, Moller B, et al. Hepatoprotective effect of tumor necrosis factor alpha blockade in psoriatic arthritis: a cross-sectional study. Ann Rheum Dis 2010;69:1148–50.

47. Curtis JR, Beukelman T, Onofrei A, et al. Elevated liver enzyme tests among patients with rheumatoid arthritis or psoriatic arthritis treated with methotrexate and/or leflunomide. Ann Rheum Dis 2010;69:43–7.

48. Bergner R, Peters L, Schmitt V, Loffler C. Leflunomide in dialysis patients with rheumatoid arthritis—A pharmakokinetic study. Clin Rheumatol 2013;32:267–70.

49. Al-Hasani H, Roussou E. Methotrexate for rheumatoid arthritis patients who are on hemodialysis. Rheumatol Int 2011;31:1545–7.

50. Maza A, Montaudie H, Sbidian E, et al. Oral cyclosporin in psoriasis: A systemic review on treatment modalities, risk of kidney toxicity and evidence for use in non-plaque psoriasis. J Eur Acad Dermatol Venereol 2011;25 Suppl 2:19–27.

51. Behrens F, Cañete JD, Olivieri I, van Kuijk AW, McHugh N, Combe B. Tumour necrosis factor inhibitor monotherapy vs combination with MTX in the treatment of PsA: a systematic review of the literature. Rheumatology (Oxford). 2015;54(5):915–26.

52. Armstrong AW, Bagel J, Van Voorhees AS, Robertson AD, Yamauchi PS. Combining biologic therapies with other systemic treatments in psoriasis: evidence-based, best-practice recommendations from the Medical Board of the National Psoriasis Foundation. JAMA Dermatol. 2015 ;151(4):432–8.

53. Paziana K, Del Monaco M, Cardonick E, Moritz M, et al. Cyclosporin use during pregnancy. Drug Safe ;36(5):279–94.

CHAPTER 29

Biologic DMARDs (TNF inhibitors)

Tristan Boyd and Arthur Kavanaugh

Introduction

Tumour necrosis factor-α inhibitors (TNFi) are highly effective therapies that have increased treatment expectations and consequently revolutionized the management of psoriatic arthritis (PsA). There are currently five TNFi approved for use in the treatment of PsA worldwide: etanercept, infliximab, adalimumab, golimumab, and certolizumab pegol (see Figure 29.1).

Biosimilar versions of several of these are also available in some countries. All TNFi are highly effective at treating the heterogeneous clinical manifestations seen in psoriatic disease and have similar safety profiles. While no head-to-head comparisons have been made, indirect comparisons have not revealed any statistically significant differences between any of the TNFi in the treatment of PsA [1]. This chapter discusses the rationale for using TNFi in the treatment of PsA, reviews clinical trial evidence for the efficacy and safety of TNFi in PsA, and outlines the most recent treatment recommendations. We conclude with a discussion of novel treatment concepts involving the use of these agents in the management of PsA.

Traditional DMARDs and PsA: unmet needs

PsA was previously likened to a mild form of seronegative rheumatoid arthritis (RA); however, it is now recognized as a distinct entity with unique clinical features. Perhaps the most striking difference between the two diseases is the significant heterogeneity seen in PsA, which can affect the axial and peripheral skeleton, entheses, skin and nails, and other organ systems, (e.g. anterior uveitis and inflammatory bowel disease). Common comorbidities (e.g. obesity, metabolic syndrome, non-alcoholic fatty liver disease, cardiovascular disease, and depression) must be taken into consideration when selecting therapy. Recently, the term 'psoriatic disease' was coined to encompass the diverse clinical spectrum that can be seen in this systemic disease [2].

Traditional disease-modifying anti-rheumatic drugs (DMARDs) have not been shown to effectively treat all the diverse clinical manifestations of psoriatic disease (e.g. axial symptoms, uveitis, enthesitis, and dactylitis); nor do they inhibit structural joint damage in peripheral joints. In contrast, TNFi effectively treat all domains of disease activity in PsA and have been shown to prevent disease progression [3, 4]. While there is a paucity of data addressing the long-term benefits of treating comorbidities in PsA, there is some evidence to suggest TNFi may prevent the progression of subclinical

atherosclerosis and reduce arterial stiffness in inflammatory arthritis [5]. There is also evidence that suggests improved response to treatment when associated comorbidities are treated: patients achieving weight loss ≥5% from baseline were shown to have improved response to TNFi with increased likelihood of achieving minimal disease activity (odds ratio 4.20, P<0.001) [6]. Thus, it is important to identify and manage comorbidities as they may influence choice of therapy and may also have implications regarding response to treatment and prognosis.

Rationale for the use of TNF inhibitors in PsA

TNF-α is a pro-inflammatory cytokine that has been found to be upregulated in psoriatic skin and synovium, and is believed to play a critical role in the pathogenesis of autoimmune inflammatory conditions, such as psoriasis and psoriatic arthritis [7–10]. TNF-α activates multiple signalling pathways resulting in increased synthesis of inflammatory mediators (e.g. interleukin-1, interleukin-6, interleukin-8, and granulocyte-monocyte colony-stimulating factor) that help promote inflammation [11]. TNF-α stimulates epidermal proliferation, contributing to the generation of psoriatic skin plaques, and also increases the expression of vascular endothelial growth factor leading to formation of new blood vessels in psoriatic skin and synovium [12]. The resulting long and tortuous vessels are characteristic of psoriatic synovium and can distinguish it from the vascular pathology typically seen in RA. TNF-α and interleukin-1β increase the production of degradative enzymes, including matrix metalloproteinases (MMPs), which can result in cartilage degradation [13, 14]. TNF-α also induces the differentiation of osteoclast precursors, which mediate bone resorption after their migration to the inflamed synovium and subchondral bone [15]. These processes can result in joint inflammation and damage, and may ultimately lead to impaired physical function and diminished quality of life.

Treatment with TNFi has been associated with a significant reduction in T-cell infiltrate in psoriatic skin lesions, as well as decreased MMP expression and macrophage infiltration in synovial tissue [16, 17]. Serum MMP-3 levels have been found to be associated with therapeutic response (i.e. high levels at baseline and their reduction after initiating therapy) to TNFi in PsA patients [18]. The significant clinical response associated with TNF-α inhibition supports the importance of this pro-inflammatory cytokine in the

TNF inhibitor Generic Name (*Trade Name*)	Structure description	Standard dosing regimen
Etanercept (Enbral®) 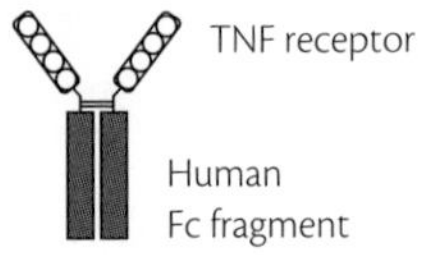 TNF receptor Human Fc fragment	Soluble receptor fusion protein composed of extracellular ligand-binding portion of TNF receptor (p75) dimerized on Fc portion of human IgG1. Interferes with endogenous TNF-α activity by binding soluble TNF-u (can also bind membrane-bound, but less efficiently than monoclonal antibodies).	50 mg SC weekly (or 25 mg SC twice weekly) (Note: dosing for skin psoriasis is 50 mg twice weekly x12 weeks, then weekly)
Infliximab (Remicade®) 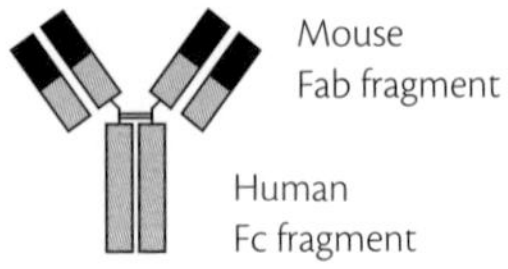 Mouse Fab fragment Human Fc fragment	Murine/human chimeric anti-TNF-α monoclonal antibody. Interferes with endogenous TNF-a activity by binding both soluble and membrane-bound TNF-α.	Initial: 5-10 mg/kg IV at weeks 0, 2, and 6 Maintenance: repeated at 8 week intervals (can be used at intervals as short as 4 weeks)
Adalimumab (Humira®) 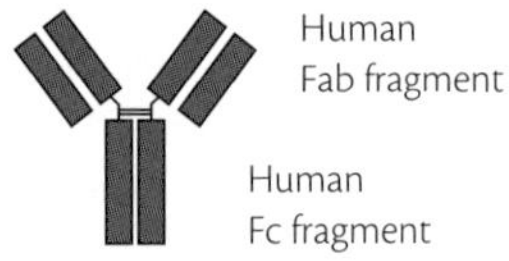 Human Fab fragment Human Fc fragment	Human monoclonal anti-TNF-α antibody. Interferes with endogenous TNF-α activity by binding soluble and membrane-bound TNF-α.	40 mg SC every 2 weeks (can be used weekly)
Golimumab (Simponi®) 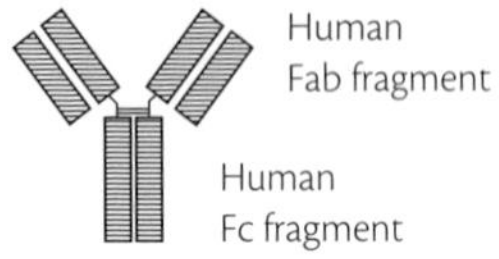 Human Fab fragment Human Fc fragment	Human monoclonal anti-TNF-α antibody. Interferes with endogenous TNF-a activity by binding soluble and membrane-bound TNF-α.	50 mg SC every 4 weeks
Certolizumab-pegol (Cimizia®) 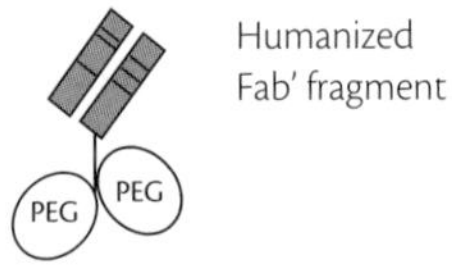 Humanized Fab' fragment PEG PEG	Humanized monoclonal antibody Fab' fragment of TNF-a coupled to polyethylene glycol (i.e., pegylated). Interferes with TNF-a activity by binding both soluble and membrane-bound TNF-α.	Initial: 400 mg SC at weeks 0, 2, and 4 Maintenance: 200 mg SC every 2 weeks (or 400 mg SC every 4 weeks)

Figure 29.1 TNF inhibitors approved for use in the treatment of psoriatic arthritis.

Fc, fragment crystallizable region; Fab. Fragment antigen-binding region; TNF, tumour necrosis factor; SC, subcutaneously; IV, intravenously; PEG, polyethylene glycol.

pathogenesis of PsA. As will be discussed further, TNFi are effective in treating all of the diverse domains of disease activity in PsA, including peripheral arthritis, axial arthritis, enthesitis, dactylitis, skin psoriasis, and nail disease, as well as other manifestations (see Figure 29.2) [3, 4].

Clinical trial data

Table 29.1 provides a summary of key randomized, placebo-controlled clinical trials involving the use of TNFi in PsA. These studies will be reviewed in more detail below. As mentioned previously, no head-to-head comparisons have been made between TNFi, but indirect comparisons have shown similar efficacy for these agents.1 In addition to looking at outcome measures for peripheral arthritis and skin psoriasis, some of these studies included analyses of enthesitis, dactylitis, function, quality of life, and patient-reported outcomes, all of which improved and were separated statistically from patients treated with placebo. Unlike traditional DMARDs, TNFi have been shown to inhibit radiographic progression in peripheral joints [19–23].

Evidence for the efficacy of TNF inhibitors in PsA

Etanercept (Enbrel®)

Etanercept is a soluble receptor fusion protein that binds to and antagonizes soluble TNF-α. It is composed of the extracellular ligand-binding portion of the TNF receptor (p75) dimerized on the Fc portion of human IgG1. For the treatment of PsA, etanercept is administered subcutaneously (SC) at a dose of 50 mg weekly, or alternatively 25 mg twice weekly.

Etanercept was initially found to be effective in treating PsA in a 12-week randomized, placebo-controlled trial that included 60 PsA patients with a mean disease duration of 9 years [24]. Patients received either etanercept, administered at a dose of 25 mg SC twice weekly, or placebo. At 12 weeks, patients treated with etanercept achieved significantly better outcomes in American College of Rheumatology 20 (ACR20), ACR50, and ACR70 responses than placebo (73, 50, and 13% vs. 13, 3, and 0%, respectively). The proportion of patients who achieved a reduction of 75% from baseline

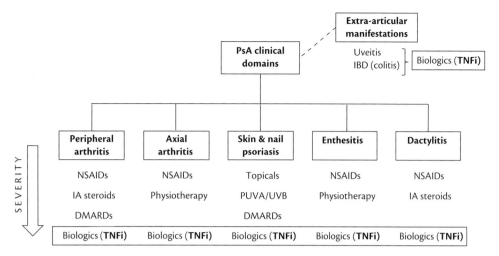

Figure 29.2 TNF inhibitors effectively treat all domains of disease activity in psoriatic arthritis.

TNF inhibitors effectively treat all signs and symptoms of inflammation in PsA. They treat extra-articular manifestations and also prevent radiographic progression in peripheral joints. Abbreviations: PsA, psoriatic arthritis; TNFi, TNF inhibitor; NSAID, nonsteroidal anti-inflammatory drug; IA, intra-articular; DMARDs, disease-modifying anti-rheumatic drugs; PUVA, psoralen and ultraviolet A; UVB, ultraviolet B.

in the psoriasis area-and-severity index (PASI75) score at 12 weeks was significantly greater in patients treated with etanercept than in those treated with placebo (26 vs 0%, P=0.0154).

A second larger study, included 205 PsA patients with a mean disease duration of 9 years [21]. Patients were randomized to receive either etanercept 25 mg SC twice weekly or placebo for 24 weeks. ACR20 response was measured at 12 weeks and was achieved by 59% of etanercept-treated patients compared with 15% of patients who received placebo (P<0.0001). These results were sustained at week 24, with continued benefit noted at week 48 in the open-label extension phase of the study, where ACR20 response was achieved in 64% of etanercept-treated patients [25]. The Psoriatic Arthritis Response Criteria (PsARC), which is a composite outcome measure that uses a modified version of the ACR joint count to be more representative of the joints involved in PsA, also demonstrated early and sustained improvement with 72% and 84% of patients achieving this response at weeks 12 and 48, respectively [26].

PASI75 response was achieved in 23% of etanercept-treated patients at week 24 compared with 3% of placebo patients (P=0.001). In the open-label extension study, PASI75 response improved to ~40% of all patients by week 12 and was maintained throughout the remainder of the study. The extension study also assessed structural damage in 169 patients and noted less prominent radiographic progression in patients treated with etanercept compared with the placebo group after 2 years of treatment [25].

Infliximab (Remicade®)

Infliximab is a mouse-human chimeric anti-TNF-α monoclonal antibody that binds to and inhibits both soluble and membrane-bound TNF-α. For the treatment of PsA, it is administered intravenously (IV) at a dose of 5 mg/kg (range 5–10 mg/kg) at weeks 0, 2, and 6 and subsequently every 8 weeks, with the possibility of shorter intervals if clinically indicated.

The efficacy of infliximab in PsA was first studied in the IMPACT trial, a phase II, randomized, double-blind, placebo-controlled study of 104 patients with PsA [27]. In the initial phase of the study, half of the patients received infliximab 5 mg/kg IV at weeks 0, 2,

6, and 14, while the other half received placebo. At week 16, 65% of patients treated with infliximab achieved ACR20 response compared with 10% in the placebo group. ACR50 and 70 responses were achieved by 46% and 29% of infliximab-treated patients, compared with 0% of patients who received placebo. In addition, 68% of patients treated with infliximab achieved PASI75 at week 16 compared with 0% in the placebo group.

After week 16, all patients received infliximab 5 mg/kg IV every 8 weeks through week 50. The response was sustained in patients treated with infliximab, with continued improvement observed in articular and dermatological manifestations. A 2-year extension study involving 78 of these patients showed maintenance of the ACR20 response criteria (62%) and PASI75 score (64%) at week 98 in patients receiving infliximab [28]. In addition, radiographic progression was inhibited with a lower rate of progression noted in the infliximab group in analyses performed at week 50 [20].

The IMPACT 2 study was a larger study evaluating the efficacy and safety of infliximab in PsA [29]. This phase III, double-blind, randomized study included 200 patients with active PsA that was unresponsive to prior therapy with traditional DMARDs. Patients were treated with IV infliximab (5 mg/kg) or placebo at weeks 0, 2, 6, 14, and 22. The primary outcome measure was ACR20 at week 14, which was achieved in 58% of patients treated with infliximab compared with 11% of patients receiving placebo (P<0.001). Patients treated with infliximab had significantly improved outcomes over placebo in PsARC (77 vs 27%) and PASI75 (64 vs 2%) responses (P<0.001 for both). In addition to dermatological and articular manifestations, this study also assessed dactylitis, enthesitis, functional status, and quality of life—all of which improved in patients treated with infliximab and separated statistically from those who received placebo. The effect of treatment was maintained through week 54, with ACR20 response achieved by 58.9% in patients who were originally randomized to receive infliximab [30]. Of note, patients who were initially randomized to receive placebo but were treated with infliximab starting at week 16 or 24 also showed significant improvement, achieving an ACR20 response of 61.4% at week 54.

Table 29.1 Summary of key randomized controlled trials of TNF inhibitors in psoriatic arthritis

Patients meeting response criteria, % (weeks)						
Agent/trial name/ reference	**Study size (n)**	**ACR20**	**ACR50**	**ACR70**	**PsARC**	**PASI75**
Etanercept						
Initial study[25]	205	59 (12)	38 (12)	12 (12)	72 (12)	38 (40)
		55 (24)	40 (24)	10 (24)	70 (24)	40 (24)
Extension study[26]	169	64 (48)	44 (48)	13 (48)	84 (48)	40 (48)
Infliximab						
IMPACT2[5]	200	58 (14)	36 (14)	15 (14)	77 (14)	64 (14)
		54 (24)	41 (24)	27 (24)	70 (24)	60 (24)
Extension study[29,30]	173	59 (54)	37 (54)	22 (54)	74 (54)	50 (54)
	104	62 (98)	45 (98)	35 (98)	67 (98)	64 (98)
Adalimumab						
ADEPT[32]	315	58 (12)	36 (12)	20 (12)	62 (12)	49 (12)
		57 (24)	39 (24)	23 (24)	60 (24)	59 (24)
Extension study[33,34]	285	59 (48)	43 (48)	28 (48)	66 (48)	58 (48)
		57 (104)	45 (104)	30 (104)	63 (104)	58 (104)
Golimumab						
GO-REVEAL[23,35,36]						
50 mg	405	51 (14)	29 (14)	10 (14)	73 (14)	40 (14)
		52 (24)	33 (24)	18 (24)	70 (24)	56 (24)
	360	67 (52)	49 (52)	36 (52)	–	62 (52)
	335	67 (104)	47 (104)	29 (104)	–	63 (104)
100 mg	405	45 (14)	30 (14)	18 (14)	72 (14)	58 (14)
		61 (24)	38 (24)	22 (24)	85 (24)	66 (24)
	360	71 (52)	51 (52)	30 (52)	–	68 (52)
	335	70 (104)	51 (104)	36 (104)	–	72 (104)
Certolizumab pegol						
RAPID-PsA[37,38]	409					
200 mg	138	58 (12)	36 (12)	25 (12)	–	47 (12)
		64 (24)	44 (24)	28 (24)	78 (24)	62 (24)
		67 (48)	49 (48)	35 (48)	–	66 (48)
400 mg	135	52 (12)	33 (12)	13 (12)	–	47 (12)
		56 (24)	40 (24)	24 (24)	77 (24)	60 (24)
		66 (48)	46 (48)	30 (48)	–	62 (48)

Abbreviations: ACR20, American College of Rheumatology 20% improvement criteria; PsARC, Psoriatic Arthritis Response Criteria; PASI75, psoriasis area-and-severity index 75% reduction.

Adalimumab (Humira®)

Adalimumab is a recombinant human anti-TNF-α monoclonal antibody that binds to and inhibits both soluble and membrane-bound TNF-α. For the treatment of PsA, it is administered at a dose of 40 mg SC every 2 weeks.

The efficacy of adalimumab was initially confirmed in a 12-week randomized-controlled trial involving 100 patients who had previously had inadequate response to traditional DMARD therapy [31]. The primary outcome was ACR20 response and was achieved in 39% of patients treated with adalimumab vs 16% of patients in the placebo arm (P = 0.012). The PsARC response also separated statistically from placebo with 51% of adalimumab-treated patients achieving this secondary outcome measure compared with 24% of patients in the placebo group

(P = 0.007). Adalimumab also improved psoriatic skin lesions in these patients.

The larger phase III study of adalimumab in PsA was called the ADEPT trial, which was a 24-week, double-blind study of adalimumab versus placebo in 315 patients with PsA [32]. Adalimumab was administered at a dose of 40 mg SC every 2 weeks. At 12 weeks, 58% of adalimumab-treated patients achieved an ACR20 response compared with 14% in the placebo arm. These results were maintained at 24 weeks. There were also improvements in quality of life and inhibition of radiographic damage in adalimumab-treated patients.

In the open-label extension study of the ADEPT trial, adalimumab showed sustained efficacy in ACR 20, 50, and 70 responses at week 48 (58.7, 42.7, and 27.8%, respectively) and week 104 (57.3, 45.2, and 29.9%, respectively) [33, 34]. The percentage of patients achieving PsARC was 65.9 and 63.5% at weeks 48 and 104, respectively. Skin response was maintained with PASI75 response of 58% at both time points. There were also sustained improvements in patient reported outcome measures, as well as inhibition of radiographic progression.

Golimumab (Simponi®)

Golimumab is a human anti-TNF-α monoclonal antibody that binds to and interferes with the activity of both soluble and membrane-bound TNF-α. For the treatment of PsA, it is administered at a dose of 50 mg SC every 4 weeks.

The phase III study of golimumab in PsA was called the GO-REVEAL study, which was a large, randomized, placebo-controlled trial involving 405 patients [35]. Patients in this study received either golimumab, administered at doses of 50 or 100 mg SC every 4 weeks, or placebo. At week 14, ACR20 response was achieved by 51% of patients receiving 50 mg and 45% of patients receiving 100 mg of golimumab compared with 9% of patients in the placebo arm (P<0.001 for both). PsARC response was achieved in 73% and 72% of patients treated with 50 and 100 mg of golimumab, respectively, compared with 24% in the placebo group (P<0.001). There was also significant skin improvement with PASI75 scores achieved by 40% (50 mg) and 58% (100 mg) of golimumab-treated patients compared with 2.5% of placebo patients (P<0.001).

Further improvement was observed in all three measures at week 24 for both doses of golimumab. In addition, improvement was noted in other efficacy end points such as ACR50 and ACR70 responses, health assessment questionnaire (HAQ) score, disease activity in 28 joints using CRP (DAS28-CRP), short form (36) health survey (SF-36 score), nail disease, and enthesitis. In the long-term extension of the GO-REVEAL study, clinical improvements were sustained at weeks 52 and 104 [22, 36]. Golimumab was also noted to inhibit structural progression in radiographic analyses of the GO-REVEAL study performed at 1 year.

Certolizumab pegol (Cimzia®)

Certolizumab pegol is a pegylated humanized anti-TNF-α antigen-binding fragment (Fab'). Certolizumab neutralizes both soluble and membrane-bound TNF-α. In contrast to other TNF-α monoclonal antibodies, it lacks an Fc region and therefore does not activate antibody-dependent, cell-mediated cytotoxicity or complement-dependent cytotoxicity. It is administered at a dose of 200 mg SC every 2 weeks, or alternatively 400 mg SC every 4 weeks.

The phase III study establishing the efficacy of certolizumab in PsA was called the RAPID-PsA study [37]. This was a 24-week randomized, double-blind, placebo-controlled trial that evaluated the efficacy of certolizumab in 409 patients with PsA. Patients had previously failed at least one DMARD, and 25% of patients had previously received treatment with a TNFi. Patients receiving certolizumab were given a loading dose of 400 mg at weeks 0, 2, and 4, followed by either 200 mg SC every 2 weeks or 400 mg SC every 4 weeks. ACR20 response at week 12 was significantly greater in patients receiving certolizumab than placebo with 58.0% and 51.9% achieving this result for certolizumab 200 mg and 400 mg, respectively, compared with 24.3% of placebo patients. Of note, clinical responses among the patients previously exposed to another TNFi were comparable to those achieved by TNFi naive patients.

At 24 weeks 62.2% of patients treated with 200 mg and 60.5% of patients treated with 400 mg of certolizumab achieved PASI75 scores compared with 15.1% of patients treated with placebo (P<0.001). Further improvements were achieved in both articular and cutaneous manifestations through week 48 of the study: at week 48, ACR20, 50, and 70 responses were 66.7, 49.3, and 34.8% (200 mg) and 65.9, 45.9, and 30.4% (400 mg), respectively [38]. PASI75 scores at week 48 were achieved by 66.7 and 61.8% of patients treated with 200 and 400 mg of certolizumab, respectively. PsARC response at 24 weeks was also significantly better in patients treated with certolizumab vs placebo: 78.3% (200 mg) and 77.0% (400 mg) compared with 33.1% in the placebo group (P<0.001). Improvements were also observed with respect to nail disease, enthesitis, and dactylitis. Radiographic progression was shown to be less at weeks 24 and 48 in patients treated with certolizumab compared with those in the placebo group [39].

Safety and tolerability

In addition to its role in autoimmune disease, TNF-α plays an important role in host defence. As a result, inhibition of TNF-α potentially increases the risk of infections. However, TNFi have been well tolerated in clinical trials, with infection rates being only slightly higher than those observed with placebo. The most commonly reported adverse effects include upper respiratory tract infections, nasopharyngitis, and injection site/infusion reactions.

Malignancy and serious infections are much less common. Clinical registry data, which provides more robust evidence regarding the long-term safety of TNFi than shorter clinical trials, have revealed no increased risk of solid tumours, but a slightly more frequent occurrence of non-melanoma skin cancers [40]. Reactivation of tuberculosis has been reported with all TNFi, but is extremely infrequent. The risk can be abated with pre-treatment screening with chest radiography, tuberculin skin tests, and/or interferon gamma release assays.

Overall in PsA TNFi have had a safety profile generally similar to traditional DMARDs, while being significantly more effective in treating all domains of disease activity. They are well tolerated by most patients and may also have a favourable cost-benefit ratio [41].

Current recommendations and clinical practice guidelines

There are two major treatment guidelines in PsA, published by the Group for Research and Assessment of Psoriasis and Psoriatic Arthritis (GRAPPA) and the European League Against Rheumatism (EULAR).

GRAPPA recommendations

In 2009, GRAPPA published treatment guidelines for PsA based on evidence from a systematic literature review as well as expert opinion from rheumatologists and dermatologists [42]. They provide recommendations for five clinical domains: peripheral arthritis, axial disease, skin and nail disease, dactylitis, and enthesitis. The guidelines take into account the extent of involvement in each domain, adopting a severity grid system to help assist in clinical decision making. Revision of these guidelines is underway in 2015 and the new guidelines will shed light on the incorporation of newer agents (e.g. the anti-IL-12/23 monoclonal antibody ustekinumab, the phosphodiesterase-4 inhibitor apremilast, and the IL-17 inhibitor secukinumab) into the treatment algorithm and how comorbidities influence treatment decisions [43].

EULAR recommendations

The initial EULAR guidelines were published in 2012 and are based on a systematic literature review as well as consensus opinion [44]. They adopt an algorithmic approach and include ten recommendations for strategies to achieve optimal outcomes in PsA, with a focus on musculoskeletal manifestations, excluding skin and nail involvement. The main focus of these guidelines is peripheral arthritis in PsA. The EULAR guidelines were updated in 2015 [45].

General consensus: when to use TNF inhibitors in PsA

Despite the proven efficacy of TNFi in treating all clinical manifestations of PsA, both the GRAPPA and EULAR recommendations suggest the use of TNFi be reserved for patients with active PsA with moderate-to-severe disease (see Figure 29.1). In general, TNFi are recommended only after an inadequate response to anti-inflammatories, corticosteroids, and traditional DMARDs, although they may be used as initial therapy under certain situations, for instance in patients with poor prognostic features (e.g. high number of involved joints, structural damage, and elevated

---

Box 29.1 Minimal disease activity criteria for psoriatic arthritis

A patient is classified as having minimal disease activity (MDA) if they meet 5 of 7 of the following criteria:

1. Tender joint count ≤ 1

2. Swollen joint count ≤ 1

3. PASI score ≤ 1 or body surface area ≤3%

4. Patient pain ≤ 15mm (VAS)

5. Patient global disease activity ≤ 20mm (VAS)

6. HAQ score ≤ 0.5

7. Tender enthesitis points ≤ 1

The MDA criteria take into account several clinical domains, recognizing the heterogeneity seen in psoriatic arthritis. They have been validated in clinical trials. Abbreviations: PASI, psoriasis activity-and-severity index; VAS, visual analogue scale; HAQ, health assessment questionnaire.

Data sourced from Coates, Fransen, and Halliwell Defining minimal disease activity in psoriatic arthritis: a proposed objective target for treatment. Annals of the Rheumatic Diseases (2010) 69:48–53.

---

inflammatory markers) or relevant extra-articular manifestations (i.e. uveitis or inflammatory bowel disease). Given the lack of superiority among TNFi, the choice of which agent to use should be based on clinical manifestations, comorbidities, and patient preference.

Novel treatment concepts involving the use of TNF inhibitors

In the last decade, effective therapies and more clearly defined treatment objectives have altered the treatment paradigm in PsA. Many treatment concepts from RA have been extrapolated to PsA, despite distinct differences in disease pathogenesis, clinical manifestations, and patient populations. Evidence is now accumulating to support some of these practices in PsA patients.

Early intervention in PsA

The importance of early initiation of therapy in PsA has become increasingly accepted due to the growing recognition that PsA is a more severe disease than previously thought. Between 40% and 60% of patients experience a severe and deforming arthritis with early radiographic changes [46–48]. In a prospective study of 129 patients with early PsA treated with traditional DMARD therapy, erosive disease was detected in 47% of patients at 2 years, despite overall clinical improvement [49]. In another study, a delay as short as 6 months from symptom onset to first rheumatologic assessment was associated with the development of peripheral joint erosions and worse functional outcome in PsA [50].

The introduction of medications, most notably TNFi, that are capable of altering the disease course in PsA has made the idea of early intervention more appealing. Because the onset of skin psoriasis precedes the onset of arthritis in more than 80% of PsA patients—often by more than a decade—there is a unique opportunity in PsA to identify and treat patients with musculoskeletal manifestations early in the disease course [3, 51].

Targeted therapy in PsA

Unlike in RA, there are no validated remission criteria for PsA. The lack of a clearly defined target on which to base treatment decisions is one of the major challenges in the management of PsA. Adopting a targeted approach to treatment in PsA has become possible as a result of two recent advances:

1. Criteria for minimal disease activity (MDA) have been developed (see Box 29.1), which include measures of disease activity in a number of clinical domains, taking into account the heterogeneity seen in PsA [52]. The MDA criteria have been validated in randomized controlled trials and observational cohorts, and have also been shown to have prognostic value: patients achieving MDA for ≥12 months had a significant reduction in progression of joint damage [53, 54]. The MDA criteria are commonly considered an acceptable therapeutic target.

2. EULAR recently published treat-to-target recommendations for spondyloarthritis, which included recommendations for PsA [55]. Remission or inactive disease in all musculoskeletal domains was considered the major treatment goal of these recommendations. Where remission was not possible, low disease activity was considered an appropriate alternative. These recommendations highlight the importance of individualized

treatment goals, incorporating extra-articular manifestations and associated comorbidities into selection of therapy.

Both the MDA criteria and the EULAR recommendations are consistent with the growing consensus that optimal treatment requires achieving the least amount of activity possible in all domains of psoriatic disease [39]. They acknowledge the importance of having a pre-specified treatment objective in order to guide adjustments to therapy accordingly.

Benefits of tight control in PsA

Unlike in RA, there has been a shortage of data demonstrating the benefits of tight control in PsA. Preliminary results of the TICOPA (Tight Control of Psoriatic Arthritis) trial suggest improved outcomes with intensive treatment in newly diagnosed PsA: patients treated using a tight control strategy achieved significantly better clinical outcomes in ACR20, 50, and 70 responses (61.8, 51.2, and 38.4% vs 44.6, 25.0, and 17.4%, respectively), PASI75 (58.7% vs 33.4%, respectively), and patient-reported outcomes at week 48 compared with those in the standard care group [56, 57].

An important consideration is that patients in the tight control group experienced more adverse effects (e.g. nausea, infections, and elevated transaminases). This may be the result of overtreatment, as it has not been established if the complete absence of disease activity is necessary to prevent the progression of joint damage in PsA. Permitting low levels of disease activity may be one possibility to overcome this dilemma.

TNF inhibitor switching

Switching from one TNFi to another is a concept that has been established in RA. While the data is more limited in PsA, there is some evidence supporting the concept of switching from one TNFi to another in PsA. Clinical trial data from the RAPID-PsA study showed comparable outcomes for certolizumab in PsA patients who had been previously exposed to TNFi and those who were TNFi-naive [37].

In addition, registry data have revealed that switching TNFi can result in clinical improvement. Data from the Norwegian DMARD (NOR-DMARD) registry suggested 20–40% of patients respond to a second TNFi, although the durability of remaining on the second TNFi was shorter [58]. Data from the Danish nationwide registry of biologic therapies (DANBIO) also revealed that switching TNFi can result in clinical improvement: after 2 years, 47% of patients who had switched TNFi achieved an ACR20 response [59]. Response rates and drug survival were both lower in patients who had switched TNFi. However, because a significant proportion of patients achieve a good clinical outcome, switching TNFi should always be considered in PsA [60].

Tapering therapy in controlled disease

There is some evidence to support tapering biologic therapy in PsA, which can be performed either by reducing the dose of the agent given, or increasing the interval of administration. In a prospective study of PsA patients who had previously had a 'complete response' to adalimumab therapy, 86.6% of patients remained in remission when the interval of administration was increased from 2 to 4 weeks [61]. Success with reducing the dose of TNFi has also been observed in axial and peripheral spondyloarthropathy [62]. While patients tapering anti-TNF therapy often remain on traditional

DMARDs, this strategy may be beneficial with respect to safety concerns and the economic burden of therapies with high costs.

Clinical outcome after discontinuation of TNFi in PsA patients who have achieved remission is uncertain. In a prospective study of patients with peripheral PsA, those receiving TNFi achieved remission (defined according to ACR remission criteria) for longer periods after discontinuation of therapy than patients treated with traditional DMARDs [63]. It should be noted, however, that relapses occurred in 49% of these patients within 12 ± 2.4 months after discontinuing treatment. Despite relapse in a significant proportion of PsA patients, they remained in remission for prolonged periods of time after discontinuation of their TNFi therapy. An intermittent treatment strategy, with periods of temporary discontinuation followed by re-initiating therapy if disease recurs, is another possibility [64]. Further study is required to assess the impact of dose reduction in domains other than peripheral arthritis, and whether certain patient characteristics can predict clinical response to lower doses of therapy.

Combination therapy

In RA, the combination of methotrexate (MTX) and anti-TNF therapy has demonstrated synergistic efficacy in clinical trials [65]. In contrast, whether PsA patients might have improved outcomes with concomitant use of MTX with TNFi has not been systematically studied. Clinical trials of TNFi in PsA have typically allowed the concomitant use of stable doses of MTX in approximately half of patients. Because all patients were required to have active disease for study entry, such a study design cannot determine if there is any additive or synergistic effect of TNFi plus MTX. A study testing this is in the planning stages in 2015.

A systematic review of 14 studies examining the use of MTX in combination with TNFi noted no improvement of clinical symptoms beyond those attained by monotherapy with the anti-TNF agent [66]. Data from registries suggests there may be some benefit to concomitant MTX use in PsA patients receiving TNFi therapy. A study of PsA patients from the NOR-DMARD registry compared patients receiving TNFi monotherapy with those receiving concomitant MTX [67]. Similar outcomes were observed in both groups; however, drug survival was longer in patients receiving combination therapy. Combinations of TNFi with other traditional DMARDs and biologics have not been systematically studied in PsA.

Alternative treatment options for treatment failures

TNFi are effective in PsA, with many patients achieving a prompt and sustained response. Nevertheless, some patients have clinical manifestations that either do not respond to TNFi or achieve less of a clinical response than desired, so called 'inadequate responders'. Two effective medications have recently been approved for use in the treatment of psoriatic arthritis: ustekinumab and apremilast. Data from phase III clinical trials has shown significant improvement in PsA signs and symptoms, skin disease, enthesitis, dactylitis, and physical function for both medications [68, 69]. Ustekinumab has also demonstrated efficacy in inhibiting progression of radiographic damage [70]. There are also several IL-17 inhibitors (secukinumab, ixekizumab, and brodalumab) in advanced phase clinical trials. These agents target the T helper 17 (Th17) cell pathway preventing the synthesis of inflammatory mediators. Available data suggest significant efficacy in treating skin psoriasis and peripheral arthritis in PsA [71–76].

Box 29.2 Key points

1. There are currently five TNF inhibitors available for the treatment of psoriatic arthritis (PsA), all of which have similar efficacy and safety problems.

2. TNF inhibitors effectively treat all disease manifestations in psoriatic arthritis.

3. Evidence-based guidelines recommend the use of TNF inhibitors for the treatment of moderate-to-severe PSA, with the worst affected domain guiding the choice of therapy.

4. There is accumulating evidence for new treatment strategies involving the use of TNF inhibitors in the management of PsA:

   - Early intervention
   - Targeted therapy—minimal disease activity (MDA) criteria
   - TNF inhibitor switching
   - Tapering or discontinuing therapy in controlled disease
   - Combination therapy

5. Alternative agents for patients who fail to adequately respond to TNF inhibitors include:

   - IL-12/23 inhibitor (ustekinumab)
   - Phosphodiesterase-4 inhibitor (apremilast)
   - IL-7 inhibitors (secukinumab, ixekizumab, and brodalumab)

Conclusion

Clinical evidence reviewed here illustrates targeting TNF-α is an effective therapeutic strategy in the treatment of PsA (see Box 29.2). All five TNFi have demonstrated significant efficacy in treating signs and symptoms of PsA, as well as inhibiting radiographic progression in peripheral joints. They are safe and effective medications that have revolutionized the approach to managing PsA.

References

1. Thorlund K, Druyts E, Avina-Zumbieta JA, et al. Anti-tumour necrosis factor (TNF) drugs for the treatment of psoriatic arthritis: an indirect comparison meta-analysis. Biologics: Targets and Therapy 2012; 6: 417–27.

2. Scarpa R, Ayala F, Caporaso N, et al. Psoriasis, psoriatic arthritis, or psoriatic disease? J Rheumatol 2006; 33: 210–12.

3. Huynh DH, Kavanaugh A. Psoriatic arthritis: current therapy and future approaches. Rheumatology (Oxford) 2015; 54: 20–8.

4. Mease P. Management of psoriatic arthritis: the therapeutic interface between rheumatology and dermatology. Curr Rheumatol Rep 2006; 8: 348–54.

5. Tam LS, Kitas GD, Gonzalez-Gay MA. Can suppression of inflammation by anti-TNF prevent progression of subclinical atherosclerosis in inflammatory arthritis? Rheumatology 2014; 53: 1108–19.

6. Di Minno MN, Peluso R, Iervolino S, et al. Weight loss and achievement of minimal disease activity in patients with psoriatic arthritis starting treatment with tumor necrosis factor alpha blockers. Ann Rheum Dis 2014; 73: 1157–62.

7. Ettehadi P, Greaves MW, Wallach D, et al. Elevated tumour necrosis factor-alpha (TNF-α) biological activity in psoriatic skin lesions. Clin Exp Immunol 1994; 96: 146–51.

8. Partsch G, Steiner G, Leeb BF, et al. Highly increased levels of tumor necrosis factor-alpha and other proinflammatory cytokines in psoriatic arthritis synovial fluid. J Rheumatol 1997; 24: 518–23.

9. Ritchlin C, Haas-Smith SA, Hicks D, et al. Patterns of cytokine production in psoriatic synovium. J Rheumatol 1998; 25: 1544–52.

10. Gottlieb AB. Clinical research helps elucidate the role of tumor necrosis factor-α in the pathogenesis of T_1-mediated immune disorders: use of targeted immunotherapeutics as pathogenic probes. Lupus 2003; 12: 190–4.

11. Choy EHS, Panayi GS. Cytokine pathways and joint inflammation in rheumatoid arthritis. New Engl J Med 2001; 344: 907–16.

12. Detmar M, Brown LF, Claffey KP, et al. Overexpression of vascular permeability factor/vascular endothelial growth factor and its receptors in psoriasis. J Exp Med 1994; 180: 1141–6.

13. Gladman DD. Psoriatic arthritis. Dermatol Ther 2009; 22: 40–55.

14. Myers A, Lakey R, Cawston TE, et al. Serum MMP-1 and TIMP-1 levels are increased in patients with psoriatic arthritis and their siblings. Rheumatology 2004; 43: 272–6.

15. Ritchlin CT, Haas-Smith SA, Li P, et al. Mechanisms of TNF-α and RANKL-mediated osteoclastogenesis and bone resorption in psoriatic arthritis. J Clin Invest 2003; 111: 821–31.

16. Goedkoop A, Kraan M, Teunissen M, et al. Early effects of tumour necrosis factor α blockade on skin and synovial tissue in patients with active psoriasis and psoriatic arthritis. Ann Rheum Dis 2004; 63: 769–73.

17. Van Kuijk AWR, Gerlag DM, Vos K, et al. A prospective, randomised, placebo-controlled study to identify biomarkers associated with active treatment in psoriatic arthritis: effects of adalimumab treatment on synovial tissue. Ann Rheum Dis 2009; 68: 1303–9.

18. Chandran V, Shen H, Pollock RA, et al. Soluble biomarkers associated with response to treatment with tumor necrosis factor inhibitors in psoriatic arthritis. J Rheumatol 2013; 40: 866–71.

19. Mease PJ, Kivitz AJ, Burch FX, et al. Etanercept treatment of psoriatic arthritis: safety, efficacy, and effect on disease progression. Arthritis Rheum 2004; 50: 2264–72.

20. Kavanaugh A, Antoni CE, Gladman D, et al. The Infliximab Multinational Psoriatic Arthritis Controlled Trial (IMPACT): results of radiographic analyses after 1 year. Ann Rheum Dis 2006; 65: 1038–43.

21. Mease PJ, Ory P, Sharp JT, et al. Adalimumab for long-term treatment of psoriatic arthritis: 2-year data from the adalimumab effectiveness in psoriatic arthritis trial (ADEPT). Ann Rheum Dis 2009; 68: 702–9.

22. Kavanaugh A, van der Heijde D, McInnis IB, et al. Golimumab in psoriatic arthritis: one-year clinical efficacy, radiographic, and safety results from a phase III, randomized, placebo-controlled trial. Arthritis Rheum 2012; 64: 2504–17.

23. Van der Heijde D, Fleischmann R, Wollenhaupt J, et al. Effect of different imputation approaches on the evaluation of radiographic progression in patients with psoriatic arthritis: results of the RAPID-PsA 24-week phase III double-blind randomised placebo-controlled study of certolizumab pegol. Ann Rheum Dis 2014; 73: 233–7.

24. Mease PJ, Goffe BS, Metz J, et al. Etanercept in the treatment of psoriatic arthritis and psoriasis: a randomized trial. Lancet 2000; 356: 385–90.

25. Mease PJ, Kivitz AJ, Burch FX, et al. Continued inhibition of radiographic progression in patients with psoriatic arthritis following 2 years of treatment with etanercept. J Rheumatol 2006; 33: 712–21.

26. Mease PJ, Antoni CE, Gladman DD, et al. Psoriatic arthritis assessment tools in clinical trials. Ann Rheum Dis 2005; 64 (Suppl II): ii49–54.

27. Antoni CE, Kavanaugh A, Kirkham B, et al. Sustained benefits of infliximab therapy for dermatologic and articular manifestations of psoriatic arthritis: results from the infliximab multinational psoriatic arthritis controlled trial (IMPACT). Arthritis Rheum 2005; 52: 1227–36.

28. Antoni CE, Kavanaugh A, Van der Heidje D, et al. Two-year efficacy and safety of infliximab treatment in patients with active psoriatic arthritis: findings of the Infliximab Multinational Psoratic Arthritis Controlled Trial (IMPACT). J Rheumatol 2008; 35: 869–76.

29. Antoni C, Krueger GG, de Vlam K, et al. Infliximab improves signs and symptoms of psoriatic arthritis: results of the IMPACT 2 trial. Ann Rheum Dis 2005; 64: 1150–7.

30. Kavanaugh A, Krueger GG, Beutler A, et al. Infliximab maintains a high degree of clinical response in patients with active psoriatic arthritis through 1 year of treatment: results from the IMPACT 2 trial. Ann Rheum Dis 2007; 66: 498–505.

31. Genovese MC, Mease PJ, Thomson GT, et al. Safety and efficacy of adalimumab in treatment of patients with psoriatic arthritis who had failed disease modifying antirheumatic drug therapy. J Rheumatol 2007; 34: 1040–50.

32. Mease PJ, Gladman DD, Ritchlin CT, et al. Adalimumab for the treatment of patients with moderately to severely active psoriatic arthritis: results of a double-blind, randomized, placebo-controlled trial. Arthritis Rheum 2005; 52: 3279–89.

33. Gladman DD, Mease PJ, Ritchlin CT, et al. Adalimumab for long-term treatment of psoriatic arthritis: forty-eight week data from the adalimumab effectiveness in psoriatic arthritis trial. Arthritis Rheum 2007; 56: 476–88.

34. Mease PJ, Ory P, Sharp JT, et al. Adalimumab for long-term treatment of psoriatic arthritis: 2-year data from the Adalimumab Effectiveness in Psoriatic Arthritis Trial (ADEPT). Ann Rheum Dis 2009; 68: 702–9.

35. Kavanaugh A, McInnes I, Mease P, et al. Golimumab, a new human tumor necrosis factor alpha antibody, administered every four weeks as a subcutaneous injection in psoriatic arthritis: twenty-four-week efficacy and safety results of a randomized, placebo-controlled study. Arthritis Rheum 2009; 60: 976–86.

36. Kavanaugh A, McInnes IB, Mease PJ, et al. Clinical efficacy, radiographic and safety findings through 2 years of golimumab treatment in patients with active psoriatic arthritis: results from a long-term extension of the randomised, placebo-controlled GO-REVEAL study. Ann Rheum Dis 2013; 72: 1777–85.

37. Mease PJ, Fleischmann R, Deodhar AA, et al. Effect of certolizumab pegol on signs and symptoms in patients with psoriatic arthritis: 24-week results of a Phase 3 double-blind randomised placebo-controlled study (RAPID-PsA). Ann Rheum Dis 2014; 73: 48–55.

38. Mease PJ, Fleischmann RM, Wollenhaupt J, et al. Effect of certolizumab pegol over 48 weeks on signs and symptoms in patients with psoriatic arthritis with and without prior tumor necrosis factor inhibitor exposure. Abstract #312. Arthritis Rheum 2013; 65: (Suppl): S132.

39. Van der Heijde D, Fleischmann R, Wollenhaupt J, et al. Effect of different imputation approaches on the evaluation of radiographic progression in patients with psoriatic arthritis: results of the RAPID-PsA 24-week phase III double-blind randomised placebo-controlled study of certolizumab pegol. Ann Rheum Dis 2014; 73: 233–7.

40. Palazzi C, D'Angelo S, Leccese P, et al. Safety of anti-tumor necrosis factor agents in psoriatic arthritis—an update. Expert Opin Drug Saf 2014; 13: 191–6.

41. Olivieri I, Mantovani LG, D'Angelo S, et al. Psoriatic arthritis: pharmacoeconomic considerations. Curr Rheumatol Rep 2009; 11: 263–9.

42. Ritchlin CT, Kavanaugh A, Gladman DD, et al. Treatment recommendations for psoriatic arthritis. Ann Rheum Dis 2009; 68: 1387–94.

43. Coates LC, Kavanaugh AF, Mease PJ, et al. GRAPPA treatment recommendations: an update from the GRAPPA 2014 annual meeting and GRAPPA meeting adjacent to the 2014 ACR meeting. J Rheumatol 2015; 42: 1052–5.

44. Gossec L, Smolen JS, Gaujoux-Viala C, et al. European League Against Rheumatism recommendations for the management of psoriatic arthritis with pharmacological therapies. Ann Rheum Dis 2012; 71: 4–12.

45. Gossec L, Smolen JS, Ramiro S, et al. European League Against Rheumatism (EULAR) recommendations for the management of psoriatic arthritis with pharmacological therapies: 2015 update. Ann Rheum Dis 2016;75(3):499–510.

46. McHugh NJ, Balachrishnan C, Jones SM. Progression of peripheral joint disease in psoriatic arthritis. Rheumatology (Oxford) 2003; 42: 778–83.

47. Gladman DD, Stafford-Brady F, Chang CH, et al. Longitudinal study of clinical and radiological progression in psoriatic arthritis. J Rheumatol 1990; 17: 809–12.

48. Sokoll KB, Helliwell PS. Comparison of disability and quality of life in rheumatoid and psoriatic arthritis. J Rheumatol 2001; 28: 1842–6.

49. Kane D, Stafford L, Bresnihan B, et al. A prospective, clinical and radiological study of early psoriatic arthritis: an early synovitis clinic experience. Rheumatology 2003; 42: 1460–8.

50. Haroon M, Gallagher P, FitzGerald O. Diagnostic delay of more than 6 months contributes to poor radiographic and functional outcome in psoriatic arthritis. Ann Rheum Dis 2015; 74: 1045–50.

51. Anandarajah AP, Ritchlin CT. The diagnosis and treatment of early psoriatic arthritis. Nat Rev Rheum 2009; 5: 634–41.

52. Coates LC, Fransen J, Helliwell PS. Defining minimal disease activity in psoriatic arthritis: a proposed objective for treatment. Ann Rheum Dis 2010; 69: 48–53.

53. Coates LC, Helliwell PS. Validation of minimal disease activity for psoriatic arthritis using interventional trial data. Arthritis Care Res 2010; 62: 965–9.

54. Coates LC, Cook R, Lee KA, et al. Frequency, predictors, and prognosis of sustained minimal disease activity in an observational psoriatic arthritis cohort. Arthritis Care Res 2010; 62: 970–6.

55. Smolen JS, Braun J, Dougados M, et al. Treating spondyloarthritis, including ankylosing spondylitis and psoriatic arthritis, to target: recommendations of an international task force. Ann Rheum Dis 2014; 73: 6–16.

56. Coates LC, Moverly A, McParland L, et al. Results of a randomized control trial comparing tight control of psoriatic arthritis (TICOPA) with standard care: tight control improves outcome. ACR meeting, San Diego, 2013. Abstract 814.

57. Coates LC. Treating to target in psoriatic arthritis. Curr Opin Rheumatol 2015; 27: 107–10.

58. Fagerli K, Lie E, van der Heijde D, et al. Switching between TNF inhibitors in psoriatic arthritis: data from the NOR-DMARD study. Ann Rheum Dis 2013; 72: 1840–4.

59. Glintborg B, Ostergaard M, Krogh NS, et al. Clinical response, drug survival, and predictors thereof among 548 patients with psoriatic arthritis who switched tumor necrosis factor α inhibitor therapy: results from the Danish Nationwide DANBIO registry. Arthritis Rheum 2013; 65: 1213–23.

60. Coates LC, Cawkwell LS, Ng NWF, et al. Sustained response to long-term biologics and switching in psoriatic arthritis: results from real life experience. Ann Rheum Dis 2008; 67: 717–9.

61. Cantini F, Niccoli L, Cassara E, et al. Sustained maintenance of clinical remission after adalimumab dose reduction in patients with early psoriatic arthritis: a long-term follow-up study. Biologics 2012; 6: 201–6.

62. Olivieri I, D'Angelo S, Padula A, et al. Can we reduce the dosage of biologics in spondyloarthritis? Autoimmun Rev 2013; 12: 691–3.

63. Cantini F, Niccoli L, Nannini C, et al. Frequency and duration of clinical remission in patients with peripheral psoriatic arthritis requiring second-line drugs. Rheumatology (Oxford) 2008; 47: 872–6.

64. Tanaka Y. Intensive treatment and treatment holiday of TNF-inhibitors in rheumatoid arthritis. Curr Opin Rheumatol 2012; 24: 319–26.

65. Kavanaugh A, Cohen S, Cush J. The evolving use of TNF inhibitors in rheumatoid arthritis. J Rheumatol 2004; 31: 1881–4.

66. Daly M, Alikhan A, Armstrong AW. Combination systemic therapies in psoriatic arthritis. J Dermatol Treat 2011; 22: 276–84.

67. Fagerli KM, Lie E, van der Heijde D, et al. The role of methotrexate co-medication in TNF-inhibitor treatment in patients with psoriatic arthritis: results from 440 patients included in the NOR-DMARD study. Ann Rheum Dis 2014; 73: 132–7.

68. McInnes IB, Kavanaugh A, Gottlieb AB, et al. Efficacy and safety of ustekinumab in patients with active psoriatic arthritis: 1 year results of the phase 3, multicenter, double-blind, placebo-controlled PSUMMIT 1 trial. Lancet 2013; 382: 780–9.

69. Kavanaugh A, Mease PJ, Gomez-Reino JJ, et al. Treatment of psoriatic arthritis in a phase 3 randomised, placebo-controlled trial with apremilast, an oral phosphodiesterase 4 inhibitor. Ann Rheum Dis 2014; 73: 1020–6.

70. Kavanaugh A, Ritchlin C, Rahman P, et al. Ustekinumab, an anti-IL-12/23 p40 monoclonal antibody, inhibits radiographic progression in patients with active psoriatic arthritis: results of an integrated analysis of radiographic data from the phase 3, multicenter, randomized, double-blind, placebo-controlled PSUMMIT-1 and PSUMMIT-2 trials. Ann Rheum Dis 2014; 73: 1000–6.

71. Langley RG, Elewski BE, Lebwohl M, et al. Secukinumab in plaque psoriasis—results of two phase 3 trials. N Engl J Med 2014; 371: 326–38.

72. Leonardi C, Matheson R, Zachariae C, et al. Anti–interleukin-17 monoclonal antibody ixekizumab in chronic plaque psoriasis. N Engl J Med 2012; 366: 1190–9.

73. Papp A, Leonardi C, Menter A, et al. Brodalumab, an anti–interleukin-17-receptor antibody for psoriasis. N Engl J Med 2012; 366: 1181–9.

74. Mease P. Inhibition of interleukin-17, interleukin-23 and the TH17 cell pathway in the treatment of psoriatic arthritis and psoriasis. Curr Opin Rheumatol 2015; 27: 127–33.

75. Van Der Heijde D, Landewe R, Mease P, et al. Secukinumab, a monoclonal antibody to interleukin-17A, provides significant and sustained inhibition of structural damage in active psoriatic arthritis regardless of prior TNF inhibitors or concomitant methotrexate: a phase 3 randomized, double-blind, placebo-controlled study. Arthritis Rheum 2014; 66 (Suppl): S424. Abstract 954.

76. Mease PJ, Genovese MC, Greenwald MW, et al. Brodalumab, an anti-IL-17RA monoclonal antibody, in psoriatic arthritis. N Engl J Med 2014; 370: 2295–306.

CHAPTER 30

Biologic treatments for psoriatic arthritis apart from TNF inhibition

Philip Mease

Introduction

The introduction of the TNF inhibitors (TNFi), the first biologics used in the treatment of rheumatologic disease, in the late 1990s greatly strengthened the ability to achieve states of low disease activity or remission for conditions such as rheumatoid arthritis (RA) and the spondyloarthritides, including psoriatic arthritis (PsA). In parts of the world where these therapies are affordable, these agents have become the gold standard for management of these diseases. However, not all patients are able to achieve or maintain such satisfactory states for a variety of reasons. Some patients may have a contraindication to use of TNFi, e.g. those with multiple sclerosis, and should not have a TNFi initiated. Others may have a 'relative' contraindication, e.g. having severe congestive heart failure, lymphoma, or living or working in an area endemic for tuberculosis or invasive fungal infections, in which case the patient or physician may be reluctant to initiate TNFi therapy. A significant number of patients do not respond to TNFi therapy. Depending what one considers a desirable response, in typical clinical trials of TNFi therapy in PsA, at least 40% do not achieve an ACR 20 response, at least 60% do not achieve an ACR 50 response, and at least 80% do not achieve an ACR 70 response by 24 weeks of treatment [1]. Reasons for primary non-response include true lack of clinical effect, intolerability, and serious adverse effects. Sometimes such a 'primary' non-responder will have a response when a second TNFi is tried, but registry data suggest that achievement of a good response is not as likely in patients who have demonstrated non-response to a trial of a first TNFi. In those who do have a satisfactory response to a first TNFi, we are learning that 'survival' on the TNFi, i.e. durability of a satisfactory response, can be quite variable, ranging from months to many years. Support for this comes from observations made in clinical registries, such as the Consortium of Rheumatology Researchers of North America (Corrona) [2], and biologic registries in countries such as Norway [3] and Denmark [4]. It appears that average 'survival' of PsA patients on TNFi is in the range of 2–4 years for the first TNFi tried and shorter duration for subsequent TNFi. Reasons for loss of effect of the TNFi appear to be multifactorial. In some, intolerability or serious adverse effects may occur with time, in others, disease activity may change and increase despite the use of the TNFi, and in others, gradual loss of effect may occur. Loss of effect may be partly due development of immunogenicity to the therapeutic protein, i.e. development of an antibody response which may wholly or partly neutralize treatment effect. This has most clearly been documented with chimeric antibody constructs such as infliximab, in which the antibody response may be directed against the murine portion of the molecule [5, 6]. Neutralizing antibodies appear to be more likely to occur in monoclonal antibody constructs compared to the soluble receptor construct exemplified by etanercept [5, 6] It is known that concomitant use of methotrexate (MTX) can inhibit antibody formation against TNFi [5, 6]. Indirect evidence that immunogenicity may shorten duration of TNFi effectiveness is derived from registry studies, in which it has been demonstrated that infliximab survival is shorter in PsA when this agent is used as monotherapy vs use in combination with MTX [2, 3]. In contrast, this difference has not been noted with etanercept, potentially resulting from less immunogenicity associated with this agent [2]. In summary, many PsA patients either do not initially achieve response or they gradually lose response to TNFi, generating a need for therapies with different mechanisms of action and demonstrated ability to modify disease activity both *de novo* and post TNFi inadequate response. Furthermore, the development of therapies with different administration frequency and improved safety profile will appeal to patient and physician preference.

Targeting the Th17 cell axis in PsA

Studies conducted in the last few years have shown that IL-23, IL-17, and IL-22, key cytokines involved in the pathway of Th17 lymphocyte activation and effector activities (Figure 30.1) [7], are richly expressed in psoriatic skin lesions and the blood and synovium of PsA patients. Their roles in pathophysiology include hyperproliferation of keratinocytes, promotion of synovitis, and activation of a variety of effector cells involved in cartilage and bone destruction [8–12]. Trials of therapeutic agents which inhibit IL-23 and IL-17, elaborated below, demonstrate significant benefit in various clinical domains of psoriasis and PsA [13–15]. These agents have demonstrated effectiveness in patients naive to anti-TNF therapy as well as patients who have experienced anti-TNFs previously, with somewhat lesser efficacy in the latter group. Between the two IL-17 inhibitors that are proceeding in development, both targeting IL-17A, clinical efficacy and safety seems similar, although there have not been any head-to-head trials.

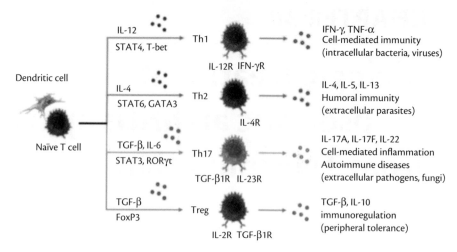

Figure 30.1 T Cell differentiation pathways.

Reproduced from Patel DD, Lee DM, Kolbinger F, et al. Effect of IL-17A blockade with secukinumab in autoimmune diseases. Ann Rheum Dis. 2013;72 Suppl 2:ii116-23 with permission from the BMJ Publishing Group.

IL-12/23 inhibition

Ustekinumab

Ustekinumab is a fully human monoclonal IgG1 antibody which binds to the common p40 subunit of IL-12 and IL-23, thus inhibiting the activity of those two cytokines and the Th1 and Th17 cell pathways which they influence. Ustekinumab is approved by the Food and Drug Administration for the treatment of psoriasis and PsA in a weight-based regimen: 45 mg for patients less than 100 kg and 90 mg for those greater than 100 kg. The drug is given subcutaneously at baseline, 4 weeks, and every 12 weeks thereafter. Efficacy in psoriasis is described in Chapter 26.

Ustekinumab was studied in two phase III trials in PsA. In PSUMMIT 1,615 patients who had inadequate response to MTX were randomized to receive 45 or 90 mg of ustekinumab vs placebo [16]. At the primary endpoint, week 24, 42.4% and 49.5% of the 45 and 90 mg treated patients achieved ACR 20 response compared to 22.8% of placebo-treated patients, which was statistically significant. Other key measures of enthesitis, dactylitis, skin and nail disease, function, and quality of life also improved. Similar rates of adverse events were noted between the groups and there were no opportunistic infections or major cardiovascular events. PSUMMIT 2 was similar in design but allowed two thirds of its subject population to have previously been treated with anti-TNF agents [17]. ACR20 response was observed in 43.7%, 43.8% and 20.2% of the 45 mg, 90 mg, and placebo treated patients in the overall population, and 36.7%, 34.5%, and 14.5% of the anti-TNF-experienced population. In a separate report in which radiographic data from the two trials was pooled, inhibition of structural damage was observed, although this benefit was driven by the MTX inadequate response population from PSUMMIT 1 rather than the subjects from PSUMMIT 2 who had been previously exposed to anti-TNF therapy [18].

IL-17 inhibition

Three IL-17 inhibitors, secukinumab, ixekizumab, and brodalumab, have been studied for the treatment of psoriasis, psoriatic arthritis, and/or ankylosing spondylitis. Secukinumab and ixekizumab are now approved for psoriasis and secukinumab for PsA and ankylosing spondylitis (AS).

Secukinumab

Secukinumab is a human monoclonal IgG1k antibody that targets IL-17A, which has recently gained Food and Drug Administration approval for psoriasis, PsA and AS. Results of psoriasis trials are reported elsewhere in this textbook.

Two phase III trials in PsA have been conducted [19, 20]. FUTURE 1 enrolled 606 patients who were randomized to an IV loading dose of secukinumab, 10 mg/kg at baseline, week 2 and 4 and then either 150 mg or 75 mg every 4 weeks from week 8 vs placebo. Thirty percent had received prior anti-TNF therapy and 60% were on concomitant methotrexate (MTX), randomized equally. At 24 weeks, the 150 mg dose arm demonstrated 50.0%, 34.7%, and 18.8% ACR 20/50/70 responses whilst the 75 mg arm demonstrated 50.5%, 30.7%, and 16.8% responses and placebo arm 17.3%, 7.4%, and 2.0% responses respectively. Key secondary measures of enthesitis, dactylitis, skin disease, radiographic evidence of inhibition of X-ray progression, function, and quality of life all separated statistically from placebo in the treatment arms compared to placebo. FUTURE 2 [20] enrolled 397 patients to receive subcutaneous secukinumab 300 mg, 150 mg, 75 mg, and placebo at weeks 1, 2, 3, 4 and every 4 weeks thereafter. Thirty-five percent had received previous anti-TNF therapy. ACR, enthesitis, dactylitis, skin, function, and quality of life responses were similar to those seen in FUTURE 1. In both studies, the two thirds of patients who had not had previous anti-TNF exposure demonstrated higher response rates than those who had previously been exposed to anti-TNF therapy. Overall serious adverse events were few and similar in frequency between the treatment and placebo arms through week 16 in both studies. In FUTURE 1, overall infection rate was slightly greater in the secukinumab arm than placebo; there were no opportunistic infections, including TB. Mild to moderate cases of cutaneous or oral candidiasis and infrequent episodes of neutropenia were noted. Both of these side-effects are felt to be related mechanistically to the inhibition of IL-17. The standard dose of secukinumab in psoriasis is 300 mg weekly for 5 weeks followed by 300 mg monthly. The dose can be lowered to 150 mg. If a PsA patient has moderate to severe psoriasis, then the usual dose is 300 mg in the same regimen as psoriasis. If the PsA patient has minimal or no psoriasis, the recommended dose is 150 mg. At the time of writing of this chapter, three year results of the FUTURE 1 trial and two year results of FUTURE 2 have been recently reported and showed sustained efficacy and no increase of adverse effects [19, 20].

Results with secukinumab in rheumatoid arthritis (RA) have not been as robust. In a phase II trial in 237 RA patients with an inadequate response to MTX, subjects receiving 25, 75, 150, and 300 mg of secukinumab demonstrated 36.0–53.7% ACR 20 response vs 34% in the placebo group; no dose arm statistically separated from placebo [21]. On the other hand, it was noted that the continuous measure, DAS28, did show statistical separation as did hs-CRP reduction. No further development of secukinumab for RA is anticipated.

Ixekizumab

Ixekizumab is an IL-17A inhibitor that has been approved for psoriasis and is in development for PsA and AS. As with secukinumab, this agent has shown a high degree of efficacy and similar safety profile in the treatment of psoriasis [22].

Phase III results through one year in PsA have recently been reported in 417 patients treated with ixekizumab 80 mg every 2 weeks or 4 weeks vs an active control arm of adalimumab every 2 weeks vs placebo [23]. At 24 weeks, ACR 20 responses were 62/58/57/30% for ixekizumab q 2 weeks/4 weeks/adalimumab/placebo; ACR 50 responses were 47/40/39/15% and ACR 70 responses were 34/23/26/6% respectively. PASI 75 responses were 80/71/54/10% respectively. Enthesitis, dactylitis, and function statistically improved with ixekizumab treatment and radiographic progression was inhibited. These results were maintained through week 52 [24]. A phase III trial in PsA patients previously treated with TNFi has not yet been reported at the time of writing of this chapter.

Ixekizumab has been studied in a phase II study in RA [25]. In this trial, 260 biologic naive and 188 patients with inadequate response to anti-TNF therapy were studied. Subcutaneous doses of 3, 10, 30, , and 180 mg of ixekizumab vs placebo were studied in the former group and 80 or 180 mg vs placebo in the latter group. At week 12 in the biologics naive group, ACR 20 responses of 45, 43, 70, 51, and 54% in the five different drug doses vs placebo response of 35%. Of these, only the 30 mg dose showed statistical significance. As was seen in the secukinumab RA study, significant response was seen in DAS28 improvement and CRP reduction. It does not appear that further development of this agent will occur in RA.

Brodalumab

Brodalumab is a human monoclonal antibody which blocks the IL-17A receptor. As in the trials of the direct IL-17A inhibitors, brodalumab has demonstrated significant efficacy in psoriasis [26].

Brodalumab was studied in a phase II study in 168 PsA patients [27]. At the 12 week primary endpoint, ACR20 response was experienced by 37 and 39% of 140 and 280 mg treated subjects vs 18% in the placebo group, statistically superior for both treatment arms. As these same patients continued into open label use of brodalumab on these same doses, ACR20 responses were observed in 51 and 64% respectively of the 140 and 280 mg treated patients. During the open label extension, two events of Grade 2 neutropenia occurred.

Brodalumab has also been studied in RA. In a phase IB ascending dose study in 40 subjects with RA, brodalumab was not more effective than placebo, a finding also demonstrated in a phase II study in RA [28, 29].

At the time of writing of this chapter, clinical trial work with brodalumab has been put on hold as a result of infrequent events of suicidal ideation and suicide noted in psoriasis clinical trials, of uncertain causal relationship.

The IL-17 inhibitors will not be studied in inflammatory bowel disease (IBD). Clinical trial experience suggests that there is no benefit for this disease and there could possibly be a signal of potential flare of IBD with IL-17 inhibition, which is a caution.

Dual TNF and IL-17 inhibitor

A novel approach to cytokine blockade is the development of antibodies which, in the same molecular platform, inhibit more than one cytokine. The concept is that such an approach may demonstrate additive or synergistic effect and be less costly than administering two different cytokine blockers simultaneously. Several dual cytokine blockers are in development and data were recently presented in PsA and RA on one of these which blocks both TNF and IL-17, known as ABT-122. In a phase II trial in 240 PsA patients, ACR 20 results at 12 weeks showed ABT-122 240 mg weekly/120 mg weekly/adalimumab 40 mg every other week/placebo results of 75/65/68/25% [30].

ACR 50 results were 53/37/38/13% and ACR 70 was demonstrated in 32/23/15/4% respectively. PASI 75 was demonstrated in 78/74/58/27% of ABT-122 240 mg/120 mg/adalimumab 40 mg/placebo respectively. Importantly, there were no serious infections in any of the treatment arms. One case of Candida infection occurred in each of the ABT-122 arms, consistent with IL-17 inhibition effect. Unlike prior trials in RA in which two different cytokine blockers were employed and serious infection rate was increased, this was not observed in this short trial. Efficacy results were superior in the ABT-122 arms of the study, particularly in the higher dose group and in psoriasis response. In a parallel study in RA, the drug was similarly safe but there was less differentiation between the effect of ABT-122 and adalimumab [31]. At the time of writing, further development of this molecule is not progressing because it was considered not to be differentiated enough from adalimumab alone. Despite this, the trial demonstrated that this novel approach to molecular development can work and be reasonably safe.

IL-23 inhibitors

IL-23 is a key cytokine involved in the differentiation and proliferation of Th17 cells, thus acting upstream from IL-17 expression and potentially capable of inhibiting the production of several different types of cytokines from Th17 cells and other immune cells, including both IL-17 and IL-22 [13, 14]. Three IL-23 inhibitors have reported results in the treatment of psoriasis, and one in PsA [15].

Guselkumab

Guselkumab is a human monoclonal antibody directed against the p19 subunit of IL-23. In a phase II study of 149 patients with PsA, 9% of whom had previously received TNFi, ACR 20/50/70 responses were seen in 58/34/14% vs 18/10/2% in the placebo group. PASI 75 responses were 79% vs 13% in guselkumab vs placebo-treated patients. Resolution of enthesitis and dactylitis were 57% and 55% in guselkumab-treated vs 29% and 17% in placebo-treated patients [32]. Further study of this agent is anticipated.

Tildrakizumab

Tildrakizumab targets the p19 subunit of IL-23. In a phase II study of 355 psoriasis patients at 12 weeks, PASI75 response was reported in 33, 64, 66, and 74% of patients receiving 5, 25, 100 and 200 mg of tildrakizumab vs 2% of patients receiving placebo in 355 patients at 12 weeks. A low rate of adverse effects was noted [33]. This agent is in development for PsA.

Risankizumab

Risankizumab is a humanized IgG1 monoclonal antibody directed against the p19 subunit of IL-23. Trials in psoriasis have shown significant efficacy, including a recent head-to-head comparison with ustekinumab, in which superiority of risankizumab was demonstrated in the 90 and 180 mg subcutaneous formulations administered at weeks 0, 4, and 16 [34]. This agent is in development for the treatment of PsA.

Co-stimulatory blockade modulating T lymphocyte function

Abatacept

Abatacept is a co-stimulatory blockade agent which inhibits T cell activation through second signal inhibition. The 'first' signal of T cell activation is the interaction between the major histocompatibility complex (MHC) and the T cell receptor (TCR). A 'second' signal is needed for full T cell activation. A number of receptor–ligand pairs act as second signals, including CD80/86 on an antigen presenting cell and CD28 on the T cell surface. The natural inhibitor of this second signal interaction is CTLA4Ig. This molecule is mimicked by abatacept, which by binding to CD80/86, inhibits CD28 binding, thus inhibiting the second signal and reducing T cell activation. Abatacept is approved for the treatment of RA. A phase II study of 170 PsA patients, using various doses of the intravenous formulation of abatacept, demonstrated significant improvement of ACR20 response [35]. Magnetic resonance imaging (MRI) study of hands or feet at 24 weeks demonstrated improved synovitis, erosion, and osteitis scores. Skin psoriasis responses were modest. A phase III study of subcutaneous abatacept in 424 PsA patients, 60% of whom had been treated with previous TNFi therapy, has been recently presented in abstract form [36]. At 24 weeks, statistically more abatacept treated than placebo treated patients (39% vs 22%) achieved ACR 20 response. Greater responses were also seen in other musculoskeletal domains with abatacept treatment; however, only modest change in psoriasis was noted.

IL-6 inhibition

Interleukin 6 (IL-6) is a pleiotropic pro-inflammatory cytokine which has a significant role in RA pathogenesis and has been demonstrated to be elevated in PsA synovitis and psoriasis skin lesions [37]. Tocilizumab, an IL-6 receptor blocker, is approved for RA. Case reports of its use in PsA have shown both positive and negative results [38].

Clazakizumab

Clazakizumab is a direct IL-6 inhibitor that has demonstrated efficacy in RA [39]. This agent was studied in a phase II trial with 165 PsA patients, 70% of whom were on background MTX [40]. ACR20 response was observed in 29/46/52/39% of patients in the placebo/25 mg/100 mg/200 mg monthly groups at the week 16 primary endpoint, which was statistically significant in the 100 mg group. PASI 75 responses were observed in 12/15/17/5% of placebo/25 mg/100 mg/200 mg groups. Improvements in enthesitis and dactylitis were most noted in the 100 mg group. The safety profile included issues expected for an IL-6 inhibiting agent, including increased risk for infection and elevation of hepatic transaminases and lipids. The demonstration of apparently greater effect in joints than skin suggests a differential role for IL-6 in the pathogenesis of synovitis as compared to psoriasis. A true dose effect was not demonstrated, given the underperformance of the highest dose group, due partly to use of non-responder imputation analysis and a greater number of adverse effects and dropouts in the higher dose group.

B lymphocyte inhibition

Rituximab, which works by ablating B lymphocytes, is approved for the treatment of RA and vasculitis. Although some B cell aggregation has been noted in PsA synovium [41, 42], B lymphocytes are not considered to be as prominent a part of the pathophysiology of PsA as RA. Small cohorts of PsA patients have been treated with rituximab [43, 44] and modest effect on arthritis but virtually no effect on skin psoriasis has been noted [45].

Conclusion

Our ability to achieve therapeutic benefit for the heterogeneous clinical aspects of PsA, including arthritis, enthesitis, dactylitis, spondylitis, and psoriasis has been significantly improved by the introduction of parenteral biologic therapies. The first introduced biologic therapies which inhibit TNFα have been able to achieve enduring states of low disease activity or remission in many, but not all patients. Further, efficacy may be lost over time due to a number of factors including issues of tolerability and safety or development of immunogenicity. Thus, it has been important to develop and test biologic agents with a different mechanism of action than TNF inhibition. Agents which have shown effectiveness in psoriasis, as well as PsA thus far tested, and have been approved for use or are in development include those which inhibit IL-12/23 (ustekinumab), IL-17 (secukinumab, ixekizumab), IL-23 (guselkumab, tildrikizumab, risankizumab), and abatacept, as well as more agents with novel mechanisms of action in the therapeutic pipeline.

References

1. Mease P. Psoriatic arthritis and spondyloarthritis assessment and management update. Curr Opin Rheumatol. 2013;25(3):287–96.
2. Mease P, Collier D, Karki N, et al. Persistence and predictors of biologic TNFi therapy among biologic naïve psoriatic arthritis patients in a US registry. Arthritis Rheum. 2014;66(S10).
3. Fagerli KM, Lie E, van der Heijde D, et al. The role of methotrexate co-medication in TNF-inhibitor treatment in patients with psoriatic arthritis: results from 440 patients included in the NOR-DMARD study. Ann Rheum Dis. 2014;73(1):132–7.
4. Jorgensen TS, Kristensen LE, Christensen R, et al. Effectiveness and drug adherence of biologic monotherapy in routine care of patients with rheumatoid arthritis: a cohort study of patients registered in the Danish biologics registry. Rheumatology (Oxford). 2015.
5. Thomas SS, Borazan N, Barroso N, et al. Comparative immunogenicity of TNF inhibitors: impact on clinical efficacy and tolerability in the

management of autoimmune diseases. A systematic review and meta-analysis. BioDrugs. 2015; 9(4):241–58.

6. Zisapel M, Zisman D, Madar-Balakirski N, et al. Prevalence of TNF-alpha blocker immunogenicity in psoriatic arthritis. J Rheumatol. 2015;42(1):73–8.

7. Patel DD, Lee DM, Kolbinger F, et al. Effect of IL-17A blockade with secukinumab in autoimmune diseases. Ann Rheum Dis. 2013;72 Suppl 2:ii116–23.

8. Frleta M, Siebert S, McInnes IB. The interleukin-17 pathway in psoriasis and psoriatic arthritis: disease pathogenesis and possibilities of treatment. Curr Rheumatol Rep. 2014;16(4):414.

9. Nestle FO, Kaplan DH, Barker J. Psoriasis. N Engl J Med. 2009;361(5):496–509.

10. Raychaudhuri SP. Role of IL-17 in psoriasis and psoriatic arthritis. Clinical reviews in allergy & immunology. 2013;44(2):183–93.

11. Jandus C, Bioley G, Rivals JP, et al. Increased numbers of circulating polyfunctional Th17 memory cells in patients with seronegative spondylarthritides. Arthritis Rheum. 2008;58(8):2307–17.

12. Suzuki E, Mellins ED, Gershwin ME, et al. The IL-23/IL-17 axis in psoriatic arthritis. Autoimmun Rev. 2014;13(4-5):496–502.

13. Tausend W, Downing C, Tyring S. Systematic review of interleukin-12, interleukin-17, and interleukin-23 pathway inhibitors for the treatment of moderate-to-severe chronic plaque psoriasis: ustekinumab, briakinumab, tildrakizumab, guselkumab, secukinumab, ixekizumab, and brodalumab. J Cutan Med Surg. 2014;18(3):156–69.

14. Leonardi CL, Gordon KB. New and emerging therapies in psoriasis. Semin Cutan Med Surg. 2014;33(2 Suppl 2):S37–41.

15. Mease PJ. Inhibition of interleukin-17, interleukin-23 and the TH17 cell pathway in the treatment of psoriatic arthritis and psoriasis. Curr Opin Rheumatol. 2015;27(2):127–33.

16. McInnes IB, Kavanaugh A, Gottlieb AB, et al. Efficacy and safety of ustekinumab in patients with active psoriatic arthritis: 1 year results of the phase 3, multicentre, double-blind, placebo-controlled PSUMMIT 1 trial. Lancet. 2013;382(9894):780–9.

17. Ritchlin C, Rahman P, Kavanaugh A, et al. Efficacy and safety of the anti-IL-12/23 p40 monoclonal antibody, ustekinumab, in patients with active psoriatic arthritis despite conventional non-biological and biological anti-tumour necrosis factor therapy: 6-month and 1-year results of the phase 3, multicentre, double-blind, placebo-controlled, randomised PSUMMIT 2 trial. Ann Rheum Dis. 2014;73(6):990–9.

18. Kavanaugh A, Ritchlin C, Rahman P, et al. Ustekinumab, an anti-IL-12/23 p40 monoclonal antibody, inhibits radiographic progression in patients with active psoriatic arthritis: results of an integrated analysis of radiographic data from the phase 3, multicentre, randomised, double-blind, placebo-controlled PSUMMIT-1 and PSUMMIT-2 trials. Ann Rheum Dis. 2014;73(6):1000–6.

19. Mease PJ, McInnes IB, Kirkham B, et al. Secukinumab inhibition of interleukin-17A in patients with psoriatic arthritis. N Engl J Med. 2015;373(14):1329–39.

20. McInnes IB, Mease PJ, Kirkham B, et al. Secukinumab, a human anti-interleukin-17A monoclonal antibody, in patients with psoriatic arthritis (FUTURE 2): a randomised, double-blind, placebo-controlled, phase 3 trial. Lancet. 2015;386(9999):1137–46.

21. Genovese MC, Durez P, Richards HB, et al. Efficacy and safety of secukinumab in patients with rheumatoid arthritis: a phase II, dose-finding, double-blind, randomised, placebo controlled study. Ann Rheum Dis. 2013;72(6):863–9.

22. Leonardi C, Matheson R, Zachariae C, et al. Anti-interleukin-17 monoclonal antibody ixekizumab in chronic plaque psoriasis. N Engl J Med. 2012;366(13):1190–9.

23. Mease PJ, van der Heijde D, Ritchlin CT, et al. Ixekizumab, an interleukin-17A specific monoclonal antibody, for the treatment of biologic-naive patients with active psoriatic arthritis: results from the 24-week randomised, double-blind, placebo-controlled and active (adalimumab)-controlled period of the phase III trial SPIRIT-P1. Ann Rheum Dis. 2017;76(1):79–87.

24. Mease P, Okada M, Kishimoto M, et al. Efficacy and safety of ixekizumab in patients with active psoriatic arthritis: 52 week results from a Phase 3 study. Arthritis Rheum. 2016 Oct;68(Supplement S10).

25. Genovese MC, Greenwald M, Cho CS, et al. A phase II randomized study of subcutaneous ixekizumab, an anti-interleukin-17 monoclonal antibody, in rheumatoid arthritis patients who were naive to biologic agents or had an inadequate response to tumor necrosis factor inhibitors. Arthritis Rheum. 2014;66(7):1693–704.

26. Papp KA, Leonardi C, Menter A, et al. Brodalumab, an anti-interleukin-17-receptor antibody for psoriasis. N Engl J Med. 2012;366(13):1181–9.

27. Mease PJ, Genovese MC, Greenwald MW, et al. Brodalumab, an anti-IL17RA monoclonal antibody, in psoriatic arthritis. N Engl J Med. 2014;370(24):2295–306.

28. Martin DA, Churchill M, Flores-Suarez L, et al. A phase Ib multiple ascending dose study evaluating safety, pharmacokinetics, and early clinical response of brodalumab, a human anti-IL-17R antibody, in methotrexate-resistant rheumatoid arthritis. Arthritis Res Ther. 2013;15(5):R164.

29. Pavelka K, Chon Y, Newmark R, et al. A randomized, double-blind, placebo-controlled, multiple-dose study to evaluate the safety, tolerability, and efficacy of brodalumab (AMG 827) in subjects with rheumatoid arthritis and an inadequate response to methotrexate (abstract 831). Arthritis Rheum. 2012;64(S362).

30. Mease P, Genovese M, Weinblatt M, et al. Safety and efficacy of ABT-122, a TNF and IL-17–targeted dual variable domain (DVD)–Ig™, in psoriatic arthritis patients with inadequate response to methotrexate: Results from a phase 2 trial. Arthritis Rheum. 2016 Oct;68(Supplement S10).

31. Genovese M, Weinblatt M, Aelion JA, et al. ABT-122, a TNF– and IL-17–targeted dual variable domain (DVD)–Ig™ in rheumatoid arthritis patients with inadequate response to methotrexate: results from a phase 2 trial. Arthritis Rheum. 2016 Oct;68(Supplement S10).

32. Deodhar A, Gottlieb A, Boehncke WH, et al. Efficacy and safety results of guselkumab, an anti-IL23 monoclonal antibody, in patients with active psoriatic arthritis over 24 weeks: A phase 2a, randomized, double-blind, placebo-controlled study. Arthritis Rheum. 2016 Oct;68(Supplement S10).

33. Papp K, Thaci D, Reich K, et al. Tildrakizumab (MK-3222), an anti-interleukin-23p19 monoclonal antibody, improves psoriasis in a phase IIb randomized placebo-controlled trial. Br J Dermatol. 2015;173(4):930–9.

34. Papp K, Menter A, Sofen H, et al. Efficacy and safety of different dose regimens of a novel selective IL-23p19 inhibitor (BI 655066) compared with ustekinumab in patients with moderate-to-severe plaque psoriasis. 73th Annual Meeting of the American Academy of Dermatology (AAD). March 2015; Late-Breaking Research in Dermatology Forums, abstract 2586.

35. Mease P, Genovese MC, Gladstein G, et al. Abatacept in the treatment of patients with psoriatic arthritis: results of a six-month, multicenter, randomized, double-blind, placebo-controlled, phase II trial. Arthritis Rheum. 2011;63(4):939–48.

36. Mease P, Gottlieb A, Van der Heidje D, et al. Abatacept in the treatment of active psoriatic arthritis: 24-week results from a phase III study. Arthritis Rheum. 2016;68(Supplement S10).

37. Fonseca JE, Santos MJ, Canhao H, et al. Interleukin-6 as a key player in systemic inflammation and joint destruction. Autoimmun Rev. 2009;8(7):538–42.

38. Costa L, Caso F, Cantarini L, et al. Efficacy of tocilizumab in a patient with refractory psoriatic arthritis. Clin Rheumatol. 2014;33(9):1355–7.

39. Mease P, Strand V, Shalamberidze L, et al. A phase II, double-blind, randomised, placebo-controlled study of BMS945429 (ALD518) in patients with rheumatoid arthritis with an inadequate response to methotrexate. Ann Rheum Dis. 2012;71(7):1183–9.

40. Mease PJ, Gottlieb A, Berman A, et al. A phase IIb, randomized, double-blind, placebo-controlled, dose-ranging, multicenter study

to evaluate the efficacy and safety of clazakizumab, an anti-IL-6 monoclonal antibody, in adults with active psoriatic arthritis. Arthritis Rheum. 2014;66(S10).

41. Celis R, Planell N, Fernandez-Sueiro JL, et al. Synovial cytokine expression in psoriatic arthritis and associations with lymphoid neogenesis and clinical features. Arthritis Res Ther. 2012; 14(2):R93.

42. Veale D, Yanni G, Rogers S, et al. Reduced synovial membrane macrophage numbers, ELAM-1 expression, and lining layer hyperplasia in psoriatic arthritis as compared with rheumatoid arthritis. Arthritis Rheum. 1993;36(7):893–900.

43. Mease PJ. Is there a role for rituximab in the treatment of spondyloarthritis and psoriatic arthritis? J Rheumatol. 2012;39(12):2235–7.

44. Mease P, Kavanaugh A, Genovese M, et al. Rituximab in psoriatic arthritis provides modest clinical improvement and reduces expression of inflammatory biomarkers in skin lesions. Arthritis Rheum. 2010;62 (Supplement 10):S818.

45. Wendling D, Dougados M, Berenbaum F, et al. Rituximab treatment for spondyloarthritis. A nationwide series: data from the AIR registry of the French Society of Rheumatology. J Rheumatol. 2012;39(12):2327–31.

CHAPTER 31

Small molecules in the treatment of psoriatic arthritis

George E. Fragoulis and Iain B. McInnes

Introduction

Psoriatic arthritis (PsA) is a chronic inflammatory arthritis affecting approximately 0.8% of the general population and occurs in about one third of psoriasis patients [1]. PsA comprises a clinical syndrome that variously presents with skin lesions, peripheral or axial (enthesial) arthritis, dactylitis, and nail lesions. The bone phenotype is distinct from other inflammatory arthropathies and includes the counterintuitive combination of erosion and new bone formation. The clinical syndrome of psoriasis and PsA is associated with clinically significant comorbidities including diabetes mellitus, cardiovascular disease, metabolic syndrome, hypertension, and psychological dysfunction [2]. Psoriasis and PsA share common pathogenetic mechanisms (Chapter 4). Briefly, upon a predisposed genetic background, including polymorphisms within and beyond the HLA complex [3], IFNα produced by plasmatocytoid dendritic cells (pDC) promotes Th1 and Th17 responses. Resident skin and synovial tissue cells, as well as osteoblasts and osteoclasts, thereafter combine with immune cell subsets to promote the lesions that comprise the histopathological features of psoriasis and PsA. Although psoriatic disease was initially thought to be only Th1 mediated, with IFNγ and TNFα being the main players [4], evidence emerging over the last decade has clearly demonstrated that the IL-23/-17 axis is in fact pivotal in disease pathogenesis.

Current treatment landscape

Treatment of PsA entails use of a variety of distinct therapeutics generally applied cognizant of the severity and tissue profile (i.e. skin, nail, entheseal, axial or peripheral joint involvement) of the disease. For mild PsA cases, non-steroidal anti-inflammatory drugs (NSAIDs) and glucocorticosteroids (intra-articular/intra-muscular, and rarely per-os) are a rational approach. The rheumatologists' armamentarium thereafter employs in the first instance non-biological disease-modifying antirheumatic drug (nbDMARDs; methotrexate, leflunomide, cyclosporine, and sulphasalazine) [5, 6]. Upon failure of DMARDs, anti-TNF treatment is generally considered the first choice option, whereupon the newly introduced anti-IL-17 and anti-IL-12/23 regimens also represent a reasonable therapeutic modality. In highly resistant cases, combination of anti-TNF and anti-IL-17 treatment may be employed [7]. Many variables confound the foregoing approach. For example, in axial disease anti-TNF treatment may be the first option prior to nbDMARDs, while in patients with severe skin involvement anti-IL-17 or 12/23 therapy may be deemed more appropriate as an early therapeutic choice.

Anti-TNF regimens occupy prime utility in most treatment algorithms for PsA e.g. 2015 EULAR Guidelines [5], although some limitations require mention, namely the relapse of PsA after their cessation [8], lack or loss of response over time in some patients, their relatively high cost, the increased risk of infections and/or tuberculosis reactivation, and their contraindication in patients with recent malignancy. Furthermore, despite the developing number of therapeutic options, a substantial number of psoriatic patients are *a priori*, or become, drug resistant. A recent study that included PsA patients initiated with a biologic or non-biologic DMARD showed that more than half of the starting cohort changed their treatment after a median time of 3–4 months [9].

The continuously emerging new discoveries in the field of psoriatic disease have provided several novel therapeutic molecular targets at the subcellular level. Herein, we describe small molecules interfering with the pathogenetic cascade (Figure 31.1) that are in the market or being assessed in clinical trials for psoriasis/PsA (Table 31.1). This chapter will complement those that define the success of biologics that target IL-12/23p40 and IL-17A that have mediated significant benefit in PsA.

Molecules approved or in phase III trials in PsA

Apremilast

Cyclic AMP (cAMP) is a critical intracellular mediator that regulates the inflammatory response [10]. Its production is defined by the equilibrium formed by the activity of adenylcyclases forming cAMP, upon their activation through G-protein coupled receptors and phosphodiesterases (PDE), that degrade cAMP to AMP [11]. There are 11 families of PDE and their expression is not only tissue specific but they are also located in different cellular compartments. PDE4 is the most specific enzyme isoform for hydrolyzing cAMP [12, 13] and has four different isotypes (A, B, C, and D) and more than 20 different isoforms [14]. It is primarily expressed in immune cells and in cell types involved in the pathogenesis of psoriasis and psoriatic arthritis such as keratinocytes, endothelial cells, and synovial cells rendering it an attractive therapeutic target. Apremilast is a small molecule that inhibits specifically PDE4, without exhibiting selectivity among PDE4 isotypes [15], leading to an increase of cAMP and subsequent activation of

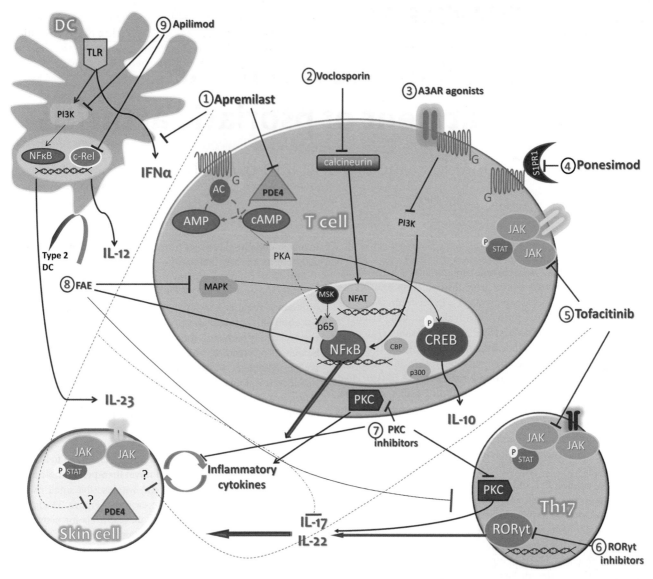

Figure 31.1 Mechanism of action of small molecules approved or investigated for the treatment of psoriasis and/or psoriatic arthritis, at a glance. 1. Apremilast inhibits PDE4, leading to the increase of cAMP, that further activates PKA. The latter activates CREB and hinders the NFκB pathway. Apremilast also reduces IFNα production by DCs and IL-17 production by Th-17 cells. 2. Voclosporin is a calcineurin inhibitor, modulating the transcription factor NFAT. 3. A3AR agonists act through the adenosine A3 receptor and suppress the PI3K-mediated activation of NFκB. 4. Ponesimod induces the internalization and degradation of S1PR1 hindering lymphocytes circulation. 5. Tofacitinib blocks signal transduction through the JAK/STAT pathway, triggered by the binding of several cytokines to their receptors. 6. RORγt inhibitors are thought to block RORγt, a key transcription factor for IL-23/IL-17 axis. 7. PKC inhibitors block PKC, thus suppressing the production of inflammatory cytokines from T cells and skin resident cells as well as IL-17 from Th17 cells. 8. FAE inhibit the translocation of or deactivate NFκB, through MSK, skew DC to type 2 subtype (see text), reduce IL-17 and IL-22 expression. 9. Apilimod: suppresses the synthesis of IL-12/23, preventing the translocation of transcription factor c-Rel and inhibiting a PI3Kinase activated via TLR pathway.

protein kinase A. The latter can interfere with the transcriptional activity of NFκB (nuclear factor kappa-light-chain-enhancer of activated B cells), inhibiting its p65 subunit by modifying the C-terminal region [16] and also phosphorylating the cAMP responsive element binding protein (CREB). The latter can in turn, recruit and sequester various cofactors that function as players in the NFκB activation pathway (e.g. p300, CREB binding protein), [17] thereby inhibiting the expression of several inflammatory cytokines and chemokines (TNFa, IFNg, IL-12, IL-23, CXCL9, CXCL10) [10] and also serving as a transcription factor for anti-inflammatory protein gene expression (e.g. IL-10).

PDE4 is implicated in arthritis processes *in vivo* and *in vitro*. In collagen type-II induced arthritis in mice, apremilast was found to improve arthritis signs, maintaining a healthy joint architecture, in a dose-dependent manner. Moreover, in a mouse model in which NK cells from psoriasis patients were xenografted in normal skin [18], the drug ameliorated clinical and histopathological features of psoriasis decreasing the expression of TNFα and of antigen-presenting and adhesion molecules in developing skin lesions. In cultured synovial cells from rheumatoid arthritis (RA) patients, apremilast inhibited the production of TNFα, IL-7, and matrix metalloproteinases [12, 19]. In psoriasis patients, it inhibited the

Table 31.1 Molecules approved or tested for the treatment of psoriasis and/or psoriatic arthritis

Molecule	Target	Phase
Apremilast (Otezla®)	Phosphodiesterase 4 (PDE4)	PS: Approved PsA: Approved
Tofacitinib (Xeljanz®)	JAK3, JAK1 > JAK2	PS: Phase III PsA: Phase III
Ponesimod	S1P1-receptor	PS: Phase II PsA: NA
Voclosporin	Calcineurin	PS: Phase III PsA: NA
Fumaric Acid Esters (Fumaderm®)	Inhibiting translocation of NFκB DCs type 2 generation MAPK/MSK pathway	PS: Phase III PsA: Phase II
Apilimod	c-Rel PI3K: PIKfyve	PS: Phase II PsA: NA
CF101	A3AR agonists	PS: II PsA: NA
Sostaurin and other PKC inhibitors	Protein Kinase C	PS: II PsA: NA
RORγt inhibitors (SR1001, T0901317, diphenylpropanamides, digoxin, ursolic acid)	RORγt	PS: NA PsA: NA

PS: Psoriasis, PsA: Psoriatic arthritis, S1P: sphingosine-1-phosphate lysophospholipid, NA: Not applicable, DC: Dendritic cells, MAPK: Mitogen activated protein kinases, MSK: Mitogen-and stress-activated protein kinases, PI3K: Phosphoinositide 3 kinase, A3AR: A3 Adenosine receptors, PKC: Protein kinase C.

expression of pro-inflammatory cytokines and chemokines from stimulated peripheral blood monocytes (PBMCs), reduced IL-17 production from T cells, IFNα production from pDCs upon TLR9 triggering, while no effects were observed in B cells or upon immunoglobulin secretion [12, 18]. Furthermore in skin lesions, transcription of genes implicated in the IL-23/-17 axis [20] was down-regulated and the infiltration rates of T cells, myeloid DCs, natural killer cells (NK) and NK-T cells were reduced in patients' dermis and epidermis, as a result of apremilast treatment.

Apremilast is Food and Drugs Administration (FDA) and European Medicines Agency (EMA) approved for the treatment of psoriasis and psoriatic arthritis. The first trial published exploring the efficacy of apremilast in psoriasis showed promising results [21], improving psoriatic patient lesions at the histological (epidermal thickness and decreased infiltrating rates of T cells and CD11 + DCs in dermis and epidermis) and clinical (Psoriasis Area Severity Index—PASI score) level. Several Phase II studies followed [22–24]. Papp et al. conducted a multicentre placebo-controlled trial showing that apremilast was efficacious at 20 mg twice daily (bid) and 30 mg bid doses as these groups, compared to placebo, exhibited favourable results, at week 16, in PASI75, Physician's Global Assesment (PGA), 36-item short form health survey (SF-36), Dermatology Life Quality Index (DLQI), Visual Analogue Scale (VAS) pruritus score, and social and physical functioning.

PASI improvement was already there from week 2 and was generally maintained through week 24 [22–24]. In a phase III multicentre placebo-controlled study (ESTEEM1), examining the efficacy and safety profile of apremilast 30 mg bid in 844 psoriasis patients, it was demonstrated that at week 16, PASI75 was achieved by 33% of apremilast-treated patients vs 5.3% of placebo. The positive results were also evident for nail and scalp psoriasis and were generally maintained through week 52 in those who continued treatment [25]. Apremilast 30 mg bid had an acceptable safety profile. Adverse events, the most common of which were diarrhoea, nausea and nasopharyngitis, were mild to moderate and did not lead to increased rates of treatment discontinuation compared to placebo [25]. Efficacy of a topical PDE4 inhibitor (AN2728) was also examined in further phase II and phase III trials [26] (ClinicalTrails.gov—NCT01300052, NCT00759161, NCT00755196).

In PsA, a phase II multicentre placebo-controlled trial, demonstrated efficacy of apremilast (20 mg bid or 40 mg daily). At week 12, 43.5% and 35.8% of active drug recipients, respectively achieved ACR20 compared to 11.8% of placebo. Patient reported outcomes, reflecting quality of life were also found to be significantly improved in both groups [27]. It is of note that favourable results were recorded irrespective of the concomitant use of methotrexate. Up to week 24, the safety profile was acceptable [28]. Promising results were confirmed in a large clinical trial programme (PALACE) comprised of four phase III studies, with open extension up to 5 years. The studies were designed with similar protocols, thereby to examine approximately 500 patients each. PALACE 1, 2, and 3 recruited patients with prior exposure to DMARDs or biologic agents and PALACE 4 those without. PALACE 1 results have been recently published. A total of 504 patients with PsA were randomized to receive 20 mg bid, 30 mg bid apremilast or placebo. At week 16, non-responders (not improved ≥20% in swollen and tender joint counts) from the placebo group were re-randomized to receive apremilast (20 mg bid or 30 mg bid) while non-responders from the apremilast groups remained under their initial treatment. At week 16, more than one third of the patients (31.3% for 20 mg group and 39.8% for 30 mg group) reached ACR20 compared to 19% of placebo [29], with the positive results being more pronounced in the biological treatment-naive patients. Minimal clinically important differences in the HAQ-DI score were achieved only in the 30 mg group [29]. At week 24, a significantly greater percentage of both apremilast-treated groups compared to placebo, achieved ACR20, ACR50, ACR70, Maastricht Ankylosing Spondylitis Enthesitis Score (MASES) score = 0, PASI50 and PASI75 and had lower disease activity, as attested by DAS-28 (CRP), modified (Psoriatic arthritis response criteria) PsARC response, and good or moderate EULAR response. Interestingly in a post-hoc analysis of PALACE 1, it was found that at week 24, IL-8, TNFα, IL-6, MIP-1β, MCP-1, and ferritin were significantly reduced in the apremilast groups, whereas TNFα levels correlated with ACR20 response [30]. Data published in an abstract support the positive results from PALACE 1 being maintained through week 104 [31, 32].

Pooled data from PALACE 1, 2, and 3 suggest that both apremilast groups, at week 16, achieved ACR20 and PASI75 in greater proportions than placebo and exhibited significantly improved disease activity and quality of life-related indices. MASES and dactylitis score were also improved [33, 34]. All positive responses, along with work productivity and work limitations which were also already improved from week 16 maintained up to week

52 [33, 35], while data available for dactylitis and enthesitis suggest that their improvement is sustained through week 104 [36]. Of note, the MASES score was improved significantly at week 24 for apremilast 30 mg group [37]. DMARD-naive patients, treated with apremilast, examined in the PALACE 4 study had significantly increased rates of ACR20 and ACR50 responses, but not ACR70 and mean % change in the HAQ-DI index, compared to placebo at week 16 [38]. Dactylitis and MASES scores were also improved with the latter reaching statistical significance for the apremilast 30 mg group [39]. Data extracted from abstract presentations support the notion that all improvements as well as mean PASI changes remained through week 104 [40].

In general, apremilast was well tolerated with gastrointestinal symptoms being most common, followed by headache, upper respiratory tract infections, and nasopharyngitis [41]. In a pooled analysis, up to week 104 from PALACE 1, 2, and 3, published in abstract form, comprising 1,493 patients, it was suggested that apremilast offers a safe profile with mild to moderate adverse events encountered more often in the first year of the treatment course not leading to treatment discontinuation in a high number of patients [41]. Notably no increase in cardiac events, malignant neoplasms, or opportunistic infections was reported. Furthermore, through week 52, apremilast was associated with weight loss, although this was not significant (being <5% from baseline for most of the patients), did not lead to treatment discontinuation and did not associate with nausea or vomiting [42]. In PALACE 4, apremilast exhibited the same acceptable safety profile and through week 104, severity and intensity of adverse events did not change [40].

The non-selectivity of apremilast for PDE4 isotypes may be responsible for its improved tolerability compared to other PDE inhibitors, especially regarding gastrointestinal adverse events [14]. Data from the PALACE trials support the proposition that apremilast needs no adjustment for weight or body mass index. Finally, although the drug appears to be safe for patients with renal or hepatic impairment it is suggested that the dose should be 30 mg daily for patients with creatinine clearance less than 30 mg/ dl [10]. There are no data supporting monitoring with special or repeated laboratory exams, since laboratory abnormalities are infrequent and reversible [41]. From the long safety data, no cases of new or reactivated tuberculosis have been described and there is no statistical significant difference in psychiatric events between apremilast and placebo groups. However due to the complex nature of psoriatic disease and its relationship with depression and suicidal behaviour, these features should be monitored closely in the post-market surveillance and in the long-term safety data [43]. The position of apremilast, in the therapeutic algorithm of PsA remains to be defined, as there are no studies comparing the efficacy of this drug with that of methotrexate. Of interest, the co-administration of these two drugs appears to be safe [29, 44]. Clinical trials comparing apremilast with anti-TNF regimens for the treatment of psoriasis are underway (ClinicalTrials.gov—NCT01690299).

JAK/STAT inhibitors

Tofacitinib

The JAK (janus kinases) family has four members, namely JAK1, JAK2, JAK3, and tyrosine-protein kinase-2 (TYK-2) [45]. JAKs are cytoplasmic tyrosine kinases possessing two phosphate-transferring domains, one with kinase activity and another, negatively regulating the first [46]. They play a crucial role in the signal transduction of various cytokines and other molecules (e.g. GM-CSF, erythropoeitin) that bind their receptors to promote immune and physiologic functions. Activated receptors recruit JAKs which are dimerized and thereafter both autophosphorylate and phosphorylate residues within the receptor. This allows the binding of members of the signal transducer and activator of transcription (STAT) family, which are also phosphorylated by JAKs. Thereafter, activated STATs translocate to the nucleus and regulate expression of various genes encoding pro-inflammatory (including Th17-related) cytokines, and proteins related to apoptosis and cell growth. Different JAK combinations can activate diverse STATs affecting the expression of a significant number of proteins [17, 47].

Tofacitinib is an orally available inhibitor of JAK3 and JAK1 and to a lesser extent of JAK2, already approved for the treatment of RA [46]. Although the mode of action of tofacitinib in psoriatic disease is not clear, data from a murine model suggest that upon triggering of Th cells with IL-6 and IL-23 tofacitinib can inhibit the expression of Th17-related cytokines (IL-17A, IL-17F, IL-22), thereby blocking the IL-23/-17 axis. In contrast, IL-17A expression was surprisingly augmented in the presence of TGF-b [48]. JAK inhibitors, most probably are also acting via modulation of other immune cells including macrophages or NK cells [49].

After a phase I dose-escalating study showed clinical and histological improvement of psoriasis patients [50], phase II trials suggested that tofacitinib might serve as an alternative therapeutic approach in psoriasis. In 197 patients randomized to receive various doses of tofacitinib or placebo, PASI75 response was significantly higher, in all body regions [51], in all treatment groups from week 4 and was maintained through week 12. Also from week 2, many patient-reported outcomes reflecting individuals' quality of life were improved [52]. Rates of adverse events, including infections, anaemia, and neutropenia, were similar across groups [53]. Concerning haematological parameters, dose-dependent reduction in hematocrit, red blood cells, polymorphonuclear cells, eosinophils, and NK cells, and the increase of B cells were reversible and tolerable in the trials' short time period and 4 weeks after off-treatment [54, 55]. Dose-dependent alterations in lipid profile were also observed. The increase in total cholesterol, high-density lipoprotein (HDL) and low-density lipoprotein (LDL) reversed after the end of treatment. In a recently published phase III trial, including two large studies with similar protocols (OPT Pivotal 1 and OPT Pivotal 2), it was demonstrated that at week 16, groups receiving tofacitinib at doses of 5mg bid or 10 mg bid had higher responses compared to placebo (PASI75; for tofacitinib 5 mg bid, 10 mg bid, and placebo; OPT Pivotal 1: 39.9%, 59.2%, and 6.2% OPT Pivotal 2: 46.0%, 59.6%, and 11.4%) while improvement was observed from week 4, already. Moreover, at week 16, significant dose dependent improvement was seen for body surface area (BSA), DLQI, and Nail Psoriasis Severity Index (NAPSI) [56]. A phase III trial comparing tofacitinib with etanercept (twice a week) for the treatment of psoriasis, showed that at week 12, tofacitinib 10 mg bid was superior to placebo and non-inferior to etanercept while the scheme of 5 mg twice daily was inferior to etanercept (PASI75: 39.5%, 63.6%, 58.8%, 5.6% and PGA response achieved: 47.1%, 68.2%, 66.3%, 15.0% for tofacitinib 5 mg, 10 mg, etanercept, and placebo, respectively). Unfortunately, no information is provided regarding arthritis features, apart from the prevalence of PsA that was approximately 20% in all groups. Rate and severity of adverse events were similar amongst groups [57].

A further phase III trial demonstrated that withdrawal of tofacitinib treatment for 16 weeks led to disease flare in more than half of psoriasis patients. Retreatment conferred recovery in about 60% of the patients of the 10 mg bid tofacitinib group. This 'loss' of therapeutic potential, although observed with other biological treatments, cannot be easily attributed to an anti-drug antibody mechanism [58]. The safety profile of tofacitinib is still an open issue. Drug-related hyperlipidaemia appears to be reversible upon treatment discontinuation and responsive to statins, while risk of herpes zoster seems to be increased compared to that of other biologic drugs, and more pronounced in Asian populations, or in those on steroids or over 65 years of age [56, 57, 59]. Furthermore, a meta-analysis showed that although in randomized controlled trials the risk for tubercuolosis (TB) is not increased for tofacitinib-treated patients, long-term extended studies demonstrated that there was a risk for TB similar to the other biological drugs [60]. It is of note that topical application of tofacitinib as well as of ruxolitinib (JAK1 and JAK2 inhibitor) has been studied in phase II trials in psoriasis, with good efficacy and safety profile in psoriasis patients [47, 61, 62].

Several trials are underway to test the optimum dose of tofacitinib, as well as the efficacy and safety of the drug in PsA patients who previously failed or relapsed in DMARD or anti-TNF treatment (ClinicalTrials.gov—NCT01976364, NCT01519089, NCT01882439, NCT01877668). Data presented in recent abstracts of these studies, suggest that tofacitinib is effective in treating active PsA. In particular, a recent study [both active (adalimumab) and placebo controlled] which recruited biologic-naive patients, non-responders to at least one conventional DMARD, found that tofacitinib (5 mg or 10 mg, twice a day) was superior to placebo achieving primary endpoints (ACR20 and changes in HAQ score) and most of the secondary endpoints at week 12. Results were maintained until month 12 [63]. In another phase III study, PsA patients recruited were non-responders to anti-TNFs and it was shown that at week 12, tofacitinib 5 mg or 10 mg, twice a day, was superior to placebo for ACR20 and ACR50. Most of the other endpoints were also achieved at week 12, including statistically significant differences in HAQ, enthesitis, and dactylitis scores and PASI75 (PASI75 difference was not statistically significant for tofacitinib 5 mg group) [64].

The safety profile was acceptable for both studies, not adding anything to what is already known from psoriasis or RA studies [63, 64].

A newly developed JAK inhibitor with selectivity for JAK3 (ASP015K) has shown favourable results with an acceptable safety profile in psoriasis patients in a phase II study [65]. The efficacy of this regimen in RA is also being currently tested (ClinicalTrials. gov—NCT01554696, NCT01565655, NCT01649999).

Bariticinib is an oral inhibitor of JAK1 and JAK2. In a phase II, placebo-controlled, dose-ranging trial, exploring the effects of baricitinib in plaque psoriasis patients it was found that at week 12, patients received 8 mg or 10 mg per day achieved PASI75 in significantly higher rates compared to placebo. Also, the 4 mg and 10 mg groups had improved DLQI scores. At week 16 and 24, the vast majority (82% and 90%, respectively) of the responders (achieved PASI75 at week 12) sustained their response. Infection related adverse events were not higher in the baricitinib group compared to placebo, while some laboratory, reversible abnormalities were noticed [66]. Several trials for the evaluation of baricitinib in RA are currently underway (ClinicalTrials.gov—NCT01721057, NCT01885078, NCT01710358).

Fumaric acid esters

The utility of fumaric acid esters in the treatment of psoriasis has been established since the 1950s. In 1994, orally administered fumaric acid esters were approved in Germany [67] and used in some European countries; they still lack approval in the UK and the United States. Although their mode of action is largely unknown, fumarates are believed to skew Th1 (and possibly Th17) to Th2 responses, mediated by hindering the translocation of NFκB, thereby inhibiting the expression of various pro-inflammatory cytokines, and also by directly enhancing Th2 responses and by inducing generation of type II DCs which produce IL-10 instead of IL-23 and IL-12 [68, 69]. It is also believed that fumarates promote T cell apoptosis and modify the expression of adhesion molecules in leukocytes [69]. Others have proposed that dimethylfumarate (DMF), a fumaric ester acid, modulates the MAPK-p38-MSK1/2 pathway. DMF inhibits the activation of MSK1 and MSK2 leading to inactivation of several transcription factors, which mediate pro-inflammatory cytokines expression, including NFκB [70]. A recent study examining the effect of DMF in the T cell responses of psoriatic patients showed that it decreased mRNA levels of IL-17, GM-CSF, and IL-22 in patients' PBMCs and decreased IFNγ expression and IFNγ and GM-CSF secretion in cultured PBMCs from both healthy individuals and psoriatic patients [67]. Furthermore, fumarate acid ester metabolites have been found to exhibit anti-proliferative and pro-differentiative effects on human keratinocytes [71].

Studies examining the efficacy of this compound in psoriasis are limited [69, 72]. Although there is a large variation between the results reported from different investigators, it seems that fumaric esters confer some improvement in psoriatic patients. In the study of Wein et al., PASI75 was achieved at 3 months by only a minority of the 80 psoriasis patients examined, while Walker et al. found that at 12 months there was a 67.2% and 66.6% improvement in the DLQI and PASI scores, respectively and in a multicentre German study, Mrowietz et al. described an 80% reduction in mean PASI at week 16 [69, 73]. Adverse events arising from use of fumaric esters are generally mild and include gastrointestinal symptoms, flushing, reversible eosinophilia, and mild lymphopenia. Surprisingly, some cases of progressive multifocal leukoencephalopathy have been described most probably related to long lasting lymphopenia [74]. In conclusion, while fumaric esters seem to be inferior to the other available treatment regimens for psoriasis, they may serve as an adjuvant in some cases. Phase II and phase III trials are conducted or are about to start examining the efficacy of a newer formulation of dymethylfumarate (FP187) in patients with psoriasis and/or PsA (ClinicalTrials.gov—NCT01230138, NCT02475304, NCT01815723).

Molecular pathways under exploration

Ponesimod

Ponesimod is an orally administered drug, affecting the number of circulating lymphocytes. The migration of the latter from secondary lymphoid organs to the circulation and target tissues is regulated, amongst other means, by the binding of the lysophospholipid sphingosine-1-phosphate (S1P) to its G protein-coupled receptor (S1PR1) [75]. Ponesimod acts as a reversible modulator of this receptor, inducing its internalization and degradation, abolishing thereby the action of S1P and diminishing the number of circulating lymphocytes [76]. Some favourable results have been generated for ponesimod, as well as for fingolimod that offers a similar mechanism of action, in the treatment of another Th17-related disease—namely multiple sclerosis [77]. In psoriasis, a phase II, dose-ranging study was reported [78]. It was found that ponesimod was effective in chronic plaque psoriasis, manifest in benefits emerging from week 16. In the 20 mg, 40 mg ponesimod, and in placebo groups, the PASI75 and PGA scores of 0 or 1 rates, were 46.0%, 48.1%, and 13.4% and 34.1%, 33.8%, and 6.0%, respectively. The responses were generally maintained until week 28 in those patients who continued treatment.

The most common adverse events observed were dose-dependent dyspnoea and reversible increase of liver function tests, sometimes leading to treatment discontinuation. Moreover, on day 1 of drug administration decrease of heart rate was recorded, which recovered gradually after 4 hours. This was most probably due to the vagomimetic effect of the drug on cardiomyocytes [79]. Interestingly, four patients have withdrawn from the protocol due to the development of second-degree heart block [76]. Although the study was not designed for this purpose, patients who also had PsA experienced more frequently pain improvement compared to placebo [78]. From indirect comparisons only, one can note that the response rates of ponesimod-treated patients were comparable to those obtained with methotrexate treatment, higher compared to those treated with apremilast and low dose tofacitinib, but lower compared to high-dose tofacitinib and anti-TNF treatment [76]. Future studies may determine its full safety profile and reveal possible therapeutic potential for PsA. To the best of our knowledge, at this time point there is no trial ongoing.

Voclosporin

Voclosporin is a novel small molecule acting in a manner similar to ciclosporin, as a calcineurin (calcium-dependent nuclear factor of activated T-cells –NFAT- phosphatase) inhibitor. Data from pharmacodynamic studies, indicate that compared to cyclosporine, voclosporin inhibits calcineurin more completely and has a different metabolic rate, exhibiting thereby a different safety profile. The latter is reinforced from animal studies [80] and trials in humans, showing that voclosporin, indirectly compared to cyclosporine, affects to a lesser extent the glomerular filtration rate (GFR), lipid profile and arterial blood pressure of treated patients [81].

Following a phase II trial [81, 82] that showed efficacy of the drug in psoriasis patients at week 12, a phase III study was conducted—451 patients were randomized to take various doses of voclosporin, twice a day or placebo. The primary endpoint (PASI75) was achieved, at week 12, in the 0.2 mg/kg, 0.3 mg/kg, 0.4 mg/kg groups and in placebo by 16%, 25%, 47% and 4%, respectively. Response was maintained up to week 24. Quality of life was also improved at week 12, as attested by DLQI and Psoriasis Disability Index (PDI) [83]. Unfortunately, the proportion of PsA patients in this cohort and/or efficacy of voclosporin in those patients is not reported. The most frequently observed adverse events were GFR reduction, upper respiratory infection, and headache. Despite the fact that adverse event rates were comparable between patient and placebo groups, some lead to the discontinuation of treatment [84] with GFR reduction being the most common cause. Although some concerns about the methodological approach of

this trial have been expressed [85] and the efficacy of voclosporin seems not to be superior to ciclosporin, the former could be used in psoriatic disease, as indirect comparison between the two drugs and data obtained from animal studies [80, 86], suggest that the former displays a better safety profile than the latter. Results from a phase III trial comparing the efficacy of voclosporin and ciclosporin in plaque psoriasis patients are awaited (ClinicalTrials.gov- NCT00408187).

Molecules postulated to have promise, that were tested but failed

Apilimod

Apilimod is a newly described 1,3,5-triazine derivative that is found to suppress the synthesis of IL-12 and IL-23. Initially, apilimod (STA-5326) was developed during screening for a potent IL-12 inhibitor [87]. It is believed that this compound acts through the prevention of nuclear translocation of the transcription factor c-Rel that regulates the genes for IL-12 and IL-23 subunits [88]. However, more recent data suggest that apilimod also binds to the class-III PI3 (phosphoinositide 3) kinase: PIKfyve. The latter is thought to phosphorylate PI3P (phosphatidylinositol 3-phosphate) in the TLR-pathway signalling [89], participating in the maintenance of the endosomal compartment, and in the production of IL-12/IL-23p40. In 2012, an open-label study was published from Wada et al., describing the clinical and histopathological benefits of this drug in psoriasis patients. Fifty-one individuals received various doses of the compound. At week 12, the 70 mg daily dosage group was found to promote histological improvement. In the affected skin, expression of IL-23p19, IL-12/-23p40 and of Th1 and Th17 cytokines and chemokines was reduced in contrast to increased levels of IL-10. The number of infiltrating DC and T cells was also reduced while the number of T and B cells in the periphery was increased. Clinical effects were mild. At week 12, PASI50 was 47% and PAS75 was only 13% with the restricted clinical efficacy attributed by the authors to the limited dose of 70 mg employed. Unfortunately, central nervous system related adverse effects have been described in higher doses (105 mg) [88]. Larger and well-designed trials are needed to investigate the role of apilimod in psoriasis and/or PsA while the results of a phase II trial for RA are expected (Clinicaltrials.gov—NCT00642629).

A3 adenosise receptors agonists

A3 adenosine receptor (A3AR) is the fourth member of the G-protein-coupled adenosine receptor family, after A1, A2A, and A2B receptors. Its involvement in inflammatory arthritis is supported by animal models showing increased expression of A3AR in synovial tissues as well as in PBMCs from adjuvant induced arthritis rats [90]. A3AR agonists have been also found to reduce pannus, fibrosis formation, cartilage and bone destruction, decrease the number of osteoclasts [91], down-regulate inflammatory cytokines and chemokines, and induce apoptosis of autoreactive T cells, mediated by downregulation of PI3K and subsequently NFκB [90, 92]. In humans, A3AR were found to be overexpressed in PBMCs of patients with RA, psoriasis, and Crohn's disease [90] in a manner dependent on the PI3K/Akt—NFκB pathway activated from TNFα and other inflammatory cytokines, A negative feedback loop, is thus formatted implying that A3AR overexpression is rather a result than a cause in the pathogenesis of immune-mediated diseases.

CF101, an A3AR agonist, has been tested in phase II trials for RA and psoriasis. In both diseases, it was well tolerated and although there was some improvement in clinical signs and symptoms, efficacy of this compound was much lower, indirectly compared to other available drugs. In a phase II psoriasis trial, PASI50 was achieved in only 35.3% of the CF101 treated group [92–94].

Protein kinase C inhibitors

The protein kinase C (PKC) family numbers 15 different members divided into three classes. PKCs under normal conditions are inactive in the cytoplasm. Upon cell activation they translocate to the cell membrane, phosphorylating serine and/or threonine residues [95]. A putative role of PKC in inflammatory arthritis is supported by murine models deficient in PKC that are protected from CIA and manifest impaired production of IL-17 and aberrant response of NFκB activation upon T cell receptor triggering [96–98]. PKCs have been found to play a major role in T cell biology (especially PKCα and PKCθ), mediating their activation and expansion as well as the production of inflammatory cytokines [99, 100]. Moreover, in RA and psoriasis patients, PKC blockade not only prevented the activation of T effector cells but also enhanced the suppressive capacity of T regulatory cells hindering IL-17 and IFNγ production and restoring their function [100, 101]. Interestingly, PKCδ, along with JAK1, STAT3, and STAT1 was found to be increased in T cells from synovial fluid in PsA patients [102]. Sotrastaurin, a non-selective PKC inhibitor (having stronger action for PKCθ, PKCα ,and PKCβ) [3], diminishes IL-17 and IFNγ production from skin resident T cells and reduces inflammatory cytokine production from PBMCs and keratinocytes from psoriasis patients [100, 103). Clinical trials at phase I and phase II supported the efficacy of sotrastaurin for psoriasis. However, the lack of significant benefits over current therapies in conjunction with the adverse events observed (attributed to the inhibition of PKCα leading to increased heart contractility] halted the further testing of the compound. Efforts are ongoing for the development of safer compounds in this target category [99].

Possible future targets

RORγt inhibitors

RORγt, belonging to the nuclear hormone receptor superfamily, is the key-transcription factor in the Th17 pathway. Controlled by the IL-6 and IL-23 activated STAT3 pathway ROTγt induces the expression of IL-17-related genes and skews the differentiation of T cells towards Th17 [104, 105]. In recent years, many RORγt inhibitors have been developed (benzenesulfoamide T0901317, diphenylpropanamides compounds) [106–108] or discovered (digoxin, ursolic acid) [109, 110], reflecting its potential for therapeutic targeting in IL-17 mediated diseases such as psoriasis, PsA, and multiple sclerosis. For example, a specific ligand for RORα and RORγt, namely SR1001, binds specifically to the ligand binding domains of the transcription factors, changing their conformational structure, leading thus to a decrease of their transcriptional activity. It was found that in mouse models, this agent could reduce IL-17A mRNA and protein expression in T17 cells and ameliorate the clinical presentation of experimental autoimmune encephalomyelitis. In human Th17 cells, it diminished IL-17 expression [111]. Recently, it has been shown that TMP778, an inverse agonist of RORγt, inhibited IL-17 expression from Tγδ cells in mice and ameliorated psoriasis like skin inflammation induced by imiquimod (a TLR7 agonist). In human samples, it blocked the Th17 differentiation and modulated the Th-17 gene signature and the IL-23 induced IL-17 production in PBMCs from psoriatic patients [112].

The application of RORγt inhibitors in clinical practice could be a double-edged sword. Since they block a critical modulator of the IL-23/-17 axis, they might be more effective than anti IL-17 targeted antibodies, but on the other hand, their usage may be accompanied by more adverse events. In consequence, their safety profile will be of great importance, given the similarities of ligand-binding domains of RORγt with other ligand-activated transcription factors (nuclear hormone receptors) [113].

Conclusion

Psoriatic spectrum disease produces a multifaceted clinical picture including skin manifestations, inflammatory arthritis, eye, and bowel manifestations, as well as metabolic and psychological disorders. An emerging understanding of its complex underlying molecular mechanisms led to the development of several different therapeutic molecules against subcellular targets. These small molecules may prove to be useful as an alternative to meet the unmet needs in PsA treatment. Though indirect comparisons of existing agents with anti-TNF treatment suggest they may have lower efficacy in terms of inflammatory arthritis, they could conceivably offer benefits, such as low immunogenicity, cost, and ease of route of administration, allowing their application after anti-TNF failure or where anti-TNF therapy is contraindicated. On the other hand, those agents thus far developed exhibit at least equal or better results compared to standard synthetic DMARDs, with the caveat though of potential additional adverse events as yet not fully defined by their relative early phase of development. Furthermore, some aforementioned drugs may prove efficient only against certain characteristics of the disease (e.g. skin, scalp, and nail involvement), offering thereby another weapon in the physician's arsenal for tailoring patient-orientated therapy [114].

References

1. Chandran V, Raychaudhuri SP. Geoepidemiology and environmental factors of psoriasis and psoriatic arthritis. J Autoimmun. 2010;34(3):J314–21.
2. Kimball AB, Gladman D, Gelfand JM, et al. National Psoriasis Foundation clinical consensus on psoriasis comorbidities and recommendations for screening. J Am Acad Dermatol. 2008;58(6):1031–42.
3. Mease PJ, Armstrong AW. Managing patients with psoriatic disease: the diagnosis and pharmacologic treatment of psoriatic arthritis in patients with psoriasis. Drugs. 2014;74(4):423–41.
4. Novelli L, Chimenti MS, Chiricozzi A, Perricone R. The new era for the treatment of psoriasis and psoriatic arthritis: perspectives and validated strategies. Autoimmun Rev. 2014;13(1):64–9.
5. Gossec L, Smolen JS, Ramiro S, et al. European League Against Rheumatism (EULAR) recommendations for the management of psoriatic arthritis with pharmacological therapies: 2015 update. Ann Rheum Dis. 2015 Dec 7.
6. Gossec L, Smolen JS, Gaujoux-Viala C, et al. European League Against Rheumatism recommendations for the management of psoriatic arthritis with pharmacological therapies. Ann Rheum Dis. 2012;71(1):4–12.

7. Cuchacovich R, Garcia-Valladares I, Espinoza LR. Combination biologic treatment of refractory psoriasis and psoriatic arthritis. J Rheumatol. 2012;39(1):187–93.

8. Chimenti MS, Graceffa D, Perricone R. Anti-TNFalpha discontinuation in rheumatoid and psoriatic arthritis: is it possible after disease remission? Autoimmun Rev. 2011;10(10):636–40.

9. Zhang HF, Gauthier G, Hiscock R, Curtis JR. Treatment patterns in psoriatic arthritis patients newly initiated on oral nonbiologic or biologic disease-modifying antirheumatic drugs. Arthritis Res Ther. 2014;16(4):420.

10. Abdulrahim H, Thistleton S, Adebajo AO, Shaw T, Edwards C, Wells A. Apremilast: a PDE4 inhibitor for the treatment of psoriatic arthritis. Expert Opin Pharmacother. 2015;16(7):1099–108.

11. Serezani CH, Ballinger MN, Aronoff DM, Peters-Golden M. Cyclic AMP: master regulator of innate immune cell function. Am J Respir Cell Mol Biol. 2008;39(2):127–32.

12. Schafer PH, Parton A, Capone L, et al. Apremilast is a selective PDE4 inhibitor with regulatory effects on innate immunity. Cell Signal. 2014;26(9):2016–29.

13. Conti M, Richter W, Mehats C, Livera G, Park JY, Jin C. Cyclic AMP-specific PDE4 phosphodiesterases as critical components of cyclic AMP signaling. J Biol Chem. 2003;278(8):5493–6.

14. Schafer P. Apremilast mechanism of action and application to psoriasis and psoriatic arthritis. Biochem Pharmacol. 2012;83(12):1583–90.

15. Mazur M, Karczewski J, Lodyga M, Zaba R, Adamski Z. Inhibitors of phosphodiesterase 4 (PDE 4): A new therapeutic option in the treatment of psoriasis vulgaris and psoriatic arthritis. J Dermatolog Treat. 2014; 26(4):326–8.

16. Takahashi N, Tetsuka T, Uranishi H, Okamoto T. Inhibition of the NF-kappaB transcriptional activity by protein kinase A. Eur J Biochem. 2002;269(18):4559–65.

17. Huynh D, Kavanaugh A. Psoriatic arthritis: current therapy and future approaches. Rheumatology (Oxford). 2015;54(1):20–8.

18. Schafer PH, Parton A, Gandhi AK, et al. Apremilast, a cAMP phosphodiesterase-4 inhibitor, demonstrates anti-inflammatory activity in vitro and in a model of psoriasis. Br J Pharmacol. 2010;159(4):842–55.

19. McCann FE, Palfreeman AC, Andrews M, et al. Apremilast, a novel PDE4 inhibitor, inhibits spontaneous production of tumour necrosis factor-alpha from human rheumatoid synovial cells and ameliorates experimental arthritis. Arthritis Res Ther. 2010;12(3):R107.

20. Gottlieb AB, Matheson RT, Menter A, et al. Efficacy, tolerability, and pharmacodynamics of apremilast in recalcitrant plaque psoriasis: a phase II open-label study. J Drugs Dermatol. 2013;12(8):888–97.

21. Gottlieb AB, Strober B, Krueger JG, et al. An open-label, single-arm pilot study in patients with severe plaque-type psoriasis treated with an oral anti-inflammatory agent, apremilast. Curr Med Res Opin. 2008;24(5):1529–38.

22. Papp K, Cather JC, Rosoph L, et al. Efficacy of apremilast in the treatment of moderate to severe psoriasis: a randomised controlled trial. Lancet. 2012;25:380(9843):738–46.

23. Papp KA, Kaufmann R, Thaci D, Hu C, Sutherland D, Rohane P. Efficacy and safety of apremilast in subjects with moderate to severe plaque psoriasis: results from a phase II, multicenter, randomized, double-blind, placebo-controlled, parallel-group, dose-comparison study. J Eur Acad Dermatol Venereol. 2013;27(3):e376–83.

24. Strand V, Fiorentino D, Hu C, Day RM, Stevens RM, Papp KA. Improvements in patient-reported outcomes with apremilast, an oral phosphodiesterase 4 inhibitor, in the treatment of moderate to severe psoriasis: results from a phase IIb randomized, controlled study. Health Qual Life Outcomes. 2013;11:82.

25. Papp K, Reich K, Leonardi CL, Kircik L, et al. Apremilast, an oral phosphodiesterase 4 (PDE4) inhibitor, in patients with moderate to severe plaque psoriasis: Results of a phase III, randomized, controlled trial (Efficacy and Safety Trial Evaluating the Effects of Apremilast in Psoriasis [ESTEEM] 1). J Am Acad Dermatol. 2015;73(1):37–49.

26. Gooderham M. Small molecules: an overview of emerging therapeutic options in the treatment of psoriasis. Skin Therapy Lett. 2013;18(7):1–4.

27. Strand V, Schett G, Hu C, Stevens RM. Patient-reported Health-related Quality of Life with apremilast for psoriatic arthritis: a phase II, randomized, controlled study. J Rheumatol. 2013;40(7):1158–65.

28. Schett G, Wollenhaupt J, Papp K, et al. Oral apremilast in the treatment of active psoriatic arthritis: results of a multicenter, randomized, double-blind, placebo-controlled study. Arthritis Rheum. 2012;64(10):3156–67.

29. Kavanaugh A, Mease PJ, Gomez-Reino JJ, et al. Treatment of psoriatic arthritis in a phase 3 randomised, placebo-controlled trial with apremilast, an oral phosphodiesterase 4 inhibitor. Ann Rheum Dis. 2014;73(6):1020–6.

30. Schafer PH, Chen P, Fang L, Wang A, Chopra R. The pharmacodynamic impact of apremilast, an oral phosphodiesterase 4 inhibitor, on circulating levels of inflammatory biomarkers in patients with psoriatic arthritis: substudy results from a phase III, randomized, placebo-controlled trial (PALACE 1). J Immunol Res. 2015;2015:906349.

31. Kavanaugh A, Adebajo A, Gladman D, et al. Long-term (104-week) efficacy and safety profile of apremilast, an oral phosphodiesterase 4 inhibitor, in patients with psoriatic arthritis: results from a phase III, randomised, controlled trial and open-label extension (PALACE 1). Ann Rheum Dis. 2015;74 (Suppl2):350.

32. Zhang F, Clancy Z, Li S, et al. Long-term impact of apremilast on physical function in patients with psoriatic arthritis using the HAQ-DI assessment. Ann Rheum Dis 2015;74 (Suppl 2):1168.

33. Kavanaugh A, Cutolo M, Mease P, et al. Apremilast, an oral phosphodiesterase 4 inhibitor, is associated with long-term (52-week) improvement in measures of disease activity in patients with psoriatic arthritis: results from 3 phase 3, randomized, controlled trials. Arthritis Rheumatol. 2014;66(Suppl):239.

34. Schett G, Mease P, Gladman D, et al. Apremilast, an oral phosphodiesterase 4 inhibitor, is associated with long-term (52-week) improvement in physical function in patients with psoriatic arthritis: results from three phase 3, randomized, controlled trials. Arthritis Rheumatol. 2013;65(Suppl):143.

35. Zhang F, Clancy Z, Li, S. Long-term work productivity improvement associated with apremilast, an oral phosphodiesterase 4 inhibitor, in patients with psoriatic arthritis: pooled analysis of 3 phase 3 studies. Ann Rheum Dis. 2015;74(Suppl2):866.

36. Gladman D, Kavanaugh A, Adebajo A, et al. Apremilast, an oral phosphodiesterase 4 inhibitor, is associated with long-term (104-week) improvements in enthesitis and dactylitis in patients with psoriatic arthritis: pooled results from three phase 3, randomized, controlled trials. Ann Rheum Dis. 2015;74(Suppl2): 133.

37. Gladman D, Mease P, Kavanaugh A, et al. Apremilast, An oral phosphodiesterase 4 inhibitor, is associated with long-term (52-week) improvements in enthesitis and dactylitis in patients with psoriatic arthritis: pooled results from three phase 3, randomized, controlled trials. Arthritis Rheumatol. 2013;65(Suppl).

38. Wells A, Adebajo A, Aelion J, et al. Apremilast, an oral phosphodiesterase 4 inhibitor, is associated with long-term (52-week) improvement in the signs and symptoms of psoriatic arthritis in DMARD-naive patients: results from a phase 3, randomized, controlled trial. Arthritis Rheumatol. 2014;66(suppl):680.

39. Edwards C, Aelion J, Adebajo A, et al. Apremilast, an oral phosphodiesterase 4 inhibitor, is associated with long-term (52-week) improvements in enthesitis and dactylitis in patients with psoriatic arthritis: results from a phase 3, randomized, controlled trial. Arthritis Rheumatol. 2014; 66(Suppl):694.

40. Wells A, Edwards C, Adebajo A, Kivitz A, Bird P, Shah K, et al. Long-term (104-week) efficacy and safety of apremilast monotherapy in DMARD-naïve patients with psoriatic arthritis: a phase 3, randomized, controlled trial and open-label extension (PALACE 4). Ann Rheum Dis. 2015;74(Suppl2):863.

41. Mease P, Adebajo A, Gladman D, et al. Long-term (104-week) safety profile of apremilast, an oral phosphodiesterase 4 inhibitor, in patients with psoriatic arthritis: pooled safety analysis of three phase 3, randomized, controlled trials. Ann Rheum Dis. 2015;74(Suppl2):355.

42. Mease P, Gladman D, Kavanaugh A, et al. Change in weight from baseline with apremilast, an oral phosphodiesterase 4 inhibitor: pooled results from 3 phase 3, randomized controlled trials. Arthritis Rheumatol. 2014;66(10 (Supplement)):s698.

43. Busa S, Kavanaugh A. Drug safety evaluation of apremilast for treating psoriatic arthritis. Expert Opin Drug Saf. 2015;14(6):979–85.

44. Liu Y, Zhou S, Nissel J, Wu A, Lau H, Palmisano M. The pharmacokinetic effect of coadministration of apremilast and methotrexate in individuals with rheumatoid arthritis and psoriatic arthritis. Clin Pharmacol Drug Dev. 2014;3(6):456–65.

45. Hansen RB, Kavanaugh A. Novel treatments with small molecules in psoriatic arthritis. Curr Rheumatol Rep. 2014;16(9):443.

46. Braun J, Kiltz U, Heldmann F, Baraliakos X. Emerging drugs for the treatment of axial and peripheral spondyloarthritis. Expert Opin Emerg Drugs. 2015;20(1):1–14.

47. Hsu L, Armstrong AW. JAK inhibitors: treatment efficacy and safety profile in patients with psoriasis. J Immunol Res. 2014;2014:283617.

48. Ghoreschi K, Jesson MI, Li X, et al. Modulation of innate and adaptive immune responses by tofacitinib (CP-690,550). J Immunol. 2011;186(7):4234–43.

49. Ghoreschi K, Gadina M. Jakpot! New small molecules in autoimmune and inflammatory diseases. Exp Dermatol. 2014;23(1):7–11.

50. Boy MG, Wang C, Wilkinson BE, et al. Double-blind, placebo-controlled, dose-escalation study to evaluate the pharmacologic effect of CP-690,550 in patients with psoriasis. J Invest Dermatol. 2009;129(9):2299–302.

51. Menter A, Papp KA, Tan H, Tyring S, Wolk R, Buonanno M. Efficacy of tofacitinib, an oral janus kinase inhibitor, on clinical signs of moderate-to-severe plaque psoriasis in different body regions. J Drugs Dermatol. 2014;13(3):252–6.

52. Mamolo C, Harness J, Tan H, Menter A. Tofacitinib (CP-690,550), an oral Janus kinase inhibitor, improves patient-reported outcomes in a phase 2b, randomized, double-blind, placebo-controlled study in patients with moderate-to-severe psoriasis. J Eur Acad Dermatol Venereol. 2014;28(2):192–203.

53. Papp KA, Menter A, Strober B, et al. Efficacy and safety of tofacitinib, an oral Janus kinase inhibitor, in the treatment of psoriasis: a phase 2b randomized placebo-controlled dose-ranging study. Br J Dermatol. 2012;167(3):668–77.

54. Strober B, Buonanno M, Clark JD, et al. Effect of tofacitinib, a Janus kinase inhibitor, on haematological parameters during 12 weeks of psoriasis treatment. Br J Dermatol. 2013;169(5):992–9.

55. Valenzuela F, Papp KA, Pariser D, et al. Effects of tofacitinib on lymphocyte sub-populations, CMV and EBV viral load in patients with plaque psoriasis. BMC Dermatol. 2015;15:8.

56. Papp KA, Menter MA, Abe M, et al. Tofacitinib, an oral Janus kinase inhibitor, for the treatment of chronic plaque psoriasis: results from two, randomised, placebo-controlled, phase 3 trials. Br J Dermatol. 2015; 173(4):949-61.

57. Bachelez H, van de Kerkhof PC, Strohal R, et al. Tofacitinib versus etanercept or placebo in moderate-to-severe chronic plaque psoriasis: a phase 3 randomised non-inferiority trial. Lancet. 2015;386:552–561.

58. Bissonnette R, Iversen L, Sofen H, et al. Tofacitinib withdrawal and retreatment in moderate-to-severe chronic plaque psoriasis: a randomized controlled trial. Br J Dermatol. 2015;172(5):1395–406.

59. Curtis JR, Xie F, Yun H, Bernatsky S, Winthrop KL. Real-world comparative risks of herpes virus infections in tofacitinib and biologic-treated patients with rheumatoid arthritis. Ann Rheum Dis. 2016;75(10):1843–7.

60. Souto A, Maneiro JR, Salgado E, Carmona L, Gomez-Reino JJ. Risk of tuberculosis in patients with chronic immune-mediated inflammatory diseases treated with biologics and tofacitinib: a systematic review and meta-analysis of randomized controlled trials and long-term extension studies. Rheumatology (Oxford). 2014;53(10):1872–85.

61. Ports WC, Khan S, Lan S, et al. A randomized phase 2a efficacy and safety trial of the topical Janus kinase inhibitor tofacitinib in the treatment of chronic plaque psoriasis. Br J Dermatol. 2013;169(1):137–45.

62. Punwani N, Scherle P, Flores R, et al. Preliminary clinical activity of a topical JAK1/2 inhibitor in the treatment of psoriasis. J Am Acad Dermatol. 2012;67(4):658–64.

63. Mease PJ, Hall S, FitzGerald O, et al. Efficacy and safety of tofacitinib, an oral janus kinase inhibitor, or adalimumab in patients with active psoriatic arthritis and an inadequate response to conventional synthetic Dmards: a randomized, placebo-controlled, phase 3 trial [abstract]. Arthritis Rheumatol 2016;68(suppl 10).

64. Gladman DD, Rigby W, Azevedo VF, et al. Efficacy and safety of tofacitinib, an oral janus kinase inhibitor, in patients with active psoriatic arthritis and an inadequate response to tumor necrosis factor inhibitors: opal beyond, a randomized, double blind, placebo-controlled, phase 3 trial [abstract]. Arthritis Rheumatol 2016;68(suppl 10).

65. Papp K, Pariser D, Catlin M, et al. A phase 2a randomized, double-blind, placebo-controlled, sequential dose-escalation study to evaluate the efficacy and safety of ASP015K, a novel Janus kinase inhibitor, in patients with moderate-to-severe psoriasis. Br J Dermatol. 2015;173(3):767–76.

66. Menter A, Disch D, Clemens J, Janes J, Papp K, W. M. A phase 2b trial of baricitinib, an oral JAK inhibitor, in patients with moderate to severe psoriasis. 2014;Volume 70(Suppl)(5):AB162.

67. Tahvili S, Zandieh B, Amirghofran Z. The effect of dimethyl fumarate on gene expression and the level of cytokines related to different T helper cell subsets in peripheral blood mononuclear cells of patients with psoriasis. Int J Dermatol. 2015;54(7):e254–60.

68. Ghoreschi K, Bruck J, Kellerer C, et al. Fumarates improve psoriasis and multiple sclerosis by inducing type II dendritic cells. J Exp Med. 2011;208(11):2291–303.

69. Wain EM, Darling MI, Pleass RD, Barker JN, Smith CH. Treatment of severe, recalcitrant, chronic plaque psoriasis with fumaric acid esters: a prospective study. Br J Dermatol. 2010;162(2):427–34.

70. Gesser B, Johansen C, Rasmussen MK, et al. Dimethylfumarate specifically inhibits the mitogen and stress-activated kinases 1 and 2 (MSK1/2): possible role for its anti-psoriatic effect. J Invest Dermatol. 2007;127(9):2129–37.

71. Helwa I, Patel R, Karempelis P, Kaddour-Djebbar I, Choudhary V, Bollag WB. The antipsoriatic agent monomethylfumarate has antiproliferative, prodifferentiative, and anti-inflammatory effects on keratinocytes. J Pharmacol Exp Ther. 2014;352(1):90–7.

72. Mrowietz U, Christophers E, Altmeyer P. Treatment of psoriasis with fumaric acid esters: results of a prospective multicentre study. German Multicentre Study. Br J Dermatol. 1998;138(3):456–60.

73. Walker F, Adamczyk A, Kellerer C, et al. Fumaderm(R) in daily practice for psoriasis: dosing, efficacy and quality of life. Br J Dermatol. 2014;171(5):1197–205.

74. Nieuwkamp DJ, Murk JL, van Oosten BW, et al. PML in a patient without severe lymphocytopenia receiving dimethyl fumarate. N Engl J Med. 2015;372(15):1474–6.

75. Piali L, Froidevaux S, Hess P, et al. The selective sphingosine 1-phosphate receptor 1 agonist ponesimod protects against lymphocyte-mediated tissue inflammation. J Pharmacol Exp Ther. 2011;337(2):547–56.

76. Ryan C, Menter A. Ponesimod—a future oral therapy for psoriasis? Lancet. 2014 Dec 6;384(9959):2006–8.

77. Olsson T, Boster A, Fernandez O, et al. Oral ponesimod in relapsing-remitting multiple sclerosis: a randomised phase II trial. J Neurol Neurosurg Psychiatry. 2014;85(11):1198–208.

78. Vaclavkova A, Chimenti S, Arenberger P, et al. Oral ponesimod in patients with chronic plaque psoriasis: a randomised, double-blind, placebo-controlled phase 2 trial. Lancet. 2014;384(9959):2036–45.

79. Peters SL, Alewijnse AE. Sphingosine-1-phosphate signaling in the cardiovascular system. Curr Opin Pharmacol. 2007;7(2):186–92.

80. Maksymowych WP, Jhangri GS, Aspeslet L, et al. Amelioration of accelerated collagen induced arthritis by a novel calcineurin inhibitor, ISA(TX)247. J Rheumatol. 2002;29(8):1646–52.

81. Bissonnette R, Papp K, Poulin Y, et al. A randomized, multicenter, double-blind, placebo-controlled phase 2 trial of ISA247 in patients with chronic plaque psoriasis. J Am Acad Dermatol. 2006;54(3):472–8.

82. Gupta AK, Langley RG, Lynde C, et al. ISA247: quality of life results from a phase II, randomized, placebo-controlled study. J Cutan Med Surg. 2008;12(6):268–75.

83. Kunynetz R, Carey W, Thomas R, Toth D, Trafford T, Vender R. Quality of life in plaque psoriasis patients treated with voclosporin: a Canadian phase III, randomized, multicenter, double-blind, placebo-controlled study. Eur J Dermatol. 2011;21(1):89–94.

84. Papp K, Bissonnette R, Rosoph L, et al. Efficacy of ISA247 in plaque psoriasis: a randomised, multicentre, double-blind, placebo-controlled phase III study. Lancet. 2008;371(9621):1337–42.

85. Naidoo P, Rambiritch V. Voclosporin (ISA247) for plaque psoriasis. Lancet. 2008;372(9642):888–9; author reply 9.

86. Aspeslet L, Freitag D, Trepanier D, et al. ISA(TX)247: a novel calcineurin inhibitor. Transplant Proc. 2001;33(1-2):1048–51.

87. Wada Y, Lu R, Zhou D, et al. Selective abrogation of Th1 response by STA-5326, a potent IL-12/IL-23 inhibitor. Blood. 2007;109(3):1156–64.

88. Wada Y, Cardinale I, Khatcherian A, et al. Apilimod inhibits the production of IL-12 and IL-23 and reduces dendritic cell infiltration in psoriasis. PLoS One. 2012;7(4):e35069.

89. Cai X, Xu Y, Cheung AK, Tomlinson RC, et al. PIKfyve, a class III PI kinase, is the target of the small molecular IL-12/IL-23 inhibitor apilimod and a player in Toll-like receptor signaling. Chem Biol. 2013;20(7):912–21.

90. Ochaion A, Bar-Yehuda S, Cohen S, et al. The anti-inflammatory target A(3) adenosine receptor is over-expressed in rheumatoid arthritis, psoriasis and Crohn's disease. Cell Immunol. 2009;258(2):115–22.

91. Rath-Wolfson L, Bar-Yehuda S, Madi L, et al. IB-MECA, an A3 adenosine receptor agonist prevents bone resorption in rats with adjuvant induced arthritis. Clin Exp Rheumatol. 2006;24(4):400–6.

92. David M, Akerman L, Ziv M, et al. Treatment of plaque-type psoriasis with oral CF101: data from an exploratory randomized phase 2 clinical trial. J Eur Acad Dermatol Venereol. 2012;26(3):361–7.

93. Borea PA, Varani K, Vincenzi F, et al. The A3 adenosine receptor: history and perspectives. Pharmacol Rev. 2015;67(1):74–102.

94. Silverman MH, Strand V, Markovits D, et al. Clinical evidence for utilization of the A3 adenosine receptor as a target to treat rheumatoid arthritis: data from a phase II clinical trial. J Rheumatol. 2008;35(1):41–8.

95. Wagner J, von Matt P, Faller B, et al. Structure-activity relationship and pharmacokinetic studies of sotrastaurin (AEB071), a promising novel medicine for prevention of graft rejection and treatment of psoriasis. J Med Chem. 2011;54(17):6028–39.

96. Healy AM, Izmailova E, Fitzgerald M, et al. PKC-theta-deficient mice are protected from Th1-dependent antigen-induced arthritis. J Immunol. 2006;177(3):1886–93.

97. Sun Z, Arendt CW, Ellmeier W, et al. PKC-theta is required for TCR-induced NF-kappaB activation in mature but not immature T lymphocytes. Nature. 2000;404(6776):402–7.

98. Tan SL, Zhao J, Bi C, et al. Resistance to experimental autoimmune encephalomyelitis and impaired IL-17 production in protein kinase C theta-deficient mice. J Immunol. 2006;176(5):2872–9.

99. George DM, Breinlinger EC, Friedman M, et al. Discovery of selective and orally bioavailable protein kinase Cθ (PKCθ) inhibitors from a fragment hit. J Med Chem. 2014;58(1):222–36.

100. He X, Koenen HJ, Smeets RL, et al. Targeting PKC in human T cells using sotrastaurin (AEB071) preserves regulatory T cells and prevents IL-17 production. J Invest Dermatol. 2014;134(4):975–83.

101. Zanin-Zhorov A, Ding Y, et al. Protein kinase C-theta mediates negative feedback on regulatory T cell function. Science. 2010;328(5976):372–6.

102. Fiocco U, Accordi B, Martini V, et al. JAK/STAT/PKCdelta molecular pathways in synovial fluid T lymphocytes reflect the in vivo T helper-17 expansion in psoriatic arthritis. Immunol Res. 2014;58(1):61–9.

103. Skvara H, Dawid M, Kleyn E, et al. The PKC inhibitor AEB071 may be a therapeutic option for psoriasis. J Clin Invest. 2008;118(9):3151–9.

104. Ciofani M, Madar A, Galan C, et al. A validated regulatory network for Th17 cell specification. Cell. 2012;151(2):289–303.

105. Suzuki E, Mellins ED, Gershwin ME, Nestle FO, Adamopoulos IE. The IL-23/IL-17 axis in psoriatic arthritis. Autoimmun Rev. 2014;13(4-5):496–502.

106. Huh JR, Littman DR. Small molecule inhibitors of RORgammat: targeting Th17 cells and other applications. Eur J Immunol. 2012;42(9):2232–7.

107. Khan PM, El-Gendy Bel D, Kumar N, et al. Small molecule amides as potent ROR-gamma selective modulators. Bioorg Med Chem Lett. 2013;23(2):532–6.

108. Kumar N, Solt LA, Conkright JJ, et al. The benzenesulfoamide T0901317 [N-(2,2,2-trifluoroethyl)-N-[4-[2,2,2-trifluoro-1-hydroxy-1-(trifluoromethyl)ethy l]phenyl]-benzenesulfonamide] is a novel retinoic acid receptor-related orphan receptor-alpha/gamma inverse agonist. Mol Pharmacol. 2010;77(2):228–36.

109. Huh JR, Leung MW, Huang P, et al. Digoxin and its derivatives suppress TH17 cell differentiation by antagonizing RORγt activity. Nature. 2011;472(7344):486–90.

110. Xu T, Wang X, Zhong B, Nurieva RI, Ding S, Dong C. Ursolic acid suppresses interleukin-17 (IL-17) production by selectively antagonizing the function of RORgamma t protein. J Biol Chem. 2011;286(26):22707–10.

111. Solt LA, Kumar N, Nuhant P, et al. Suppression of TH17 differentiation and autoimmunity by a synthetic ROR ligand. Nature. 2011;472(7344):491–4.

112. Skepner J, Ramesh R, Trocha M, et al. Pharmacologic inhibition of RORγt regulates Th17 signature gene expression and suppresses cutaneous inflammation in vivo. J Immunol. 2014;192(6):2564–75.

113. Isono F, Fujita-Sato S, Ito S. Inhibiting RORγt/Th17 axis for autoimmune disorders. Drug Discov Today. 2014;19(8):1205–11.

114. Felquer ML, Soriano ER. New treatment paradigms in psoriatic arthritis: an update on new therapeutics approved by the U.S. Food and Drug Administration. Curr Opin Rheumatol. 2015;27(2):99–106.

CHAPTER 32

Treatment algorithm and treat to target

Laura C. Coates, Arthur Kavanaugh, and Christopher T. Ritchlin

Treatment algorithms

Treatment of psoriatic arthritis (PsA) is a complex undertaking due to the potential heterogeneity of disease presentation and course, involvement of multiple domains in a single patient and the high prevalence of patients who develop bone damage. The evidence supporting the efficacy and safety of therapies in PsA is reviewed in detail in Chapters 26 to 31. However, in clinical practice treating physicians are eager for information on how best to use these therapies. Unfortunately the published research in this area in PsA is extremely limited.

Step up vs Step down approaches

A common differentiation between treatment strategies in rheumatoid arthritis (RA) is whether they utilize a step up or a step down approach. In a step up approach, one therapy is initiated, before moving onto additional therapies either in combination or in sequence if the initial single therapy is unsuccessful. In contrast, in the step down approach, combination therapies are prescribed and if patients achieve treatment goals these can be gradually tapered and even discontinued. In RA, a step down approach with initial intensive therapy has been shown to be beneficial both with combination standard disease-modifying antirheumatic drugs (DMARDs) and also with early use of biologics. Of note, however, possibly due to considerations including cost and potential toxicities, in clinical practice, a step up approach is followed for most RA patients. In PsA, at present there has not been comparable research investigating and comparing these various strategies. The potential benefits of early combination or aggressive treatment strategies need to be established initially in randomized controlled trials (RCT) where the overall potential benefits as well as the associated potential risks of the various treatment approaches can be elucidated.

The EULAR guidelines for the management of PsA use a step up approach and were approved by expert committee consensus [1]. They include five overarching principles for the management of PsA patients and ten specific recommendations on therapy of PsA with a related algorithm. They recommend initial use of single DMARDs, followed by a second DMARD either in series or in combination or an escalation to biologic therapy if poor prognostic markers are present. They performed a comprehensive literature review of therapies in PsA but treatment recommendations were largely based on expert opinion and consensus due to the lack of high quality studies from which relevant data could be obtained to address key clinical questions.

In particular, no PsA studies performed to date have systematically addressed whether patients should receive DMARDs prior to treatment with biologics and whether combination DMARDs are effective. In this void, many experts emphasize that treatment decisions must be individualized but influenced by markers of prognosis to influence therapeutic choices. This strategy is reinforced in the EULAR guidelines where biologics can be prescribed earlier in patients when activity in certain disease domains is unresponsive to DMARDs (e.g. enthesitis or axial disease) and in patients with peripheral arthritis who have poor prognostic markers. Given the lack of evidence for early combination therapy and the potential risk of side-effects from therapy, a step up approach probably remains the best option for most patients at this time. The poor prognostic markers of disease to stratify treatment decisions in PsA that are evidence-based include polyarticular disease, functional impairment, previous joint damage, and previous use of corticosteroids. From observational data, we know that active inflammation in joints predicts future progression of joint damage suggesting that treating inflammation effectively at an early stage could prevent damage. Unfortunately, however, there is no direct evidence to date that inclusion of these factors into any treatment strategy improves patient outcomes. Nevertheless, these risk factors remain the best indicators of a poor prognosis prompting consideration of early treatment escalation. The final key feature of the EULAR guidelines is that they recommend treating patients to a 'target' which is assessed every 3–6 months. This target is remission or at least low disease activity but no specific guidance is provided regarding specific outcomes and cut offs [1].

Does early treatment improve outcome?

Evidence indicates that the diagnosis of PsA may be delayed for a significant number of patients. Also, studies of psoriasis cohorts, for example among patients followed in dermatology offices, often identify undiagnosed PsA [2, 3]. In recent years, observational data from a number of cohorts have shown that delay in diagnosis, and subsequent delay in therapy, can negatively impact patients' outcome [4–6]. The Swedish early PsA registry examined predictors of improved disease activity outcomes at 5-year follow-up and found that a shorter duration of symptoms prior to diagnosis was one of the significant factors [4]. In the Bath cohort, Tillett et al. identified that delay in diagnosis of over 12 months was a significant predictor of functional impairment at 10 years [5]. Haroon et al. studied 283 patients with PsA and compared many outcomes for those patients with delayed diagnosis. Patients with over 6 months of symptoms prior to diagnosis were more likely to have erosive peripheral joint disease, arthritis mutilans, joint deformity, functional impairment, and sacroiliitis, and were significantly less likely to achieve a drug-free remission [6].

Given this strong observational evidence, it seems likely that early intervention with therapies could improve ultimate patient outcome. As with most questions in therapeutic strategies in PsA, this has not been directly addressed to date in RCTs or in other types of research. One study though did address this question in patients with recent onset PsA who were randomized to immediate treatment with methotrexate or to nonsteroidal anti-inflammatory drugs (NSAIDs) for 3 months and then started on methotrexate. The study was small (n=35) and open label but did not find a significant difference in outcome at 6 months. An improvement in tender and swollen joint counts was seen at 3 months in those patients taking methotrexate, but there was no significant difference in most of the outcome measures between methotrexate or NSAIDs alone at the 3-month time-point [7] and unfortunately outcomes were not assessed beyond the 6-month time-point. Therefore this study with several flaws in study design does not contradict the hypothesis that early intervention can improve outcome given that the dose of methotrexate, sample size, open label format, and observational period were not optimal for addressing the question. The only other indirect evidence of early therapy is the RESPOND trial, an open label study that randomized PsA patients to receive methotrexate 15 mg weekly with or without infliximab infusions. The study showed a significant difference between infliximab and methotrexate compared to methotrexate alone using the ACR20 at 16 weeks, but also showed very high responses in both the methotrexate alone and the methotrexate and infliximab arms [8] that were much higher than would be expected in trials of established PsA. Part of the reason for this high response rate is likely to be that the study is open label so the patients were aware that all of them were receiving therapy. Obviously one must be cautious when directly comparing these results to other methotrexate or TNF inhibitor studies, but they may suggest a better outcome with both a DMARD and a biologic in early, DMARD naive disease.

Treat to target

EULAR review of treating to target in SpA

The concept of tight control or treating to target was developed in rheumatology in RA following studies identifying the link between inflammation and damage in this condition. The pivotal study which showed the benefit of treating to target was the Tight Control of RA (TICORA) study where a significant benefit after 18 months of therapy was observed despite only using conventional DMARDs and corticosteroids. Patients in the tight control arm who continued to have a disease activity score >2.4 at their monthly visits had their DMARD therapy escalated and were given systemic or intra-articular steroids. At the end of the study, 82% of tight control patients met the EULAR good response compared to 44% of controls (P<0.0001) [9]. In addition to the TICORA study, two other large RA RCTs demonstrated a similar benefit for treating to target. The CAMERA study treated recent onset

RA with methotrexate either prescribed by rheumatologists in standard care or using a computer-generated algorithm based on disease activity [10]. In established RA, similar improvements associated with treating to target were reported in a cluster randomized Dutch study [11]. Based in part on these publications, the concept of treating to a pre-specified target was adopted into the design of many RA therapeutic trials and this approach is strongly advocated for newly diagnosed RA patients [12].

In PsA, data support a link between inflammation and damage. Analysis of the Toronto cohort demonstrated that active inflamed joints predict future joint damage, both clinically [13] and radiographically [14]. Indeed, it has been shown that inflammation in a particular joint predicts later damage within that joint in the same cohort [15]. Following the success in RA, the concept of treat to target was addressed in the spondyloarthritides (SpA). A large literature review was performed in 2011 by EULAR to identify research relevant to treat to target in SpA [16]. They were principally looking for 'strategic studies that compared a therapy steered towards a pre-specified treatment target versus a conventional non-steered approach'. However, their inclusion criteria included any study where therapy was altered based on the achievement of a pre-specified target. At the time, they were unable to identify studies in any of the SpAs, including PsA, that compared a treat to target to a conventional treatment approach. They did find a small number of studies where treatment was changed based on a pre-specified target, although they had no comparator arm. The majority of patients who were included in a treat to target format were found in three RCTs of TNF inhibitors in PsA. Three large RCTs with infliximab [17], adalimumab [18], and golimumab [19] included a plan in the study protocol for an escalation of treatment if pre-specified targets were not met. In the adalimumab and golimumab studies, this constituted an 'early escape' arm where patients at a set timepoint (12 or 16 weeks respectively), still in the double-blind portion of the study could be re-randomized to potentially increase therapy if a certain reduction in their disease activity was not met. In IMPACT 2, patients who had had no response or who had lost effect over the course of the study could increase their dose to 10 mg/kg after 38 weeks. In the infliximab and adalimumab studies, therapy was escalated for patients who did not show a 20% reduction in joint count, and in the golimumab study this reduction was 10%.

One further study looking at TNF inhibitors in PsA used an escalation in infliximab therapy (by shortening the interval between doses) if patients did not reach a 30% reduction in their active joint counts. However, this study only included 16 patients [20]. In another PsA study the efficacy of sulfasalazine was examined and doses could be increased if patients did not show a reduction of 40% in the number of active joints at 3 months [21].

Two studies examined the efficacy of infliximab in a mixture of SpA patients. In the first study by Cherouvim et al., patients with AS and PsA were treated with 3 mg/kg infliximab infusions. The patients with PsA were required to have at least three tender and three swollen joints for inclusion and response was measured as a 40% reduction in the patient global assessment of disease activity at 14 weeks. Infliximab infusions were increased to 4 weekly if this target was not met [22]. In the second study by Collantes et al., patients also had their infliximab infusions increased in frequency if they did not respond; response was defined as BASDAI<4 or normal inflammatory markers. Only two PsA patients were included in the study and both of these patients were classified as responders based on these criteria [23]; however, data on their baseline or follow-up peripheral joint activity was not available. It is possible that they could have had active PsA despite a BASDAI <4 and normal inflammatory markers.

Deciding on a target for treatment in PsA

One of the issues raised by the EULAR literature review and subsequent recommendations on treatment to target in SpA [24] was the difficulty in identifying an appropriate target. The EULAR taskforce recommended remission as the main target for all SpA with low disease activity as an alternative target [24]. Unfortunately at that time, there were no remission criteria validated in PsA and this is still the case. One of the key challenges is the heterogeneity of disease presentation in PsA and ensuring that a potential target would work for most patients. The majority of patients with PsA demonstrate disease involvement in more than one domain, with co-existent skin and musculoskeletal symptoms. However, disease activity in skin and musculoskeletal domains do not correlate at disease presentation and a differential skin and joint response to therapy is quite common particularly with agents that inhibit the IL-23-17 pathway [25, 26].

The EULAR taskforce carefully considered these issues and put forth the following recommendations. First, within the overarching principles, treatment targets should be based on a shared decision between the rheumatologist and patient, ensuring that individual patients have input in therapeutic selection. Then within the specific recommendations, the choice of target was discussed. Specifically treatment targets should be individualized according to the current clinical manifestations of the disease and validated measures of musculoskeletal disease activity (arthritis, dactylitis, enthesitis, axial disease) should be included. For PsA specifically, they also stated that cutaneous manifestations should also be considered [24].

Potential targets in PsA

The best validated criteria defining low disease activity/remission to date are the 'minimal disease activity' (MDA) criteria for PsA [27]. The MDA criteria require assessment of articular disease (a 68/66 joint count), enthesitis, skin disease (PASI or BSA), and patient reported measures (visual analogue score (VAS) for pain and global disease activity and the Health Assessment Questionnaire (HAQ)for function). These criteria do not provide a disease activity score, only the definition of a low disease state (Table 25.2). They have been validated in observational cohorts showing responsiveness to change, agreement with treatment decisions, and reduced progression of joint damage [28]. In RCT data they have been shown to differentiate between drug and placebo and correlate with other outcome measures. They also show association with radiographic outcome suggesting a prognostic value [29]. The criteria are relatively quick and feasible to perform but expressed as a binary (MDA or not) outcome and do not provide a level of disease activity or response.

The Group for Research and Assessment of Psoriasis and Psoriatic Arthritis (GRAPPA) have developed and tested a number of composite measures which answer these limitations (Table 32.1) [30, 31]. The composite psoriatic disease activity index (CPDAI) was developed by FitzGerald based on the GRAPPA grid [32] and assesses disease activity and impact in five domains: joints, skin,

Table 32.1 Multivariable logistic regression analysis for the effect of treatment on the primary endpoint and key secondary endpoints at 48 weeks post-randomisation in the TICOPA study (ITT population with multiple imputation)

Outcome measure	OR	Lower 95% CI	Upper 95% CI	P value
ACR20	1.91	1.03	3.55	0.0392
ACR50	2.36	1.25	4.47	0.0081
ACR70	2.64	1.32	5.26	0.0058
PASI75	2.92	1.51	5.65	0.0015

Data sourced from Coates, Laura C, et al. Effect of Tight Control of Inflammation in Early Psoriatic Arthritis (TICOPA): A UK Multicentre, Open-Label, Randomised, Controlled Trial. Lancet 386(10012):2489–2498.

entheses, dactylitis, and axial disease [30]. It provides a composite score of 0–15 but also allows easy identification of which domains are active. Both the psoriatic arthritis disease activity score (PASDAS) and GRAPPA Composite exercise (GRACE) index were developed as part of an international GRAPPA exercise where new composite measures were derived from over 500 sets of data. Both measures include physician and patient reported outcome measures combined into a composite index. The calculation of both indices is more complex than other measures but easily performed using a computer spreadsheet.

All three of these instruments (CPDAI, PASDAS, and GRACE) are composite disease activity measures and have proposed response levels and cut-offs for disease activity based on physician and patient opinion [33]. The cut-offs for low, moderate, and high disease activity were developed using patient and physician VAS scores as anchors and were compared with average scores of those who were having their treatment escalated and those who were not. The proposed cut-offs now give a combined response measure assessing change from baseline and absolute final score, analogous to the EULAR responses in RA. These measures are derived from patient data, provide an overall assessment of disease activity across the domains, and provide both a measure of disease activity at one timepoint and response over time. However, they do take slightly longer to perform in clinic than the MDA criteria and require a more complex calculation. This limits their feasibility in time-pressed clinics.

The other measure under development in PsA is the Disease Activity in Psoriatic Arthritis (DAPSA) [34]. This measure is identical to the disease activity in reactive arthritis (DAREA) score which was renamed as it was found to correlate with important domains in PsA patients in a principal component analysis. This includes a 68/66 joint count, patient pain, and patient global disease activity VAS and C-reactive protein. They are simply added up allowing easy calculation of the score. Potential response measures for the DAPSA were developed in the GRAPPA paper above and there has also been a recent publication looking at separate cut-offs for disease activity levels and response [35]. Unfortunately, whilst this measure is feasible to perform and easy to calculate in clinic, it only assesses articular disease and thus provides a very limited assessment of psoriatic disease manifestations. The time advantage offered by a simple articular measure is lost when additional measures of skin, enthesitis, dactylitis, and axial involvement would also be required to ensure that a proper assessment of disease activity is made.

All of these measures include a 68/66 joint count to assess arthritis. This measure was recommended for assessment of peripheral arthritis by the GRAPPA/OMERACT group as it provides a comprehensive assessment of disease [36]. Some studies, using data from RCTs of biologic therapies, have shown that reduced joint counts and their associated composite measures such as the DAS28 can perform well and be responsive to change [37, 38]. However, two caveats are important to consider regarding the use of reduced joint counts in clinical practice. First, while these studies showed that reduced joint counts were responsive to change, concerns were raised that some swollen or tender joints were not assessed. If treatment is to be tailored to a specific disease state such as remission or MDA, rather than a response such as a 50% reduction, then a full evaluation of all involved joints is key. Secondly, this observation is specific to the subset of patients that were included in the biologic studies. Most patients had joint counts of around 20 at baseline and very few oligoarthritis patients are included. When looking at reduced joint counts in oligoarthritis, a significant proportion of disease is missed by reduced joint counts [39].

The Tight Control of PsA study (TICOPA)

At the 2013 ACR Annual Meeting, the first study of treat to target in spondyloarthritis was presented and was published in 2015 [40]. This study would have met the primary search in the EULAR literature review of treat to target in SpA: 'strategic studies that compared a therapy steered towards a prespecified treatment target versus a conventional non-steered approach'. The Tight Control of Psoriatic Arthritis (TICOPA) study recruited 206 patients with recent onset PsA. They were randomized 1:1 to tight control or standard care. Patients in the tight control arm were reviewed 4-weekly by the research rheumatologists and if they did not fulfil the MDA criteria they had their treatment escalated (Figure 32.1). The study used a treatment algorithm of methotrexate, combination DMARDs, and biologics in a step up design. Patients in the standard care arm were reviewed every 12 weeks and were treated by their usual rheumatologist. There were no limitations on their care, except compliance with UK National Institute for Health and Clinical Excellence (NICE) criteria for the use of TNF inhibitors in PsA which was standard across both trial arms [41].

The primary outcome of the trial was ACR20 the odds of achieving ACR20 at 48 weeks were significantly higher in the tight control arm (OR 1.91, P=.0392) using intention to treat analysis. The odds of achieving ACR50, ACR70, and PASI75 were all significantly higher for the tight control group (see Table 32.1). If anything, it appears that the difference is more marked at more stringent levels of response (e.g. ACR70) suggesting a marked improvement in disease activity. Improvements were also seen in patient reported outcomes including physical function (HAQ) and quality of life (PsQOL), and also BASDAI and BASFI for those with axial disease.

No difference in the radiographic progression between the two arms was detected but the mean change in the modified van der Heijde-Sharp score was zero in both groups. This is in contrast to many more recent RCTs in PsA where the TNF inhibitors and other biologic agents have shown a reduction in radiographic progression compared to placebo. One of the reasons for this is that the TICOPA trial consisted of two active treatment arms and did not have a placebo. The vast majority of patients in the standard care arm, as well as the tight control arm, received active therapy with corticosteroids, DMARDs, and biologics. The other key difference is the type of PsA patients included in the TICOPA trial. The trial recruited all new PsA patients with evidence of active arthritis, enthesitis, or axial disease, and did not require a minimum joint count for inclusion. Around 30% of the patients had oligoarthritis and therefore the chances of these patients showing progression on a modified Sharp-van der Heijde score are much lower.

The tight control arm was associated with increased rates of adverse events and serious adverse events which may be due to the more rapid escalation of DMARD therapy [42]. Patients in the tight control arm received higher doses of methotrexate with all

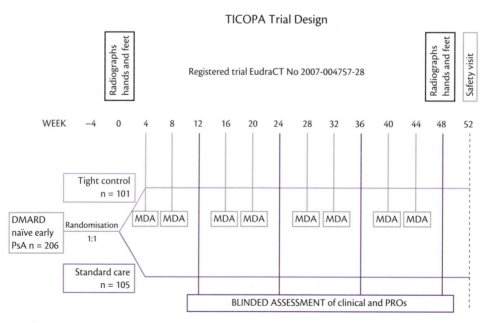

Figure 32.1 TICOPA trial design.

patients receiving at least 15 mg/week by week 12 of the study (90% received at least 20 mg/week, 82% received 25 mg/week). At the end of the study around half of the patients in the standard care group remained on monotherapy methotrexate, whilst only one quarter of those in the tight control group were on this treatment. There was a higher usage of combination DMARDs (24% vs 11%) and biologics (37% vs 7%) in the tight control arm compared to those in standard care.

A cost-effectiveness analysis was included in the TICOPA trial. The mean cost per patient in the tight control group was approximately twice that of the patients in the standard care group (£4198 vs £2000). Using mean quality-adjusted-life-years, the study found an incremental cost-effectiveness ratio of £53,948 per quality-adjusted life-year. This is significantly higher than often quoted threshold for cost per QALY of $50000 or around £30,000. The excess costs in the tight control arm were accounted for predominantly by drug costs (increased prescription of biologics) and rheumatology visit costs which were attended every 4 weeks throughout the trial period. Sensitivity analyses were performed to account for a reduction in visits once patients were consistently in MDA and did yield levels of around £30,000. As a result of this publication, the latest update of the EULAR Recommendations for the Management of PsA, presented at the 2015 EULAR meeting in Rome, have recommended that a treat to target approach is used for the management of PsA [43]. Further research is required to assess feasibility of this in practice, and the outcomes that will be seen when this is performed routinely in clinic.

What about comorbidities and other related conditions?

The potential treatment targets discussed above focus on the musculoskeletal and cutaneous manifestations of PsA but for many patients the disease has significant ramifications in other systems. As part of the spondyloarthritis family, patients with PsA are known to have an increased risk of having concomitant uveitis and inflammatory bowel disease. These manifestations clearly fall outside of the composite measures introduced so far. However, when considering therapy for an individual patient, activity in these domains is likely to impact on drug choice and may drive therapeutic escalation if the disease activity is severe in these areas. The EULAR recommendations for treat to target in SpA reinforce this stating that extra-articular manifestations should be considered. These manifestations may also require input from outside the rheumatology and dermatology specialities. Although not evidence-based, the potential importance of a multi-disciplinary approach appears clear to help ensure optimal treatment for the patient. Given that biologic therapies, such as the TNF inhibitors, may impact these comorbidities, careful selection of a drug that could treat both core PsA domains as well as these other related diseases should be considered.

Other key comorbidities seen in PsA are also likely to influence treatment options. In a cohort of patients with established PsA, 44% had metabolic syndrome [44] and both metabolic syndrome and insulin resistance were associated with PsA disease severity. Whilst it is thought that the inflammation seen in psoriasis and PsA is driving the development of insulin resistance and endothelial dysfunction [45], no evidence is available to support the concept that aggressive treatment of inflammation can impact the progression

of metabolic disorders also referred to as the 'psoriatic march' [45]. To further complicate matters, elements of the metabolic syndrome can complicate the selection of PsA treatments and impact their efficacy and safety.

The use of corticosteroids for the rapid control of inflammation in PsA, even if given intra-articularly, can have an impact on blood glucose levels which may have implications for those with insulin resistance or diabetes. Certain DMARDs are relatively contraindicated with elements of the metabolic syndrome. There are concerns about the risk of hypertension developing or worsening with the use of both cyclosporine and leflunomide, limiting their use particularly in the long term. Finally, the most commonly prescribed DMARD for PsA is methotrexate which is metabolized in the liver. Given the central adiposity and fatty liver disease seen in patients with psoriasis and PsA, it is to be expected that fewer patients will be able to tolerate this drug without an increase in their liver function tests. Moreover, hepatic fibrosis was noted to progress rapidly on serial liver biopsies in psoriasis patients with obesity or diabetes [46].

More recent research in PsA has highlighted the importance of obesity in terms of drug response. The prevalence of obesity in PsA has been reported as 45% with 81% categorized as overweight or obese [47]. A longitudinal study of patients with PsA starting on TNF inhibitors showed that those who were obese were significantly less likely to achieve the MDA state suggesting a worse outcome [48] and this was corroborated by the Toronto group who also showed a lower MDA rate in obese patients [49]. Whilst successful intervention leading to weight loss is difficult, the same group showed that weight loss of at least 5% was associated with a higher rate of achievement of MDA after 6 months on therapy. A clear 'dose-response' curve was seen with even higher rates of MDA in those who lost 5–10% and over 10% of their body mass [50]. This most recent study highlights the importance of holistic care of patients with PsA and suggests an additional reason for overweight patients with PsA to consider weight loss.

How should these treatment algorithms be adopted in clinical practice?

Given the current evidence, and the balance between efficacy and safety, it seems that a step up approach to the management of patients with PsA should be recommended. The evidence for early aggressive combination therapy is lacking and there are legitimate concerns about the safety of co-prescription of multiple DMARDs. Cost issues are also important to the consideration of treatment strategies. Current treatment recommendations suggest some subgroups where early use of biologics is justified including those subtypes of disease with poor response to DMARDs and those with poor prognostic factors [1]. The key when planning therapy is a full and accurate assessment of disease activity addressing both musculoskeletal and skin manifestations of PsA as well as presence of comorbidities. This ensures that the best treatment is selected and minimizes potentially harmful effects on patients. Non-pharmacologic therapies, such as physiotherapy and joint protection devices, can be of value in some patients. In addition, adjunctive therapies such as simple analgesics and NSAIDs are used by many patients, sometimes on an intermittent basis.

The translation of a treat to target approach from the TICOPA study and EULAR recommendations into clinical practice requires the same assessment of multiple domains of disease with utilization of a pre-specified target. The selection of an optimal target is complex, but at present the most efficient and evidence-based target is the MDA criteria for PsA. They were used in the only PsA treat to target RCT published to date and this approach was shown to improve both musculoskeletal and skin manifestations [40]. These criteria do not function as a disease activity measure just giving a binary outcome, but they are the most feasible assessment with inclusion of all key domains. The criteria also require physicians to perform a specific assessment of joint counts, enthesitis, and skin which can then be used to make treatment decisions. Indeed, the new 2015 EULAR recommendations for the management of PsA recommend this approach [43]. Another major barrier in PsA therapy is adherence to therapies. In the rheumatologic database of Danish biologics registry, DANBIO the median drug survival of the first anti-TNF agent prescribed was 2.9 years and 1-year and 2-year drug survival rates were 70% and 57%, respectively [51]. Most patients stopped therapy due to lack of treatment effect. In a multivariate analysis, elevated CRP, male sex, and younger age were significantly associated with longer drug survival. A better understanding of the factors that underlie drug discontinuation is definitely important in order to tailor any treat to target strategy.

The management of patients with significant musculoskeletal and skin manifestations requires a multi-speciality team with a strong working relationship between rheumatologists and dermatologists. Beyond these manifestations, other key specialists caring for uveitis, inflammatory bowel disease, metabolic syndrome, and psychological issues may also be required to work together to ensure the best care for individual patients. Attention to obesity may be of particular importance given that reports have demonstrated that weight loss is associated with improved clinical responses in PsA [52]. The multi-speciality team need to assess all aspects of a patient's disease, plan care with multidisciplinary input and optimize outcomes across the board.

References

1. Gossec L, Smolen JS, Gaujoux-Viala C, et al. European League Against Rheumatism recommendations for the management of psoriatic arthritis with pharmacological therapies. Ann Rheum Dis, 2012;71(1):4–12.
2. Coates LC, Aslam T, Al Balushi F, et al. Comparison of three screening tools to detect psoriatic arthritis in patients with psoriasis (CONTEST study). Br J Dermatol, 2013;168(4):802–7.
3. Gladman DD, et al. Development and initial validation of a screening questionnaire for psoriatic arthritis: the Toronto Psoriatic Arthritis Screen (ToPAS). Ann Rheum Dis, 2009;68(4): p. 497–501.
4. Theander E, Husmark T, Alenius GM, et al. Early psoriatic arthritis: short symptom duration, male gender and preserved physical functioning at presentation predict favourable outcome at 5-year follow-up. Results from the Swedish Early Psoriatic Arthritis Register (SwePsA). Ann Rheum Dis, 2014; 73(2):407–13.
5. Tillett W, Jadon D, Shaddick G, et al. Smoking and delay to diagnosis are associated with poorer functional outcome in psoriatic arthritis. Ann Rheum Dis, 2013;72(8):1358–61.
6. Haroon M, Gallagher P, Fitzgerald O. Diagnostic delay of more than 6 months contributes to poor radiographic and functional outcome in psoriatic arthritis. Ann Rheum Dis, 2015; 74(6):1045–50.
7. Scarpa R, Peluso R, Atteno M, et al. The effectiveness of a traditional therapeutical approach in early psoriatic arthritis: results of a pilot randomised 6-month trial with methotrexate. Clin Rheumatol, 2008;27(7): 823–6.
8. Baranauskaite A, Raffayová H, Kungurov NV, et al. Infliximab plus methotrexate is superior to methotrexate alone in the treatment of psoriatic arthritis in methotrexate-naive patients: the RESPOND study. Ann Rheum Dis, 2012:71(4):541–8.
9. Grigor C, Capell H, Stirling A, et al. Effect of a treatment strategy of tight control for rheumatoid arthritis (the TICORA study): a single-blind randomised controlled trial. Lancet, 2004;364(9430): 263–9.
10. Verstappen SM, Jacobs JW, van der Veen MJ, et al. Intensive treatment with methotrexate in early rheumatoid arthritis: aiming for remission. Computer Assisted Management in Early Rheumatoid Arthritis (CAMERA, an open-label strategy trial). Ann Rheum Dis, 2007;66(11):1443–9.
11. Fransen J, Moens HB, Speyer I, van Riel PL. Effectiveness of systematic monitoring of rheumatoid arthritis disease activity in daily practice: a multicentre, cluster randomised controlled trial. Ann Rheum Dis, 2005;64(9):1294–8.
12. National Institute for Health and Clinical Excellence, The management of rheumatoid arthritis in adults. 2009.
13. Gladman, D.D. and V.T. Farewell, Progression in psoriatic arthritis: role of time varying clinical indicators. J Rheumatol, 1999;26(11):2409–13.
14. Bond SJ, Farewell VT, Schentag CT, Gladman DD. Predictors for radiological damage in psoriatic arthritis: results from a single centre. Ann Rheum Dis, 2007;66(3):370–6.
15. Cresswell L, Chandran V, Farewell VT, Gladman DD, et al. Inflammation in an individual joint predicts damage to that joint in psoriatic arthritis. Ann Rheum Dis, 2011;70(2):305–8.
16. Schoels MM, Braun J, Dougados M, et al. Treating axial and peripheral spondyloarthritis, including psoriatic arthritis, to target: results of a systematic literature search to support an international treat-to-target recommendation in spondyloarthritis. Ann Rheum Dis, 2014;73(1):238–42.
17. Kavanaugh A, Krueger GG, Beutler A, et al. Infliximab maintains a high degree of clinical response in patients with active psoriatic arthritis through 1 year of treatment: results from the IMPACT 2 trial. Ann Rheum Dis, 2007;66(4):498–505.
18. Mease PJ, Ory P, Sharp JT, et al. Adalimumab for long-term treatment of psoriatic arthritis: 2-year data from the Adalimumab Effectiveness in Psoriatic Arthritis Trial (ADEPT). Ann Rheum Dis, 2009;68(5):702–9.
19. Kavanaugh A, McInnes I, Mease P, et al. Golimumab, a new human tumor necrosis factor alpha antibody, administered every four weeks as a subcutaneous injection in psoriatic arthritis: Twenty-four-week efficacy and safety results of a randomized, placebo-controlled study. Arthritis Rheum, 2009;60(4):976–86.
20. Feletar M, Brockbank JE, Schentag CT, Lapp V, Gladman DD. Treatment of refractory psoriatic arthritis with infliximab: a 12 month observational study of 16 patients. Ann Rheum Dis, 2004;63(2):156–61.
21. Rahman P, Gladman DD, Cook RJ, Zhou Y, Young G. The use of sulfasalazine in psoriatic arthritis: a clinic experience. J Rheumatol, 1998;25(10):1957–61.
22. Cherouvim EP, Zintzaras E, Boki KA, Moutsopoulos HM, Manoussakis MN. Infliximab therapy for patients with active and refractory spondyloarthropathies at the Dose of 3 mg/kg: a 20-month open treatment. J Clin Rheumatol, 2004;10(4):162–8.
23. Collantes-Estevez E, Muñoz-Villanueva MC, Zarco P, et al. Effectiveness of reducing infliximab dose interval in non-responder patients with refractory spondyloarthropathies. An open extension of a multicentre study. Rheumatology (Oxford), 2005;44(12):1555–8.
24. Smolen JS, Braun J, Dougados M, et al. Treating spondyloarthritis, including ankylosing spondylitis and psoriatic arthritis, to target: recommendations of an international task force. Ann Rheum Dis, 2014;73(1):6–16.
25. Mease PJ, Genovese MC, Greenwald MW, et al. Brodalumab, an anti-IL17RA monoclonal antibody, in psoriatic arthritis. N Engl J Med, 2014;370(24):2295–306.
26. Papp KA, Leonardi C, Menter A, et al. Brodalumab, an anti-interleukin-17-receptor antibody for psoriasis. N Engl J Med, 2012;366(13):1181–9.

27. Coates LC, Fransen J, Helliwell PS. Defining minimal disease activity in psoriatic arthritis: a proposed objective target for treatment. Ann Rheum Dis, 2010;69(1):48–53.

28. Coates LC, Cook R, Lee KA, Chandran V, Gladman DD. Frequency, predictors, and prognosis of sustained minimal disease activity in an observational psoriatic arthritis cohort. Arthritis Care Res (Hoboken), 2010;62(7):970–6.

29. Coates LC, Helliwell PS. Validation of minimal disease activity for psoriatic arthritis using interventional trial data. Arthritis Care Res, 2010;62(2):965–69.

30. Mumtaz A, Gallagher P, Kirby B, et al. Development of a preliminary composite disease activity index in psoriatic arthritis. Ann Rheum Dis, 2011;70(2):272–7.

31. Helliwell PS, FitzGerald O, Fransen J, et al. The development of candidate composite disease activity and responder indices for psoriatic arthritis (GRACE project). Ann Rheum Dis, 2013;72(6):986–91.

32. Ritchlin CT, Kavanaugh A, Gladman DD, et al. Treatment recommendations for psoriatic arthritis. Ann Rheum Dis, 2009;68(9):1387–94.

33. Helliwell PS, FitzGerald O, Fransen J. Composite disease activity and responder indices for psoriatic arthritis: a report from the GRAPPA 2013 meeting on development of cutoffs for both disease activity states and response. J Rheumatol, 2014;41(6):1212–7.

34. Schoels M, Aletaha D, Funovits J, Kavanaugh A, Baker D, Smolen JS. Application of the DAREA/DAPSA score for assessment of disease activity in psoriatic arthritis. Ann Rheum Dis, 2010;69(8):1441–7.

35. Schoels MM, Aletaha D, Alasti F, Smolen JS. Disease activity in psoriatic arthritis (PsA): defining remission and treatment success using the DAPSA score. Ann Rheum Dis, 2016;75(5):811–8.

36. Gladman DD, Mease PJ, Strand V, et al. Consensus on a core set of domains for psoriatic arthritis. J Rheumatol, 2007;34(5):1167–70.

37. Englbrecht M, Wang Y, Ronneberger M, et al. Measuring joint involvement in polyarticular psoriatic arthritis: an introduction of alternatives. Arthritis Care Res (Hoboken), 2010;62(7):977–83.

38. Fransen J, Antoni C, Mease PJ, et al. Performance of response criteria for assessing peripheral arthritis in patients with psoriatic arthritis: analysis of data from randomised controlled trials of two tumour necrosis factor inhibitors. Ann Rheum Dis, 2006;65(10):1373–8.

39. Coates LC, FitzGerald O, Gladman DD, et al. Reduced joint counts misclassify patients with oligoarticular psoriatic arthritis and miss significant numbers of patients with active disease. Arthritis Rheum, 2013;65(6):1504–9.

40. Coates LC, Moverley AR, McParland L, et al. Effect of tight control of inflammation in early psoriatic arthritis (TICOPA): a UK multicentre, open-label, randomised controlled trial. Lancet, 2015;386(10012):2489–98.

41. Coates LC, Navarro-Coy N, Brown SR, et al. The TICOPA protocol (TIght COntrol of Psoriatic Arthritis): a randomised controlled trial to compare intensive management versus standard care in early psoriatic arthritis. BMC Musculoskelet Disord, 2013;14:101.

42. Coates LC, Moverley AR, McParland L, et al. Results of a randomised controlled trial comparing tight control of early psoriatic arthritis (TICOPA) with standard care: tight control improves outcome. Arthritis Rheum, 2013;65(10):S346.

43. Gossec L, Smolen JS, Ramiro S, et al. European League Against Rheumatism (EULAR) recommendations for the management of psoriatic arthritis with pharmacological therapies: 2015 update. Ann Rheum Dis, 2016;75(3):499–510.

44. Haroon M, Gallagher P, Heffernan E, FitzGerald O. High prevalence of metabolic syndrome and of insulin resistance in psoriatic arthritis is associated with the severity of underlying disease. J Rheumatol, 2014;41(7):1357–65.

45. Boehncke WH, Boehncke S, Tobin AM, Kirby B. The 'psoriatic march': a concept of how severe psoriasis may drive cardiovascular comorbidity. Exp Dermatol, 2011;20(4):303–7.

46. Rosenberg P, Urwitz H, Johannesson A, et al. Psoriasis patients with diabetes type 2 are at high risk of developing liver fibrosis during methotrexate treatment. J Hepatol, 2007;46(6):1111–8.

47. Labitigan M, Bahče-Altuntas A, Kremer JM, et al. Higher rates and clustering of abnormal lipids, obesity, and diabetes mellitus in psoriatic arthritis compared with rheumatoid arthritis. Arthritis Care Res (Hoboken), 2014;66(4):600–7.

48. di Minno MN, Peluso R, Iervolino S, et al. Obesity and the prediction of minimal disease activity: a prospective study in psoriatic arthritis. Arthritis Care Res (Hoboken), 2013;65(1):141–7.

49. Eder L, Thavaneswaran A, Chandran V, Cook RJ, Gladman DD. Obesity is associated with a lower probability of achieving sustained minimal disease activity state among patients with psoriatic arthritis. Ann Rheum Dis, 2015;74(5):813–7.

50. Tillett W, Adebajo A, Brooke M, et al. Patient involvement in outcome measures for psoriatic arthritis. Curr Rheumatol Rep, 2014;16(5):418.

51. Glintborg B, Ostergaard M, Krogh NS, et al. Clinical response, drug survival, and predictors thereof among 548 patients with psoriatic arthritis who switched tumor necrosis factor alpha inhibitor therapy: results from the Danish Nationwide DANBIO Registry. Arthritis Rheum, 2013;65(5):1213–23.

52. Di Minno MN, Peluso R, Iervolino S, et al. Weight loss and achievement of minimal disease activity in patients with psoriatic arthritis starting treatment with tumour necrosis factor alpha blockers. Ann Rheum Dis, 2014;73(6):1157–62.

Future directions

CHAPTER 33

Recent progress in psoriatic arthritis and areas for further research

Oliver FitzGerald and Dafna Gladman

There has been very significant progress made in the past 10 to 15 years in how we diagnose, assess, and treat our patients with PsA. Up until the turn of the century, there were many who doubted the existence of PsA arguing that it was a rheumatoid-like arthropathy, perhaps complicated by psoriasis but not a distinct entity. Outcome measures and assessment tools were simply borrowed from rheumatoid arthritis (RA) and treatment strategies were also largely borrowed from RA with very sparse PsA-specific clinical trial information available.

The pivotal advances over the past 10 years would certainly include the following though this list is not exhaustive:

1) **Development of the CASPAR Classification Criteria.** Now generally accepted as being the criteria to be used when enrolling patients in studies or in clinical trials, the development of these criteria ensures that there is some uniformity among the patients being studied with a reduced opportunity to recruit patients who do not have PsA. As there are no diagnostic criteria and as yet no diagnostic test for PsA, the CASPAR Criteria are now the standard classification criteria required for clinical or treatment studies (see Chapter 20 for greater detail).

2) **Agreement on core outcome measures**. The agreement relating to the core domains and instruments to be used in PsA clinical trials was a major development achieved by the GRAPPA Group at the OMERACT Meeting in Malta 2006 (see Chapter 23 for more detail). Whilst these outcome measures are now included in PsA randomized controlled trials (RCTs), the OMERACT/GRAPPA Meeting in 2014 recommended that the outcome measures should be revised in order to incorporate greater patient involvement. The revised outcome measures were presented at the OMERACT/GRAPPA Meeting at Whistler, Canada earlier this year following considerable patient input with a new core set approved by the OMERACT delegates. Work is continuing to develop the appropriate instruments with which to measure the new domains.

3) **Development of assessment tools.** A number of assessment tools have been developed specifically to measure some of the features of PsA. These assessment tools include the patient global assessment, the Leeds Enthesitis Index and the Leeds Dactylitis Index. Tools to measure patient-related measures such as impact of disease have also been developed with the Psoriatic Arthritis Impact of Disease (PsAID) involving patients at every stage of the process. In terms of composite measures, the ACR20 and the disease activity in 28 joints using CRP (DAS28-CRP), both developed for RA, remain the standard measures used in RCTs. This situation is slowly changing, however, with the development of more appropriate composite tools which have been devised specifically for PsA patients and which attempt to reflect all of the ways in which patients might be affected by their disease. These composite tools have shown responsiveness in clinical trial data sets and the minimal disease activity (MDA) criteria have been shown to be a useful target for treatment in the recently reported TICOPA study. With the development of new core outcome measures, it is likely that these composite tools will need further refinement (see Chapters 23 and 25 for more detail).

4) **Improved understanding of PsA genetics.** With the development of sequence-based genetic typing and the CASPAR Criteria to ensure uniformity of patients studied, there has been improved understanding of the genetic basis of this disease. Studies have shown a clear difference across the HLA region in the percentage of patients with HLAC06 comparing those patients with PsA with those who have psoriasis but no musculoskeletal features. Furthermore, additional B-antigen associations emerge in those patients with PsA, such as *HLA-B*27, HLA-B*39*, or *HLA-B*08*. Apart from contributing to disease susceptibility, it would appear that the presence of specific genotypes also contributes to clinical features, such as the duration between the onset of psoriasis and PsA, or specific patterns of disease involvement, such as the presence of symmetrical or asymmetrical sacroiliitis. Outside of the HLA region, genome-wide association studies have identified additional genes of interest, some of which are shared with psoriasis but others which appear to be specifically upregulated in those with PsA (see Chapters 5 and 6 for more detail).

5) **Identification of the importance of both TNFα and IL-17 in driving disease leading to 'game changing' treatment options.** The identification of cytokines such as TNFα and IL-17

at sites of tissue involvement (both skin and joint) in PsA coupled with evidence of polymorphisms in genes involved in both the TNF and IL-17 pathways has led to the understanding that both of these pathways may be key to driving disease in PsA (see Chapter 7 for more detail). Confirming this concept, drugs targeting both the TNFα and IL-17 pathways have proven highly effective in controlling disease features which for many patients can lead to significant clinical improvements with slowing of radiographic damage (see Chapters 29, 30 and 31 for more detail). In the past, at best we looked for some slowing of the disease process but with the range of treatment options now available, we can look to target either remission or minimal disease activity in most of our PsA patients. Unfortunately, not everybody responds to these treatments and, additionally, those who do show some response may continue to have significant inflammation across the various domains of involvement.

Research agenda

Of course there are a number of questions which remain and which are the focus of ongoing research. These key questions include:

1) **Further development of a new core outcome set with appropriate instruments.** Together with a number of patient research partners this work is well under way and it is hoped that the new core outcome set and instruments can be approved at the OMERACT Meeting in 2018.

2) **Refinement of composite measures and their inclusion in randomized control trials.** Once the new core outcome set together with instruments is approved, the composite measures can be appropriately refined and the results tested in further RCTs. It is expected that these measures will include a greater emphasis on patient-related outcomes.

3) **Development of remission criteria.** With remission as the new treatment target, it will be important to develop and validate PsA-specific remission criteria. At present, the best validated treatment target is MDA. The MDA criteria will likely require revision with the development of the new core outcome set and while the MDA is a patient-acceptable state, ongoing inflammation possibly resulting in damage may persist. The development of validated remission criteria would be welcome particularly as treatment outcomes improve.

4) **Development of biomarkers which may improve patient identification, patient assessment prediction and prediction of treatment response.** It is unlikely that a single biomarker will be identified and validated as being sufficiently robust to distinguish, for example, those patients who will develop joint damage from those will not. More likely a panel of biomarkers will be developed which together, perhaps, with clinical and genetic features will help separate out patients with PsA from those with other forms of arthritis, will prove better at assessing disease activity than our current acute phase makers, will be able to accurately predict those patients developing joint damage, and which will help identify at baseline those more likely to respond to a specific treatment strategy. A number of groups, many working in collaboration, are using novel technologies such as proteomics to address these important questions. It is hoped that these biomarker panels and algorithms will emerge soon ready for testing and validation in larger patient cohorts.

Index

Notes Tables, figures and boxes are indicated by an italic *t*, *f* and *b* following the page number *vs.* indicates a comparison or differential diagnosis

Abbreviations used

DIP joint   distal interphalangeal joint
DMARDs   disease modifying anti-rheumatic drugs
MRI   magnetic resonance imaging
NSAIDs   non-steroidal anti-inflammatory drugs
PIP joint   proximal interphalangeal joint
sDMARDs   ynthetic disease modifying anti-rheumatic drugs

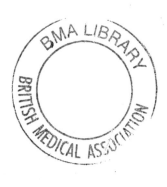